Immunotherapy, Tumor Microenvironment and Survival Signaling

Immunotherapy, Tumor Microenvironment and Survival Signaling

Editor

Vita Golubovskaya

MDPI • Basel • Beijing • Wuhan • Barcelona • Belgrade • Manchester • Tokyo • Cluj • Tianjin

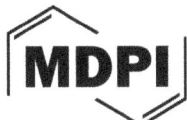

Editor
Vita Golubovskaya
Research and Business
Development, Promab
Biotechnologies, USA
Department of Medicine,
University of Oklahoma, USA

Editorial Office
MDPI
St. Alban-Anlage 66
4052 Basel, Switzerland

This is a reprint of articles from the Special Issue published online in the open access journal *Cancers* (ISSN 2072-6694) (available at: https://www.mdpi.com/journal/cancers/special_issues/ITMSS).

For citation purposes, cite each article independently as indicated on the article page online and as indicated below:

LastName, A.A.; LastName, B.B.; LastName, C.C. Article Title. *Journal Name* **Year**, *Volume Number*, Page Range.

ISBN 978-3-0365-4419-9 (Hbk)
ISBN 978-3-0365-4420-5 (PDF)

Cover image courtesy of Vita Golubovskaya

© 2022 by the authors. Articles in this book are Open Access and distributed under the Creative Commons Attribution (CC BY) license, which allows users to download, copy and build upon published articles, as long as the author and publisher are properly credited, which ensures maximum dissemination and a wider impact of our publications.

The book as a whole is distributed by MDPI under the terms and conditions of the Creative Commons license CC BY-NC-ND.

Contents

About the Editor vii

Preface to "Immunotherapy, Tumor Microenvironment and Survival Signaling" ix

Vita Golubovskaya
Editorial on Special Issue "Immunotherapy, Tumor Microenvironment and Survival Signaling"
Reprinted from: Cancers 2022, 14, 91, doi:10.3390/cancers14010091 1

Vita Golubovskaya, Hua Zhou, Feng Li, Michael Valentine, Jinying Sun, Robert Berahovich, Shirley Xu, Milton Quintanilla, Man Cheong Ma, John Sienkiewicz, Yanwei Huang and Lijun Wu
Novel CD37, Humanized CD37 and Bi-Specific Humanized CD37-CD19 CAR-T Cells Specifically Target Lymphoma
Reprinted from: Cancers 2021, 13, 981, doi:10.3390/cancers13050981 5

Sripathi M. Sureban, Robert Berahovich, Hua Zhou, Shirley Xu, Lijun Wu, Kai Ding, Randal May, Dongfeng Qu, Edwin Bannerman-Menson, Vita Golubovskaya and Courtney W. Houchen
DCLK1 Monoclonal Antibody-Based CAR-T Cells as a Novel Treatment Strategy against Human Colorectal Cancers
Reprinted from: Cancers 2020, 12, 54, doi:10.3390/cancers12010054 19

Zhiyun Cao, Nathaniel Weygant, Parthasarathy Chandrakesan, Courtney W. Houchen, Jun Peng and Dongfeng Qu
Tuft and Cancer Stem Cell Marker DCLK1: A New Target to Enhance Anti-Tumor Immunity in the Tumor Microenvironment
Reprinted from: Cancers 2020, 12, 3801, doi:10.3390/cancers12123801 37

Joslyn L. Mangal, Jamie L. Handlos, Arezoo Esrafili, Sahil Inamdar, Sidnee Mcmillian, Mamta Wankhede, Riccardo Gottardi and Abhinav P. Acharya
Engineering Metabolism of Chimeric Antigen Receptor (CAR) Cells for Developing Efficient Immunotherapies
Reprinted from: Cancers 2021, 13, 1123, doi:10.3390/cancers13051123 55

Bianca Simon, Dennis C. Harrer, Beatrice Schuler-Thurner, Gerold Schuler and Ugur Uslu
Arming T Cells with a gp100-Specific TCR and a CSPG4-Specific CAR Using Combined DNA- and RNA-Based Receptor Transfer
Reprinted from: Cancers 2019, 11, 696, doi:10.3390/cancers11050696 73

Robert Berahovich, Xianghong Liu, Hua Zhou, Elias Tsadik, Shirley Xu, Vita Golubovskaya and Lijun Wu
Hypoxia Selectively Impairs CAR-T Cells In Vitro
Reprinted from: Cancers 2019, 11, 602, doi:10.3390/cancers11050602 87

Mouldy Sioud, Solveig Pettersen, Ieva Ailte and Yngvar Fløisand
Targeted Killing of Monocytes/Macrophages and Myeloid Leukemia Cells with Pro-Apoptotic Peptides
Reprinted from: Cancers 2019, 11, 1088, doi:10.3390/cancers11081088 103

Shin-Yi Liu, Wen-Chien Huang, Hung-I Yeh, Chun-Chuan Ko, Hui-Ru Shieh, Chung-Lieh Hung, Tung-Ying Chen and Yu-Jen Chen
Sequential Blockade of PD-1 and PD-L1 Causes Fulminant Cardiotoxicity—From Case Report to Mouse Model Validation
Reprinted from: *Cancers* **2019**, *11*, 580, doi:10.3390/cancers11040580 123

Vito Longo, Oronzo Brunetti, Amalia Azzariti, Domenico Galetta, Patrizia Nardulli, Francesco Leonetti and Nicola Silvestris
Strategies to Improve Cancer Immune Checkpoint Inhibitors Efficacy, Other Than Abscopal Effect: A Systematic Review
Reprinted from: *Cancers* **2019**, *11*, 539, doi:10.3390/cancers11040539 141

María Julia Lamberti, Annunziata Nigro, Vincenzo Casolaro, Natalia Belén Rumie Vittar and Jessica Dal Col
Damage-Associated Molecular Patterns Modulation by microRNA: Relevance on Immunogenic Cell Death and Cancer Treatment Outcome
Reprinted from: *Cancers* **2021**, *13*, 2566, doi:10.3390/cancers13112566 161

Maximilian Haist, Henner Stege, Stephan Grabbe and Matthias Bros
The Functional Crosstalk between Myeloid-Derived Suppressor Cells and Regulatory T Cells within the Immunosuppressive Tumor Microenvironment
Reprinted from: *Cancers* **2021**, *13*, 210, doi:10.3390/cancers13020210 181

Tilahun Ayane Debele, Cheng-Fa Yeh and Wen-Pin Su
Cancer Immunotherapy and Application of Nanoparticles in Cancers Immunotherapy as the Delivery of Immunotherapeutic Agents and as the Immunomodulators
Reprinted from: *Cancers* **2020**, *12*, 3773, doi:10.3390/cancers12123773 215

Hana Sahinbegovic, Tomas Jelinek, Matous Hrdinka, Juli R. Bago, Marcello Turi, Tereza Sevcikova, Amina Kurtovic-Kozaric, Roman Hajek and Michal Simicek
Intercellular Mitochondrial Transfer in the Tumor Microenvironment
Reprinted from: *Cancers* **2020**, *12*, 1787, doi:10.3390/cancers12071787 239

Karan Mediratta, Sara El-Sahli, Vanessa D'Costa and Lisheng Wang
Current Progresses and Challenges of Immunotherapy in Triple-Negative Breast Cancer
Reprinted from: *Cancers* **2020**, *12*, 3529, doi:10.3390/cancers12123529 251

Marilina García-Aranda and Maximino Redondo
Immunotherapy: A Challenge of Breast Cancer Treatment
Reprinted from: *Cancers* **2019**, *11*, 1822, doi:10.3390/cancers11121822 285

Raoud Marayati, Colin H. Quinn and Elizabeth A. Beierle
Immunotherapy in Pediatric Solid Tumors—A Systematic Review
Reprinted from: *Cancers* **2019**, *11*, 2022, doi:10.3390/cancers11122022 303

Sandra Gessani and Filippo Belardelli
Immune Dysfunctions and Immunotherapy in Colorectal Cancer: The Role of Dendritic Cells
Reprinted from: *Cancers* **2019**, *11*, 1491, doi:10.3390/cancers11101491 321

Evangelos Koustas, Panagiotis Sarantis, Georgia Kyriakopoulou, Athanasios G. Papavassiliou and Michalis V. Karamouzis
The Interplay of Autophagy and Tumor Microenvironment in Colorectal Cancer—Ways of Enhancing Immunotherapy Action
Reprinted from: *Cancers* **2019**, *11*, 533, doi:10.3390/cancers11040533 339

About the Editor

Vita Golubovskaya, Phd

Associate Professor Vita Golubovskaya is a director of research and business development at *Promab Biotechnologies*, leading research concerning novel anticancer immunotherapies including CAR-T and CAR-NK cell therapy. She has more than 20 years of experience in the fields of cancer research, oncology and immunology. Previously, Dr. Golubovskaya was a research associate professor at the Roswell Park Cancer Institute and a research professor at the University of Buffalo, SUNY, Buffalo, NY. Dr. Golubovskaya has authored more than 90 publications, 30 patents and several book chapters. She was awarded the Susan Komen Grant for Breast Cancer, as well as the NCI NIH and STTR grants. Dr. Golubovskaya served as a Guest Editor in *Frontiers in Bioscience, Vaccines, Anti-Cancer Agents in Medicinal Chemistry* and *Cancers*. She is an active member of AACR.

Preface to "Immunotherapy, Tumor Microenvironment and Survival Signaling"

Immunotherapy, Tumor Microenvironment and Survival Signaling

The book is based on the Cancers journal Special Issue entitled "Immunotherapy, Tumor Microenvironment and Survival Signaling", and focuses on important problems concerning tumors and tumor microenvironment interactions, as well as novel immunotherapies such as CAR-T cell therapy. Immunotherapies have recently shown remarkable results in the treatment of cancer patients. However, there are still many questions that remain to be solved in regards to more effective therapies, such as the tumor heterogeneous profile, tumor microenvironment, tumor survival epigenetic and genetic pathways, all of which make patients resistant to the presently available treatments for cancer.

This book demonstrates different approaches to overcome the challenges faced by immunotherapies due to suppressive tumor microenvironment. This book includes 18 papers that can be divided into three chapters: 1. novel immunotherapies; 2. targeting tumor microenvironment and novel approaches; 3. targeting tumors and tumor microenvironment in different types of cancer.

Novel Immunotherapies

Recently, a novel type of immunotherapy, CAR-T cell therapy, has demonstrated excellent and exciting efficacy in leukemia, lymphoma and multiple myeloma. CD19 and BCMA-CAR-T cell therapies have been approved by the FDA to treat patients with the above diseases. There are still several challenges for CAR-T cells, such as targeting solid tumors with a repressive microenvironment, resistance to CAR-T cell therapy due to the loss of antigens or other mechanisms, persistency of CAR-T cells, etc. One of the approaches presented in the paper used to overcome potential CD19 loss during treatment with CD19 CAR-T cells is the use of novel CD37 and CD37-CD19-CAR-T cells.

Another group presented novel DCLK1 (Doublecortin-like kinase 1) antibody and DCLK-1-CAR-T cells, which target colorectal cancers. The authors also demonstrated that DCLK1 is a marker of tuft cells (TC) and cancer stem cells (CSCs), suggesting that DCLK1-positive TCs participate in the initiation and progression of inflammation-associated cancer.

The different approaches were discussed in regards to generating metabolically fit CAR-T cells to overcome immune-suppressive tumor microenvironment. Different enzymes or protein regulators of metabolism were presented, able to be modulated to increase the efficacy of T cells. One of the approaches is to induce the expression of PPAR-gamma coactivator 1-α (PGC1-α), which controls mitochondrial biogenesis and increases the efficacy of T cells. Another approach is to generate the CAR-T cell secreting antioxidant catalase enzyme to overcome hypoxic tumor microenvironment. Several other approaches are highlighted, including CAR-T cells engineered to effect glycolysis, glutaminolysis and other metabolic pathways

An original approach to overcome potential antigen loss during immunotherapy was described, where the authors engineered T cells with a gp100 antigen (also known as premelanosome protein, PMEL-specific TCR) and a CSPG4 (chondroitin sulfate proteoglycan 4, also known as melanoma-associated chondroitin sulfate proteoglycan, MCSP, or high-molecular-weight melanoma-associated antigen, HMW-MAA)-specific CAR. This represents a novel approach in immunotherapy needing future expansion and optimization for used in clinic.

Targeting Tumor Microenvironment and Novel Approaches

It is well known that the solid tumor microenvironment is hypoxic when treated with a high level of TGF–repressing immunotherapy. The hypoxic tumor microenvironment is present not only in the case of solid tumors, but also in bone marrow niches where B cells reside. One of the reports studied the effect of hypoxia on the function of CAR-T cells, and detected that hypoxia impaired CAR-T cell expansion, differentiation and cytokine production. This novel study could allow to generate better equipped CAR-T cells to overcome the effects of a hypoxic tumor microenvironment.

Most tumors are surrounded and infiltrated by TAMs (tumor-associated macrophages) that promote tumor motility, angiogenesis, metastasis and repress T cell functions and inhibit the effect of chemo- or immunotherapies. An interesting study delivered special lytic proapoptotic peptides to block TAMs, eliminating circulating monocytes and macrophages.

One of the approaches to block tumors and tumor microenvironment is to use antibodies to block programmed cell death 1 (PD-1) or its ligand 1 (PD-L1). One of the reports demonstrated that the sequential use of PD-1 and PD-L1 antibodies could cause cardiotoxicity in patients with brain metastatic lung adenocarcinoma.

Another report reviewed different agents to improve checkpoint inhibitor efficacy in clinic. The authors reported that while in melanoma and non-small cell lung cancer the use of immune checkpoint inhibitors resulted in a high efficacy, the response rate in other tumors, such as gastrointestinal cancers, breast cancer, sarcomas, and other genitourinary cancers, remained low. Several strategies were discussed that could improve efficacy, such as the use of predictive factors of response (for example, PD-L1 expression, tumor mutational burden and clinical factors), a combination therapy approach, the use of different drugs such as microbiota modulators, antiangiogenic agents, small molecules and oncolytic viruses, and drugs targeting coinhibitory receptors.

An interesting review focused on the role of microRNA in the modulation of damage-associated molecular patterns modulation (DAMP) immunogenic cell death (ICD), which is triggered by several ICD inducers released into the tumor microenvironment and plays a major role in stimulating the antitumor response. The exposure of DAMP, such as calreticulin, ATP, Hsps and HMGB1, confers adjuvanticity to cancer cell death. The authors reviewed the main microRNA that targets DAMPs such as Hsp 70, Hsp 90, HMGB1 and calreticulin.

Another review summarized the interactions and crosstalk between myeloid-derived suppressor cells and regulatory T cells within the immunosuppressive tumor microenvironment. The authors reviewed the role of beta-integrins, metabolic pathways and cell–cell interactions.

An interesting review focused on nanoparticles in cancer immunotherapy as the delivery agents of immunotherapeutic agents, as well as immunomodulators. The authors discussed nanoimmunotherapy, targeting the microenvironment with different nanoparticle-based agents and overviewed future directions and challenges of this novel promising field.

Another interesting review focused on the novel mechanism of intercellular mitochondria transfer in both solid and hematological cancers. The mitochondria transfer can change metabolic pathways and affect the microenvironment and drug resistance mechanisms in different types of cancers.

Targeting Tumors and Tumor Microenvironment in Different Types of Cancer

Several reviews concentrated on the interplay between targeting tumors and the tumor microenvironment in different types of cancer, such as triple-negative breast cancer, breast, pediatric and colorectal cancer.

The role of dendritic cells was reviewed in the immunotherapy of colorectal cancer. Novel strategies to combine DC vaccination with checkpoint inhibitors introduce novel perspectives for the attainment of a more effective treatment of the disease.

The role of autophagy in the regulation of the tumor microenvironment in colorectal cancer was discussed, and the specific mechanism by which autophagy is implicated in immune responses during CRC tumorigenesis was described in the context of anticancer therapy.

Conclusions

This Special Issue demonstrated the complex interactions between tumors and the tumor microenvironment, reviewed the cross-talk and interplay between them and provided best strategies to overcome challenges in targeting tumors with a repressive immune environment. The reports provided future directions in regards to increasing the number of available anticancer therapies.

Vita Golubovskaya
Editor

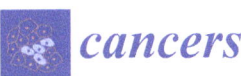

Editorial

Editorial on Special Issue "Immunotherapy, Tumor Microenvironment and Survival Signaling"

Vita Golubovskaya

Promab Biotechnologies, 2600 Hilltop Drive, Richmond, CA 94806, USA; vita.gol@promab.com

1. Novel Immunotherapies

Recently, novel types of immunotherapies such as CAR-T cell therapy demonstrated efficacy in leukemia, lymphoma, and multiple myeloma [1–3]. CD19 and BCMA-CAR-T cell therapies were approved by FDA to treat patients with the above diseases. There are still several challenges for CAR-T cell therapy, including safe and effective antigen targets for solid tumors, overcoming a suppressive tumor microenvironment, and loss of antigen expression, among others [4,5].

One of the approaches to overcome potential CD19 loss during treatment with CD19 CAR-T cells was presented in a paper with novel CD37 and CD37-CD19-CAR-T cells [6]. The authors generated a novel CD37 antibody and engineered both novel Cd37-CAR-T cells and bispecific CD37-CD19-CAR-T cells that effectively targeted CD19+CD37+ lymphoma in vitro and in vivo [6].

Another group presented novel DCLK1 (doublecortin-like kinase 1) antibody and DCLK-1-CAR-T cells targeting colorectal cancers [7]. The authors demonstrated that DCLK1 was a marker of tuft cells (TC) and cancer stem cells (CSCs) and suggested that DCLK1-positive TCs participated in the initiation and progression of inflammation-associated cancer [8].

In another report, the authors reviewed different approaches to generate metabolically fit CAR-T cells to overcome the immune-suppressive tumor microenvironment [9]. Since it is known that metabolic pathways can control T cell proliferation, expansion, differentiation, and function, the authors describe different enzymes or protein regulators of metabolism that can be modulated to increase the efficacy of CAR-T cells [9]. One of the approaches is to induce expression of PPAR-gamma coactivator 1-α (PGC1-α), which controls mitochondrial biogenesis and results in an increased efficacy of T cells. Another approach is to generate CAR-T cells which secrete the antioxidant enzyme catalase to overcome the hypoxic tumor microenvironment [9]. Several other approaches are highlighted with CAR-T cells engineered to effect glycolysis, glutaminolysis, and the pentose phosphate pathway.

In an original approach to overcome potential antigen loss during immunotherapy, the authors engineered T cells with anti gp100 TCR antigen targeting PMEL (premelanosome protein) and anti-CSPG4 CAR targeting chondroitin sulfate proteoglycan 4 (also known as melanoma-associated chondroitin sulfate proteoglycan, MCSP, or high molecular weight melanoma-associated antigen, HMW-MAA) [10]. These armed T cells were generated with stable lentiviral delivery of gp100 TCR and transient delivery of CSPG4-CAR using RNA electroporation [10]. This represents a novel approach in immunotherapy which needs further optimization to be used in clinics.

2. Novel Approaches Targeting the Tumor Microenvironment

It is well known that the solid tumor microenvironment is hypoxic with high level of TGF-β which represses immunotherapy. Hypoxia is present in the case of solid tumors and in bone marrow niche where B cells reside [11]. One report studied the effect of hypoxia on function of CAR-T cells and found that hypoxia impaired CAR-T cell expansion and affected differentiation and cytokine production [12].

Citation: Golubovskaya, V. Editorial on Special Issue "Immunotherapy, Tumor Microenvironment and Survival Signaling". *Cancers* 2022, 14, 91. https://doi.org/10.3390/cancers14010091

Received: 23 November 2021
Accepted: 15 December 2021
Published: 24 December 2021

Publisher's Note: MDPI stays neutral with regard to jurisdictional claims in published maps and institutional affiliations.

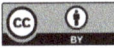

Copyright: © 2021 by the author. Licensee MDPI, Basel, Switzerland. This article is an open access article distributed under the terms and conditions of the Creative Commons Attribution (CC BY) license (https://creativecommons.org/licenses/by/4.0/).

Most tumors are surrounded and infiltrated by TAM (tumor associated macrophages) that promote tumor motility, angiogenesis, metastasis, repress T cell functions, and inhibit the effect of chemo- or other immunotherapies [13]. The authors delivered special lytic proapoptotic peptides to block TAMs, eliminate circulating monocytes and macrophages [13].

One of the approaches to block tumors and tumor microenvironment players is to use antibodies to block programmed cell death 1 (PD-1) or its ligand 1 (PD-L1). One of the reports demonstrated that sequential use of PD-1 and PD-L1 antibodies can cause cardiotoxicity in patient with brain metastatic lung adenocarcinoma [14]. Thus, the authors conclude that the combinatory use of PD-1 and PD-L1 blockade, either sequentially or concurrently, should be used carefully to avoid cardiotoxicity [14].

Another report reviewed different agents to improve checkpoint inhibitor efficacy in clinic [15]. The authors report that while in melanoma and non-small cell lung cancer using immune checkpoint inhibitors results in a high efficacy, the response rate in other tumors, such as gastrointestinal cancers, breast cancer, sarcomas, and some genitourinary cancers remains low [15]. Several strategies are discussed that can improve efficacy such as use of predictive factors of the response (for example PD-L1 expression, tumor mutational burden, and clinical factors), combination therapy approach, use in addition to abscopal effect of radiotherapy other drugs such as microbiota modulators, anti-angiogenic agents, small molecules, and oncolytic viruses (drugs targeting co-inhibitory receptors) [15].

Another review focuses on the role of microRNA in the modulation of damage-associated molecular patterns (DAMP) [16]. Immunogenic cell death (ICD) which is triggered by several ICD-inducers released into tumor microenvironment plays a major role in stimulating anti-tumor response [16]. The exposure of DAMP such as calreticulin, ATP, Hsps and HMGB1 confers adjuvanticity to cancer cell death [16]. The authors review the main microRNA that target DAMPs such as Hsp 70, Hsp 90, HMGB1, calreticulin [16].

Another report summarizes interactions and crosstalk between myeloid-derived suppressor cells and regulatory T cells within the immunosuppressive tumor microenvironment [17]. The authors review role of beta-integrins, metabolic pathways, and cell-cell interactions as modulators of this cross-talk [17].

Another review focused on nanoparticles in cancer immunotherapy as the delivery agent of immunotherapeutic agents and as the immunomodulators [18]. The authors discussed nano-immunotherapy, targeting microenvironment with different nanoparticle-based agents, and overviewed future directions and challenges of this novel promising field [18].

Another review presented new mechanism of intercellular mitochondria transfer in both solid and hematological cancers [19]. The mitochondria transfer can change metabolic pathways and affect microenvironment and drug resistance mechanisms in different types of cancers.

3. Targeting Tumors and Tumor Microenvironment in Different Types of Cancer

Several reviews concentrated on targeting tumors and interplay with tumor microenvironment in different types of cancer such as triple negative breast cancer [20], breast cancer [21], pediatric cancer [22], and colorectal cancer [23,24].

The challenges in treating triple negative breast cancer patients with immune checkpoint inhibitors (ICI) are partly attributed to dysregulated angiogenesis, resulting in hypoxic tumor microenvironment, increased production of VEGF, EGF, and PDGF, thereby stimulating angiogenesis and metastasis [20]. Other challenges are long non-coding RNAs and microsatellite instability that cause immunosuppression and affect the efficacy of ICI [20]. Since there is limited T-cell infiltration in most breast cancers, the development of novel strategies to enhance sufficient lymphocyte infiltration, as well as to generate de novo T-cell responses that overcome the immunosuppressive tumor environment, may be the key to the success of this kind of therapy in breast cancer patients [21].

The role of dendritic cells is reviewed in immunotherapy of colorectal cancer [23]. New strategies to combine DC vaccination with check-point inhibitors open perspectives for a more effective treatment of disease [23].

The role of autophagy in the regulation of the tumor microenvironment for colorectal cancer, the specific mechanism by which autophagy is implicated in immune responses during CRC tumorigenesis, and the context of anticancer therapy is reviewed in [24].

4. Conclusions

This issue demonstrated the complex interaction between tumors and tumor microenvironment, reviewed cross talk and interplay between them, and provided the best strategies for overcoming challenges in targeting tumors with repressive immune environment. The reports provided future directions in increasing anticancer therapies.

Conflicts of Interest: The author declares no conflict of interest.

References

1. Shin, E.-C. Cancer immunotherapy: Special issue of BMB Reports in 2021. *BMB Rep.* **2021**, *54*, 1. [CrossRef] [PubMed]
2. Ding, L.; Hu, Y.; Huang, H. Novel progresses of chimeric antigen receptor (CAR) T cell therapy in multiple myeloma. *Stem Cell Investig.* **2021**, *8*, 1. [CrossRef] [PubMed]
3. Eshhar, Z.; Waks, T.; Gross, G. The Emergence of T-Bodies/CAR T Cells. *Cancer J.* **2014**, *20*, 123–126. [CrossRef] [PubMed]
4. Razavi, A.; Keshavarz-Fathi, M.; Pawelek, J.; Rezaei, N. Chimeric antigen receptor T-cell therapy for melanoma. *Expert Rev. Clin. Immunol.* **2021**, *17*, 209–223. [CrossRef]
5. Schneider, D.; Xiong, Y.; Wu, D.; Hu, P.; Alabanza, L.; Steimle, B.; Mahmud, H.; Anthony-Gonda, K.; Krueger, W.; Zhu, Z.; et al. Trispecific CD19-CD20-CD22–targeting duoCAR-T cells eliminate antigen-heterogeneous B cell tumors in preclinical models. *Sci. Transl. Med.* **2021**, *13*, 586. [CrossRef]
6. Golubovskaya, V.; Zhou, H.; Li, F.; Valentine, M.; Sun, J.; Berahovich, R.; Xu, S.; Quintanilla, M.; Ma, M.C.; Sienkiewicz, J.; et al. Novel CD37, Humanized CD37 and Bi-Specific Humanized CD37-CD19 CAR-T Cells Specifically Target Lymphoma. *Cancers* **2021**, *13*, 981. [CrossRef] [PubMed]
7. Sureban, S.M.; Berahovich, R.; Zhou, H.; Xu, S.; Wu, L.; Ding, K.; May, R.; Qu, D.; Bannerman-Menson, E.; Golubovskaya, V.; et al. DCLK1 Monoclonal Antibody-Based CAR-T Cells as a Novel Treatment Strategy against Human Colorectal Cancers. *Cancers* **2019**, *12*, 54. [CrossRef]
8. ZCao, Z.; Weygant, N.; Chandrakesan, P.; Houchen, C.W.; Peng, J.; Qu, D. Tuft and Cancer Stem Cell Marker DCLK1: A New Target to Enhance Anti-Tumor Immunity in the Tumor Microenvironment. *Cancers* **2020**, *12*, 3801. [CrossRef]
9. Mangal, J.; Handlos, J.; Esrafili, A.; Inamdar, S.; Mcmillian, S.; Wankhede, M.; Gottardi, R.; Acharya, A. Engineering Metabolism of Chimeric Antigen Receptor (CAR) Cells for Developing Efficient Immunotherapies. *Cancers* **2021**, *13*, 1123. [CrossRef]
10. Simon, B.; Harrer, D.C.; Schuler-Thurner, B.; Schuler, G.; Uslu, U. Arming T Cells with a gp100-Specific TCR and a CSPG4-Specific CAR Using Combined DNA- and RNA-Based Receptor Transfer. *Cancers* **2019**, *11*, 696. [CrossRef] [PubMed]
11. Irigoyen, M.; Garcia-Ruiz, J.C.; Berra, E. The hypoxia signalling pathway in haematological malignancies. *Oncotarget* **2017**, *8*, 36832–36844. [CrossRef]
12. Berahovich, R.; Liu, X.; Zhou, H.; Tsadik, E.; Xu, S.; Golubovskaya, V.; Wu, L. Hypoxia Selectively Impairs CAR-T Cells In Vitro. *Cancers* **2019**, *11*, 602. [CrossRef] [PubMed]
13. Sioud, M.; Pettersen, S.; Ailte, I.; Fløisand, Y. Targeted Killing of Monocytes/Macrophages and Myeloid Leukemia Cells with Pro-Apoptotic Peptides. *Cancers* **2019**, *11*, 1088. [CrossRef] [PubMed]
14. Liu, S.-Y.; Huang, W.-C.; Yeh, H.-I.; Ko, C.-C.; Shieh, H.-R.; Hung, C.-L.; Chen, T.-Y.; Chen, Y.-J. Sequential Blockade of PD-1 and PD-L1 Causes Fulminant Cardiotoxicity-From Case Report to Mouse Model Validation. *Cancers* **2019**, *11*, 580. [CrossRef]
15. Longo, V.; Brunetti, O.; Azzariti, A.; Galetta, D.; Nardulli, P.; Leonetti, F.; Silvestris, N. Strategies to Improve Cancer Immune Checkpoint Inhibitors Efficacy, Other Than Abscopal Effect: A Systematic Review. *Cancers* **2019**, *11*, 539. [CrossRef] [PubMed]
16. Lamberti, M.; Nigro, A.; Casolaro, V.; Vittar, N.R.; Col, J.D. Damage-Associated Molecular Patterns Modulation by microRNA: Relevance on Immunogenic Cell Death and Cancer Treatment Outcome. *Cancers* **2021**, *13*, 2566. [CrossRef]
17. Haist, M.; Stege, H.; Grabbe, S.; Bros, M. The Functional Crosstalk between Myeloid-Derived Suppressor Cells and Regulatory T Cells within the Immunosuppressive Tumor Microenvironment. *Cancers* **2021**, *13*, 210. [CrossRef] [PubMed]
18. Debele, T.A.; Yeh, C.-F.; Su, W.-P. Cancer Immunotherapy and Application of Nanoparticles in Cancers Immunotherapy as the Delivery of Immunotherapeutic Agents and as the Immunomodulators. *Cancers* **2020**, *12*, 3773. [CrossRef]
19. Sahinbegovic, H.; Jelinek, T.; Hrdinka, M.; Bago, J.R.; Turi, M.; Sevcikova, T.; Kurtovic-Kozaric, A.; Hajek, R.; Simicek, M. Intercellular Mitochondrial Transfer in the Tumor Microenvironment. *Cancers* **2020**, *12*, 1787. [CrossRef]
20. Mediratta, K.; El-Sahli, S.; D'Costa, V.; Wang, L. Current Progresses and Challenges of Immunotherapy in Triple-Negative Breast Cancer. *Cancers* **2020**, *12*, 3529. [CrossRef]

21. García-Aranda, M.; Redondo, M. Immunotherapy: A Challenge of Breast Cancer Treatment. *Cancers* **2019**, *11*, 1822. [CrossRef] [PubMed]
22. Marayati, R.; Quinn, C.H.; Beierle, E.A. Immunotherapy in Pediatric Solid Tumors—A Systematic Review. *Cancers* **2019**, *11*, 2022. [CrossRef] [PubMed]
23. Gessani, S.; Belardelli, F. Immune Dysfunctions and Immunotherapy in Colorectal Cancer: The Role of Dendritic Cells. *Cancers* **2019**, *11*, 1491. [CrossRef] [PubMed]
24. Koustas, E.; Sarantis, P.; Kyriakopoulou, G.; Papavassiliou, A.G.; Karamouzis, M.V. The Interplay of Autophagy and Tumor Microenvironment in Colorectal Cancer—Ways of Enhancing Immunotherapy Action. *Cancers* **2019**, *11*, 533. [CrossRef]

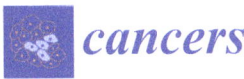

Article

Novel CD37, Humanized CD37 and Bi-Specific Humanized CD37-CD19 CAR-T Cells Specifically Target Lymphoma

Vita Golubovskaya [1,*], Hua Zhou [1], Feng Li [1,2], Michael Valentine [1], Jinying Sun [1], Robert Berahovich [1], Shirley Xu [1], Milton Quintanilla [1], Man Cheong Ma [1], John Sienkiewicz [1], Yanwei Huang [1] and Lijun Wu [1,3,*]

1. Promab Biotechnologies, 2600 Hilltop Drive, Richmond, CA 94806, USA; hua.zhou@promab.com (H.Z.); feng.li@promab.com (F.L.); michael.valentine@promab.com (M.V.); sunnie.sun@promab.com (J.S.); robert.berahovich@promab.com (R.B.); shirley.xu@promab.com (S.X.); milton.quintanilla@promab.com (M.Q.); iris.ma@promab.com (M.C.M.); john.sienkiewicz@promab.com (J.S.); yanwei.huang@promab.com (Y.H.)
2. Biology and Environmental Science College, Hunan University of Arts and Science, Changde 415000, China
3. Forevertek Biotechnology, Janshan Road, Changsha Hi-Tech Industrial Development Zone, Changsha 410205, China
* Correspondence: vita.gol@promab.com (V.G.); john@promab.com (L.W.); Tel.: +510-974-0697 (V.G.)

Citation: Golubovskaya, V.; Zhou, H.; Li, F.; Valentine, M.; Sun, J.; Berahovich, R.; Xu, S.; Quintanilla, M.; Ma, M.C.; Sienkiewicz, J.; et al. Novel CD37, Humanized CD37 and Bi-Specific Humanized CD37-CD19 CAR-T Cells Specifically Target Lymphoma. Cancers 2021, 13, 981. https://doi.org/10.3390/cancers13050981

Academic Editor: Samuel C. Mok

Received: 22 January 2021
Accepted: 22 February 2021
Published: 26 February 2021

Publisher's Note: MDPI stays neutral with regard to jurisdictional claims in published maps and institutional affiliations.

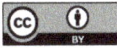

Copyright: © 2021 by the authors. Licensee MDPI, Basel, Switzerland. This article is an open access article distributed under the terms and conditions of the Creative Commons Attribution (CC BY) license (https://creativecommons.org/licenses/by/4.0/).

Simple Summary: Chimeric antigen receptor (CAR) T cell therapy represents a major advancement in cancer treatment. Recently, FDA approved CAR-T cells directed against the CD19 protein for treatment of leukemia and lymphoma. In spite of impressive clinical responses with CD19-CAR-T cells, some patients demonstrate disease relapse due to either antigen loss, cancer heterogeneity or other mechanisms. Novel CAR-T cells and targets are important for the field. This report describes novel CD37, humanized CD37 and bispecific humanized CD37-CD19-CAR-T cells targeting both CD37 and CD19. The study demonstrates that these novel CAR-T cells specifically targeted either CD37 positive or CD37 and CD19-positive cells with endogenous and exogenous protein expression and provides a basis for future clinical studies.

Abstract: CD19 and CD37 proteins are highly expressed in B-cell lymphoma and have been successfully targeted with different monotherapies, including chimeric antigen receptor (CAR)-T cell therapy. The goal of this study was to target lymphoma with novel CD37, humanized CD37, and bi-specific humanized CD37-CD19 CAR-T cells. A novel mouse monoclonal anti-human CD37 antibody (clone 2B8D12F2D4) was generated with high binding affinity for CD37 antigen (KD = 1.6 nM). The CD37 antibody specifically recognized cell surface CD37 protein in lymphoma cells and not in multiple myeloma or other types of cancer. The mouse and humanized CD37-CAR-T cells specifically killed Raji and CHO-CD37 cells and secreted IFN-gamma. In addition, we generated bi-specific humanized hCD37-CD19 CAR-T cells that specifically killed Raji cells, CHO-CD37, and Hela-CD19 cells and did not kill control CHO or Hela cells. Moreover, the hCD37-CD19 CAR-T cells secreted IFN-gamma against CD37-positive and CD19-positive target CHO-CD37, Hela-CD19 cells, respectively, but not against CD19 and CD37-negative parental cell line. The bi-specific hCD37-CD19 significantly inhibited Raji xenograft tumor growth and prolonged mouse survival in NOD scid gamma mouse (NSG) mouse model. This study demonstrates that novel humanized CD37 and humanized CD37-CD19 CAR-T cells specifically targeted either CD37 positive or CD37 and CD19-positive cells and provides a basis for future clinical studies.

Keywords: chimeric antigen receptor; CAR-T cells; CD37; CD19; immunotherapy; cell therapy; tumor antigen; lymphoma

1. Introduction

Chimeric antigen receptor (CAR) T cell therapy is an exciting and novel area of immuno-oncology research [1–3]. CAR-T cells have been tested against several targets for hematological cancers, such as CD19, CD20, CD22, CD123, BCMA, and others in clinical trials [4–13]. Novel approaches and targets are being developed to overcome challenges to existing cell therapies, such as loss of antigen, an immunosuppressive tumor microenvironment, and limited persistence of CAR-T cells [4,12,14–17]. Recently, novel anti-CD37 CAR-T cell therapy was developed for lymphoma patients [18,19].

CD37 is highly expressed in many hematological cancers, such as non-Hodgkin's lymphoma (NHL), diffuse large B-cell lymphoma (DLBCL), chronic lymphocytic leukemia (CLL), acute lymphocytic leukemia (ALL), and in some peripheral and cutaneous T cell lymphomas [20–22], and absent or weakly expressed in multiple myeloma and Hodgkin's lymphoma [23]. CD37 is a 40–52 kDa heavily glycosylated member of the transmembrane 4 superfamily (TM4SF) of tetraspanin proteins [24,25]. CD37 plays a role in integrin, AKT, PI3-Kinase-dependent survival, and apoptotic signaling, motility, immune response signaling via activation of dendritic cell migration [25,26].

CD37 expressing cancers have been targeted with several antibody-based therapies, including Fc engineered antibodies (BI836826), drug or radio immunoconjugates (maytansinoid DM1 IMGN529; monomethyl auristatin E, AGS67E, and (^{177}Lu) Betalutin), DuoHexaBody-CD37, and single-chain variable fragments (ScFv) (Otlertuzumab/TRU-016), either alone or in combination with rituximab, chemotherapy, or other agents [22,27–32].

Recently, FDA-approved CD19-CAR-T cells (Kymriah (tisagenlecleucel) and Yescarta (axicabtagene ciloleucel) have successfully treated patients with CD19+ B-cell leukemias [8,33]. However, the relapse due to loss of the CD19 antigen via alternative splicing or mutations leading to loss of the protein transmembrane domain has been observed [34,35]. To improve the efficacy of CAR-T cells in case of loss of antigen, dual, tandem, or bispecific CAR-T cells were generated which target two different antigens, such as CD19/CD20 [36,37]; CD19/CD22 [38,39]; CD19/CD123 [40].

This report demonstrates the efficacy of three novel CAR-T cells derived from CD37 antibody, clone 2B8D12F2D4: mouse CD37, humanized hCD37 CAR-T cells, and bispecific hCD37-CD19 CAR-T cells against lymphoma. Data show effective and specific targeting of lymphoma cells expressing CD37 in vitro, and decreased tumor burden, and increased median survival in a xenograft model in vivo, providing a solid basis for future clinical studies.

2. Results

2.1. CD37 Antibody Clone 2B8D12F2D4 Binds Specifically and Selectively with High Affinity to CD37 Antigen

Several murine anti-human CD37 mAbs were isolated from hybridoma and screened for binding to recombinant human CD37-Maltose binding protein (MBP)-His antigen (Figure 1A) and seven other unrelated proteins (Figure 1B). CD37 antibody, clone 2B8D12F2D4, hereafter referred to as 2B8, specifically bound to CD37 antigen and did not bind to any of the other proteins tested. (Figure 1B). To detect the affinity of the CD37 antibody, a kinetic surface plasmon resonance experiment was performed on a Biacore with CD37-His protein. The CD37 antibody bound to CD37 antigen with high affinity, with binding constant KD of 1.65 nM (Figure 1C).

To detect binding of CD37 antibody on the cell surface, we transfected human embryonic kidney, HEK-293 cells either with CD37 antigen plasmid or with negative control CD18 plasmid and showed specific binding of CD37 antibody 2B8 clone to CD37 in HEK-293-CD37 cells but not in control HEK293-CD18 or HEK293 cells (Figure 1D). In addition, Fluorescence Activated Cell Sorting, FACS analysis with Raji lymphoma cells demonstrated positive staining with CD37 antibody but not with other K562 leukemia cells or multiple myeloma RPMI8226, colon cancer Lovo cells, breast cancer MCF-7, or MDA-231 cells (Figure 1E). In addition, the CD37 antibody detected CD37 antigen in three primary leukemia samples (Supplementary Figure S1). This shows that the CD37 antibody specifically binds CD37 in lymphoma cells with endogenous expression of CD37 but not in other types of cancer. To additionally test the specificity of the CD37 antibody, we tested CHO-CD37 and CHO cells (Figure 1F).

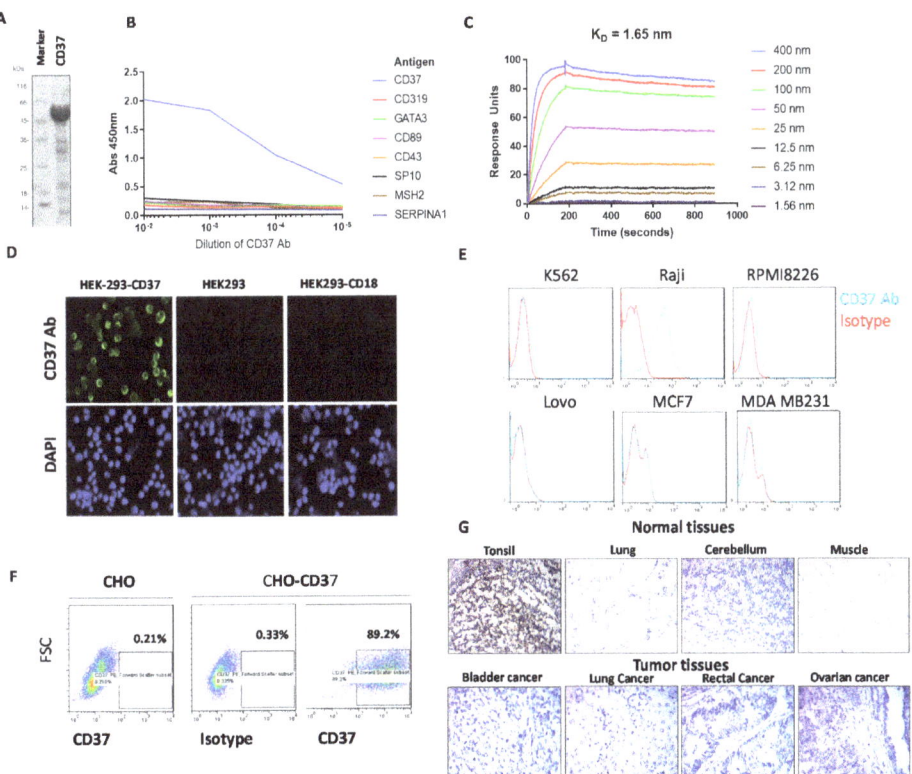

Figure 1. (**A**). Recombinant CD37 extracellular domain protein used for enzyme-linked immunosorbent assay, ELISA assay. The CD37 protein had C-terminal Maltose Binding Protein, MBP and His tag. SDS (sodium dodecyl sulfate) gel shows 56 kDa CD37 protein. (**B**). ELISA shows binding of CD37 antibody 2B8D12F2D4 (2B8) clone to CD37 protein and no binding to other unrelated control proteins. (**C**). Surface plasmon resonance kinetic data collected on Biacore with anti-CD37 2B8 antibody bound to mouse capture chip and titration of CD37-His. KD of 1.65 nm was measured from two independent experiments. (**D**). Immunostaining shows binding of CD37 2B8 clone antibody to CD37 antigen in HEK293-CD37 cells but not in HEK293-CD18 and HEK293 cells. Indirect immunofluorescence microscopy was performed with anti-CD37 2B8 followed by Goat-Anti-mouse IgG Alexa 488 (top row) and counterstained with DAPI (4′,6-diamidino-2-phenylindole) nuclear stain (bottom row). (**E**). FACS shows positive staining of CD37 2B8 antibody in CD37-positive Raji cells but not in other cancer cell lines. (**F**). FACS with CD37 antibody shows specific detection of cell surface CD37 in CHO-CD37 cells but not in CHO cells. (**G**). Indirect immunohistochemistry was performed on health (upper panel) and tumor (lower panel) adult tissue sections with anti-CD37 2B8 staining, followed by anti-mouse HRP (horseradish peroxidase). Positive staining was observed in tonsil, a lymphoid tissue, but not in normal lung, cerebellum, or muscle. Negative staining was observed in representative tumor samples.

We show that CD37 antibody has negative FACS staining in CHO cells but high staining in CHO-CD37 cells (Figure 1F). There was also negative staining with IgG1 isotype control in CHO-CD37 cells (Figure 1F). These and the above data demonstrate 2B8 bound to surface-expressed CD37 and not to other surface proteins.

Immunohistochemical staining (IHC) demonstrated low or negative staining in many normal tissues (esophagus, stomach, rectum, thyroid, kidney, lung, muscle, brain) (Supplementary Table S1) but increased staining in tonsils where lymphocytes were present (Figure 1G, upper panel). There was also negative staining in most types of cancer tumors (ovarian, lung, cervical, bladder, lung, prostate, rectal, gastric cancer) (Figure S1) (Figure 1G, lower panel).

Thus, the specific binding of CD37 to extracellular CD37 antigen in lymphoma cells makes this novel antibody suitable for CAR generation.

2.2. CD37-CAR-T Cells Specifically Target CD37-Positive Cells

We generated CAR with CD37 2B8 ScFv with a CD28 costimulatory domain and CD3 zeta activation domain (Figure 2A). The CD37-CAR-T cells were >70% CAR-positive after transduction with CD37-CAR lentivirus (Figure 2B). Then CD37-CAR-T cells were tested in Real-time cytotoxicity assay (RTCA) using target CD37-positive CHO-CD37 and CD37-negative CHO cells. CD37-CAR-T cells killed CHO-CD37 cells but did not kill CHO cells (Figure 2C, upper panels). Cytotoxicity was significantly higher for CD37 CAR-T cells than T cells or mock CAR-T cells (Figure 2C, bottom panels). IFN-γ released by CD37 CAR-T cells in response to CHO-CD37 target cells was significantly higher than in response to CHO cells (Figure 2D). Significantly higher secreted levels of IFN-gamma by CD37-CAR-T cells were detected with CD37-positive Raji cells than with CD37-negative K562 cells (Figure 2E). Thus, novel CD37 2B8 ScFv-CAR-T cells are effective and specific against CD37-positive target cells with exogenous and endogenous expression of CD37.

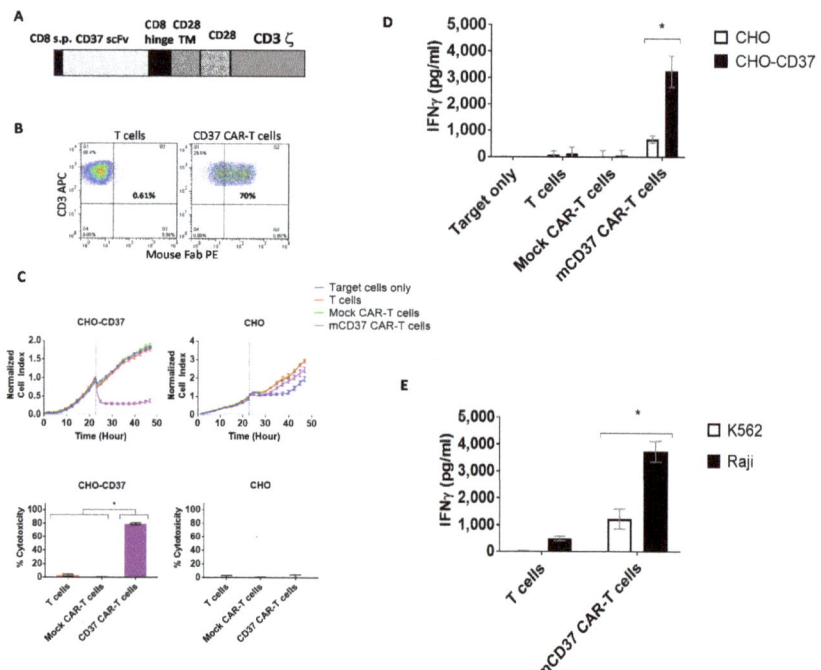

Figure 2. The specific CD37-chimeric antigen receptor (CAR)-T cell activity against CD37-positive cells in vitro. (**A**). The structure of CD37-CAR. The mouse ScFv (single-chain variable fragment) was used with CD8 hinge, CD28 transmembrane/costimulatory domains, and CD3 zeta activation domain. CD8 s.p-CD8 alpha signaling peptide; TM-transmembrane. (**B**). FACS with mouse F(ab)2 antibody (mFAB) detected CAR-positive cells. (**C**). Real-time cytotoxicity assay (RTCA) showed specific killing activity of CD37-CAR-T cells against CHO-CD37 cells but not CHO cells (upper panels). Lower panels: Percent cytotoxicity calculated at the end of the experiment. Significantly high cytotoxicity was observed against CHO-CD37 for CD37-CAR-T cells. $p < 0.0001$, One-Way ANOVA followed by Sidak multiple comparisons test. (**D**). Interferon-gamma (IFN-γ) secretion by CD37-CAR-T cells against CHO-CD37 cells is significantly higher than against CHO cells. asterisk *, $p < 0.0001$, two-way ANOVA $p < 0.0001$, followed by Tukey's multiple comparison test. (**E**). Secretion of IFN-gamma by CD37-CAR-T cells is significantly higher with Raji cells than with CD37-negative K562 cells. asterisk *, $p < 0.005$, mCD37 CAR-T cells with Raji cells versus same CAR-T cells with K562 cells, Student's t-test.

2.3. Humanized CD37-CAR-T Cells Specifically Target CD37-Positive Cells

We humanized CD37 VH and VL, as described in Materials and Methods, and generated lentiviral humanized CD37 CAR with a 4-1BB costimulatory domain and CD3 activation domain, called hCD37 CAR (Figure 3A). Surface expression of the CAR was detected by FACS with both anti-mouse Fab (72% positive) and anti-Human Fab (92% positive) (Figure 3B). In real-time cytotoxicity assay against CHO-CD37 and CHO cells, humanized anti-CD37 CAR-T cells effectively killed CHO-CD37 cells and demonstrated limited or no killing of CHO cells (Figure 3C). Cytotoxicity of humanized CD37 CAR-T cells against CHO-CD37 (95.3% ± 0.8%) was significantly higher than non-transduced T cells (17.5% ± 1.3%) or mock CAR-T cells (Figure 3D). The hCD37-CAR-T cells secreted significantly higher levels of IFN-gamma with CD37-positive target cells than with CD37-negative cells (Figure 3E). Thus, humanized CD37-CAR-T cells specifically target CD37-positive cells.

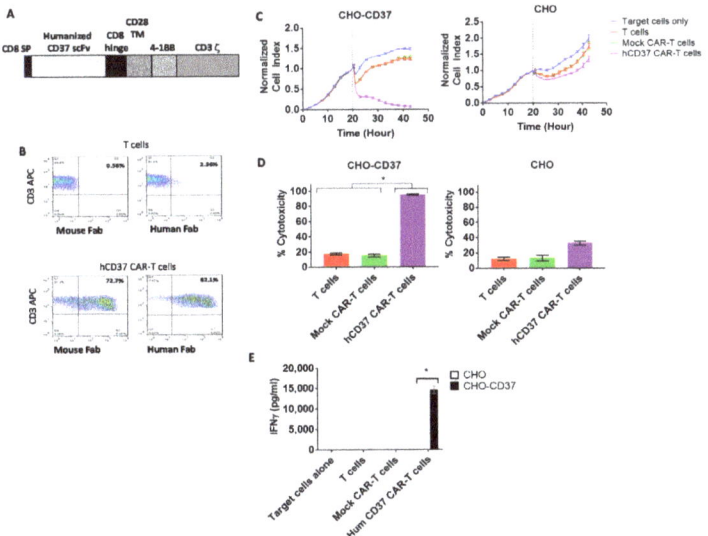

Figure 3. The humanized CD37-CAR-T cells specifically target CD37-positive cells. (**A**). The structure of humanized CD37-CAR-T cells. The structure includes CD8 signaling peptide; humanized CD37 ScFv, CD8 hinge, CD28 TM (transmembrane domain); 41BB domain; CD3 zeta activation domain. (**B**). FACS with mouse and human FAB detected CAR-positive cells. (**C**). Humanized CD37 CAR-T cells killed CHO-CD37-positive cells and did not kill CHO cells. (**D**). Quantification of cytotoxicity shows significantly higher killing by CD37CAR-T cells in CHO-CD37 cells than Mock and T cells. *, hCD37 CAR-T cells with CHO-CD37 cells versus T and Mock CAR-T cells, $p < 0.0001$, One-Way ANOVA followed by Dunnett's Multiple Comparison Test. (**E**). hCD37-CAR-T cells secrete significantly higher IFN-gamma with CHO-CD37 cells than with CHO cells. *, $p < 0.05$, IFN-gamma of humanized Hum CD37 CAR-T cells with CHO-CD37 cells versus same CAR-T cells with CHO cells by Student's t-test.

2.4. Bispecific Humanized CD37-CD19 CAR-T Cells Specifically Target CD37-Positive Cells

Next, we tested the efficacy of bi-specific humanized hCD37-CD19 CAR-T cells in vitro. To generate bi-specific humanized CD37-CD19 CAR-T cells, we used the following design as shown in Figure 4A with humanized CD37 ScFv and mouse CD19 FM63 ScFv [41]. These CAR-T cells had a surface expression of CAR as detected by FACS with anti-mouse and anti-human Fab antibodies (not shown). Real-time cytotoxicity assays were performed against CHO-CD37 and CHO cells (Figure 4B) and against Hela-CD19 and Hela cells (Figure 4C). Killing by bispecific hCD37-CD19 CAR-T cells was compared to CAR-T cells expressing monospecific hCD37 CAR or CD19 CAR. Bi-specific hCD37-CD19 CAR-T cells killed CHO-CD37 as effective as single hCD37-CAR-T cells and did not kill CHO cells (Figure 4B).

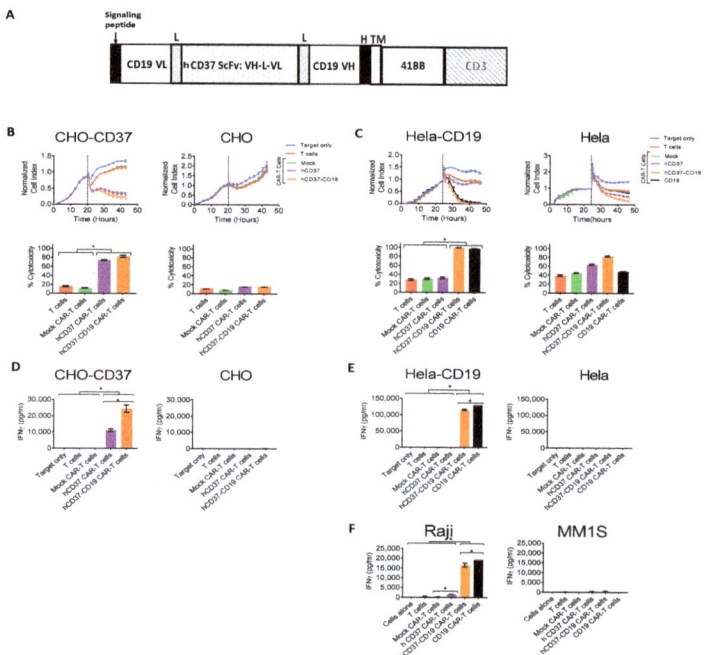

Figure 4. Bi-specific hCD37-CD19-CAR-T cells specifically target CD37-positive and CD19-positive cells. (**A**). The structure of bi-specific CD37-CD19 CAR-T cells. VL-light chain; VH-heavy chain; ScFv-single chain variable fragment; L-linker; H-hinge; TM, transmembrane domain. (**B**). RTCA activity of hCD37-CD19-CAR-T cells with CHO-CD37 cells (left) and CHO cells (right). Cytotoxicity of bispecific CD37-CD19 CAR-T cells against CHO-CD37 cells was significantly higher than that of humanized CD37 CAR-T cells, *, $p < 0.0001$, hCD37 and hCD37-CD19-CAR-T cells with CHO-CD37 cells vs T and Mock CAR-T cells, One-Way ANOVA followed by Sidak's multiple comparison test $p = 0.0006$. (**C**). RTCA activity of hCD37-CD19-CAR-T cells with Hela-CD19 cells (left) and Hela cells (right). Quantification of RTCA at the end time point is shown under the RTCA plots. * $p < 0.0001$, * hCD37-CD19 CAR-T cells and CD19 CAR-T cells with Hela-CD19 cells vs T cells, Mock CAR-T cells, CD37 CAR-T cells by One-Way ANOVA followed by Sidak's multiple comparison as in B. (**D**). IFN-gamma secretion by hCD37-CD19-CAR-T cells was significantly higher with CHO-CD37 cells than with CHO cells. * $p < 0.0001$, CD37, hCD37-CD19 CAR-T cells vs other groups with CHO-CD37 cells by One-way ANOVA followed by Tukey's test. (**E**). IFN-gamma secretion by CD37-CAR-T cells was significantly higher with Hela-CD19 cells than with Hela cells, * $p < 0.05$, hCD37-CD19 and CD19 CAR-T cells with Hela-CD19 cells vs other groups with Raji cells, Student's t-test. (**F**). IFN gamma secretion by hCD37-CD19-CAR-T cells against Raji cells was significantly higher than with CD37-negative multiple myeloma MM1S cells, $p < 0.001$, * hCD37, hCD37-CD19 and CD19 CAR-T cells with Raji cells vs Mock CAR-T cell groups with Raji cells by Tukey's test.

The hCD37-CD19 CAR-T cells also killed Hela-CD19 target cells and did not kill Hela cells (Figure 4C). As expected, single hCD37-CAR-T cells did not kill Hela-CD19 cells. The hCD37-CD19 CAR-T cells and hCD37-CAR-T cells secreted significantly higher levels of IFN-gamma against CHO-CD37 cells versus CHO cells (Figure 4D). Both hCD37-CD19 and CD19-CAR-T cells secreted significantly higher levels of IFN-gamma against Hela-CD19 target cells but not against Hela cells (Figure 4E).

In separate coculture experiments, IFN-γ release against Raji cells or MM1s cells was measured (Figure 4F). Both CD37-CD19 CAR-T cells and CD19 CAR-T cells had significantly more IFN-γ release than humanized CD37 CAR-T cells, mock CAR-T cells, and non-transduced T cells ($p < 0.0001$, Tukey's test) (Figure 4F). The secretion of IFN-gamma was significantly higher for CD37-CD19-CAR-T cells against Raji cells than against MM1S cells.

Thus, hCD37-CD19 CAR-T cells demonstrate high and specific efficacy against CD37 and CD19-positive target cells in vitro.

2.5. Humanized CD37-CD19 CAR-T Cells Inhibit Raji Lymphoma Xenograft Tumor Growth and Prolong Mice Survival

At first, we tested the efficacy of CD37-CAR-T cells in vivo and performed survival analysis using a Raji-xenograft tumor model after an injection of mouse CD37-CAR-T cells and humanized CD37-CAR-T cells (Figure S2). Mouse and humanized CD37-CAR-T cells prolonged mouse survival as well as CD19-CAR-T cells (Supplementary Figure S2).

To test the efficacy of the bispecific humanized CD37-CD19 CAR-T cells in vivo, Nod Scid Gamma, NSG mice were injected with 5×10^5 Raji-Luc cells followed 24 h later with 1×10^7 humanized CD37-CD19 CAR-T cells, mock CAR-T cells, or vehicle. Tumor luminescence was detected in mice treated with mock CAR-T cells or vehicle but not in mice treated with CD37-CD19 CAR-T cells (Figure 5A). Tumor luminescence in CD37-CD19 CAR-T cell treated mice was significantly lower than in mock CAR-T cell treated mice (Figure 5B). Survival of CD37-CD19 CAR-T cell treated group was significantly longer (≥ 75 days) (log–rank test $p < 0.0001$) than vehicle (18 days) and mock CAR-T cell treated groups (Figure 5C). Thus, humanized CD37 CAR-T cells and bi-specific hCD37-CD19 CAR-T cells are efficacious in the model in vivo.

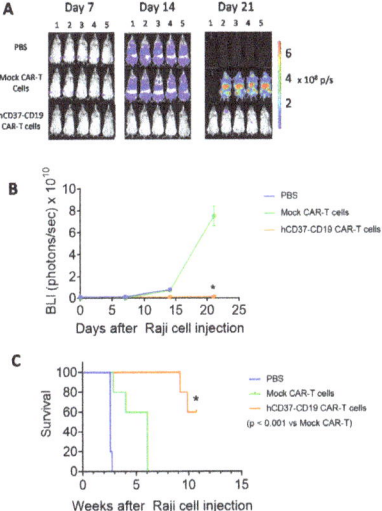

Figure 5. hCD37-CD19-CAR-T cells significantly block Raji xenograft tumor growth in vivo. (**A**). In vivo imaging of Raji tumors in mice on days 7, 14, and 21 following Raji-Luc+ cells injection with the vehicle, mock-CAR-T cells, or bispecific CD37-CD19 CAR-T cell-treated groups ($n = 5$ each). (**B**). Tumor luminescence flux from In Vivo Imaging System, IVIS imaging. Vehicle-treated mice had died by day 14. * $p < 0.05$, hCD37-CD19 CAR-T cells vs. Mock CAR-T cells, Student's t-test. (**C**). hCD37-CD19-CAR-T cells significantly prolong mouse survival in the Raji xenograft model. Kaplan–Myer curve is shown, $p < 0.05$, log–rank test hCD37-CD19 CAR-T cell-treated vs. Mock CAR-T cell-treated group.

3. Discussion

The present report demonstrates the efficacy of novel CD37-CAR-T cells and bispecific hCD37-CD19 CAR-T cells in vitro and in vivo. The novel CD37 antibody clone 2B8 was specific for the CD37 extracellular domain and bound with high affinity.

Standard of care for Non-Hodgkin lymphoma may include chemotherapy combined with anti-CD20 Ab (Rituximab) [21]. Relapse frequently occurs, demanding novel approaches. CD37 has been identified as a possible target for NHL immunotherapy. Anti-CD37-radioimmunoconjugates [27], duaHexabody CD37R0 [32], CD37 chimeric antibody (BI 836826) [29], and recently, CAR-T cells [18,19] have been tested.

The CD37-CAR-T cell therapy is especially important during lymphoma relapse when CD19 antigen is lost in lymphoma by either alternative splicing or other mechanisms, such as mutations [18]. Thus, CD37-CAR-T cells can improve the outcome of CD19-negative relapsed lymphoma patients. Bi-specific CD37-CD19 CAR-T cells can be important to increase the efficacy of CD19-CAR-T cells and also important in case of CD37 antigen loss due to missense mutations or other mechanisms [42].

The CD19-CD37 CAR-T cells were described by [19], but they had a different structure than described in this report. The CD37-CD19 CAR design presented here is similar to the CD19-CD22 CAR design described by [39]. In the future, clinical studies will show the advantages of each CAR. In addition, this study shows that humanized CD37-CD19 CAR-T cells effectively blocked lymphoma growth in vivo that can be advantageous in case of downregulation of either CD19 or CD37 pathways or for more efficient targeting of both antigens. Moreover, humanized CD37 ScFv can also be used for the development of other approaches, such as antibody conjugates or bispecific antibodies.

Interestingly, IFN-gamma secreted by CD19-CAR-T cells was higher than by hCD37-CAR-T cells. The differences by CAR-T cells in the secretion of IFN-gamma can be explained by 3D conformation of antigen, distance to the membrane of the antibody epitope, and other mechanisms. The lower secretion of IFN-gamma by CD37-CAR-T cells can be important for potentially reducing of cytokine release storm (CRS) in the clinic.

Since lymphoma tumors are heterogeneous and surrounded by a microenvironment that can block immune response functions [43], the combination therapy of CAR-T cells with checkpoint inhibitors, checkpoint blocking antibodies with agonist antibodies inducing an immune response, or with small molecules can overcome these barriers. Tumor-associated macrophages (TAM)s were also reported to block immune responses in leukemia and lymphoma, and novel therapies needed to repress TAM in combination with targeting lymphoma cells [44]. Thus, future combination therapies can be tested in preclinical and clinical studies that target both the tumor and tumor microenvironment.

The novel CD37, humanized CD37, and CD37-CD19 CAR-T cells provide a basis for future clinical studies.

4. Materials and Methods

4.1. Cell Lines, Antibodies, Recombinant Proteins

Raji, RPMI8226, H929, MM1S, K562, CHO, MCF-7, MDA-231, and Lovo cell lines were purchased from the ATCC (Manassas, VA, USA) and cultured either in DMEM (GE Healthcare, Chicago, IL, USA) or in RPMI-1640 medium (ThermoFisher, Waltham, MA, USA) containing 10% FBS (AmCell, Mountain View, CA, USA). CHO-CD37 cells were purchased from BPS Bioscience (San Diego, CA, USA) and cultured in Ham's F12K medium containing 10% Fetal Bovine Serum, FBS and 1 mg/mL geneticin (ThermoFisher). Hela-CD37 were generated by transducing Hela cells with CD37 lentivirus. Human peripheral blood mononuclear cells (PBMC) from whole blood obtained in the Stanford Hospital Blood Center, Stanford, according to IRB-approved protocol (#13942), were isolated by density sedimentation over Ficoll-Paque (GE Healthcare, San Ramon, CA, USA).

CD37 antibody clone 2B8D12F2D4 was from Promab, (Richmond, CA, USA). Control monoclonal CD37 antibody was from Biolegend (San Diego, CA, USA). Recombinant proteins CD37, CD318, GATA3, CD89, CD43, SP10, MSH2, SERPINA1 were obtained from

Promab (Richmond, CA, USA). For ELISA with CD37 and other proteins, HRP labeled anti-Mouse IgG was used from Sigma-Aldrich (St Louis, MO, USA) (Cat#: A0168). Human serum and goat anti-mouse (Fab)2 or anti-human (Fab)2, CD3 antibodies for FACS were from Jackson Immunoresearch (West Grove, PA, USA).

4.2. Generation of CD37 Antibody, Clone 2B8D12F2D4

Six-eight weeks old BALB/c mice were immunized by subcutaneous injection, with the recombinant fusion CD37 extracellular domain (109–242 amino-acids of isoform 1 (P11049-1) with C-terminal MBP (Maltose binding protein) and 6× His (histidine) tags. For hybridoma generation, the immunized mice splenocytes were fused with SP2/0 myeloma cells using PEG (Polyethylene glycol) and then hypoxanthine (HAT) medium selection. Hybridomas were diluted to obtain single clones on 96-well plates and then were screened by ELISA for the selection of positive clones against the immunogen and unrelated tagged proteins. Several positive hybridoma clones were further cultured and expanded to produce anti-CD37 antibodies. The supernatants of these antibody clones were collected, purified through the Protein G affinity capture column, and analyzed by ELISA, Western, and FACS. The positive clone 2B8D12F2D4 (called 2B8) was selected for VH and VL sequencing and CAR generation.

4.3. CAR Lentiviral Construct Design

The codon-optimized sequence ScFv based on CD37, clone 2B8D12F2D4 VH and VL was synthesized in Integrated DNA Technologies (IDT) (San Diego, CA, USA) as a Gblock and subcloned into second-generation CAR sequence with either CD28 costimulatory domain for mouse CD37-CAR-T cells or 4-1BB costimulatory domain for humanized CD37 and bispecific hCD37-CD19 CAR-T cells and CD3 zeta activation domains. The CAR was subcloned into 3^d generation lentivirus under either EF1 (with CD28 costimulatory domain CAR) or MNDU3 promoter (with 41BB costimulatory domain CAR). Mock CAR-T cells without ScFv (TF tagged)-CD28-CD3 CAR-T cells were used as Mock CAR-T cells [10].

4.4. Humanization of CD37

Humanization of CD37 VH and VL was performed as described before [12,45] by grafting mouse complementarity-determining regions (CDRs) with humanized framework sequences [46].

4.5. CAR Lentivirus

2.5×10^7 HEK293FT cells (Thermo Fisher) were seeded on 0.01% gelatin-coated 15 cm plates and cultured overnight in DMEM, 2% FBS, 1xpen/strep, and then transfected with the pPACKH1 Lentivector Packaging mix (System Biosciences, Palo Alto, CA, USA) and 10 μg of the lentiviral vector using the NanoFect transfection reagent NF100 (Alstem, Richmond, CA, USA). The next day the medium was replaced with fresh medium, and 48 h later, the lentivirus-containing medium was collected. The medium was cleared of cell debris by centrifugation at $2100 \times g$ for 30 min. The virus particles were collected by centrifugation at $112,000 \times g$ for 60 min at 4 °C using a SW28.1 rotor, suspended in serum-free DMEM medium, aliquoted, and frozen at −80 °C.

4.6. CAR-T Cells

PBMC were suspended at 1×10^6 cells/mL in AIM V-AlbuMAX medium (ThermoFisher) containing 10% FBS and 10 ng/mL IL-2 (ThermoFisher), mixed with an equal number (1:1 ratio) of CD3/CD28 Dynabeads (ThermoFisher), and cultured in non-treated 24-well plates (0.5 mL per well). At 24 and 48 h, lentivirus was added to the cultures. The T cells proliferated over the next 10–12 days, the cells were counted every 2–3 days, and fresh medium with 10 ng/mL IL-2 was added to the cultures to maintain the cell density at 1–2×10^6 cells/mL.

4.7. Flow Cytometry (FACS)

To measure CAR expression, 0.25 million cells were suspended in 100 µL of buffer (PBS (phosphate buffered saline) containing 2 mM EDTA pH 8 and 0.5% BSA) and incubated on ice with 1 µL of human serum for 10 min. Diluted primary antibody biotin-conjugated goat anti-mouse (Fab)2 or anti-human (Fab)2 was used with cells for 30 min at 4 °C, and after washing, the secondary antibody was added with APC-conjugated mouse α-human CD3 antibody and PE-conjugated streptavidin at 1:100 dilution for 30 min incubation at 4 °C. The cells were rinsed with 3 mL of washing buffer, then stained for 10 min with 7-AAD, suspended in the buffer, and acquired on a FACSCalibur (BD Biosciences, San Jose, CA, USA). Cells were analyzed first for light scatter versus 7-AAD staining, then the 7-AAD$^-$ live gated cells were plotted for anti-CD3 staining versus CAR$^+$ staining with anti-(Fab)2 antibodies.

4.8. Cytotoxicity (RTCA)

Adherent target cells (CHO-CD37; CHO; Hela-CD37 or Hela) were seeded into 96-well E-plates (Acea Biosciences, San Diego, CA, USA) at 1×10^4 cells per well and monitored in culture overnight with the impedance-based real-time cell analysis (RTCA) xCELLigence system (Acea Biosciences). The next day, the medium was removed and replaced with AIM V-AlbuMAX medium containing 10% FBS $\pm$ 1×10^5 effector cells (CAR-T cells or non-transduced T cells) in triplicate. The cells in the E-plates were monitored for another 24–48 h with the RTCA system, and impedance was plotted over time. Cytotoxicity was calculated as (impedance of target cells without effector cells—impedance of target cells with effector cells) × 100/impedance of target cells without effector cells.

4.9. Affinity Measurement Using SPR Biacore Assay

Anti-CD37 antibody 2B8 clone affinity for CD37 antigen was measured in duplicate experiments on Biacore 3000 using an anti-mouse IgG coated CM5 chip for anti-CD37 antibody 2B8 capture and an activated reference surface. Following Anti-CD37 antibody 2B8 capture in degassed pH 7.4 HEPES (4-(2-hydroxyethyl)-1-piperazineethanesulfonic acid) buffered saline with 0.005% (w/v) Tween-20 and 3 min stabilization, duplicate serial dilutions of extracellular domain of CD37, CD37-His protein (Prospec, Rehovot, Israel) were injected for 3 min association phase kinetics followed by 15 min dissociation and surface regeneration with pH 1.7 10 mM glycine. The average KD was detected in nM.

4.10. ELISA for Detection IFN-Gamma

Nonadherent target cells (Raji, MM1S, K562) were cultured with the effector cells (CAR-T cells or non-transduced T cells) at a 1:1 ratio (1×10^4 cells each) in U-bottom 96-well plates with 200 µL of AIM V-AlbuMAX medium containing 10% FBS, in triplicate. After 16 h, the top 150 µL of the medium was transferred to V-bottom 96-well plates and centrifuged at 300 g for 5 min to pellet any residual cells. The top 120 µL of supernatant was transferred to a new 96-well plate and analyzed by ELISA for human IFN-γ levels using a kit from R&D Systems (Minneapolis, MN, USA) according to the manufacturer's protocol. The supernatant after RTCA with adherent target cells was collected and analyzed as above.

4.11. Mouse Tumor Xenograft Model and Imaging

Six-week-old male NSG mice (Jackson Laboratories, Bar Harbor, ME, USA) were housed in accordance with the Institutional Animal Care and Use Committee (IACUC) (# LUM-001). Each mouse was injected subcutaneously on day 0 with 100 µL of 5×10^5 Raji-luciferase positive cells in sterile serum-free medium. The next day 1×10^7 CAR-T cells in serum-free medium were injected intravenously. Imaging was done using Raji-luciferase positive cells after luciferin injection with Xenogen Ivis System. Quantification was done by measuring photons/sec signals. A Kaplan–Myer survival curve was done based on mice survival data.

4.12. Immunohistochemistry (IHC)

Tumor tissue sections (4 μm) were deparaffinized in xylenes twice for 10 min, then hydrated in graded alcohols and rinsed in PBS. Antigen retrieval was performed for 20 min in a pressure cooker using 10 mM citrate buffer, pH 6.0. The sections were cooled, rinsed with PBS, incubated in a 3% H_2O_2 solution for 10 min, and rinsed with PBS. The tissue sections were incubated in goat serum for 20 min and then incubated with primary CD37 antibody. Then sections were rinsed with PBS, incubated with biotin-conjugated goat anti-mouse IgG for 10 min, rinsed with PBS, incubated with streptavidin-conjugated peroxidase for 10 min, and rinsed with PBS. Finally, the sections were incubated in DAB (3,3'Diaminobenzidine) substrate solution for 2–5 min, immersed in tap water, counterstained with hematoxylin, rinsed with water, and dehydrated in graded alcohols and xylenes. Coverslips were mounted with glycerin. Images were acquired on a Motic DMB5-2231PL microscope with Images Plus 2.0 software (Motic, Xiamen, China).

4.13. Statistical Analysis

Data were analyzed and plotted with Prism software (GraphPad V7, San Diego, CA, USA). Comparisons between two groups were performed by unpaired Student's *t*-test; one or two-way ANOVA, followed by Sidak or Dunnett's tests for multiple comparisons. The *p*-value < 0.05 was considered significant.

5. Conclusions

This study demonstrates that novel CD37, humanized CD37, and humanized CD37-CD19 CAR-T cells specifically targeted CD19 and CD37 positive cells and provides the basis for future clinical studies.

6. Patents

The patent application was filed based on the work reported in this manuscript.

Supplementary Materials: The following are available online at https://www.mdpi.com/2072-6694/13/5/981/s1, Figure S1: FACS with CD37 antibody (clone 2B8) shows positive staining in three patient-derived leukemia samples. Figure S2: Mouse and humanized CD37 CAR-T cells significantly block Raji xenograft tumor growth in vivo. Table S1: IHC staining with CD37 antibody (clone 2B8) in different normal and tumor tissues.

Author Contributions: Conceptualization, V.G. and L.W.; Methodology, M.V.; H.Z.; F.L.; R.B.; S.X.; J.S. (Jinying Sun); J.S. (John Sienkiewicz); Y.H.; M.Q.; M.C.M. Software, M.V.; H.Z.; R.B.; Validation, M.V., H.Z. Formal Analysis, V.G.; Investigation, R.B.; H.Z.; M.V.; F.L. Resources, L.W.; Data Curation, M.V.; Writing—Original Draft Preparation, V.G.; Writing—Review & Editing, V.G.; M.V.; L.W. Visualization, V.G.; Supervision, V.G.; Project Administration, V.G., L.W.; Funding Acquisition, L.W. All authors have read and agreed to the published version of the manuscript.

Funding: This research was funded by Promab Biotechnologies.

Institutional Review Board Statement: Not applicable.

Informed Consent Statement: Not applicable.

Data Availability Statement: Data is contained within the article or Supplementary Materials.

Acknowledgments: The authors would like to acknowledge Promab's Hybridoma Facility for help in generating CD37 monoclonal antibody (Changsha, China) and Ed Lim for help with animal experiments.

Conflicts of Interest: Wu is CEO of Promab Biotechnologies, and the co-authors are employees of Promab Biotechnologies.

References

1. Eshhar, Z.; Gross, G. Chimeric T cell receptor which incorporates the anti-tumour specificity of a monoclonal antibody with the cytolytic activity of T cells: A model system for immunotherapeutical approach. *Br. J. Cancer Suppl.* **1990**, *10*, 27–29.
2. Eshhar, Z.; Waks, T.; Gross, G. The emergence of T-bodies/CAR T cells. *Cancer J.* **2014**, *20*, 123–126. [CrossRef] [PubMed]
3. Maus, M.V.; Grupp, S.A.; Porter, D.L.; June, C.H. Antibody-modified T cells: CARs take the front seat for hematologic malignancies. *Blood* **2014**, *123*, 2625–2635. [CrossRef] [PubMed]
4. Maus, M.V.; June, C.H. Making Better Chimeric Antigen Receptors for Adoptive T-cell Therapy. *Clin. Cancer Res.* **2016**, *22*, 1875–1884. [CrossRef] [PubMed]
5. Golubovskaya, V.; Wu, L. Different Subsets of T Cells, Memory, Effector Functions, and CAR-T Immunotherapy. *Cancers* **2016**, *8*, 36. [CrossRef]
6. Klebanoff, C.A.; Yamamoto, T.N.; Restifo, N.P. Immunotherapy: Treatment of aggressive lymphomas with anti-CD19 CAR T cells. *Nat. Rev. Clin. Oncol.* **2014**, *11*, 685–686. [CrossRef] [PubMed]
7. Locke, F.L.; Davila, M.L. Regulatory challenges and considerations for the clinical application of CAR-T cell anti-cancer therapy. *Expert Opin. Biol. Ther.* **2017**, *17*, 659–661. [CrossRef]
8. Locke, F.L.; Ghobadi, A.; Jacobson, C.A.; Miklos, D.B.; Lekakis, L.J.; Oluwole, O.O.; Lin, Y.; Braunschweig, I.; Hill, B.T.; Timmerman, J.M.; et al. Long-term safety and activity of axicabtagene ciloleucel in refractory large B-cell lymphoma (ZUMA-1): A single-arm, multicentre, phase 1-2 trial. *Lancet Oncol.* **2019**, *20*, 31–42. [CrossRef]
9. Locke, F.L.; Neelapu, S.S.; Bartlett, N.L.; Siddiqi, T.; Chavez, J.C.; Hosing, C.M.; Ghobadi, A.; Budde, L.E.; Bot, A.; Rossi, J.M.; et al. Phase 1 Results of ZUMA-1: A Multicenter Study of KTE-C19 Anti-CD19 CAR T Cell Therapy in Refractory Aggressive Lymphoma. *Mol. Ther.* **2017**, *25*, 285–295. [CrossRef]
10. Valentine, M.; Li, L.; Zhou, H.; Xu, S.; Sun, J.; Liu, C.; Harto, H.; Berahovich, R.; Golubovskaya, V.; Wu, L. Transferrin epitope-CD19-CAR-T cells effectively kill lymphoma cells in vitro and in vivo. *Front. Biosci.* **2020**, *25*, 270–282.
11. Berahovich, R.; Xu, S.; Zhou, H.; Harto, H.; Xu, Q.; Garcia, A.; Liu, F.; Golubovskaya, V.M.; Wu, L. FLAG-tagged CD19-specific CAR-T cells eliminate CD19-bearing solid tumor cells in vitro and in vivo. *Front. Biosci.* **2017**, *22*, 1644–1654.
12. Berahovich, R.; Zhou, H.; Xu, S.; Wei, Y.; Guan, J.; Guan, J.; Harto, H.; Fu, S.; Yang, K.; Zhu, S.; et al. CAR-T Cells Based on Novel BCMA Monoclonal Antibody Block Multiple Myeloma Cell Growth. *Cancers* **2018**, *10*, 323. [CrossRef]
13. Tettamanti, S.; Biondi, A.; Biagi, E.; Bonnet, D. CD123 AML targeting by chimeric antigen receptors: A novel magic bullet for AML therapeutics? *Oncoimmunology* **2014**, *3*, e28835. [CrossRef]
14. Davila, M.L.; Bouhassira, D.C.; Park, J.H.; Curran, K.J.; Smith, E.L.; Pegram, H.J.; Brentjens, R. Chimeric antigen receptors for the adoptive T cell therapy of hematologic malignancies. *Int. J. Hematol.* **2014**, *99*, 361–371. [CrossRef]
15. Dotti, G.; Gottschalk, S.; Savoldo, B.; Brenner, M.K. Design and development of therapies using chimeric antigen receptor-expressing T cells. *Immunol. Rev.* **2014**, *257*, 107–126. [CrossRef]
16. Fesnak, A.; Lin, C.; Siegel, D.L.; Maus, M.V. CAR-T Cell Therapies from the Transfusion Medicine Perspective. *Transfus. Med. Rev.* **2016**, *30*, 139–145. [CrossRef] [PubMed]
17. Golubovskaya, V.M.; Berahovich, R.; Xu, Q.; Zhou, H.; Xu, S.; Guan, J.; Harto, H.; Li, L.; Wu, L. GITR domain inside CAR co-stimulates activity of CAR-T cells against cancer. *Front. Biosci.* **2018**, *23*, 2245–2254. [CrossRef]
18. Koksal, H.; Dillard, P.; Josefsson, S.E.; Maggadottir, S.M.; Pollmann, S.; Fane, A.; Blaker, Y.N.; Beiske, K.; Huse, K.; Kolstad, A.; et al. Preclinical development of CD37CAR T-cell therapy for treatment of B-cell lymphoma. *Blood Adv.* **2019**, *3*, 1230–1243. [CrossRef] [PubMed]
19. Scarfo, I.; Ormhoj, M.; Frigault, M.J.; Castano, A.P.; Lorrey, S.; Bouffard, A.A.; van Scoyk, A.; Rodig, S.J.; Shay, A.J.; Aster, J.C.; et al. Anti-CD37 chimeric antigen receptor T cells are active against B- and T-cell lymphomas. *Blood* **2018**, *132*, 1495–1506. [CrossRef]
20. Bertoni, F.; Stathis, A. Staining the target: CD37 expression in lymphomas. *Blood* **2016**, *128*, 3022–3023. [CrossRef]
21. de Winde, C.M.; Elfrink, S.; van Spriel, A.B. Novel Insights into Membrane Targeting of B Cell Lymphoma. *Trends Cancer* **2017**, *3*, 442–453. [CrossRef]
22. Payandeh, Z.; Noori, E.; Khalesi, B.; Mard-Soltani, M.; Abdolalizadeh, J.; Khalili, S. Anti-CD37 targeted immunotherapy of B-Cell malignancies. *Biotechnol. Lett.* **2018**, *40*, 1459–1466. [CrossRef]
23. Schwartz-Albiez, R.; Dorken, B.; Hofmann, W.; Moldenhauer, G. The B cell-associated CD37 antigen (gp40-52). Structure and subcellular expression of an extensively glycosylated glycoprotein. *J. Immunol.* **1988**, *140*, 905–914. [PubMed]
24. Witkowska, M.; Smolewski, P.; Robak, T. Investigational therapies targeting CD37 for the treatment of B-cell lymphoid malignancies. *Expert Opin. Investig. Drugs* **2018**, *27*, 171–177. [CrossRef]
25. Gartlan, K.H.; Wee, J.L.; Demaria, M.C.; Nastovska, R.; Chang, T.M.; Jones, E.L.; Apostolopoulos, V.; Pieretsz, G.A.; Hickey, M.J.; van Spriel, A.B.; et al. Tetraspanin CD37 contributes to the initiation of cellular immunity by promoting dendritic cell migration. *Eur. J. Immunol.* **2013**, *43*, 1208–1219. [CrossRef]
26. Lapalombella, R.; Yeh, Y.Y.; Wang, L.; Ramanunni, A.; Rafiq, S.; Jha, S.; Staubli, J.; Lucas, D.M.; Mani, R.; Herman, S.E.; et al. Tetraspanin CD37 directly mediates transduction of survival and apoptotic signals. *Cancer Cell* **2012**, *21*, 694–708. [CrossRef] [PubMed]
27. Blakkisrud, J.; Holtedahl, J.E.; Londalen, A.; Dahle, J.; Bach-Gansmo, T.; Holte, H.; Nygaard, S.; Kolstad, A.; Stokke, C. Biodistribution and Dosimetry Results from a Phase 1 Trial of Therapy with the Antibody-Radionuclide Conjugate (177)Lu-Lilotomab Satetraxetan. *J. Nucl. Med.* **2018**, *59*, 704–710. [CrossRef] [PubMed]

28. Hicks, S.W.; Lai, K.C.; Gavrilescu, L.C.; Yi, Y.; Sikka, S.; Shah, P.; Kelly, M.E.; Lee, J.; Lanieri, L.; Ponte, J.F.; et al. The Antitumor Activity of IMGN529, a CD37-Targeting Antibody-Drug Conjugate, Is Potentiated by Rituximab in Non-Hodgkin Lymphoma Models. *Neoplasia* **2017**, *19*, 661–671. [CrossRef] [PubMed]
29. Kroschinsky, F.; Middeke, J.M.; Janz, M.; Lenz, G.; Witzens-Harig, M.; Bouabdallah, R.; La Rosee, P.; Viardot, A.; Salles, G.; Kim, S.J.; et al. Phase I dose escalation study of BI 836826 (CD37 antibody) in patients with relapsed or refractory B-cell non-Hodgkin lymphoma. *Investig. New Drugs* **2020**, *5*, 1472–1482. [CrossRef] [PubMed]
30. Maaland, A.F.; Heyerdahl, H.; O'Shea, A.; Eiriksdottir, B.; Pascal, V.; Andersen, J.T.; Kolstad, A.; Dahle, J. Targeting B-cell malignancies with the beta-emitting anti-CD37 radioimmunoconjugate (177)Lu-NNV003. *Eur. J. Nucl. Med. Mol. Imaging* **2019**, *46*, 2311–2321. [CrossRef]
31. van der Horst, H.J.; Oostindie, S.C.; Cillessen, S.; Gelderloos, A.T.; Overdijk, M.B.; Nijhof, I.S.; Zweegman, S.; Chamuleau, M.E.D.; Breij, E.C.W.; Mutis, T. Potent Preclinical Efficacy of DuoHexaBody-CD37 in B-Cell Malignancies. *Hemasphere* **2021**, *5*, e504. [CrossRef]
32. Oostindie, S.C.; van der Horst, H.J.; Kil, L.P.; Strumane, K.; Overdijk, M.B.; van den Brink, E.N.; van den Brakel, J.H.N.; Rademaker, H.J.; van Kessel, B.; van den Noort, J.; et al. DuoHexaBody-CD37((R)), a novel biparatopic CD37 antibody with enhanced Fc-mediated hexamerization as a potential therapy for B-cell malignancies. *Blood Cancer J.* **2020**, *10*, 30. [CrossRef] [PubMed]
33. June, C.H.; O'Connor, R.S.; Kawalekar, O.U.; Ghassemi, S.; Milone, M.C. CAR T cell immunotherapy for human cancer. *Science* **2018**, *359*, 1361–1365. [CrossRef]
34. Abramson, J.S.; Lunning, M.; Palomba, M.L. Chimeric Antigen Receptor T-Cell Therapies for Aggressive B-Cell Lymphomas: Current and Future State of the Art. *Am. Soc. Clin. Oncol. Educ. Book* **2019**, *39*, 446–453. [CrossRef]
35. Ruella, M.; June, C.H. Chimeric Antigen Receptor T cells for B Cell Neoplasms: Choose the Right CAR for You. *Curr. Hematol. Malig. Rep.* **2016**, *11*, 368–384. [CrossRef] [PubMed]
36. Schneider, D.; Xiong, Y.; Wu, D.; Nlle, V.; Schmitz, S.; Haso, W.; Kaiser, A.; Dropulic, B.; Orentas, R.J. A tandem CD19/CD20 CAR lentiviral vector drives on-target and off-target antigen modulation in leukemia cell lines. *J. Immunother. Cancer* **2017**, *5*, 42. [CrossRef] [PubMed]
37. Zah, E.; Lin, M.Y.; Silva-Benedict, A.; Jensen, M.C.; Chen, Y.Y. T Cells Expressing CD19/CD20 Bispecific Chimeric Antigen Receptors Prevent Antigen Escape by Malignant B Cells. *Cancer Immunol. Res.* **2016**, *4*, 498–508. [CrossRef] [PubMed]
38. Dai, H.; Wu, Z.; Jia, H.; Tong, C.; Guo, Y.; Ti, D.; Han, X.; Liu, Y.; Zhang, W.; Wang, C.; et al. Bispecific CAR-T cells targeting both CD19 and CD22 for therapy of adults with relapsed or refractory B cell acute lymphoblastic leukemia. *J. Hematol. Oncol.* **2020**, *13*, 30. [CrossRef]
39. Fry, T.J.; Shah, N.N.; Orentas, R.J.; Stetler-Stevenson, M.; Yuan, C.M.; Ramakrishna, S.; Wolters, P.; Martin, S.; Delbrook, C.; Yates, B.; et al. CD22-targeted CAR T cells induce remission in B-ALL that is naive or resistant to CD19-targeted CAR immunotherapy. *Nat. Med.* **2018**, *24*, 20–28. [CrossRef]
40. Ruella, M.; Barrett, D.M.; Kenderian, S.S.; Shestova, O.; Hofmann, T.J.; Perazzelli, J.; Klichinsky, M.; Aikawa, V.; Nazimuddin, F.; Kozlowski, M.; et al. Dual CD19 and CD123 targeting prevents antigen-loss relapses after CD19-directed immunotherapies. *J. Clin. Investig.* **2016**, *126*, 3814–3826. [CrossRef]
41. Kochenderfer, J.N.; Feldman, S.A.; Zhao, Y.; Xu, H.; Black, M.A.; Morgan, R.A.; Wilson, W.H.; Rosenberg, S.A. Construction and preclinical evaluation of an anti-CD19 chimeric antigen receptor. *J. Immunother.* **2009**, *32*, 689–702. [CrossRef] [PubMed]
42. Elfrink, S.; de Winde, C.M.; van den Brand, M.; Berendsen, M.; Roemer, M.G.M.; Arnold, F.; Janssen, L.; van der Schaaf, A.; Jansen, E.; Groenen, P.; et al. High frequency of inactivating tetraspanin C D37 mutations in diffuse large B-cell lymphoma at immune-privileged sites. *Blood* **2019**, *134*, 946–950. [CrossRef]
43. Anagnostou, T.; Ansell, S.M. Immunomodulators in Lymphoma. *Curr. Treat. Options Oncol.* **2020**, *21*, 28. [CrossRef]
44. Li, Y.; You, M.J.; Yang, Y.; Hu, D.; Tian, C. The Role of Tumor-Associated Macrophages in Leukemia. *Acta Haematol.* **2020**, *143*, 112–117. [CrossRef] [PubMed]
45. Golubovskaya, V.; Berahovich, R.; Zhou, H.; Xu, S.; Harto, H.; Li, L.; Chao, C.C.; Mao, M.M.; Wu, L. CD47-CAR-T Cells Effectively Kill Target Cancer Cells and Block Pancreatic Tumor Growth. *Cancers* **2017**, *9*, 139. [CrossRef] [PubMed]
46. Almagro, J.C.; Fransson, J. Humanization of antibodies. *Front. Biosci.* **2008**, *13*, 1619–1633. [PubMed]

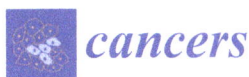

Article

DCLK1 Monoclonal Antibody-Based CAR-T Cells as a Novel Treatment Strategy against Human Colorectal Cancers

Sripathi M. Sureban [1,2,*], Robert Berahovich [3], Hua Zhou [3], Shirley Xu [3], Lijun Wu [3], Kai Ding [2], Randal May [1,2], Dongfeng Qu [1,2], Edwin Bannerman-Menson [1], Vita Golubovskaya [3] and Courtney W. Houchen [1,2,4,*]

1. COARE Holdings Inc., Oklahoma, OK 73104, USA; randal-may@ouhsc.edu (R.M.); dongfeng-qu@ouhsc.edu (D.Q.); eddie@bannermanmenson.com (E.B.-M.)
2. Department of Internal Medicine, Digestive Diseases and Nutrition Section, The University of Oklahoma Health Science Center, Oklahoma, OK 73014, USA; kai-ding@ouhsc.edu
3. ProMab Biotechnologies Inc., Richmond, CA 94806, USA; Robert.berahovich@promab.com (R.B.); huazhou369@gmail.com (H.Z.); shirley.xu@promab.com (S.X.); john@promab.com (L.W.); vita.gol@promab.com (V.G.)
4. Veterans Affairs Medical Center, Oklahoma, OK 73104, USA
* Correspondence: sripathi@coarebiotechnology.com (S.M.S.); courtney-houchen@ouhsc.edu (C.W.H.); Tel.: +1-405-271-5428 (S.M.S. & C.W.H.)

Received: 9 October 2019; Accepted: 16 December 2019; Published: 23 December 2019

Abstract: CAR-T (chimeric antigen receptor T cells) immunotherapy is effective in many hematological cancers; however, efficacy in solid tumors is disappointing. Doublecortin-like kinase 1 (DCLK1) labels tumor stem cells (TSCs) in genetic mouse models of colorectal cancer (CRC). Here, we describe a novel CAR-T targeting DCLK1 (CBT-511; with our proprietary DCLK1 single-chain antibody variable fragment) as a treatment strategy to eradicate CRC TSCs. The cell surface expression of DCLK1 and cytotoxicity of CBT-511 were assessed in CRC cells (HT29, HCT116, and LoVo). LoVo-derived tumor xenografts in NOD Scid gamma (NSG™) mice were treated with CBT-511 or mock CAR-T cells. Adherent CRC cells express surface DCLK1 (two-dimensional, 2D). A 4.5-fold increase in surface DCLK1 was observed when HT29 cells were grown as spheroids (three-dimensional, 3D). CBT-511 induced cytotoxicity (2D; $p < 0.0001$), and increased Interferon gamma (IFN-γ) release in CRC cells (2D) compared to mock CAR-T ($p < 0.0001$). Moreover, an even greater increase in IFN-γ release was observed when cells were grown in 3D. CBT-511 reduced tumor growth by approximately 50 percent compared to mock CAR-T. These data suggest that CRC cells with increased clonogenic capacity express increased surface DCLK1. A DCLK1-targeted CAR-T can induce cytotoxicity in vitro and inhibit xenograft growth in vivo.

Keywords: DCLK1; CAR-T; tumor stem cells; immunotherapy; clonogenicity

1. Introduction

Colorectal cancer (CRC) is the third leading cause of cancer-related deaths in the U.S. [1]. For individuals diagnosed with stage IV of the disease, the five-year survival rate is just 12% [1]. A growing body of evidence suggests that cancer stem cells (CSCs) play a critical role in the initiation, progression, and metastatic spread of cancer [2,3]. In solid tumor cancers, including CRCs, the tumor attempts to either evade the anti-tumor immune system or emit inhibitory signals to suppress immune effector cells and limit their anti-tumorigenic activity [4,5].

Immunotherapy has been remarkably successful for treating solid tumor cancers due to its unique ability to inhibit immune system checkpoint proteins (e.g., PD-1, PD-L1, CTLA4) and reactivate the host's anti-tumor immunity [6]. Mechanistically, these checkpoint inhibitors enable cytotoxic CD8$^+$ T cells to attack and destroy cancer cells [6]. However, the efficacy of these inhibitors as a monotherapy or in combination with other therapeutics varies considerably and is largely dependent on tumor type and individual patient characteristics [7]. In addition, the composition, pH, and metabolic activity within the tumor microenvironment (TME) are additional factors that can influence the effectiveness of these agents [8]. Infiltrating T lymphocytes that invade the TME and exert cytotoxic effects within the tumor have been shown to correlate with increased efficacy and improved survival rate in several cancers [8,9]. However, the efficacy again varies greatly between patient populations and the type of tumor being targeted.

The CSC hypothesis is based on findings that solid tumor cancers, including CRCs, are derived from a rare population of long lived, relatively quiescent, self-renewing cancer cells that are able to differentiate into every individual epithelial cell type within the tumor mass [10,11]. These cells are also able to differentiate into non-epithelial cell types via a process called epithelial-mesenchymal transition (EMT) [3,12–16]. This process facilitates TSC entry into the blood stream prior to dissemination and uptake into distant organs where they re-epithelialized through a process known as mesenchymal-epithelial transition (MET) [17]. Although the molecular mechanisms that regulate these highly integrative processes are under investigation, their contribution to advanced CRC-related mortality is clear. Inhibition of protooncogenic processes within the TSCs, as well as TSC eradication and inactivation, are crucial for successful anti-cancer treatments [10,11,18]. Recent studies have demonstrated that increased expression of EMT transcription factors and CSC-related proteins in human CRC tissues are strongly associated with unfavorable clinicopathological manifestations and poor patient outcomes [18]. Given the aggressive nature of CRC tumors and their high rate(s) of recurrence or metastasis, EMT-and CSC-related proteins may provide novel therapeutic targets for the treatment of CRC [10,11,18].

Doublecortin-like kinase 1 (DCLK1) is a microtubule-associated kinase that regulates EMT and is associated with microRNAs known to regulate tumor growth and progression [19–24]. A compelling study published in Nature Genetics utilizing the $Dclk1^{CreErt2}$ mouse model demonstrated that Dclk1 specifically marks TSCs that continuously produce tumor progeny in the polyps of $Apc^{Min/+}$ mice. In addition, specific ablation of Dclk1$^+$ TSCs resulted in marked polyp regression and no intestinal damage [25]. This landmark study was the first to identify Dclk1 as a marker that can distinguish normal gastrointestinal epithelial cells from TSCs and to demonstrate that normal intestinal Dclk1 expressing epithelial cells are not required for normal homeostatic function [25]. In another study, quiescent Dclk1$^+$ tuft cells served as colon cancer-initiating cells following loss of Apc and in the presence of inflammation in a $Dclk1^{CreErt}$ mouse model [26]. In human CRC tumors, elevated levels of DCLK1 are associated with higher rates of recurrence and mortality [27]. Therefore, strategies directed at eliminating DCLK1-expressing TSCs have the potential to mitigate CRC-related morbidity, recurrence, and metastasis and improve survival in patients afflicted by this insidious disease.

Immunotherapy using CAR-T (T cells modified with chimeric antigen receptor) is recognized as an increasingly effective therapy for the treatment of hematologic malignancies [28–30]. However, its efficacy in treating solid tumor malignancies has been less promising [31]. Several hypotheses have been generated that may explain this treatment disparity: a hypoxic TME that reduces CD8$^+$ cytotoxic T cell viability, tumor associated induction of innate immunosuppression, and solid tumor-based physical impediments that prevent T cell cytotoxicity against the tumor [32–35]. These solid tumor-associated features are not encountered during systemic administration of CAR-T therapies used for hematologic malignancies [32–35]. CAR-T therapy is an exciting new treatment modality in which a patient's CD8$^+$ T cell population is removed and re-engineered to create a new population of chimeric T cells. The cells are designed to include an extracellular antigen-binding domain targeting tumor-specific antigens expressed on the surface of cancer cells [36,37]. This personalized approach to cancer therapy enables a patient's own T cells to be programmed to attack and eliminate their specific cancer. Typically, the tumor antigen specific targeting region is a single-chain antibody variable fragment (ScFv) fused to a hinge, transmembrane domain, and co-stimulatory domains (CD28, 4-1BB, CD27 or others) to stimulate the immune response, as well as a CD3ζ activation domain [38–43].

In this report, we demonstrate that the proprietary humanized DCLK1 ScFv sequence can be used to detect cell surface expression of the extracellular DCLK1 (human isoforms 2 and 4) on several CRC cell lines. Furthermore, we demonstrate that HT29 cells grown in three-dimensional (3D) matrices exhibit a 4.5-fold increase in cell surface DCLK1 expression compared to cells grown in two-dimensional (2D). These data support our hypothesis that the TSC population can be targeted using a DCLK1-specific CAR-T. Here, we report that, in collaboration with ProMab Inc., we have developed a novel CAR-T based on the DCLK1 ScFv containing a CD28 transmembrane and co-stimulatory domain and CD3ζ activation domain [39–46]. CAR-T cells generated using DCLK1 ScFv (CBT-511) demonstrated ~20% CAR expression and significantly induced CRC cell cytotoxicity. Compared to mock CAR-T treatments, CBT-511 significantly induced Interferon gamma (IFN-γ) production in CRC cells grown in 2D and 3D matrices, indicating that the CAR-T cells are able to successfully bind/interact with CRC cells (HT29, HCT116, and LoVo). Finally, CBT-511 treatment resulted in significant inhibition of LoVo CRC cells-derived tumor xenograft growth in NSG™ mice. These data taken together strongly suggest that DCLK1 CAR-T can be developed to specifically target TSCs in CRC and perhaps other solid tumors. This paper represents the first demonstration of a DCLK1-directed CAR-T formulation.

2. Results

2.1. DCLK1 mAb CBT-15 Has High Binding Affinity to DCLK1

Of the four DCLK1 isoforms (1–4), isoforms 2 and 4 are highly upregulated in cancers, whereas isoforms 1 and 3 are not [47–49]. Our proprietary DCLK1 mAb, CBT-15, recognizes a 13 amino acid sequence (extracellular domain) of the tumor-specific DCLK1 isoforms 2 and 4 with a binding affinity of < 1 nM Kd. We previously reported that targeting renal cell carcinoma TSCs with CBT-15 resulted in xenograft growth arrest and EMT inhibition [47]. Here, we have generated a humanized version of CBT-15 (hCBT-15) and demonstrated its ability to recognize the extracellular domain of DCLK1. Using flow cytometry, we analyzed several cancer cell lines with hCBT-15.

When HT29 human CRC cells were grown in 2D matrices, approximately 9% of the total population were positive for surface DCLK1 (Figure 1A). However, when grown in 3D matrices, the HT29 cells developed a spheroid-like morphology and cell sorting revealed a striking increase in surface DCLK1 to 45% of the cells (Figure 1A,B). Interestingly, when HCT-116 and LoVo cells when grown in 2D matrices, we observed 20% and 22% of cells expressing surface DCLK1, respectively. However, when grown in 3D matrices, no significant increase in cell surface DCLK1 expression was observed (Figure 1C–F). These data taken together suggest that HT29 cells with high clonogenic capacity express a marked increase in cell surface DCLK1 expression. This is not surprising, as DCLK1 marks TSCs in intestinal adenomas and targeting them resulted in complete abrogation of the adenomas [25]. Furthermore, this also provides a strong rationale to utilize the cell surface expression of DCLK1 to deliver anti-cancer payloads or for developing DCLK1-based CAR-T therapy. Interestingly, we did not observe any increases in cell surface expression in HCT116 or LoVo cells when grown in 3D. Although this finding was unsuspected, those two cell lines exhibited approximately two-fold more cell surface DCLK1 than HT29 cells grown on adherent slides.

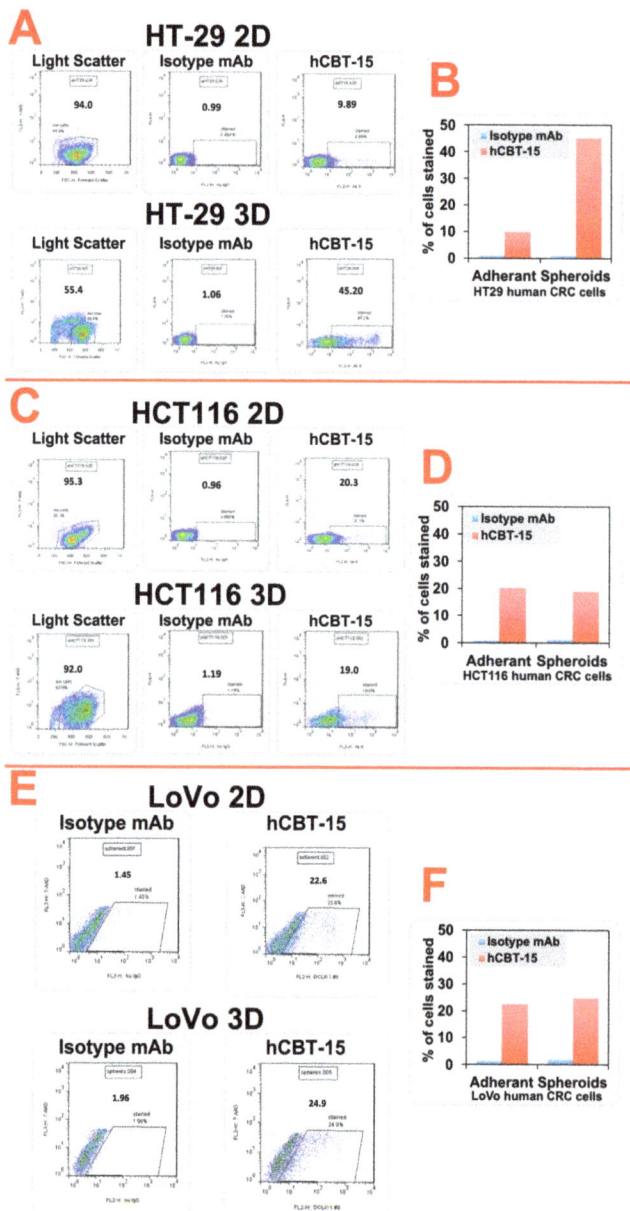

Figure 1. Doublecortin-like kinase 1 (DCLK1) surface expression in human colorectal cancer cell lines. HT29, human colorectal cancer (CRC) cells were grown in adherent 2D tissue culture plates and as 3D spheroids. These cells were disassociated and subjected to Fluorescence-activated cell sorting (FACS) using humanized DCLK1 mAb (hCBT-15). HT29 cells grown in 2D culture demonstrated extracellular DCLK1 expression on 9.89% of cells (**A**—Top panel). HT29 cells grown in 3D matrices demonstrated extracellular DCLK1 expression on 45% of cells (**A**—bottom panel). The quantitative expression is represented in the bar graph (**B**). (**C,D**): HCT116, grown in 2D demonstrated DCLK1 extracellular expression on 20% and 3D demonstrated DCLK1 extracellular on 19.5% of cells. (**E,F**): LoVo, grown in 2D demonstrated DCLK1 extracellular expression on 22% of cells and 3D demonstrated DCLK1 extracellular on 25% of cells.

2.2. DCLK1 Is Upregulated in Human CRC and CBT-15 Specifically Recognizes DCLK1 in CRC

Our previous studies demonstrated that DCLK1 is highly upregulated in human CRCs and that this upregulation is associated with poor clinical outcomes [27]. As part of the validation of CBT-15, we used a tissue microarray containing human CRC tissues and adjacent normal tissues and immunohistochemistry (IHC) to assess levels of DCLK1. DCLK1 expression was increased in human CRC tissues compared to adjacent normal (Figure 2A). This data is relatively consistent with our previous reports using an anti-DCLK1 polyclonal antibody (Abcam, Cambridge, MA, USA, catalog # ab31704) [21,23]. Additionally, we have immunostained several human tissues (normal and cancer) with CBT-15 (DCLK1 mAb). There was increased expression of DCLK1 in human cancers (Kidney, CRC, Liver, Esophagus, Bladder, Cervix, Uterus, Rectal, Lung, Ovary, Melanoma, and Breast) compared to human normal tissues (Supplementary Figure S1). To measure DCLK1 mRNA expression and determine if the levels correlated with patient survival, we analyzed the Illumina HiSeqV2 RNA-sequencing The Cancer Genome Atlas (TCGA) database. We observed a significant increase in overall and recurrence-free survival in patients with low DCLK1 expression and reduced overall and recurrence-free survival in patients with high DCLK1 expression (Figure 2B). Interestingly, patients with high DCLK1 had increasing amounts of EMT-related transcription factors (e.g., SNAI1, TWIST1, ZEB1, ZEB2 and Vimentin; Figure 2C). These data taken together suggest that high DCLK1 is associated with increased EMT transcription factors within the human CRC tissues. Furthermore, increased DCLK1 RNA (isoforms 2 and 4) was associated with increased expression of programmed cell death-ligand 1 (PD-L1) and PD-L2 mRNAs, suggesting that patients with high DCLK1 may be more responsive to immune check point inhibitors (Figure 2D,E; $p < 0.01$).

2.3. CBT-511, CAR-T Cells Generated with DCLK1 CBT-15 Antibody ScFv, Recognizes DCLK1 Protein

Using the ScFv of the hCBT-15 DCLK1 mAb, we created a second-generation DCLK1-based CAR-T cell (CBT-511; ProMab biotechnologies, Richmond, CA, USA) (Figure 3A) [39,41–43]. CBT-511 has DCLK1 ScFv fused to a CD28 transmembrane domain and co-stimulatory domain with a CD8 hinge. CBT-511 also contains a CD3zeta activation domain (Figure 3A). CAR-T cells generated using DCLK1 ScFv expanded in vitro and demonstrated ~20% CAR expression when analyzed by Fluorescence-activated cell sorting (FACS) using F(ab)2 antibody compared to non-transduced T cells (Figure 3B). These data demonstrate that DCLK1 CAR-T cells had sufficient DCLK1 CAR expression and were used in further experiments.

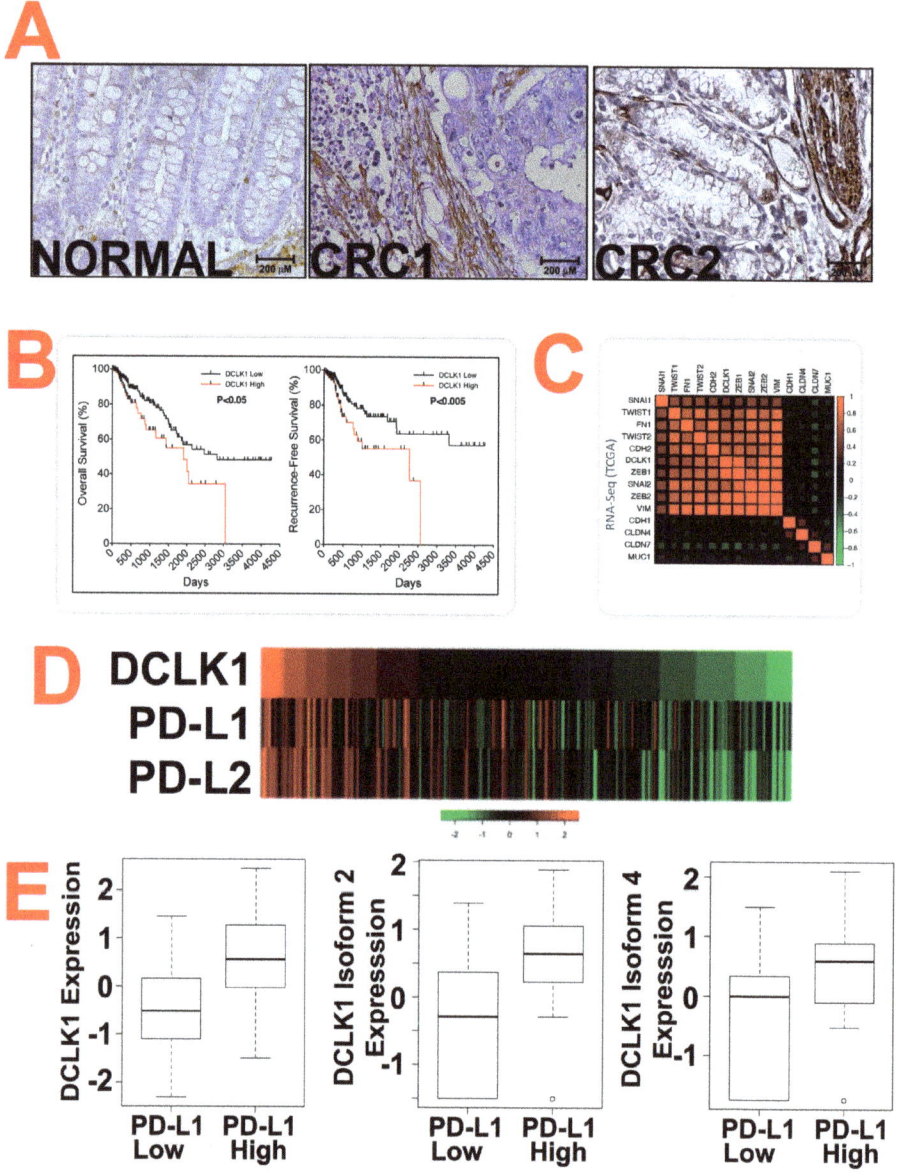

Figure 2. Doublecortin-like kinase 1 (DCLK1) expression in human colorectal cancer patient tissues. (**A**) Human colorectal cancer (CRC) tissues and adjacent normal tissues were subjected to immunohistochemical analyses for DCLK1 using hCBT-15 mAb. Representative images are presented. Scale bars are presented at the image. (**B**) The Cancer Genome Atlas (TCGA) data was generated using Illumina HiSeqV2 RNA-sequencing data and was sorted for overall survival of the patients with low or high DCLK1 expression. (**C**) Moreover, TCGA data was generated and sorted for the expression of various epithelial-mesenchymal transition (EMT)-related transcription factors in the samples with low or high DCLK1 expression indicating that EMT and DCLK1 expression is correlated with poor overall survival. (**D**) Heatmap of the TCGA analyses for DCLK1 and immunomodulating checkpoints proteins programmed cell death-ligand 1 (PD-L1) and PD-L2. (**E**) TCGA data were sorted for samples with low or high PD-L1 expression. The samples with high PD-L1 had increased expression of DCLK1, cancer stem cells (CSCs)-associated DCLK1 isoform 2 and isoform 4 ($p < 0.01$ for all comparisons).

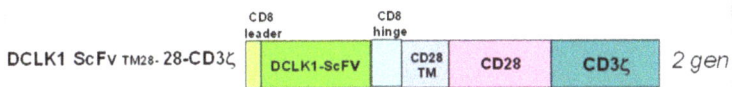

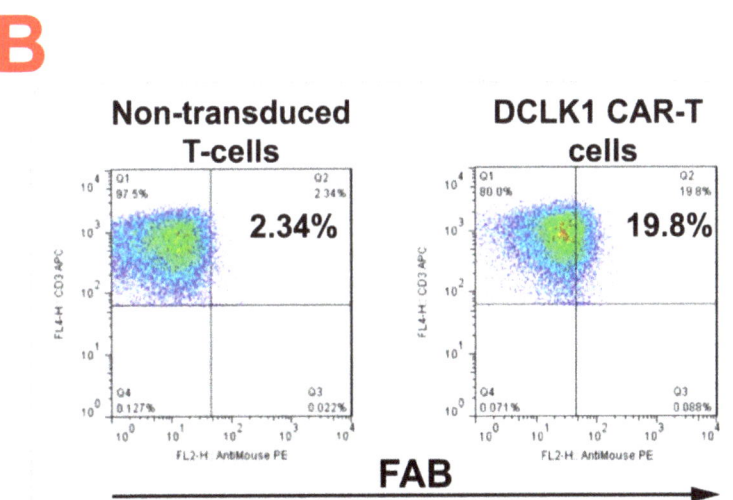

Figure 3. Expression of chimeric antigen receptors (CARs) in Doublecortin-like kinase 1 (DCLK1) CAR-T cells (CBT-511). (**A**) The illustration represents the structure of DCLK1-CAR (CBT-511). The second-generation CAR with DCLK1 ScFv, CD28 co-stimulatory domain, and CD-3zeta activation domain was generated. (**B**) Expression of DCLK1-CAR in T cells transduced with lentiviral DCLK1-CAR by Fluorescence-activated cell sorting (FACS) with F(ab)2 antibody. CBT-511 cells were effectively transduced with DCLK1-CAR and expression of CAR (~20%) was confirmed by FACS with F(ab)2 antibody.

2.4. CBT-511 Effectively Kills CRC Cells and Induces the Secretion of IFN-γ

In real-time cytotoxicity assays (RTCA), CRC cells grown in 2D were co-cultured with effector cells (DCLK1 CAR-T cells or mock CAR-T cells) at dilutions of 10:1 and 20:1 (effector cells: CRC cells). Additionally, based on our previous experience and recent published reports an E:T 10:1 and 20:1 are optimal [39,42,43]. The CRC cells were monitored for another one to two days with the RTCA xCELLigence system (Acea Biosciences, San Diego, CA, USA), and impedance were plotted over time and cytolysis were calculated. At 72h, DCLK1 CAR-T cells (10:1 dilution) effectively killed ~30% of HT29 cells and 23% of HCT116 cells (Figure 4A,B). However, at 20:1 dilution, DCLK1 CAR-T cells killed nearly 100% of HT29 cells, 60% of HCT116, and 78% of LoVo cells (Figure 4A–C). These data suggest that DCLK1 CAR-T cells effectively kill CRC cells grown in 2D at 20:1 dilution. In order to demonstrate the effects of CBT-511 on IFN-γ release, we performed co-culture experiment similar to RTCA. IFN-γ release is the best measure of CAR-T interaction with target cells that results in cytotoxicity of the cancer cells. CAR-T cells were co-cultured with CRC cells grown in 2D culture system and in 3D matrices as spheroids separately. The supernatant from these experiments were collected and subjected to IFN-γ release assay using enzyme-linked immunosorbent assay (ELISA). Treatment of HT29 cells grown in 2D with CBT-511 resulted in a dramatic release of IFN-γ as compared to mock CAR-T cells (~25 versus 0 pg/mL; $p < 0.01$). However, treatment of HT29 cells grown in 3D with CBT-511 resulted in an even higher IFN-γ release (~32 pg/mL versus 0 pg/mL; $p < 0.01$; Figure 4D). Treatment of HCT116 cells grown in 2D with CBT-511 resulted in a dramatic release of IFN-γ as compared to mock CAR-T cells (~150 versus 0 pg/mL; $p < 0.01$). However, treatment of HCT116 cells grown in 3D with CBT-511 resulted in an even higher IFN-γ release (~250 pg/mL versus 0 pg/mL; $p < 0.01$; Figure 4D). In LoVo cells however, we did not observe a similar pattern of IFN-γ release. In 2D, there was ~50 pg/mL of IFN-γ release with CBT-511 treatments; however, in cells treated with mock CAR-T treatments, there was 35 pg/mL of IFN-γ release (Figure 4E). Whereas in 3D, there was ~90 pg/mL of IFN-γ release with CBT-511 treatments and in mock CAR-T treatments there was ~50 pg/mL of IFN-γ release (Figure 4E). These data taken together suggest that although DCLK1 CAR-T cells induced IFN-γ release as expected, the mock CAR-T cells also induced IFN-γ release indicating a non-specific IFN-γ response in LoVo cells. These data suggest that hDCLK1-specific CAR-T cells successful bind to CRC cells and induce IFN-γ secretion consistent with CAR-T cells-induce cytotoxicity.

2.5. CBT-511 Blocks Subcutaneous LoVo CRC Cells-Derived Xenograft Tumor Growth In Vivo

To confirm the in vivo efficacy of DCLK1 CAR-T cells in CRC cell lines, we generated LoVo CRC cell line-derived tumor xenografts in NSG™ mice. Although we did not observe a significant increase in cell surface DCLK1 expression in LoVo cells grown in 3D compared to cells grown in 2D, we observed a 23% extracellular DCLK1 expression at baseline in adherent cells (2D). This level of expression is significantly higher than observed in many cancer cell lines (data not shown) and higher than HT29 cells (9%) in 2D. This may explain the robust cytotoxicity seen in CRC cell lines grown in adherent conditions. We chose to evaluate the effects of the DCLK1 CAR-T in LoVo cells, because this colorectal cancer cell line is derived from the distant metastatic lesion of a 56-year old patient with a histologically confirmed adenocarcinoma of the colon. Furthermore, the cell line has been well characterized and has been used extensively to evaluate the effects of drugs on colony formation and clonogenicity [50]. Moreover, the cell line is reported to have oncogenic activation of cMYC and RAS [51] that have been associated with DCLK1 [22,52]. Tumor-bearing mice were given intravenous (i.v.) injections of DCLK1 CAR-T or mock CAR-T cells (1×10^7 cells/mice/dose) every week for three weeks (days 7, 14, and 21 post-cell implantations; Figure 5A). The tumor growth and animal body weights were measured every week until day 45. The mice were euthanized and tumors were extracted and final volumes were measured. Mice treated with CBT-511 had a significant reduction in tumor size compared to those given mock CAR-T treatments (mean tumor volume of mock CAR-T versus DCLK1 CAR-T = 2123 versus 1216 mm^3 with a $p = 0.02$; Figure 5B). These data taken together indicate that DCLK1-based CAR-T cells when administered i.v. significantly inhibited CRC tumor growth. Additionally, there was no significant difference in animal body weights between the CBT-511-treated and mock-CAR-T-treated animals (Figure 5C). Based on this in vivo experiment, these data taken together strongly suggests that DCLK1 CAR-T treatments did not have any obvious toxicity in the mice.

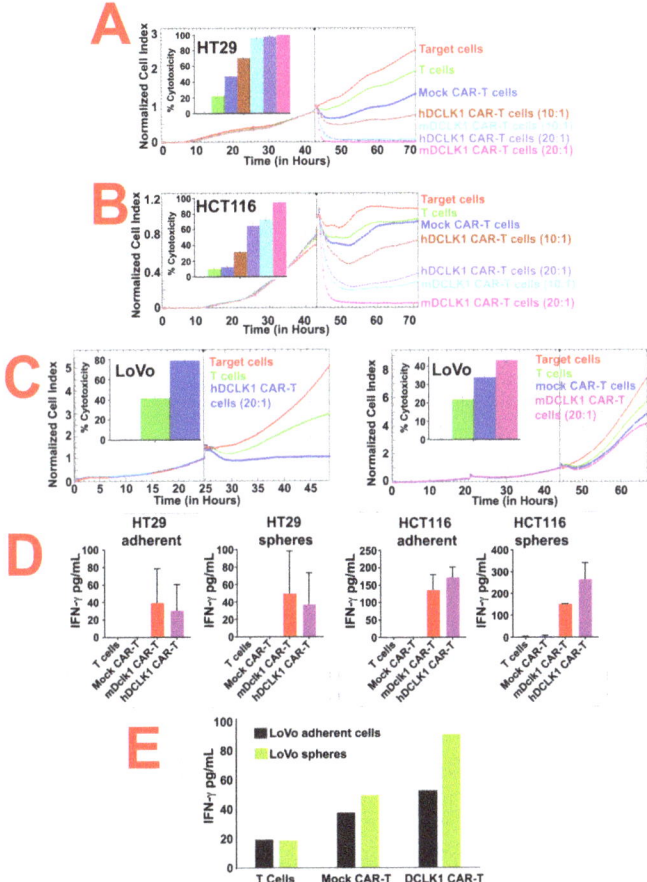

Figure 4. CBT-511 treatment induced colorectal cancer (CRC) cell cytotoxicity and secretion of Interferon gamma (IFN-γ). Human CRC cells (HT29, HCT116, and LoVo) were subjected to real-time cytotoxicity assays (RTCA). Doublecortin-like kinase 1 (DCLK1) CAR-T cells effectively killed HT29 cells compared to mock CAR-T or T cells alone (**A–C**). Bar graphs in (**A,B**): Cytotoxicity of human DCLK1 (hDCLK1)-CAR-T and mouse Dclk1 (mDCLK1)-CAR-T cells versus T cells and Mock-CAR-T cells. The quantitation of RTCA from three independent experiments is shown. All pairwise comparisons were significant ($p < 0.0001$), except for Mock CAR-T cells versus T cells ($p = 0.9363$) and hDCLK-1-CAR-T cells 20:1 versus mDCLK-1-CAR-T cells 10:1 ($p = 0.0703$). Bar graphs in (**C**): All pairwise comparisons were significant ($p < 0.05$), except for Mock CAR-T cells versus T cells ($p = 0.2017$) and Mock CAR-T cells versus mDclk-1-CAR-T cells ($p = 0.3769$). All p-values were adjusted using Tukey's method. (**D**) Treatment of HT29 cells grown in 2D with CBT-511 resulted in a dramatic release of IFN-γ (~25 pg/mL) as compared to mock CAR-T cells (0 pg/mL; $p < 0.01$). However, treatment of HT29 cells grown in 3D with CBT-511 resulted in an even higher IFN-γ release (~32 pg/mL versus 0 pg/mL; $p < 0.01$) compared to mock CAR-T. Similar treatment of HCT116 cells with CBT-511 resulted in increased IFN-γ release grown in 2D culture (150 pg/mL) compared to mock CAR-T (0 pg/mL). However, treatment of HCT116 cells grown in 3D with CBT-511 resulted in an even higher IFN-γ release (~250 pg/mL) compare to mock CAR-T (0 pg/mL; $p < 0.01$). (**E**) Treatment of LoVo cells with CBT-511 resulted in increased IFN-γ release grown in 2D culture (~50 pg/mL) compared to mock CAR-T (~30 pg/mL). However, treatment of LoVo cells grown in 3D with CBT-511 resulted in an even higher IFN-γ release (~95 pg/mL) compare to mock CAR-T (50 pg/mL). These data taken together suggests that CBT-511 is more active against CRC cells grown in 3D culture consistent with the increased clonogenic capacity of Tumor stem cells (TSCs).

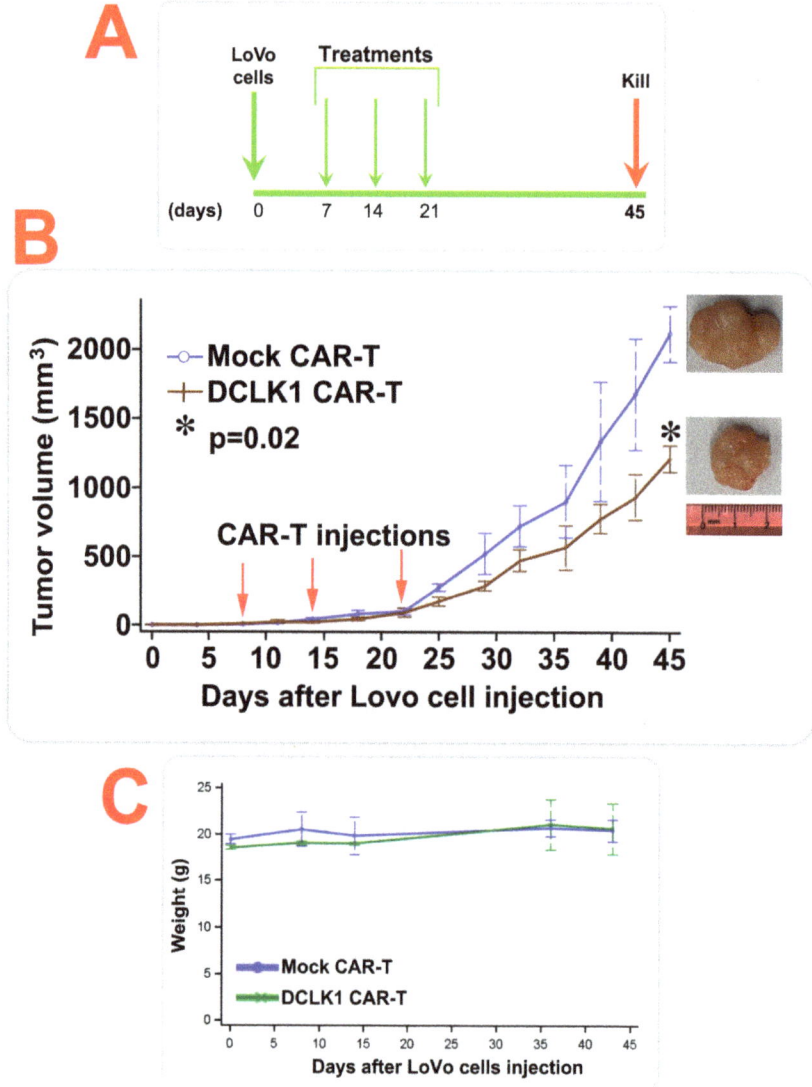

Figure 5. CBT-511 treatment reduced LoVo, human colorectal cancer (CRC) cell-line induced tumor xenograft growth. (**A**) LoVo, human CRC cells were injected subcutaneously into NOD Scid gamma (NSG™) mice and the tumors were allowed to grow. On days 7, 14, and 21 post-cell implantations, the mice were injected intravenous (*i.v.*) with either Doublecortin-like kinase 1 (DCLK1) CAR-T or mock CAR-T cells (1 × 10^7 cells/mice). Tumor volumes were measured and all the mice were weighted during the experiment period. (**B**) CBT-511 treatment resulted in a significant (* $p = 0.02$) decreased tumor xenograft growth compared to treatment with mock CAR-T cells. The mice treated with CBT-511 had smaller tumors compared to mock CAR-T treated mice. (**C**) There were no significant differences in the animal weights between CBT-511 and mock CAR-T treated mice.

3. Discussion

Advanced CRC remains an extraordinarily difficult cancer to treat. CRC is the third-leading cause of cancer death in the U.S. It represents an enormous challenge and has a poor overall survival (~12% 5-year overall survival (OS); Stage IV CRC). Novel therapeutic approaches designed to eradicate metastatic dissemination of CRC cells would fill a major gap in successful therapy.

Adoptive T cell-based immunotherapy has the potential to improve patient outcomes due to the ability of cytotoxic T cells that target the tumor epithelium, penetrate the TME, and eliminate the tumor. CAR-T cell therapy builds upon this approach by using the patient's own T cells to activate, proliferate, and destroy tumor cells. This is accomplished by engineering the T cells to express a specific tumor-related antigen that is recognized by the extracellular targeting region of the CAR-T. In this report, we describe a novel CSC-directed CAR-T that specifically binds to the extracellular regions of the TSC protein DCLK1 expressed in CRC. Using LoVo CRC cells derived from metastatic tissue from a patient with adenocarcinoma of the colon, we demonstrate that CAR-T cells expressing the ScFv region of a humanized mAb directed at isoforms 2 and 4 of human DCLK1 (hCBT-15) reduced LoVo colon cancer xenograft growth by greater than 42 percent compared to mock CAR-T controls. This occurred without any weight loss or obvious adverse effect of CAR-T cells compared to controls.

One major determinant of successful CAR-T therapy is the specificity of the mAb, and as such the ScFv regions used to generate the CAR-T against the cell surface expression of the target antigen. With respect to DCLK1 surface expression, many cancer cell lines express low levels of extra cellular isoforms 2 and 4 (e.g., BxPC3 and MIA PaCa-2 pancreatic cancer cell lines); however, in this report, we describe three cancer cell lines that express greater than 9 percent DCLK1 cell surface expression at baseline: HT29, HCT116, and LoVo cells. This level of expression was sufficient to allow CAR-T cells at 20:1 dilution to exhibit significant real time cytotoxicity. However, our overall hypothesis is that the clonogenic capacity of the CSC population is the true target of successful immunotherapy. When CRC cell lines were subsequently grown in 3D culture systems in order isolate the clonogenic population, we observed a marked increase in the expression of extracellular DCLK1 isoforms in HT29 cells (from 9 to 45%). Interestingly, we did not observe a similar increase in HCT116 or LoVo cancer cells. However, baseline expression in these two cell lines was higher than that observed in the HT29 cell line. We predict that in 3D clonogenic culture systems, we select for more undifferentiated stem-like cells [53]. HCT116 and LoVo cells had relatively higher expression of surface DCLK1 when grown in 2D compared to HT29. Although these findings are under investigation in our laboratory, tumorspheres have more undifferentiated cells that express surface DCLK1 compared to cells grown in 2D. Moreover, in these cell lines, we did not observe an increase in DCLK1 cell surface expression when grown in 3D. We speculate that LoVo cells have a more mesenchymal-like phenotype [54] and may express sufficient DCLK1 to promote tumorigenesis, whereas HT29 cells, which appear to be of a more epithelial phenotype, require a less differentiated state in order to demonstrate increased DCLK1 expression on the surface. LoVo cells, according to recent reports, generally express more vimentin than E-cadherin, suggesting a more mesenchymal phenotype compared to HCT116 or HT29 [54]. Nevertheless, studies are underway to assess the sensitivity of clonogenic cells to CAR-T based cytotoxicity.

Our in vitro studies using HT29, HCT116, and LoVo cells cultured in 3D matrices revealed a significant increase in IFN-γ release, a surrogate measure of cytotoxicity, compared to cells grown in 2D with a 19.8 percent DCLK1 CAR expression. However, we are fully aware that further studies are needed to fully assess cytokine release and accurate cytotoxicity of the specific clonogenic cells (CSC) within spheroids. In future studies, we intend to reclone the DCLK1 ScFv into a vector containing the MND U3 promoter. In preliminary studies, this promoter resulted in a nearly three-fold increase in cell surface CAR expression compared to the EF1 promoter we used in this report [55]. These data support our overall hypothesis that the clonogenic population of tumor cells may represent an ideal target for DCLK1 driven CAR-T therapy. Because DCLK1 cell surface expression is increased on a diverse range of TSCs, the need for highly specific CAR-T cells may be reduced. It is important for us to emphasize that unlike traditional extracellular antigens that are upregulated in tumors but undetectable in normal tissues, DCLK1 is highly upregulated in tumor cells and expressed at low levels in normal tissues. However, the specific TSC population and progeny are the targets of DCLK1 CAR-T therapy. Furthermore, because DCLK1 is not expressed on normal stem cells, the risk for off-target serious adverse effects may be reduced [25]. One particular advantage of a DCLK1-based anti-TSC strategy is that although DCLK1 marks TSCs, it is not expressed on normal LGR5$^+$ stem cells Thus, DCLK1 is the first and only TSC marker that can distinguish between normal cells from TSCs [25].

Analysis of the TCGA database of patients with CRC revealed that elevated levels of DCLK1 mRNA transcripts compared to normal adjacent tissue was associated with a poor prognosis and reduced OS. Conversely, patients with low DCLK1 expression levels exhibited an increase in overall and recurrence-free survival. At the protein level, tissue microarray of patients with CRC had increased levels of DCLK1 compared to normal adjacent tissues. These data illustrate the potential importance of targeting DCLK1 to eliminate and perhaps inactivate the TSC population in CRC [19,21–24].

Low levels of DCLK1 are associated with increased OS and recurrence free survival and are associated with low expression of EMT transcription factors. These data suggest that reduction of DCLK1 and DCLK1 expressing cells may be an important goal of CRC therapies aimed at reducing EMT factors to improve OS outcomes [19,21–24]. We previously demonstrated that interruption of DCLK1 signaling blocked EMT and inhibited the invasion and migration of cancer cells [20,22–24]. Furthermore, siRNA-mediated knockdown of DCLK1 has been shown to upregulate anti EMT, miR-200 family of microRNAs with downregulation of transcription factors—ZEB1, SNAIL and SLUG [19–22].

A major study by Maliar et al., demonstrated that a CAR-T construct targeting the putative CSC protein CD24 in pancreatic ductal adenocarcinoma (PDAC) improved overall survival (OS) and reduced metastasis in orthotopic patient-derived xenografts and in CAPAN-1-derived xenografts. In separate experiments, treatment with Her2/neu CAR-T cells also resulted in improved OS, and tumor eradication in xenograft models [56]. However, the anti Her2/neu CAR-T cells only demonstrated significant efficacy when epidermal growth factor receptor (EGFR) was highly expressed in the majority of cells within the tumor, whereas anti-CD24 CAR-T was successful despite low levels of CD-24 expression within the tumor. These data taken together illustrate that targeting CSCs can display similar efficacies to CAR-Ts targeting antigens expressed on rapidly proliferating tumor cell populations. The studies presented above support our rationale for targeting a highly specific TSC antigen for the treatment of CRC and perhaps other solid tumors.

4. Materials and Methods

4.1. Cells, Primary Tissues

CRC cell lines HT29, HCT116, and LoVo were purchased from the ATCC (Manassas, VA, USA) and cultured in RPMI-1640 medium (ThermoFisher, Waltham, MA, USA) containing 10% Fetal Bovine Serum (FBS) (AmCell, Mountain View, CA, USA). Human peripheral blood mononuclear cells (PBMC) were isolated from whole blood obtained in the Stanford Hospital Blood Center (Stanford University) according to Institutional Review Board (IRB)-approved protocol (#13942). PBMC were isolated by density sedimentation over Ficoll-Paque (GE Healthcare, Chicago, IL, USA).

4.2. Monoclonal Antibody

DCLK1-targeted monoclonal antibody (CBT-15 mAb), DCLK1 mAb analogue (previously reported, see [47,48]), and isotype control mAb were generated as previously described. Binding affinity of CBT-15 was confirmed by enzyme-linked immunosorbent assay (ELISA) using full-length DCLK1 [47,48,57].

4.3. Generation of CAR-Encoding Lentivirus

DNA encoding the DCLK1 CAR was synthesized and subcloned into a third-generation lentiviral vector, Lenti CMV-MCS-EF1a-puro by Syno Biological (Beijing, China) [39,42]. Ten million growth-arrested HEK293FT cells (ThermoFisher) were seeded into T75 flasks. Cells were cultured overnight and transfected using the CalPhos Transfection Kit (Takara, Mountain View, CA, USA) and pPACKH1 Lentivector Packaging Mix (System Biosciences, Palo Alto, CA, USA) containing 10 µg of the lentiviral vector. The media was changed the following day and 48 h later, media containing the lentivirus was collected and clarified by centrifugation at 2100× g for 30 min. The virus particles were collected by centrifugation at 112,000× g for 100 min, suspended in AIM V medium, aliquoted, and frozen at −80 °C. The titers of the virus preparations were determined by quantitative Reverse transcription polymerase chain reaction (RT-PCR)using the Lenti-X qRT-PCR kit (Takara) according to the manufacturer's protocol and the 7900HT thermal cycler (ThermoFisher). The lentiviral titers were >1 × 10^8 plaque forming units (pfu)/mL [39,42].

4.4. Generation and Expansion of CAR-T Cells

PBMCs were suspended at 1 × 10^6 cells/mL in AIM V-AlbuMAX medium (ThermoFisher) containing 10% FBS and 10 ng/mL IL-2 (ThermoFisher), mixed with an equal number (1:1 ratio) of CD3/CD28 Dynabeads (ThermoFisher), and cultured in non-treated 24-well plates (0.5 mL per well) [39,42]. At 24 and 48 h, lentivirus was added to the cultures at a multiplicity of infection (MOI) of 5 along with 1 µL of TransPlus transduction enhancer (AlStem, San Francisco, CA, USA). As the T cells proliferated over the next 10–12 days, the cells were counted every 2–3 days and spent media was replaced with fresh media containing 10 ng/mL IL-2 was added to maintain the cell density at 1 to 3 × 10^6 cells/mL [39,42].

4.5. Flow Cytometry

To measure CAR expression, 0.25 million cells were suspended in 100 µL of buffer (Phosphate-buffered saline (PBS) containing 2 mM Ethylenediaminetetraacetic acid (EDTA) pH 8 and 0.5% Bovine serum albumin (BSA)) and incubated on ice with 1 µL of human serum (Jackson Immunoresearch, West Grove, PA, USA) for 10 min. Then, 0.3 µg of biotinylated human DCLK1 protein (AcroBiosystems, Newark, DE, USA) was added and the cells were incubated on ice for 30 min. Cells were rinsed with 3 mL of buffer and suspended in 100 µL of buffer. Next, 1 µL of phycoerythrin (PE)-conjugated streptavidin (BD Biosciences, San Jose, CA, USA), 1 µL of allophycocyanin (APC)-labeled anti-CD3 (BioLegend, San Diego, CA, USA) and 2 µL of 7-aminoactinomycin D (7-AAD) solution (BioLegend) were added to the cells and incubated on ice for 30 min [39,42]. The cells were rinsed with 3 mL of buffer and suspended in buffer and acquired on a FACSCalibur (BD Biosciences). Cells were analyzed first for light scatter versus 7-AAD staining, and the 7-AAD⁻ live gated cells were plotted for anti-CD3 staining versus DCLK1 protein staining [39,42].

4.6. Cytokine Induction Assay

Target cells (HT29, HCT116, and LoVo) were cultured with the effector cells (CAR-T cells or non-transduced T cells) at a 10:1 ratio (E:T; 1 × 10^4 cells each) in U-bottom 96-well plates with 200 µL of AIM V-AlbuMAX medium containing 10% FBS, in triplicate. After 16 h, the top 150 µL of medium was transferred to V-bottom 96-well plates and centrifuged at 300 × g for 5 min to pellet any residual cells. The top 120 µL of supernatant was transferred to a new 96-well plate and analyzed by ELISA for human IFN-γ levels using a kit from R&D Systems (Minneapolis, MN, USA) according to the manufacturer's protocol. Additionally, based on our previous experience and published report an E:T 10:1 and 20:1 are optimal for cytokine induction and cytotoxicity [39,42,43].

4.7. Real-Time Cytotoxicity Assay (RTCA)

Adherent target cells (HT29, HCT116, and LoVo) were seeded into 96-well E-plates (Acea Biosciences, San Diego, CA, USA) at 1 × 10^4 cells per well and monitored in culture overnight using impedance-based real-time cell analysis (RTCA) xCELLigence system (Acea Bio). The next day, the media was removed and replaced with AIM V-AlbuMAX medium containing 10% FBS ± 1 × 10^5 effector cells (CAR-T cells or non-transduced T cells), in triplicate. The cells in the E-plates were monitored for another 24–48 h with the RTCA system, and impedance was plotted over time. Cytolysis was calculated as follows: (impedance of target cells without effector cells-impedance of target cells with effector cells) × 100/impedance of target cells without effector cells.

4.8. Mouse Xenograft Study

Six-week old male NSG™ mice (Jackson Laboratories, Bar Harbor, ME, USA) were housed and manipulated in strict accordance with the Institutional Animal Care and Use Committee (IACUC). All animal experiments were performed at Joint Innovation Park Animal Facility, Richmond, CA according to approved IACUC protocol. Each mouse was injected subcutaneously (both sides of the flanks; $n = 3$ mice with six tumors in each group) on day 0 with 100 µL of 1×10^7 LoVo cells/mice separately. CAR-T cells (CBT-511 or mock CAR-T cells) were injected intravenously (1×10^7 cells/mice each day) on days 7 or 14 and 21. Tumor sizes were measured with calipers twice weekly and tumor volume (in mm^3) was determined using the formula $W^2L/2$, where W is tumor width and L is tumor length until day 45. At the end of the studies, tumors were excised and final volumes measured.

4.9. Statistical Analysis

Data were analyzed and plotted using Prism software (GraphPad, San Diego, CA, USA). Comparisons between two groups were performed by unpaired Student's t-test. Comparisons between three or more groups were performed by one-way ANOVA or two-way ANOVA followed by Tukey's or Sidak's post hoc test. The difference with $p < 0.05$ was considered significant.

5. Conclusions

Together, these results indicate that DCLK1-targeted CAR-T immunotherapy provides a novel mechanism for eliminating the cell of origin and perhaps the metastatic progeny in CRC. This study is the first of its kind to demonstrate the therapeutic utility of a CAR-T directed against a TSC-specific antigen for the treatment of CRC. The results of this study may lead to the development of novel TSC-directed CAR-T therapies for CRC and perhaps other solid tumor cancers.

6. Patents

This work is part of a provisional patent application filed by COARE Biotechnology Inc.

Supplementary Materials: The following are available online at http://www.mdpi.com/2072-6694/12/1/54/s1, Figure S1: DCLK1 expression in human tissues.

Author Contributions: Conception and design of the study, S.M.S., C.W.H., and V.G.; generation, collection, assembly, analysis, and/or interpretation of data S.M.S., R.B., H.Z., S.X., L.W., V.G., K.D., R.M., and C.W.H.; drafting or revision of the manuscript S.M.S., V.G., E.B.-M., and C.W.H.; approval of the final version of the manuscript S.M.S., R.B., H.Z., S.X., L.W., V.G., K.D., D.Q., R.M., E.B.-M., and C.W.H. All authors have read and agreed to the published version of the manuscript.

Funding: This study was supported by grants awarded to SMS (1R43CA174025-01A1 and 2R44CA174025-02) and CWH (5R01CA214017-03) from the National Cancer Institute.

Acknowledgments: We would like to thank Nathaniel Weygant (the University of Oklahoma HSC, OK, USA) for help with TCGA analyses. We would like to thank Denise Briggs for editorial help.

Conflicts of Interest: S.M.S., D.Q., R.M., E.B.-M., and C.W.H. have ownership interests in COARE Holdings Inc. All the other authors have no conflict of interest.

References

1. American-Cancer-Society. What is the Survival Rates for Colorectal Cancer by Stage? Available online: http://www.cancer.org/cancer/colonandrectumcancer/detailedguide/colorectal-cancer-survival-rates (accessed on 23 June 2019).
2. Jordan, C.T.; Guzman, M.L.; Noble, M. Cancer stem cells. *N. Engl. J. Med.* **2006**, *355*, 1253–1261. [CrossRef] [PubMed]

3. Clarke, M.F.; Dick, J.E.; Dirks, P.B.; Eaves, C.J.; Jamieson, C.H.; Jones, D.L.; Visvader, J.; Weissman, I.L.; Wahl, G.M. Cancer stem cells-perspectives on current status and future directions: AACR Workshop on cancer stem cells. *Cancer Res.* **2006**, *66*, 9339–9344. [CrossRef] [PubMed]
4. Beatty, G.L.; Gladney, W.L. Immune escape mechanisms as a guide for cancer immunotherapy. *Clin. Cancer Res.* **2015**, *21*, 687–692. [CrossRef] [PubMed]
5. Markman, J.L.; Shiao, S.L. Impact of the immune system and immunotherapy in colorectal cancer. *J. Gastrointest. Oncol.* **2015**, *6*, 208–223. [CrossRef]
6. Menon, S.; Shin, S.; Dy, G. Advances in cancer immunotherapy in solid tumors. *Cancers* **2016**, *8*, 106. [CrossRef]
7. Yan, X.; Zhang, S.; Deng, Y.; Wang, P.; Hou, Q.; Xu, H. Prognostic factors for checkpoint inhibitor based immunotherapy: An update with new evidences. *Front. Pharmacol.* **2018**, *9*, 1050. [CrossRef]
8. Kouidhi, S.; Ben Ayed, F.; Benammar Elgaaied, A. Targeting tumor metabolism: A new challenge to improve immunotherapy. *Front. Immunol.* **2018**, *9*, 353. [CrossRef]
9. Noble, F.; Mellows, T.; McCormick Matthews, L.H.; Bateman, A.C.; Harris, S.; Underwood, T.J.; Byrne, J.P.; Bailey, I.S.; Sharland, D.M.; Kelly, J.J.; et al. Tumour infiltrating lymphocytes correlate with improved survival in patients with oesophageal adenocarcinoma. *Cancer Immunol. Immunother.* **2016**, *65*, 651–662. [CrossRef]
10. Fan, F.; Samuel, S.; Evans, K.W.; Lu, J.; Xia, L.; Zhou, Y.; Sceusi, E.; Tozzi, F.; Ye, X.C.; Mani, S.A.; et al. Overexpression of snail induces epithelial-mesenchymal transition and a cancer stem cell-like phenotype in human colorectal cancer cells. *Cancer Med.* **2012**, *1*, 5–16. [CrossRef]
11. Wang, Y.; Liu, Y.; Lu, J.; Zhang, P.; Wang, Y.; Xu, Y.; Wang, Z.; Mao, J.H.; Wei, G. Rapamycin inhibits FBXW7 loss-induced epithelial-mesenchymal transition and cancer stem cell-like characteristics in colorectal cancer cells. *Biochem. Biophys. Res. Commun.* **2013**, *434*, 352–356. [CrossRef]
12. Brabletz, S.; Bajdak, K.; Meidhof, S.; Burk, U.; Niedermann, G.; Firat, E.; Wellner, U.; Dimmler, A.; Faller, G.; Schubert, J.; et al. The ZEB1/miR-200 feedback loop controls Notch signalling in cancer cells. *EMBO J.* **2011**, *30*, 770–782. [CrossRef] [PubMed]
13. Krantz, S.B.; Shields, M.A.; Dangi-Garimella, S.; Munshi, H.G.; Bentrem, D.J. Contribution of epithelial-to-mesenchymal transition and cancer stem cells to pancreatic cancer progression. *J. Surg. Res.* **2012**, *173*, 105–112. [CrossRef] [PubMed]
14. Wang, Z.; Li, Y.; Kong, D.; Banerjee, S.; Ahmad, A.; Azmi, A.S.; Ali, S.; Abbruzzese, J.L.; Gallick, G.E.; Sarkar, F.H. Acquisition of epithelial-mesenchymal transition phenotype of gemcitabine-resistant pancreatic cancer cells is linked with activation of the notch signaling pathway. *Cancer Res.* **2009**, *69*, 2400–2407. [CrossRef] [PubMed]
15. Wellner, U.; Schubert, J.; Burk, U.C.; Schmalhofer, O.; Zhu, F.; Sonntag, A.; Waldvogel, B.; Vannier, C.; Darling, D.; zur Hausen, A.; et al. The EMT-activator ZEB1 promotes tumorigenicity by repressing stemness-inhibiting microRNAs. *Nat. Cell Biol.* **2009**, *11*, 1487–1495. [CrossRef]
16. Lamouille, S.; Xu, J.; Derynck, R. Molecular mechanisms of epithelial-mesenchymal transition. *Nat. Rev. Mol. Cell Biol.* **2014**, *15*, 178–196. [CrossRef]
17. Brabletz, T. EMT and MET in metastasis: Where are the cancer stem cells? *Cancer Cell* **2012**, *22*, 699–701. [CrossRef]
18. Choi, J.E.; Bae, J.S.; Kang, M.J.; Chung, M.J.; Jang, K.Y.; Park, H.S.; Moon, W.S. Expression of epithelial-mesenchymal transition and cancer stem cell markers in colorectal adenocarcinoma: Clinicopathological significance. *Oncol. Rep.* **2017**, *38*, 1695–1705. [CrossRef]
19. Sureban, S.M.; Madhoun, M.F.; May, R.; Qu, D.; Ali, N.; Fazili, J.; Weygant, N.; Chandrakesan, P.; Ding, K.; Lightfoot, S.A.; et al. Plasma DCLK1 is a marker of hepatocellular carcinoma (HCC): Targeting DCLK1 prevents HCC tumor xenograft growth via a microRNA-dependent mechanism. *Oncotarget* **2015**, *6*, 37200–37215. [CrossRef]
20. Sureban, S.M.; May, R.; Lightfoot, S.A.; Hoskins, A.B.; Lerner, M.; Brackett, D.J.; Postier, R.G.; Ramanujam, R.; Mohammed, A.; Rao, C.V.; et al. DCAMKL-1 regulates epithelial-mesenchymal transition in human pancreatic cells through a miR-200a-dependent mechanism. *Cancer Res.* **2011**, *71*, 2328–2338. [CrossRef]
21. Sureban, S.M.; May, R.; Mondalek, F.G.; Qu, D.; Ponnurangam, S.; Pantazis, P.; Anant, S.; Ramanujam, R.P.; Houchen, C.W. Nanoparticle-based delivery of siDCAMKL-1 increases microRNA-144 and inhibits colorectal cancer tumor growth via a Notch-1 dependent mechanism. *J. Nanobiotechnol.* **2011**, *9*, 40. [CrossRef]

22. Sureban, S.M.; May, R.; Qu, D.; Weygant, N.; Chandrakesan, P.; Ali, N.; Lightfoot, S.A.; Pantazis, P.; Rao, C.V.; Postier, R.G.; et al. DCLK1 regulates pluripotency and angiogenic factors via microRNA-dependent mechanisms in pancreatic cancer. *PLoS ONE* **2013**, *8*, e73940. [CrossRef] [PubMed]
23. Sureban, S.M.; May, R.; Ramalingam, S.; Subramaniam, D.; Natarajan, G.; Anant, S.; Houchen, C.W. Selective blockade of DCAMKL-1 results in tumor growth arrest by a Let-7a MicroRNA-dependent mechanism. *Gastroenterology* **2009**, *137*, 649–659. [CrossRef] [PubMed]
24. Sureban, S.M.; May, R.; Weygant, N.; Qu, D.; Chandrakesan, P.; Bannerman-Menson, E.; Ali, N.; Pantazis, P.; Westphalen, C.B.; Wang, T.C.; et al. XMD8-92 inhibits pancreatic tumor xenograft growth via a DCLK1-dependent mechanism. *Cancer Lett.* **2014**, *351*, 151–161. [CrossRef] [PubMed]
25. Nakanishi, Y.; Seno, H.; Fukuoka, A.; Ueo, T.; Yamaga, Y.; Maruno, T.; Nakanishi, N.; Kanda, K.; Komekado, H.; Kawada, M.; et al. Dclk1 distinguishes between tumor and normal stem cells in the intestine. *Nat. Genet.* **2013**, *45*, 98. [CrossRef] [PubMed]
26. Westphalen, C.B.; Asfaha, S.; Hayakawa, Y.; Takemoto, Y.; Lukin, D.J.; Nuber, A.H.; Brandtner, A.; Setlik, W.; Remotti, H.; Muley, A.; et al. Long-lived intestinal tuft cells serve as colon cancer-initiating cells. *J. Clin. Invest.* **2014**, *124*, 1283–1295. [CrossRef] [PubMed]
27. Weygant, N.; Ge, Y.; Qu, D.; Kaddis, J.S.; Berry, W.L.; May, R.; Chandrakesan, P.; Bannerman-Menson, E.; Vega, K.J.; Tomasek, J.J.; et al. Survival of patients with gastrointestinal cancers can be predicted by a surrogate microRNA signature for cancer stem-like cells marked by dclk1 kinase. *Cancer Res.* **2016**, *76*, 4090–4099. [CrossRef] [PubMed]
28. Maus, M.V. Designing CAR T cells for glioblastoma. *Oncoimmunology* **2015**, *4*, e1048956. [CrossRef]
29. Gross, G.; Waks, T.; Eshhar, Z. Expression of immunoglobulin-T-cell receptor chimeric molecules as functional receptors with antibody-type specificity. *Proc. Natl. Acad. Sci. USA* **1989**, *86*, 10024–10028. [CrossRef]
30. Gross, G.; Eshhar, Z. Therapeutic potential of T cell chimeric antigen receptors (CARs) in cancer treatment: Counteracting off-tumor toxicities for safe CAR T cell therapy. *Annu. Rev. Pharmacol. Toxicol.* **2016**, *56*, 59–83. [CrossRef]
31. Abken, H. Adoptive therapy with CAR redirected T cells: The challenges in targeting solid tumors. *Immunotherapy* **2015**, *7*, 535–544. [CrossRef]
32. Lanitis, E.; Dangaj, D.; Irving, M.; Coukos, G. Mechanisms regulating T-cell infiltration and activity in solid tumors. *Ann. Oncol.* **2017**, *28*, xii18–xii32. [CrossRef] [PubMed]
33. Maimela, N.R.; Liu, S.; Zhang, Y. Fates of CD8+ T cells in tumor microenvironment. *Comput. Struct. Biotechnol. J.* **2019**, *17*, 1–13. [CrossRef] [PubMed]
34. Martinez, M.; Moon, E.K. CAR T cells for solid tumors: New strategies for finding, infiltrating, and surviving in the tumor microenvironment. *Front. Immunol.* **2019**, *10*, 128. [CrossRef] [PubMed]
35. Yan, L.; Liu, B. Critical factors in chimeric antigen receptor-modified T-cell (CAR-T) therapy for solid tumors. *Onco Targets Ther.* **2019**, *12*, 193–204. [CrossRef] [PubMed]
36. Miliotou, A.N.; Papadopoulou, L.C. CAR T-cell therapy: A new era in cancer immunotherapy. *Curr. Pharm. Biotechnol.* **2018**, *19*, 5–18. [CrossRef]
37. Brown, C.E.; Mackall, C.L. CAR T cell therapy: Inroads to response and resistance. *Nat. Rev. Immunol.* **2019**, *19*, 73–74. [CrossRef]
38. Cheadle, E.J.; Gornall, H.; Baldan, V.; Hanson, V.; Hawkins, R.E.; Gilham, D.E. CAR T cells: Driving the road from the laboratory to the clinic. *Immunol. Rev.* **2014**, *257*, 91–106. [CrossRef]
39. Berahovich, R.; Zhou, H.; Xu, S.; Wei, Y.; Guan, J.; Guan, J.; Harto, H.; Fu, S.; Yang, K.; Zhu, S.; et al. CAR-T cells based on novel BCMA monoclonal antibody block multiple myeloma cell growth. *Cancers* **2018**, *10*, 323. [CrossRef]
40. Golubovskaya, V.M.; Berahovich, R.; Xu, Q.; Zhou, H.; Xu, S.; Guan, J.; Harto, H.; Li, L.; Wu, L. GITR domain inside CAR co-stimulates activity of CAR-T cells against cancer. *Front. Biosci.* **2018**, *23*, 2245–2254. [CrossRef]
41. Golubovskaya, V. CAR-T cell therapy: From the bench to the bedside. *Cancers* **2017**, *9*, 150. [CrossRef]
42. Golubovskaya, V.; Berahovich, R.; Zhou, H.; Xu, S.; Harto, H.; Li, L.; Chao, C.C.; Mao, M.M.; Wu, L. CD47-CAR-T Cells Effectively Kill Target Cancer Cells and Block Pancreatic Tumor Growth. *Cancers* **2017**, *9*, 139. [CrossRef] [PubMed]
43. Berahovich, R.; Xu, S.; Zhou, H.; Harto, H.; Xu, Q.; Garcia, A.; Liu, F.; Golubovskaya, V.M.; Wu, L. FLAG-tagged CD19-specific CAR-T cells eliminate CD19-bearing solid tumor cells in vitro and in vivo. *Front. Biosci.* **2017**, *22*, 1644–1654.

44. Berahovich, R.; Liu, X.; Zhou, H.; Tsadik, E.; Xu, S.; Golubovskaya, V.; Wu, L. Hypoxia selectively impairs CAR-T Cells in vitro. *Cancers* **2019**, *11*, 602. [CrossRef] [PubMed]
45. Golubovskaya, V.; Wu, L. Different subsets of T cells, memory, effector functions, and CAR-T immunotherapy. *Cancers* **2016**, *8*, 36. [CrossRef]
46. Xu, Q.; Harto, H.; Berahovich, R.; Xu, S.; Zhou, H.; Golubovskaya, V.; Wu, L. Generation of CAR-T cells for cancer immunotherapy. *Methods Mol. Biol.* **2019**, *1884*, 349–360. [CrossRef]
47. Ge, Y.; Weygant, N.; Qu, D.; May, R.; Berry, W.L.; Yao, J.; Chandrakesan, P.; Zheng, W.; Zhao, L.; Zhao, K.L.; et al. Alternative splice variants of DCLK1 mark cancer stem cells, promote self-renewal and drug-resistance, and can be targeted to inhibit tumorigenesis in kidney cancer. *Int. J. Cancer* **2018**, *143*, 1162–1175. [CrossRef]
48. Qu, D.; Weygant, N.; Yao, J.; Chandrakesan, P.; Berry, W.L.; May, R.; Pitts, K.; Husain, S.; Lightfoot, S.; Li, M.; et al. Overexpression of DCLK1-AL increases tumor cell invasion, drug resistance, and KRAS activation and can be targeted to inhibit tumorigenesis in pancreatic cancer. *J. Oncol.* **2019**, *2019*, 6402925. [CrossRef]
49. Sarkar, S.; Popov, V.L.; O'Connell, M.R.; Stevenson, H.L.; Lee, B.S.; Obeid, R.A.; Luthra, G.K.; Singh, P. A novel antibody against cancer stem cell biomarker, DCLK1-S, is potentially useful for assessing colon cancer risk after screening colonoscopy. *Lab. Investig.* **2017**, *97*, 1245–1261. [CrossRef]
50. Mu, L.; Huang, K.; Hu, Y.; Yan, C.; Li, X.; Tao, D.; Gong, J.; Qin, J. Small-sized colorectal cancer cells harbor metastatic tumor-initiating cells. *Oncotarget* **2017**, *8*, 107907–107919. [CrossRef]
51. Ahmed, D.; Eide, P.W.; Eilertsen, I.A.; Danielsen, S.A.; Eknaes, M.; Hektoen, M.; Lind, G.E.; Lothe, R.A. Epigenetic and genetic features of 24 colon cancer cell lines. *Oncogenesis* **2013**, *2*, e71. [CrossRef]
52. Ji, D.; Zhan, T.; Li, M.; Yao, Y.; Jia, J.; Yi, H.; Qiao, M.; Xia, J.; Zhang, Z.; Ding, H.; et al. Enhancement of sensitivity to chemo/radiation therapy by using miR-15b against DCLK1 in colorectal cancer. *Stem Cell Rep.* **2018**, *11*, 1506–1522. [CrossRef] [PubMed]
53. Turano, M.; Costabile, V.; Cerasuolo, A.; Duraturo, F.; Liccardo, R.; Delrio, P.; Pace, U.; Rega, D.; Dodaro, C.A.; Milone, M.; et al. Characterisation of mesenchymal colon tumour-derived cells in tumourspheres as a model for colorectal cancer progression. *Int. J. Oncol.* **2018**, *53*, 2379–2396. [CrossRef] [PubMed]
54. Bao, Y.; Lu, Y.; Wang, X.; Feng, W.; Sun, X.; Guo, H.; Tang, C.; Zhang, X.; Shi, Q.; Yu, H. Eukaryotic translation initiation factor 5A2 (eIF5A2) regulates chemoresistance in colorectal cancer through epithelial mesenchymal transition. *Cancer Cell Int.* **2015**, *15*, 109. [CrossRef] [PubMed]
55. Larson, S.M.; Truscott, L.C.; Chiou, T.T.; Patel, A.; Kao, R.; Tu, A.; Tyagi, T.; Lu, X.; Elashoff, D.; De Oliveira, S.N. Pre-clinical development of gene modification of haematopoietic stem cells with chimeric antigen receptors for cancer immunotherapy. *Hum. Vaccines Immunother.* **2017**, *13*, 1094–1104. [CrossRef]
56. Maliar, A.; Servais, C.; Waks, T.; Chmielewski, M.; Lavy, R.; Altevogt, P.; Abken, H.; Eshhar, Z. Redirected T cells that target pancreatic adenocarcinoma antigens eliminate tumors and metastases in mice. *Gastroenterology* **2012**, *143*, 1375–1384. [CrossRef]
57. Weygant, N.; Qu, D.; May, R.; Chandrakesan, P.; Ge, Y.; Ryan, C.D.; An, G.; Schlosser, M.J.; Bannerman-Menson, E.; Houchen, C.W. Systemic delivery of CBT-15G DCLK1-targeted monoclonal antibody dramatically decreases tumorigenesis in a xenograft model of pancreatic cancer. *Cancer Res.* **2016**, *76*, Am2016–Am2577.

© 2019 by the authors. Licensee MDPI, Basel, Switzerland. This article is an open access article distributed under the terms and conditions of the Creative Commons Attribution (CC BY) license (http://creativecommons.org/licenses/by/4.0/).

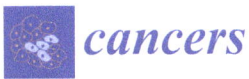

Review

Tuft and Cancer Stem Cell Marker DCLK1: A New Target to Enhance Anti-Tumor Immunity in the Tumor Microenvironment

Zhiyun Cao [1,2,3,†], Nathaniel Weygant [1,2,3,†], Parthasarathy Chandrakesan [4,5,6], Courtney W. Houchen [4,5,6], Jun Peng [1,2,3,*] and Dongfeng Qu [4,5,6,*,‡]

1. Academy of Integrative Medicine, Fujian University of Traditional Chinese Medicine, Fuzhou 350122, China; caozhiyun0824@163.com (Z.C.); nweygant@gmail.com (N.W.)
2. Fujian Key Laboratory of Integrative Medicine in Geriatrics, Fujian University of Traditional Chinese Medicine, Fuzhou 350122, China
3. Key Laboratory of Integrative Medicine of Fujian Province University, Fujian University of Traditional Chinese Medicine, Fuzhou 350122, China
4. Department of Medicine, University of Oklahoma Health Sciences Center, Oklahoma City, OK 73104, USA; parthasarathy-chandrakesan@ouhsc.edu (P.C.); Courtney-Houchen@ouhsc.edu (C.W.H.)
5. Peggy and Charles Stephenson Cancer Center, Oklahoma City, OK 73104, USA
6. Department of Veterans Affairs Medical Center, Oklahoma City, OK 73104, USA
* Correspondence: pjunlab@hotmail.com (J.P.); Dongfeng-Qu@ouhsc.edu (D.Q.); Tel.: +86-(0591)-2286-1303 (J.P.); +1-(405)-271-2175 (D.Q.); Fax: +86-(0591)-2286-1157 (J.P.); +1-(405)-271-5450 (D.Q.)
† These authors contribution is equally to this work.
‡ Current address: Department of Medicine, Digestive Diseases and Nutrition, The University of Oklahoma Health Science Center, 975 NE 10th St BRC1266, Oklahoma City, OK 73104, USA.

Received: 28 October 2020; Accepted: 14 December 2020; Published: 17 December 2020

Simple Summary: Doublecortin-like kinase 1 (DCLK1) is a tumor stem cell marker in colon, pancreatic, and potentially other cancers that has received wide attention recently. Aside from its role as a tuft cell marker in normal tissue and as a tumor stem cell marker in cancer, previous studies have demonstrated that silencing DCLK1 functionally reduces stemness, epithelial mesenchymal transition (EMT), and tumorigenesis in cancers. More recently, DCLK1's role in regulating the inflammatory, pre-cancer, and tumor microenvironment including its ability to modulate immune cell mechanisms has started to come into focus. Importantly, clinically viable therapeutic means of targeting DCLK1 have finally become available in the form of kinase inhibitors, monoclonal antibodies, and chimeric antigen receptor T cells (CAR-T). Herein, we comprehensively review the mechanistic role of DCLK1 in the tumor microenvironment, assess the potential for targeting DCLK1 in colon, pancreatic and renal cancer.

Abstract: Microtubule-associated doublecortin-like kinase 1 (DCLK1) is an accepted marker of tuft cells (TCs) and several kinds of cancer stem cells (CSCs), and emerging evidence suggests that DCLK1-positive TCs participate in the initiation and formation of inflammation-associated cancer. DCLK1-expressing CSCs regulate multiple biological processes in cancer, promote resistance to therapy, and are associated with metastasis. In solid tumor cancers, tumor epithelia, immune cells, cancer-associated fibroblasts, endothelial cells and blood vessels, extracellular matrix, and hypoxia all support a CSC phenotype characterized by drug resistance, recurrence, and metastasis. Recently, studies have shown that DCLK1-positive CSCs are associated with epithelial-mesenchymal transition, angiogenesis, and immune checkpoint. Emerging data concerning targeting DCLK1 with small molecular inhibitors, monoclonal antibodies, and chimeric antigen receptor T-cells shows promising effects on inhibiting tumor growth and regulating the tumor immune microenvironment. Overall, DCLK1 is reaching maturity as an anti-cancer target and therapies directed against it may have potential against CSCs directly, in remodeling the tumor microenvironment, and as immunotherapies.

Keywords: DCLK1; tuft cells; cancer stem cells; microenvironment; immunotherapies

---

1. Introduction

Microtubule-associated doublecortin-like kinase 1 (DCLK1) was originally thought to be a brain-specific protein before 2006 [1] when Giannakis et al. first reported DCLK1 as a potential marker of stem-like cells of the small intestine [2]. However, further research has identified these cells as differentiated tuft cells (TCs) possessing a variety of unique molecular and functional characteristics [3]. DCLK1+ tuft cells of the gastrointestinal tract are characterized by microvilli and may be long-lived and display self-renewal or progenitor functionality under some conditions [4–6]. Importantly, they regulate the immune microenvironment through IL-25/IL-17RB signaling in order to affect epithelial repair after injury, and may initiate inflammation-associated tumorigenesis after mutation [7–12]. In 2008, the Houchen group proposed that DCLK1 is a specific marker protein for intestinal adenoma stem cells [13], which brought attention to DCLK1 in cancer research and was the first of a series of research reports providing evidence that it might be an effective target for oncology drug development. To date, DCLK1 has been demonstrated to be a relatively selective marker of several kinds of cancer stem-like cells or cancer stem cells (CSCs) including in colon, breast, pancreas, kidney, and esophageal cancers [14–17]. After twenty years of research, DCLK1 is accepted as a specific marker of TCs and several kinds of CSCs, and is well known for its ability to regulate tumor growth, invasion, metastasis, epithelial-mesenchymal transition (EMT), pluripotency, angiogenesis, and pro-survival signaling [18–21].

CSCs are an important subpopulation of cells in the immunosuppressive tumor microenvironment (TME), which in turn provides a niche to support stem cell characteristics including self-renewal, differentiation, and immunosuppressive cell recruitment. Tumors create an immunosuppressive microenvironment by secreting a variety of chemokines and cytokines which may recruit tumor associated macrophages (TAM), tumor associated neutrophils (TAN), myeloid derived suppressor cells (MDSC), and other regulatory immune cells. TAM and TAN differentiate from polarized macrophages and neutrophils respectively, and remodel the TME to support tumor growth and angiogenesis [22]. TAM have been shown to promote the degradation of extracellular matrix and secrete exosomes containing mRNA and miRNA which ultimately promote tumor invasion and metastasis. Both TAM and CD4+ T-cells secrete tumor necrosis factor alpha (TNF-α) and up-regulate NF-κB signal pathway to induce the expression of EMT transcription factors Snail and Twist [23]. Moreover, they enhance transforming growth factor-β (TGF-β) signaling to promote the self-renewal of CSCs [24]. Presently, CSCs are considered a key driver of chemotherapy resistance, recurrence, and metastasis. Recent work shows that DCLK1 promotes CSC self-renewal and drug-resistance and can be targeted to inhibit tumorigenesis in kidney cancer [25]. Furthermore, several recent studies show that DCLK1 affects tumor growth and metastasis via regulating TAM and immune checkpoint. Finally, monoclonal antibodies and chimeric antigen receptor T-Cells (CAR-T) based on DCLK1 have demonstrated potential as novel cancer immunotherapies [26–28]. Herein we review key advances in the understanding of DCLK1 and DCLK1+ TCs function in the context of the tumor and immune microenvironment and discuss future directions for DCLK1-based research and development.

2. Function of DCLK1-Expressing Gastrointestinal Tuft Cells

TCs are present above the +4 position of the intestinal crypt and in the villus where they function as a chemosensory and secretory cell type. Additionally, TCs are found in the respiratory tract, salivary gland, gallbladder, pancreatic duct, auditory tube, urethra, and thymus [29–33]. The majority within the intestinal epithelium express DCLK1, and accumulating evidence suggests that DCLK1+ tuft cells take part in a diffuse chemosensory system where they serve a sentinel function to detect chemical signals in the microenvironment and orchestrate the repair of local epithelial tissue [12]. For instance,

TCs located in the lung, colon and stomach epithelium can sense alterations to pH, nutrients, or the microbiota using taste receptors including GTP-binding protein α-gustducin and transient receptor potential cation channel subfamily M member 5 (TRPM5), or regulate capillary resistance to hypoxia by inducing an epithelial response via secretion of IL-25, leading to the activation of innate lymphoid type 2 cells (ILC2) and IL-13 secretion [34–37]. Using a transgenic intestinal epithelium specific DCLK1 knockout mouse model (Villin^{Cre};Dclk1$^{fl/fl}$), May et al. reported that DCLK1 deletion in tuft cells resulted in altered gene expression in pathways for epithelial growth, stemness, barrier function, and taste reception signaling further suggesting its importance in TCs [9]. Furthermore, several studies have reported that DCLK1-expressing TCs secrete various kinds of regulatory molecules such as leukotrienes, prostaglandins, nitric oxide and IL-25, which lead to ILC2 and LGR5+ stem cell-mediated tuft and goblet cell differentiation in chronic inflammation and injury [35,38]. This is a key emerging area of interest that will provide new knowledge about the inflammatory, pre-cancer, and tumor microenvironments as well as immune–tumor interactions as they relate to tumorigenesis and progression.

There is strong evidence that DCLK1 expression in TCs play an important functional role in epithelial repair processes of the gut. Intestinal epithelium-specific knockout of DCLK1 (Vil^{Cre};Dclk1$^{flox/flox}$) leads to increased severity of injury and death in mouse whole body irradiation and dextran sulfate sodium (DSS)-induced colitis models [6,9,39]. A recent study expounded on this idea more directly. Yi et al. reported the deletion of DCLK1 in the mucin-type O-glycan deficient model of ulcerative colitis (UC) resulted in greater severity of disease characterized by enhanced mucosal thickening and increased inflammatory cell infiltration. They found that in the absence of DCLK1, epithelial proliferative responses to chronic inflammation were impaired. However, the deletion of DCLK1 did not affect the numbers of intact TCs. These results indicate that DCLK1 expression is a regulator of TC activation status, despite not being involved in TC expansion [10]. Moreover, this function has consequences to the entire intestinal epithelial response to injury as supported by previous findings [6,9,39]. Although these findings are highly suggestive, further studies will be necessary to fully determine the exact mechanisms by which DCLK1 in TCs regulate this response.

DCLK1-expressing TC expansion has been observed in human Barrett's esophagus, chronic gastritis in transgenic mice, rat gastric mucosa and intestinal neoplasia [14,40,41]. While TCs are not usually proliferative, it appears that mutations acquired by stem cells or progenitors can be passed on to TCs, which might then interconvert into tumor initiating cells under inflammatory or injurious conditions. Alternatively, putative "long-lived" TCs might acquire and maintain mutations, finally initiating tumorigenesis after a secondary insult such as colitis [6]. During the early stages of tumorigenesis, DCLK1+ TC expansion is observed in the gastrointestinal niche where they interact with neurons and promote tumorigenesis by secreting acetylcholine to stimulate enteric nerves. Notably, intestinal epithelial cells can express acetylcholine receptors to activate Wnt signaling and regulate the differentiation of intestinal epithelial cells which may be required for tumorigenesis [42]. Using lineage tracing mouse models, Nakanishi et al. and Westphalen et al. concurrently demonstrated the DCLK1+ TC's cell-of-origin status in Wnt-driven tumorigenesis. In the Nakanishi study, the Apc$^{Min/+}$ model of intestinal polyposis was crossed with a Dclk1$^{Cre-ERT}$ mouse to generate lineage tracing (Apc$^{Min/+}$;Dclk1$^{Cre-ERT}$;R26^{LacZ}) and diptheria-toxin receptor TC-specific deletion (Apc$^{Min/+}$;Dclk1$^{Cre-ERT}$;iDTR) mice. Dclk1+ TC-based lineage tracing specifically traced the entirety of the adenoma in these mice. In comparison, an intestinal stem cell marker Lgr5-based model traced the entirety of the normal epithelium and the polyp. Moreover, deletion of DCLK1+ TCs using the diptheria-toxin receptor model resulted in a complete collapse of polyps within days [43]. The Westphalen study made use of an alternative Dclk1^{Cre} model which was crossed to an Apc$^{flox/flox}$ mouse. In this model, spontaneous tumorigenesis did not occur. However, lineage tracing experiments demonstrated a small, but abnormally long-lived, population of DCLK1+ TCs in the intestinal epithelium. In conditions of colitis induced chemically via DSS, these long-lived TCs gave rise to tumors with a severe adenocarcinoma-like phenotype [6]. Importantly, this study was the first to ascertain the existence of multiple functionally unique populations of TCs. This finding has now been confirmed by single-cell RNA-Sequencing studies which identified a separate immunomodulatory population of TCs [44].

In summary, DCLK1-expressing TCs play an important role in stimulating gastrointestinal epithelial stem cells in the microenvironment and contributing to cancer progression [45]. Moreover, studying the two distinct subpopulations of TCs separately may clarify their dual-role in epithelial restitution and tumorigenesis. Promisingly, specific markers for each TC subtype have already been identified [44]. Finally, limited evidence suggests that DCLK1-expressing intestinal TCs in the gut can promote tumor progression in hepatocellular carcinoma (HCC) through activating alternative macrophages in tumor microenvironment via secreting IL-25 [46]. This distant signaling functionality across the gut-liver axis adds an interesting new dimension to understanding the role of TCs.

3. Function of DCLK1+ Acinar and Tuft Cells in Pancreatitis and Pancreatic Cancer

In the pancreas, DCLK1 is a marker of a population of pancreatic cancer-initiating cells, some of which have morphological and molecular features of gastrointestinal TCs [47]. However, DCLK1 also notably marks pancreatic acinar cells, which are a likely source of tumorigenesis through the acinar-ductal metaplasia process. Genetic lineage tracing experiments show that Dclk1+ pancreatic epithelial cells are necessary for pancreatic regeneration following injury and chronic inflammation. Moreover, KRAS mutation in Dclk1+ pancreatic epithelial cells leads to pancreatic cancer in the presence of induced pancreatitis [43]. In pancreatic tumors, it has recently been shown that immune cell-derived IL-17 regulates the development of TCs via increased expression of DCLK1, POU domain class 2 transcription factor 3 (POU2F3), aldehyde dehydrogenase 1 family member A1 (ALDH1A1), and IL17RC [48]. Intriguingly, DCLK1 kinase inhibitor can inhibit DCLK1+ organoids derived from pancreatic ductal adenocarcinoma patient tumors, indicating that DCLK1 activity and perhaps DCLK1+ TCs or acinar cells are a potential target for pancreatic ductal adenocarcinoma [49]. Although the underlying signaling mechanisms of DCLK1+ epithelial cell-mediated tumorigenesis require further elaboration, DCLK1 and DCLK1+ epithelial cells such as TCs are likely to be a target for new classes of immunotherapies and TME-remodeling drugs in gastrointestinal tract cancers.

4. Interactions between DCLK1 and the Tumor Microenvironment

CSCs depend on the surrounding microenvironment to maintain immune evasion, EMT, drug efflux, DNA repair, signaling pathway regulation, metabolic reprogramming, and epigenetic reprogramming to enhance tumor metastasis, multi-drug resistance and antitumor immunity [50]. Hypoxia is a key regulator of the TME and evidence indicates that DCLK1-positive colorectal cancer cells have increased stemness in hypoxic conditions [51]. Hypoxia famously induces CSCs to express hypoxia inducible factor (HIF) which is a key factor in inducing vascular endothelial growth factor (VEGF) and angiogenesis, which in turn further fuel CSCs. Knockdown of DCLK1 with siRNA or downregulation of DCLK1 with a kinase inhibitor (XMD8-92) results in decreased expression of angiogenic markers/VEGF receptors (VEGFR1 and VEGFR2) and EMT-related transcription factors ZEB1, ZEB2, Snail and Slug [19,52] in pancreatic tumor xenografts. Hypoxia can also be increased epigenetically by histone lysine demethylase 3A (KDM3A) overexpression in pancreatic cancer cells, which leads to increased expression of DCLK1. Knockdown of KDM3A in this context results in reduced invasion, spheroid formation, and orthotopic tumor formation [53]. Finally, in renal cell carcinoma, siRNA-mediated knockdown of DCLK1 significantly sensitized co-cultured endothelial cells to the vascular endothelial growth factor receptor (VEGFR) inhibitor sunitinib in an in vitro angiogenesis assay, demonstrating that expression of DCLK1 on neoplastic cells directly modulates this component of the tumor microenvironment. However, further studies will be needed to determine if this effect is direct [17]. Together these results link the activity of DCLK1, hypoxia, and angiogenesis and further research should be promising.

EMT and CSCs are both linked by key biological characteristics, such as resistance to cytotoxic T lymphocytes (CTLs) and reliance on TGF-β signaling pathway [54]. Microenvironmental changes, such as hypoxia, induce CSCs and in turn CSCs maintain plasticity in their niche via inflammation, EMT, and hypoxia through various signaling pathways [55]. Strong evidence demonstrates that DCLK1 is a regulator of EMT in gastric, colorectal, pancreatic, breast, renal, and other cancers [56,57]. EMT is defined as cellular phenotypic changes from epithelial to mesenchymal type with high expression of N-cadherin and Vimentin [58], and is further associated with TGF-β signaling pathway and functional migration, invasion, metastasis, extracellular matrix (ECM) alteration, apoptosis and drug resistance [59]. Enhanced EMT features after exposure to inflammatory cytokines (i.e., TGF-β, interferon gamma (IFN-γ) and TNF-α) can impact proliferation, differentiation and apoptosis of natural killer cells (NKs) and T and B cells [60], suggesting the importance of EMT in the tumor immune microenvironment. Indeed, evidence suggests that blocking TGF-β signaling may sensitize tumors to immune checkpoint inhibitors [61], and checkpoint ligand programmed cell death 1 (PD-1) ligand (PD-L1) is frequently upregulated in EMT-high tumors.

Additionally, miRNAs are known to play an important role in regulating EMT [62]. Members of miR-200 family directly inhibit ZEB1/ZEB2 activity and overexpression of the miR-200 family can suppress EMT and sensitize cancer cells to chemotherapeutic agents [63]. Knockdown of DCLK1 expression leads to down-regulation of miR-200a, miR-144, and miR-let7a along with downregulation of EMT-associated transcription factors ZEB1, ZEB2, Snail, Slug, and Twist in human pancreatic and colon cancer cells [20,64]. Therefore, DCLK1-mediated EMT could be a target in decreasing HIF levels to regulate angiogenesis and suppress migration by inhibiting cell-to-cell adhesion. Moreover, targeting DCLK1-mediated EMT to regulate TGF-β pathway may alter resistance to CTLs and other anti-tumor immune cells. Blocking DCLK1-mediated EMT also may damage CSC homeostatic processes through several correlated signaling pathways. A study using lung cancer models showed that downregulation of miR-200 family members and upregulation of ZEB1 not only drive EMT, but also lead to upregulation of the PD-L1 in association with exhaustion of intratumoral CD8+ T lymphocytes, which ultimately promotes metastasis [65]. These results suggest that targeting DCLK1-mediated EMT may increase PD-L1 regulated CD8+ T lymphocyte infiltration via regulation of the miR-200 family. Indeed, some evidence shows that DCLK1 marked CSCs support growth, metastasis, and escape from eradication in the tumor microenvironment [25,66,67]. These results are not the only ones demonstrating a relationship between DCLK1 and miRNA activity. Razi et al. showed that DCLK1 is expressed at higher levels in colorectal cancer (CRC) tissue compared to pre-cancerous polyps and that it is inversely correlated with the expression of functional tumor suppressor miRNAs miR-137 and miR-15a. The combined effect of miR-137/miR-15a loss could be significant in CRC as loss of the first is associated with more severe pathological characteristics, and loss of the second has anti-apoptotic, pro-proliferative, and pro-invasive effects [68].

Another key area of focus for DCLK1's role in the tumor microenvironment involves its basic activity in cell signal transduction. Unlike other prominent target kinases, little is known about DCLK1's ligands, interacting proteins, and substrates. This perhaps results from the difficulty in studying DCLK1's complex isoforms, two of which are initiated from an upstream CpG-island regulated promoter (alpha-promoter) and another two of which are initiated from a downstream TATA-box promoter (beta-promoter). However, strides in understanding DCLK1's basic molecular function have been made in recent years. Notably, DCLK1 has been identified as a potential RAS effector and activator in multiple studies, and DCLK1 expression in pancreatic cancer patients is correlated with RAS downstream signaling pathways ERK, PI3K, and MTOR [49,69–71]. DCLK1-AL (transcribed from the α-promoter and characterized by a lengthened C-terminus) can complex with RAS and increase GTP-bound active RAS [71].

Kato et al. showed that loss of the G9a (EHMT2) histone methyl transferase results in a decrease in the number of Dclk1-positive cells and correlated reduction in Erk phosphorylation in mouse pancreatic intraepithelial neoplasia (mPanIN) lesions of a pancreatic cancer mouse model [70], which concurs with findings in the Dclk1^{Cre};Kras$^{LSL-G12D}$ model of pancreatic tumorigenesis [69]. Ferguson et al. also provided evidence for the importance of the interaction between DCLK1 and ERK in a subset of KRAS-mutant pancreatic cancers [49]. In regards to substrates of DCLK1, Liu et al. used the novel and specific inhibitor DCLK1-IN-1 as a tool to identify several candidates including ERK2, GSK3B, CDK1, CDK2, CHK1, and PKACA. Additional potential substrates in nucleic acid processing such as CDK11, MATR3, and DNA topoisomerase 2-beta (TOP2B) were also identified and phosphopeptides including TOP2B, CDK11B, and MATR3 were significantly decreased after treatment with DCLK1-IN-1. Pathway analysis suggested substrate involvement in RNA processing, insulin signaling, ErbB signaling, proteoglycan synthesis, and maintenance of focal adhesion and tight junction pathways [72]. Finally, Koizumi et al. experimentally identified MAP7D1 (microtubule-associated protein 7 domain containing 1) as a substrate of DCLK1 in cortical neurons and the phosphomimetic MAP7D1 fully rescued the impaired callosal axon elongation in neurons after DCLK1 knockdown [73]. All together, these findings are some of the first to unravel DCLK1's complex molecular mechanisms and may have implications for future translational research and biomarker development.

5. Regulation of Immune Checkpoint and Macrophage Polarization by DCLK1

The tumor immune microenvironment (TIME) refers to the microenvironment as it relates to immune cells including: infiltrated-excluded TIME in which there is a relative lack of cytotoxic T lymphocytes in the core location of the tumor; infiltrated–inflamed TIME in which infiltration occurs to a large degree with expression of immune negative regulatory receptor PD-1 of CTLs and inhibitory PD-L1 of leukocytes; and tertiary lymphoid structure TIME, which contains a large number of lymphocytes, including initial and activated T-cells, regulatory T-cells, B cells, and dendritic cells [74]. Overexpression of PD-L1 on tumor cells inhibits the activation of immune cells by binding PD-1 on the surface of T cells after a T-cell receptor binds to cancer cells to promote PD-1 expression. PD-1 and PD-L1 antibodies can block PD-1/PD-L1 co-inhibition signaling and relieve the inhibition of T cells and induce their cytotoxicity. A recent study reported that DCLK1 regulates the level of PD-L1 expression by affecting the corresponding expression level of yes-associated protein (YAP) in the Hippo pathway in pancreatic tumors [26]. These findings concur with others in renal cancer which also show a direct relationship between DCLK1 and PD-L1 expression [26]. CSCs maintain TME stemness as well as increase angiogenesis, which is associated with reduced recognition of T cells and evasion of the immune system via lack of T-cell recognition [75]. PD-L1 perhaps has a key role in helping DCLK1-positive CSCs to evade the immune system, leading to an immune suppressive microenvironment. Moreover, this process may be linked to DCLK1 regulatory activity on EMT, as the EMT process is also strongly associated with immune checkpoint [76].

In the TME, TAMs can serve an anti-tumorigenic or pro-tumorigenic role depending on their status. Typically, the M1 pro-inflammatory macrophage status is correlated to tumor suppression, while the M2 anti-inflammatory/tissue-repair status promotes tumor progression and metastasis. CSCs can secrete various cytokines and chemokines to recruit TAMs to infiltrate the tumor and maintain the M2 phenotype. In turn, M2 macrophages activate STAT3 signaling via secreting IL-6 and epidermal growth factor to increase the expression of Sox2 and enhance the tumorigenic potential of CSCs. In addition, M2 macrophages can also secrete TGF-β to induce EMT and maintain stemness. Overexpression of DCLK1 has been related to worse clinical prognosis via increasing immune and stromal components in colon and gastric cancer patients, and DCLK1 affects multiple immune cell types such as TAMs and Treg and notably inhibits CD8+ T-cells by increasing inhibitor proteins TGF-β1 and chemokine (C-X-C motif) ligand 12 (CXCL12) and their receptors [77]. A recent study demonstrated that overexpression of DCLK1-AL in pancreatic tumor cells can lead to polarization of M1-macrophages towards an M2-phenotype characterized by secretion of chemokines and cytokines such as IL-6, IL-10, and CXCL12, which enhance tumor cell migration, invasion, and self-renewal [28]. In addition, DCLK1-AL induced M2-macrophages inhibited CD8+ T-cell proliferation and Granzyme-B activation, resulting in immunosuppression. Interestingly, silencing DCLK1 caused macrophages to retain the M1 phenotype and abrogated the M2-macrophage ability to enhance aggressiveness and self-renewal in pancreatic cancer cells. Together, these findings suggest that DCLK1 is a promising target to enhance antitumor effect through regulating TIME in some types of cancer (Figure 1).

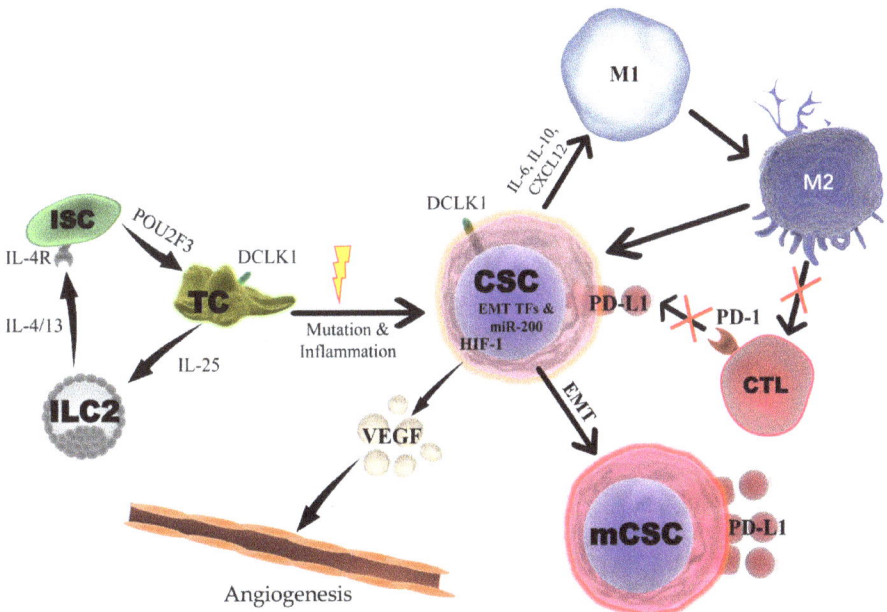

Figure 1. Potential Role of DCLK1 and DCLK1+ Cells in the Intestinal Tumor Microenvironment. DCLK1+ tuft cells (TC) will recruit innate lymphoid type-2 cells (ILC2) by secreting IL-25 which in turn reprograms intestinal stem cells (ISC) through IL4/13-IL4R signaling to express transcription factor POU2F3 leading to TC hyperplasia. In the presence of mutation and inflammation, DCLK1+ TCs can be converted to cancer stem cells (CSC) and initiate a tumor. Under hypoxia, DCLK1+ CSCs may induce angiogenesis by upregulation of HIF-1 and secretion of VEGF. Furthermore, DCLK1+ CSCs promote EMT via the miR-200 family leading to metastatic CSCs (mCSC) with high levels of PD-L1. DCLK1+ CSCs further regulate the immune tumor microenvironment by polarization of M1 macrophages towards an M2 status by secreting IL-6, IL-10 and CXCL12, which leads to inhibition of T-cell proliferation and activation. DCLK1-positive CSCs also express programmed death ligand 1 (PD-L1) expression to inhibit CD8/PD1++ CTL function.

6. Development of DCLK1-Targeted Therapeutic Agents and Biologics

The recent discovery of new CSC surface markers and functional membrane proteins has led to suitable candidate targets such as CD13 and α3β1 for hepatocellular carcinoma (HCC) and bladder cancer, respectively [78,79]. DCLK1 is an optimal target as it represents a more specific CSC marker for colorectal, pancreatic, and possibly other cancers such as gastric cancer, esophageal cancer, breast cancer and renal carcinoma. A small molecule kinase inhibitor, LRRK2-IN-1, was first reported to regulate DCLK1-mediated stemness and EMT by suppressing DCLK1 kinase activity in colorectal and pancreatic cancer [80]. LRRK2-IN-1 impaired cell proliferation, induced apoptosis, and decreased colony formation capacity in cholangiocarcinoma primary cells. Interestingly, it was also shown that DCLK1 marks a subpopulation of LGR5+ and CD133+ CSC-like cells in cholangiocarcinoma, suggesting its potential as a target in this disease [81]. However, LRRK2-IN-1 has notable activity against ERK5 and sub-optimal properties for in vivo delivery. Recently a more specific and in vivo-compatible inhibitor, DCLK1-IN-1, was developed to target the DCLK1 kinase domain based on chemo-proteomic profiling and structure-activity based design. Importantly, this inhibitor showed significant activity against clinically relevant DCLK1+ patient-derived pancreatic ductal adenocarcinoma organoids [49]. Additionally, DCLK1-IN-1 was shown to be effective in CRC using kinase-modified engineered DCLK1 in the DLD-1 cell line [72]. Further studies are needed using DCLK1-IN-1 and other specific DCLK1 kinase inhibitors, and an assessment of its ability to influence anti-tumor immunity is especially desirable as the clinical use of kinase inhibitors in conjunction with immune checkpoint therapies is emerging [82].

Overexpression of DCLK1-AL induces the expression of aldehyde dehydrogenase, stimulates CSC self-renewal, and enhances resistance to FDA-approved receptor tyrosine kinase inhibitors (sunitinib/sorafenib) and mammalian target of rapamyoin inhibitors (everolimus/temsirolimus) in renal cell carcinoma (RCC), suggesting its value as a target in this cancer. A novel monoclonal antibody (CBT-15) was developed to target DCLK1's extracellular C-terminus and effectively blocked RCC tumorigenesis in an RCC xenograft model [25]. Notably, DCLK1 variants containing the extracellular domain show restricted expression in normal tissue but overexpression in tumor tissue. CBT-15 also showed a significant effect in inhibiting tumor growth in vivo in mouse models of pancreatic cancer [71]. Another DCLK1-targeted mAb, DCLK1-87, stains tissue regions with CSC-marker ALDH expression in CRC, and CRC patients bearing tumors with low tissue staining intensity from this mAb showed improved survival [83].

Utilizing well-characterized CSC markers makes it possible to develop CAR-T cells with the potential to eliminate CSCs. As a CAR-T target, DCLK1 single-chain antibody variable fragment (CBT-511), showed a prominent cytotoxic effect against tumor cells and reduced tumor growth in CRC [27]. CBT-511 also increased IFN-γ release in CRC cells (2D and 3D). It has been reported previously that CSCs decrease the number of activated dendritic cells which is accompanied by decreased secretion of IL-10, IL-12 and IFN-γ cytokines, resulting in the inhibition of proliferation and differentiation of immature T lymphocytes [84]. Further investigation of DCLK1-targeted CAR-T in this context is warranted (Table 1).

Table 1. Investigational targeted therapies against doublecortin-like kinase 1.

Name of Drug	Class of Drug	DCLK1 Affinity	Other Significant Targets	Cancer Types Tested	Level of Evidence	Functional Target of Drug	Author (Year)	PMID
LRRK2-IN-1	Kinase inhibitor	<60 nM	LRRK2, ERK5	CRC, PDAC, CCA	In vitro, in vivo, and ex vivo	Stemness, proliferation, migration, invasion, apoptosis, cell cycle, DNA damage, EMT and tumor growth	Weygant et al. (2014) [80] Kawamura et al. (2017) [68] Nevi et al. (2020) [81] Suehiro et al. (2018) [86]	24885928 29048622 32978808 30396941
XMD8-92	Kinase inhibitor	< 100 nM	ERK5, DCLK2	Mesothelioma, PDAC	In vitro and in vivo	Stemness, EMT, angiogenesis, proliferation and tumor growth	Sureban et al. (2014) [52] Wang et al. (2017) [87]	24880079 28560410
DCLK1-IN-1	Kinase inhibitor	< 60 nM	DCLK2	PDAC, CRC	In vitro and ex vivo	Proliferation, invasion and stemness	Ferguson et al. (2020) [49] Ferguson et al. (2020) [88]	32251410 32530623
NP-siDCAMKL-1	Nanoparticle-encapsulated siRNA	N/A	None	CRC, HCC, PDAC	In vitro and in vivo	Tumor growth	Sureban et al. (2011) [64] Sureban et al. (2015) [89] Sureban et al. (2013) [19]	21929751 26468984 24040120
CBT-15	Monoclonal antibody	<1 nM	None	PDAC, RCC	In vitro and in vivo	ADCC and tumor growth	Ge et al. (2018) [25] Qu et al. (2019) [71]	29577227 31467540
DCLK1–HA–PEG-PLGA	Bifunctional-antibody/nanoparticle conjugate	N/A	CD44	Breast cancer	In vitro and in vivo		Qiao et al. (2016) [90]	27994463
CBT-511	Chimeric antigen receptor T-cells	<1 nM	None	CRC	In vitro and in vitro	Proliferation and tumor growth	Sureban et al. (2019) [27]	31878090

7. Future Directions for DCLK1 Research and Drug Development

Although traditional radiotherapy and chemotherapy have therapeutic effects on tumors, clinical data show that CSCs are resistant to chemotherapy and radiotherapy, which is a key reason for tumor metastasis and recurrence. Therefore, it is desirable to develop specific and effective targeted therapies against CSCs. DCLK1 is a promising therapeutic target as shown by studies using kinase inhibitor, mAb or CAR-T. However, further studies of DCLK1-expressing TCs and their biological effect in normal conditions and in initiating cancer will be needed to safely target DCLK1. Furthermore, exploration of DCLK1's relationship to other biological aspects are sorely needed.

Under hypoxia, DCLK1 overexpression induces stemness, but the intermediary mechanisms remain unknown. Hypoxia is known to protect CSCs from chemotherapy and radiation therapy-mediated damage in the TME, and to induce angiogenesis by secreting VEGF and recruiting monocytes, macrophages, macrophages and endothelial cells. Moreover, it limits the proliferation and activation of cytotoxic CD8+ T-cells, activates WNT and Notch signaling pathways to maintain self-renewal, and induces TGF-β signaling to promote EMT. Although DCLK1 is upregulated in angiogenesis and regulates chemotherapy resistance and cancer stemness by WNT signaling, knowledge of the effect of DCLK1 on hypoxia-driven immune cells, endothelial cells, blood vessels, and ECM remains limited [91]. Prior studies show that hypoxia induce CSCs to different metabolic phenotypes including glycolysis for the quiescent M state and oxidative phosphorylation for the proliferative E-state to enhance chemoresistance and acquire other stem-cell characteristics [92–94]. Strong evidence shows that the metabolism of CSCs is context-dependent and reliant on glycolysis or mitochondrial oxidative metabolism [95–100]. Currently, conventional therapies such as chemotherapy and radiotherapy have a low effect on CSCs because of increased expression of drug transporters, maintenance of a slow dividing state (quiescence), and efficient DNA repair mechanisms. Metabolic phenotypes are directly related with CSC dividing state and it is thought that targeting CSC metabolism may be an effective way to eliminate chemo-resistance and tumor relapse. One interesting study showed that Doublecortin-like (a splice-variant produced from DCLK1's alpha promoter) knockdown is associated with reduced mitochondrial activity which significantly decreases tumor growth by regulating cytochrome c oxidase activity and ATP synthesis in neuroblastoma tumor xenografts. Another study showed that glycolysis promotes the expression of DCLK1 and maintains the CSC and EMT phenotypes via low reactive oxygen species levels in chemo-resistant pancreatic cancer cells [101]. Tumor microenvironmental factors including hypoxia, glucose deprivation, low pH, oxygen stress, and others are key in promoting CSC selection of metabolic pathways leading to metastasis or drug-resistance [102]. Metabolic alterations may cause cells to acquire stem-cell-like characteristics, and DCLK1+ TCs are long-lived and quiescent before they are activated by injury. Recent studies demonstrate that targeting oxidative phosphorylation may inhibit CSC metabolic processes and proliferation in some cancers [103]. Switching metabolic phenotypes of CSCs and TCs by enhancing oxidative phosphorylation to inhibit their tumorigenesis or tumor growth may be a feasible direction for further study. Future studies should focus on whether targeting DCLK1 to regulate metabolic processes or targeting metabolic activity of DCLK1+ TCs or CSCs may be a viable focus for therapy.

Targeting the TIME has already resulted in remarkable achievements including CAR-T and CAR-NK technologies that can potentially kill CSCs. The composition of immune cells in the tumor microenvironment will affect their response to specific immunotherapies and alter antigen presentation and macrophage polarization. Inhibition of IL-6 secretion from TAMs can inhibit the activation of CSCs to improve therapy, and overexpression of immune checkpoint ligand PD-L1 on CSCs blocks the cytotoxic CD8+ T-cell response [104]. Although existing data is relatively limited, DCLK1 has shown promising prospects in the above areas and a full assessment of DCLK1's impact on immune checkpoint and pro-tumor macrophages is warranted.

8. Conclusions

DCLK1+ TCs are closely related with tumor initiation and chronic inflammatory diseases. Currently, the TC biological effect on cancer initiation and progression is not fully understood. Although CSCs drive chemotherapy and radiotherapy failures, there is still no effective therapeutic strategy against them. Due to these limitations, targeting the tumor microenvironment provides a prospective option for cancer treatment. However, in different tumor types or different developmental stages of the tumor, the interaction between CSCs and the microenvironment varies and will complicate developing these therapeutic strategies. Finding a reliable molecular target is crucial, and DCLK1 is one such potential marker that should be pursued in this context. DCLK1 is a multifaceted target due to several isoforms with variable functions and cellular localization. However, new evidence of their various roles is emerging. Importantly, efforts are underway to determine how DCLK1 functions within the TC to promote the response to injury, including how it modulates the immune microenvironment and how it balances this role with potential pro-tumorigenic signaling. When sufficient knowledge is gained, a variety of DCLK1-specific targeting modalities are already available for translation including specific kinase inhibitors and targeted monoclonal antibodies and CAR-T therapies.

Author Contributions: Conceptualization: Z.C., N.W., J.P. and D.Q.; writing—original draft preparation: Z.C., N.W. and D.Q.; writing—review and editing, P.C., C.W.H. and J.P.; visualization: Z.C. and N.W.; supervision: D.Q.; project administration: J.P. and D.Q.; funding acquisition: D.Q. and C.W.H. All authors have read and agreed to the published version of the manuscript.

Funding: This work was funded by an NIH R50 grant to D.Q. (R50CA233186) and two NIH R01 grants to C.W.H. (5R01CA214017 and 1R01DK119495).

Conflicts of Interest: C.W.H., D.Q., and N.W. are inventors on a patent for CBT-15 DCLK1-targeted monoclonal antibodies. C.W.H. is an inventor on a patent for CBT-511 DCLK1-targeted CAR-T. C.W.H. is an inventor on a patent for nanoparticle-encapsulated DCLK1-targeted siRNAs.

References

1. Des Portes, V.; Pinard, J.M.; Billuart, P.; Vinet, M.C.; Koulakoff, A.; Carrié, A.; Gelot, A.; Dupuis, E.; Motte, J.; Berwald-Netter, Y.; et al. A novel CNS gene required for neuronal migration and involved in X-linked subcortical laminar heterotopia and lissencephaly syndrome. *Cell* **1998**, *92*, 51–61. [CrossRef]
2. Giannakis, M.; Stappenbeck, T.S.; Mills, J.C.; Leip, D.G.; Lovett, M.; Clifton, S.W.; Ippolito, J.E.; Glasscock, J.I.; Arumugam, M.; Brent, M.R.; et al. Molecular properties of adult mouse gastric and intestinal epithelial progenitors in their niches. *J. Biol. Chem.* **2006**, *281*, 11292–11300. [CrossRef] [PubMed]
3. Gerbe, F.; Brulin, B.; Makrini, L.; Legraverend, C.; Jay, P. DCAMKL-1 expression identifies Tuft cells rather than stem cells in the adult mouse intestinal epithelium. *Gastroenterology* **2009**, *137*, 2179–2180, author reply 2180–2181. [CrossRef] [PubMed]
4. Chandrakesan, P.; May, R.; Qu, D.; Weygant, N.; Taylor, V.E.; Li, J.D.; Ali, N.; Sureban, S.M.; Qante, M.; Wang, T.C.; et al. Dclk1+ small intestinal epithelial tuft cells display the hallmarks of quiescence and self-renewal. *Oncotarget* **2015**, *6*, 30876–30886. [CrossRef]
5. Leppanen, J.; Helminen, O.; Huhta, H.; Kauppila, J.H.; Miinalainen, I.; Ronkainen, V.P.; Saarnio, J.; Lehenkari, P.P.; Karttunen, T.J. Doublecortin-like kinase 1-positive enterocyte—A new cell type in human intestine. *APMIS* **2016**, *124*, 958–965. [CrossRef] [PubMed]
6. Westphalen, C.B.; Asfaha, S.; Hayakawa, Y.; Takemoto, Y.; Lukin, D.J.; Nuber, A.H.; Brandtner, A.; Setlik, W.; Remotti, H.; Muley, A.; et al. Long-lived intestinal tuft cells serve as colon cancer-initiating cells. *J. Clin. Investig.* **2014**, *124*, 1283–1295. [CrossRef] [PubMed]
7. Middelhoff, M.; Westphalen, C.B.; Hayakawa, Y.; Yan, K.S.; Gershon, M.D.; Wang, T.C.; Quante, M. Dclk1-expressing tuft cells: Critical modulators of the intestinal niche? *Am. J. Physiol. Liver Physiol.* **2017**, *313*, G285–G299. [CrossRef]
8. Goto, N.; Fukuda, A.; Yamaga, Y.; Yoshikawa, T.; Maruno, T.; Maekawa, H.; Inamoto, S.; Kawada, K.; Sakai, Y.; Miyoshi, H.; et al. Lineage tracing and targeting of IL17RB(+) tuft cell-like human colorectal cancer stem cells. *Proc. Natl. Acad. Sci. USA* **2019**, *116*, 12996–13005. [CrossRef]

9. May, R.; Qu, D.; Weygant, N.; Chandrakesan, P.; Ali, N.; Lightfoot, S.A.; Li, L.; Sureban, S.M.; Houchen, C.W. Brief report: Dclk1 deletion in tuft cells results in impaired epithelial repair after radiation injury. *Stem Cells* **2014**, *32*, 822–827. [CrossRef]
10. Yi, J.; Bergstrom, K.; Fu, J.; Shan, X.; McDaniel, J.M.; McGee, S.; Qu, D.; Houchen, C.W.; Liu, X.; Xia, L. Dclk1 in tuft cells promotes inflammation-driven epithelial restitution and mitigates chronic colitis. *Cell Death Differ.* **2019**, *26*, 1656–1669. [CrossRef]
11. Aladegbami, B.; Barron, L.; Bao, J.; Colasanti, J.; Erwin, C.R.; Warner, B.W.; Guo, J. Epithelial cell specific Raptor is required for initiation of type 2 mucosal immunity in small intestine. *Sci. Rep.* **2017**, *7*, 5580. [CrossRef]
12. Chandrakesan, P.; May, R.; Weygant, N.; Qu, D.; Berry, W.L.; Sureban, S.M.; Ali, N.; Rao, C.; Huycke, M.; Bronze, M.S.; et al. Intestinal tuft cells regulate the ATM mediated DNA Damage response via Dclk1 dependent mechanism for crypt restitution following radiation injury. *Sci. Rep.* **2016**, *6*, 37667. [CrossRef]
13. May, R.; Riehl, T.E.; Hunt, C.; Sureban, S.M.; Anant, S.; Houchen, C.W. Identification of a novel putative gastrointestinal stem cell and adenoma stem cell marker, doublecortin and CaM kinase-like-1, following radiation injury and in adenomatous polyposis coli/multiple intestinal neoplasia mice. *Stem Cells* **2008**, *26*, 630–637. [CrossRef] [PubMed]
14. Vega, K.J.; May, R.; Sureban, S.M.; Lightfoot, S.A.; Qu, D.; Reed, A.; Weygant, N.; Ramanujam, R.; Souza, R.; Madhoun, M.; et al. Identification of the putative intestinal stem cell marker doublecortin and CaM kinase-like-1 in Barrett's esophagus and esophageal adenocarcinoma. *J. Gastroenterol. Hepatol.* **2012**, *27*, 773–780. [CrossRef]
15. May, R.; Sureban, S.M.; Hoang, N.; Riehl, T.E.; Lightfoot, S.A.; Ramanujam, R.; Wyche, J.H.; Anant, S.; Houchen, C.W. Doublecortin and CaM kinase-like-1 and leucine-rich-repeat-containing G-protein-coupled receptor mark quiescent and cycling intestinal stem cells, respectively. *Stem Cells* **2009**, *27*, 2571–2579. [CrossRef] [PubMed]
16. May, R.; Sureban, S.M.; Lightfoot, S.A.; Hoskins, A.B.; Brackett, D.J.; Postier, R.G.; Ramanujam, R.; Rao, C.V.; Wyche, J.H.; Anant, S.; et al. Identification of a novel putative pancreatic stem/progenitor cell marker DCAMKL-1 in normal mouse pancreas. *Am. J. Physiol. Liver Physiol.* **2010**, *299*, G303–G310. [CrossRef] [PubMed]
17. Weygant, N.; Qu, D.; May, R.; Tierney, R.M.; Berry, W.L.; Zhao, L.; Agarwal, S.; Chandrakesan, P.; Chinthalapally, H.R.; Murphy, N.T.; et al. DCLK1 is a broadly dysregulated target against epithelial-mesenchymal transition, focal adhesion, and stemness in clear cell renal carcinoma. *Oncotarget* **2015**, *6*, 2193–2205. [CrossRef]
18. Westphalen, C.B.; Quante, M.; Wang, T.C. Functional implication of Dclk1 and Dclk1-expressing cells in cancer. *Small GTPases* **2017**, *8*, 164–171. [CrossRef]
19. Sureban, S.M.; May, R.; Qu, D.; Weygant, N.; Chandrakesan, P.; Ali, N.; Lightfoot, S.A.; Pantazis, P.; Rao, C.V.; Postier, R.G.; et al. DCLK1 regulates pluripotency and angiogenic factors via microRNA-dependent mechanisms in pancreatic cancer. *PLoS ONE* **2013**, *8*, e73940. [CrossRef]
20. Sureban, S.M.; May, R.; Lightfoot, S.A.; Hoskins, A.B.; Lerner, M.; Brackett, D.J.; Postier, R.G.; Ramanujam, R.; Mohammed, A.; Rao, C.V.; et al. DCAMKL-1 regulates epithelial-mesenchymal transition in human pancreatic cells through a miR-200a-dependent mechanism. *Cancer Res.* **2011**, *71*, 2328–2338. [CrossRef]
21. Ito, H.; Tanaka, S.; Akiyama, Y.; Shimada, S.; Adikrisna, R.; Matsumura, S.; Aihara, A.; Mitsunori, Y.; Ban, D.; Ochiai, T.; et al. Dominant Expression of DCLK1 in Human Pancreatic Cancer Stem Cells Accelerates Tumor Invasion and Metastasis. *PLoS ONE* **2016**, *11*, e0146564. [CrossRef]
22. Kitamura, T.; Qian, B.Z.; Pollard, J.W. Immune cell promotion of metastasis. *Nat. Rev. Immunol.* **2015**, *15*, 73–86. [CrossRef] [PubMed]
23. Chanmee, T.; Ontong, P.; Konno, K.; Itano, N. Tumor-associated macrophages as major players in the tumor microenvironment. *Cancers* **2014**, *6*, 1670–1690. [CrossRef] [PubMed]
24. Smith, A.L.; Robin, T.P.; Ford, H.L. Molecular pathways: Targeting the TGF-β pathway for cancer therapy. *Clin. Cancer Res.* **2012**, *18*, 4514–4521. [CrossRef] [PubMed]
25. Ge, Y.; Weygant, N.; Qu, D.; May, R.; Berry, W.L.; Yao, J.; Chandrakesan, P.; Zheng, W.; Zhao, L.; Zhao, K.L.; et al. Alternative splice variants of DCLK1 mark cancer stem cells, promote self-renewal and drug-resistance, and can be targeted to inhibit tumorigenesis in kidney cancer. *Int. J. Cancer* **2018**, *143*, 1162–1175. [CrossRef] [PubMed]

26. Yan, R.; Li, J.; Zhou, Y.; Yao, L.; Sun, R.; Xu, Y.; Ge, Y.; An, G. Inhibition of DCLK1 down-regulates PD-L1 expression through Hippo pathway in human pancreatic cancer. *Life Sci.* **2020**, *241*, 117150. [CrossRef] [PubMed]
27. Sureban, S.M.; Berahovich, R.; Zhou, H.; Xu, S.; Wu, L.; Ding, K.; May, R.; Qu, D.; Bannerman-Menson, E.; Golubovskaya, V.; et al. DCLK1 Monoclonal Antibody-Based CAR-T Cells as a Novel Treatment Strategy against Human Colorectal Cancers. *Cancers* **2019**, *12*, 54. [CrossRef] [PubMed]
28. Chandrakesan, P.; Panneerselvam, J.; May, R.; Weygant, N.; Qu, D.; Berry, W.R.; Pitts, K.; Stanger, B.Z.; Rao, C.V.; Bronze, M.S.; et al. DCLK1-Isoform2 Alternative Splice Variant Promotes Pancreatic Tumor Immunosuppressive M2-Macrophage Polarization. *Mol. Cancer Ther.* **2020**, *19*, 1539–1549. [CrossRef]
29. Luciano, L.; Reale, E.; Ruska, H. On a "chemoreceptive" sensory cell in the tachea of the rat. *Z. fur Zellforsch. Mikrosk. Anat.* **1968**, *85*, 350–375. [CrossRef]
30. Chang, L.Y.; Mercer, R.R.; Crapo, J.D. Differential distribution of brush cells in the rat lung. *Anat. Rec.* **1986**, *216*, 49–54. [CrossRef]
31. Luciano, L.; Reale, E. Brush cells of the mouse gallbladder. A correlative light- and electron-microscopical study. *Cell Tissue Res.* **1990**, *262*, 339–349. [CrossRef] [PubMed]
32. Krasteva, G.; Hartmann, P.; Papadakis, T.; Bodenbenner, M.; Wessels, L.; Weihe, E.; Schütz, B.; Langheinrich, A.C.; Chubanov, V.; Gudermann, T.; et al. Cholinergic chemosensory cells in the auditory tube. *Histochem. Cell Biol.* **2012**, *137*, 483–497. [CrossRef] [PubMed]
33. Sato, A.; Miyoshi, S. Fine structure of tuft cells of the main excretory duct epithelium in the rat submandibular gland. *Anat. Rec.* **1997**, *248*, 325–331. [CrossRef]
34. Hass, N.; Schwarzenbacher, K.; Breer, H. A cluster of gustducin-expressing cells in the mouse stomach associated with two distinct populations of enteroendocrine cells. *Histochem. Cell Biol.* **2007**, *128*, 457–471. [CrossRef]
35. Sbarbati, A.; Bramanti, P.; Benati, D.; Merigo, F. The diffuse chemosensory system: Exploring the iceberg toward the definition of functional roles. *Prog. Neurobiol.* **2010**, *91*, 77–89. [CrossRef] [PubMed]
36. Schütz, B.; Jurastow, I.; Bader, S.; Ringer, C.; von Engelhardt, J.; Chubanov, V.; Gudermann, T.; Diener, M.; Kummer, W.; Krasteva-Christ, G.; et al. Chemical coding and chemosensory properties of cholinergic brush cells in the mouse gastrointestinal and biliary tract. *Front. Physiol.* **2015**, *6*, 87. [CrossRef]
37. Gerbe, F.; Sidot, E.; Smyth, D.J.; Ohmoto, M.; Matsumoto, I.; Dardalhon, V.; Cesses, P.; Garnier, L.; Pouzolles, M.; Brulin, B.; et al. Intestinal epithelial tuft cells initiate type 2 mucosal immunity to helminth parasites. *Nature* **2016**, *529*, 226–230. [CrossRef]
38. Nadjsombati, M.S.; McGinty, J.W.; Lyons-Cohen, M.R.; Jaffe, J.B.; DiPeso, L.; Schneider, C.; Miller, C.N.; Pollack, J.L.; Nagana Gowda, G.A.; Fontana, M.F.; et al. Detection of Succinate by Intestinal Tuft Cells Triggers a Type 2 Innate Immune Circuit. *Immunity* **2018**, *49*, 33–41.e37. [CrossRef]
39. Qu, D.; Weygant, N.; May, R.; Chandrakesan, P.; Madhoun, M.; Ali, N.; Sureban, S.M.; An, G.; Schlosser, M.J.; Houchen, C.W. Ablation of Doublecortin-Like Kinase 1 in the Colonic Epithelium Exacerbates Dextran Sulfate Sodium-Induced Colitis. *PLoS ONE* **2015**, *10*, e0134212. [CrossRef]
40. Kikuchi, M.; Nagata, H.; Watanabe, N.; Watanabe, H.; Tatemichi, M.; Hibi, T. Altered expression of a putative progenitor cell marker DCAMKL1 in the rat gastric mucosa in regeneration, metaplasia and dysplasia. *BMC Gastroenterol.* **2010**, *10*, 65. [CrossRef]
41. Okumura, T.; Ericksen, R.E.; Takaishi, S.; Wang, S.S.; Dubeykovskiy, Z.; Shibata, W.; Betz, K.S.; Muthupalani, S.; Rogers, A.B.; Fox, J.G.; et al. K-ras mutation targeted to gastric tissue progenitor cells results in chronic inflammation, an altered microenvironment, and progression to intraepithelial neoplasia. *Cancer Res.* **2010**, *70*, 8435–8445. [CrossRef] [PubMed]
42. Labed, S.A.; Wani, K.A.; Jagadeesan, S.; Hakkim, A.; Najibi, M.; Irazoqui, J.E. Intestinal Epithelial Wnt Signaling Mediates Acetylcholine-Triggered Host Defense against Infection. *Immunity* **2018**, *48*, 963–978. [CrossRef]
43. Nakanishi, Y.; Seno, H.; Fukuoka, A.; Ueo, T.; Yamaga, Y.; Maruno, T.; Nakanishi, N.; Kanda, K.; Komekado, H.; Kawada, M.; et al. Dclk1 distinguishes between tumor and normal stem cells in the intestine. *Nat. Genet.* **2013**, *45*, 98–103. [CrossRef] [PubMed]
44. Haber, A.L.; Biton, M.; Rogel, N.; Herbst, R.H.; Shekhar, K.; Smillie, C.; Burgin, G.; Delorey, T.M.; Howitt, M.R.; Katz, Y.; et al. A single-cell survey of the small intestinal epithelium. *Nature* **2017**, *551*, 333–339. [CrossRef] [PubMed]

45. Konishi, M.; Hayakawa, Y.; Koike, K. Role of Muscarinic Acetylcholine Signaling in Gastrointestinal Cancers. *Biomedicines* **2019**, *7*, 58. [CrossRef] [PubMed]
46. Friedrich, M.; Jasinski-Bergner, S.; Lazaridou, M.-F.; Subbarayan, K.; Massa, C.; Tretbar, S.; Mueller, A.; Handke, D.; Biehl, K.; Bukur, J.; et al. Tumor-induced escape mechanisms and their association with resistance to checkpoint inhibitor therapy. *Cancer Immunol. Immunother.* **2019**. [CrossRef]
47. Bailey, J.M.; Alsina, J.; Rasheed, Z.A.; McAllister, F.M.; Fu, Y.Y.; Plentz, R.; Zhang, H.; Pasricha, P.J.; Bardeesy, N.; Matsui, W.; et al. DCLK1 marks a morphologically distinct subpopulation of cells with stem cell properties in preinvasive pancreatic cancer. *Gastroenterology* **2014**, *146*, 245–256. [CrossRef]
48. Zhang, Y.; Zoltan, M.; Riquelme, E.; Xu, H.; Sahin, I.; Castro-Pando, S.; Montiel, M.F.; Chang, K.; Jiang, Z.; Ling, J.; et al. Immune Cell Production of Interleukin 17 Induces Stem Cell Features of Pancreatic Intraepithelial Neoplasia Cells. *Gastroenterology* **2018**, *155*, 210–223. [CrossRef]
49. Ferguson, F.M.; Nabet, B.; Raghavan, S.; Liu, Y.; Leggett, A.L.; Kuljanin, M.; Kalekar, R.L.; Yang, A.; He, S.; Wang, J.; et al. Discovery of a selective inhibitor of doublecortin like kinase 1. *Nat. Chem. Biol.* **2020**, *16*, 635–643. [CrossRef]
50. Weygant, N.; Ge, Y.; Westphalen, C.B.; Ma, W.W.; Vega, K.J. Role of the Microenvironment in Gastrointestinal Tumors. *J. Oncol.* **2019**, *2019*, 2153413. [CrossRef]
51. Li, L.; Bellows, C.F. Doublecortin-like kinase 1 exhibits cancer stem cell-like characteristics in a human colon cancer cell line. *Chin. J. Cancer Res.* **2013**, *25*, 134–142. [CrossRef] [PubMed]
52. Sureban, S.M.; May, R.; Weygant, N.; Qu, D.; Chandrakesan, P.; Bannerman-Menson, E.; Ali, N.; Pantazis, P.; Westphalen, C.B.; Wang, T.C.; et al. XMD8-92 inhibits pancreatic tumor xenograft growth via a DCLK1-dependent mechanism. *Cancer Lett.* **2014**, *351*, 151–161. [CrossRef] [PubMed]
53. Dandawate, P.; Ghosh, C.; Palaniyandi, K.; Paul, S.; Rawal, S.; Pradhan, R.; Sayed, A.A.A.; Choudhury, S.; Standing, D.; Subramaniam, D.; et al. The Histone Demethylase KDM3A, Increased in Human Pancreatic Tumors, Regulates Expression of DCLK1 and Promotes Tumorigenesis in Mice. *Gastroenterology* **2019**, *157*, 1646–1659. [CrossRef] [PubMed]
54. Terry, S.; Chouaib, S. EMT in immuno-resistance. *Oncoscience* **2015**, *2*, 841–842. [CrossRef] [PubMed]
55. Plaks, V.; Kong, N.; Werb, Z. The cancer stem cell niche: How essential is the niche in regulating stemness of tumor cells? *Cell Stem Cell* **2015**, *16*, 225–238. [CrossRef] [PubMed]
56. Liu, Z.Q.; He, W.F.; Wu, Y.J.; Zhao, S.L.; Wang, L.; Ouyang, Y.Y.; Tang, S.Y. LncRNA SNHG1 promotes EMT process in gastric cancer cells through regulation of the miR-15b/DCLK1/Notch1 axis. *BMC Gastroenterol.* **2020**, *20*, 156. [CrossRef] [PubMed]
57. Liu, W.; Wang, S.; Sun, Q.; Yang, Z.; Liu, M.; Tang, H. DCLK1 promotes epithelial-mesenchymal transition via the PI3K/Akt/NF-κB pathway in colorectal cancer. *Int. J. Cancer* **2018**, *142*, 2068–2079. [CrossRef]
58. Tanabe, S.; Quader, S.; Cabral, H.; Ono, R. Interplay of EMT and CSC in Cancer and the Potential Therapeutic Strategies. *Front. Pharmacol.* **2020**, *11*, 904. [CrossRef]
59. Peixoto, P.; Etcheverry, A.; Aubry, M.; Missey, A.; Lachat, C.; Perrard, J.; Hendrick, E.; Delage-Mourroux, R.; Mosser, J.; Borg, C.; et al. EMT is associated with an epigenetic signature of ECM remodeling genes. *Cell Death Dis.* **2019**, *10*, 205. [CrossRef]
60. Ricciardi, M.; Zanotto, M.; Malpeli, G.; Bassi, G.; Perbellini, O.; Chilosi, M.; Bifari, F.; Krampera, M. Epithelial-to-mesenchymal transition (EMT) induced by inflammatory priming elicits mesenchymal stromal cell-like immune-modulatory properties in cancer cells. *Br. J. Cancer* **2015**, *112*, 1067–1075. [CrossRef]
61. Mariathasan, S.; Turley, S.J.; Nickles, D.; Castiglioni, A.; Yuen, K.; Wang, Y.; Kadel, E.E., III; Koeppen, H.; Astarita, J.L.; Cubas, R.; et al. TGFβ attenuates tumour response to PD-L1 blockade by contributing to exclusion of T cells. *Nature* **2018**, *554*, 544–548. [CrossRef] [PubMed]
62. Lou, Y.; Diao, L.; Cuentas, E.R.; Denning, W.L.; Chen, L.; Fan, Y.H.; Byers, L.A.; Wang, J.; Papadimitrakopoulou, V.A.; Behrens, C.; et al. Epithelial-Mesenchymal Transition Is Associated with a Distinct Tumor Microenvironment Including Elevation of Inflammatory Signals and Multiple Immune Checkpoints in Lung Adenocarcinoma. *Clin. Cancer Res.* **2016**, *22*, 3630–3642. [CrossRef] [PubMed]
63. Fischer, K.R.; Durrans, A.; Lee, S.; Sheng, J.; Li, F.; Wong, S.T.; Choi, H.; El Rayes, T.; Ryu, S.; Troeger, J.; et al. Epithelial-to-mesenchymal transition is not required for lung metastasis but contributes to chemoresistance. *Nature* **2015**, *527*, 472–476. [CrossRef] [PubMed]

64. Sureban, S.M.; May, R.; Mondalek, F.G.; Qu, D.; Ponnurangam, S.; Pantazis, P.; Anant, S.; Ramanujam, R.P.; Houchen, C.W. Nanoparticle-based delivery of siDCAMKL-1 increases microRNA-144 and inhibits colorectal cancer tumor growth via a Notch-1 dependent mechanism. *J. Nanobiotechnol.* **2011**, *9*, 40. [CrossRef] [PubMed]
65. Chen, L.; Gibbons, D.L.; Goswami, S.; Cortez, M.A.; Ahn, Y.H.; Byers, L.A.; Zhang, X.; Yi, X.; Dwyer, D.; Lin, W.; et al. Metastasis is regulated via microRNA-200/ZEB1 axis control of tumour cell PD-L1 expression and intratumoral immunosuppression. *Nat. Commun.* **2014**, *5*, 5241. [CrossRef] [PubMed]
66. Ong, B.A.; Vega, K.J.; Houchen, C.W. Intestinal stem cells and the colorectal cancer microenvironment. *World J. Gastroenterol.* **2014**, *20*, 1898–1909. [CrossRef]
67. Oliveras-Ferraros, C.; Vazquez-Martin, A.; Cuyas, E.; Corominas-Faja, B.; Rodriguez-Gallego, E.; Fernandez-Arroyo, S.; Martin-Castillo, B.; Joven, J.; Menendez, J.A. Acquired resistance to metformin in breast cancer cells triggers transcriptome reprogramming toward a degradome-related metastatic stem-like profile. *Cell Cycle* **2014**, *13*, 1132–1144. [CrossRef]
68. Razi, S.; Sadeghi, A.; Asadi-Lari, Z.; Tam, K.J.; Kalantari, E.; Madjd, Z. DCLK1, a promising colorectal cancer stem cell marker, regulates tumor progression and invasion through miR-137 and miR-15a dependent manner. *Clin. Exp. Med.* **2020**. [CrossRef]
69. Westphalen, C.B.; Takemoto, Y.; Tanaka, T.; Macchini, M.; Jiang, Z.; Renz, B.W.; Chen, X.; Ormanns, S.; Nagar, K.; Tailor, Y.; et al. Dclk1 Defines Quiescent Pancreatic Progenitors that Promote Injury-Induced Regeneration and Tumorigenesis. *Cell Stem Cell* **2016**, *18*, 441–455. [CrossRef]
70. Kato, H.; Tateishi, K.; Fujiwara, H.; Ijichi, H.; Yamamoto, K.; Nakatsuka, T.; Kakiuchi, M.; Sano, M.; Kudo, Y.; Hayakawa, Y.; et al. Deletion of Histone Methyltransferase G9a Suppresses Mutant Kras-driven Pancreatic Carcinogenesis. *Cancer Genom. Proteom.* **2020**, *17*, 695–705. [CrossRef]
71. Qu, D.; Weygant, N.; Yao, J.; Chandrakesan, P.; Berry, W.L.; May, R.; Pitts, K.; Husain, S.; Lightfoot, S.; Li, M.; et al. Overexpression of DCLK1-AL Increases Tumor Cell Invasion, Drug Resistance, and KRAS Activation and Can Be Targeted to Inhibit Tumorigenesis in Pancreatic Cancer. *J. Oncol.* **2019**, *2019*, 6402925. [CrossRef] [PubMed]
72. Liu, Y.; Ferguson, F.M.; Li, L.; Kuljanin, M.; Mills, C.E.; Subramanian, K.; Harshbarger, W.; Gondi, S.; Wang, J.; Sorger, P.K.; et al. Chemical Biology Toolkit for DCLK1 Reveals Connection to RNA Processing. *Cell Chem. Biol.* **2020**, *27*, 1229–1240. [CrossRef] [PubMed]
73. Koizumi, H.; Fujioka, H.; Togashi, K.; Thompson, J.; Yates, J.R., 3rd; Gleeson, J.G.; Emoto, K. DCLK1 phosphorylates the microtubule-associated protein MAP7D1 to promote axon elongation in cortical neurons. *Dev. Neurobiol* **2017**, *77*, 493–510. [CrossRef] [PubMed]
74. Binnewies, M.; Roberts, E.W.; Kersten, K.; Chan, V.; Fearon, D.F.; Merad, M.; Coussens, L.M.; Gabrilovich, D.I.; Ostrand-Rosenberg, S.; Hedrick, C.C.; et al. Understanding the tumor immune microenvironment (TIME) for effective therapy. *Nat. Med.* **2018**, *24*, 541–550. [CrossRef]
75. Bruttel, V.S.; Wischhusen, J. Cancer stem cell immunology: Key to understanding tumorigenesis and tumor immune escape? *Front. Immunol.* **2014**, *5*, 360. [CrossRef]
76. Koh, Y.W.; Han, J.H.; Haam, S. Expression of PD-L1, cancer stem cell and epithelial-mesenchymal transition phenotype in non-small cell lung cancer. *Pathology* **2020**. [CrossRef]
77. Wu, X.; Qu, D.; Weygant, N.; Peng, J.; Houchen, C.W. Cancer Stem Cell Marker DCLK1 Correlates with Tumorigenic Immune Infiltrates in the Colon and Gastric Adenocarcinoma Microenvironments. *Cancers* **2020**, *12*, 274. [CrossRef]
78. Haraguchi, N.; Ishii, H.; Mimori, K.; Tanaka, F.; Ohkuma, M.; Kim, H.M.; Akita, H.; Takiuchi, D.; Hatano, H.; Nagano, H.; et al. CD13 is a therapeutic target in human liver cancer stem cells. *J. Clin. Investig.* **2010**, *120*, 3326–3339. [CrossRef]
79. Li, C.; Du, Y.; Yang, Z.; He, L.; Wang, Y.; Hao, L.; Ding, M.; Yan, R.; Wang, J.; Fan, Z. GALNT1-Mediated Glycosylation and Activation of Sonic Hedgehog Signaling Maintains the Self-Renewal and Tumor-Initiating Capacity of Bladder Cancer Stem Cells. *Cancer Res.* **2016**, *76*, 1273–1283. [CrossRef]
80. Weygant, N.; Qu, D.; Berry, W.L.; May, R.; Chandrakesan, P.; Owen, D.B.; Sureban, S.M.; Ali, N.; Janknecht, R.; Houchen, C.W. Small molecule kinase inhibitor LRRK2-IN-1 demonstrates potent activity against colorectal and pancreatic cancer through inhibition of doublecortin-like kinase 1. *Mol. Cancer* **2014**, *13*, 103. [CrossRef]

81. Nevi, L.; Di Matteo, S.; Carpino, G.; Zizzari, I.; Safarikia, S.; Ambrosino, V.; Costantini, D.; Overi, D.; Giancotti, A.; Monti, M.; et al. DCLK1, a putative novel stem cell marker in human cholangiocarcinoma. *Hepatology* **2020**. [CrossRef] [PubMed]

82. Ragavan, M.; Das, M. Systemic Therapy of Extensive Stage Small Cell Lung Cancer in the Era of Immunotherapy. *Curr. Treat. Options Oncol.* **2020**, *21*, 64. [CrossRef] [PubMed]

83. Dai, T.; Hu, Y.; Lv, F.; Ozawa, T.; Sun, X.; Huang, J.; Han, X.; Kishi, H.; Muraguchi, A.; Jin, A. Analysis of the clinical significance of DCLK1(+) colorectal cancer using novel monoclonal antibodies against DCLK1. *OncoTargets Ther.* **2018**, *11*, 5047–5057. [CrossRef] [PubMed]

84. Szaryńska, M.; Olejniczak, A.; Kobiela, J.; Łaski, D.; Śledziński, Z.; Kmieć, Z. Cancer stem cells as targets for DC-based immunotherapy of colorectal cancer. *Sci. Rep.* **2018**, *8*, 12042. [CrossRef] [PubMed]

85. Kawamura, D.; Takemoto, Y.; Nishimoto, A.; Ueno, K.; Hosoyama, T.; Shirasawa, B.; Tanaka, T.; Kugimiya, N.; Harada, E.; Hamano, K. Enhancement of cytotoxic effects of gemcitabine by Dclk1 inhibition through suppression of Chk1 phosphorylation in human pancreatic cancer cells. *Oncol Rep.* **2017**, *38*, 3238–3244. [CrossRef]

86. Suehiro, Y.; Takemoto, Y.; Nishimoto, A.; Ueno, K.; Shirasawa, B.; Tanaka, T.; Kugimiya, N.; Suga, A.; Harada, E.; Hamano, K. Dclk1 inhibition cancels 5-FU-induced cell-cycle arrest and decreases cell survival in colorectal cancer. *Anticancer Res.* **2018**, *38*, 6225–6230. [CrossRef]

87. Wang, H.; Dai, Y.Y.; Zhang, W.Q.; Hsu, P.C.; Yang, Y.L.; Wang, Y.C.; Chan, G.; Au, A.; Xu, Z.D.; Jiang, S.J.; et al. DCLK1 is correlated with MET and ERK5 expression, and associated with prognosis in malignant pleural mesothelioma. *Int. J. Oncol.* **2017**, *51*, 91–103. [CrossRef]

88. Ferguson, F.M.; Liu, Y.; Harshbarger, W.; Huang, L.; Wang, J.; Deng, X.; Cappuzzi, S.J.; Muratov, E.N.; Tropsha, A.; Muthuswamy, S.; et al. Synthesis and structure-activity relationships of DCLK1 kinase inhibitors based on a 5,11-dihydro-6H-benzo[e]pyrimido[5,4-b][1,4]diazepin-6-one scaffold. *J. Med. Chem.* **2020**, *63*, 7817–7826. [CrossRef]

89. Sureban, S.M.; Madhoun, M.F.; May, R.; Qu, D.; Ali, N.; Fazili, J.; Weygant, N.; Chandrakesan, P.; Ding, K.; Lightfoot, S.A.; et al. Plasma DCLK1 is a marker of hepatocellular carcinoma (HCC): Targeting DCLK1 prevents HCC tumor xenograft growth via a microRNA-dependent mechanism. *Oncotarget* **2015**, *6*, 37200–37215. [CrossRef]

90. Qiao, S.; Zhao, Y.; Geng, S.; Li, Y.; Hou, X.; Liu, Y.; Lin, F.H.; Yao, L.; Tian, W. A novel double-targeted nondrug delivery system for targeting cancer stem cells. *Int. J. Nanomed.* **2016**, *11*, 6667–6678. [CrossRef]

91. Jia, W.; Deshmukh, A.; Mani, S.A.; Jolly, M.K.; Levine, H. A possible role for epigenetic feedback regulation in the dynamics of the epithelial-mesenchymal transition (EMT). *Phys. Biol.* **2019**, *16*, 066004. [CrossRef] [PubMed]

92. Luo, M.; Shang, L.; Brooks, M.D.; Jiagge, E.; Zhu, Y.; Buschhaus, J.M.; Conley, S.; Fath, M.A.; Davis, A.; Gheordunescu, E.; et al. Targeting Breast Cancer Stem Cell State Equilibrium through Modulation of Redox Signaling. *Cell Metab.* **2018**, *28*, 69–86.e66. [CrossRef]

93. Vazquez, F.; Lim, J.H.; Chim, H.; Bhalla, K.; Girnun, G.; Pierce, K.; Clish, C.B.; Granter, S.R.; Widlund, H.R.; Spiegelman, B.M.; et al. PGC1α expression defines a subset of human melanoma tumors with increased mitochondrial capacity and resistance to oxidative stress. *Cancer Cell* **2013**, *23*, 287–301. [CrossRef] [PubMed]

94. Zhang, G.; Frederick, D.T.; Wu, L.; Wei, Z.; Krepler, C.; Srinivasan, S.; Chae, Y.C.; Xu, X.; Choi, H.; Dimwamwa, E.; et al. Targeting mitochondrial biogenesis to overcome drug resistance to MAPK inhibitors. *J. Clin. Investig.* **2016**, *126*, 1834–1856. [CrossRef] [PubMed]

95. Feng, W.; Gentles, A.; Nair, R.V.; Huang, M.; Lin, Y.; Lee, C.Y.; Cai, S.; Scheeren, F.A.; Kuo, A.H.; Diehn, M. Targeting unique metabolic properties of breast tumor initiating cells. *Stem Cells* **2014**, *32*, 1734–1745. [CrossRef] [PubMed]

96. Song, K.; Kwon, H.; Han, C.; Zhang, J.; Dash, S.; Lim, K.; Wu, T. Active glycolytic metabolism in CD133(+) hepatocellular cancer stem cells: Regulation by MIR-122. *Oncotarget* **2015**, *6*, 40822–40835. [CrossRef] [PubMed]

97. Emmink, B.L.; Verheem, A.; Van Houdt, W.J.; Steller, E.J.; Govaert, K.M.; Pham, T.V.; Piersma, S.R.; Borel Rinkes, I.H.; Jimenez, C.R.; Kranenburg, O. The secretome of colon cancer stem cells contains drug-metabolizing enzymes. *J. Proteom.* **2013**, *91*, 84–96. [CrossRef] [PubMed]

98. Liao, J.; Qian, F.; Tchabo, N.; Mhawech-Fauceglia, P.; Beck, A.; Qian, Z.; Wang, X.; Huss, W.J.; Lele, S.B.; Morrison, C.D.; et al. Ovarian cancer spheroid cells with stem cell-like properties contribute to tumor generation, metastasis and chemotherapy resistance through hypoxia-resistant metabolism. *PLoS ONE* **2014**, *9*, e84941. [CrossRef]
99. Zhou, Y.; Zhou, Y.; Shingu, T.; Feng, L.; Chen, Z.; Ogasawara, M.; Keating, M.J.; Kondo, S.; Huang, P. Metabolic alterations in highly tumorigenic glioblastoma cells: Preference for hypoxia and high dependency on glycolysis. *J. Biol. Chem.* **2011**, *286*, 32843–32853. [CrossRef]
100. Viale, A.; Pettazzoni, P.; Lyssiotis, C.A.; Ying, H.; Sánchez, N.; Marchesini, M.; Carugo, A.; Green, T.; Seth, S.; Giuliani, V.; et al. Oncogene ablation-resistant pancreatic cancer cells depend on mitochondrial function. *Nature* **2014**, *514*, 628–632. [CrossRef]
101. Zhao, H.; Duan, Q.; Zhang, Z.; Li, H.; Wu, H.; Shen, Q.; Wang, C.; Yin, T. Up-regulation of glycolysis promotes the stemness and EMT phenotypes in gemcitabine-resistant pancreatic cancer cells. *J. Cell. Mol. Med.* **2017**, *21*, 2055–2067. [CrossRef] [PubMed]
102. Chiche, J.; Brahimi-Horn, M.C.; Pouysségur, J. Tumour hypoxia induces a metabolic shift causing acidosis: A common feature in cancer. *J. Cell. Mol. Med.* **2010**, *14*, 771–794. [CrossRef] [PubMed]
103. Dzobo, K.; Senthebane, D.A.; Ganz, C.; Thomford, N.E.; Wonkam, A.; Dandara, C. Advances in Therapeutic Targeting of Cancer Stem Cells within the Tumor Microenvironment: An Updated Review. *Cells* **2020**, *9*, 1896. [CrossRef] [PubMed]
104. Lee, Y.; Shin, J.H.; Longmire, M.; Wang, H.; Kohrt, H.E.; Chang, H.Y.; Sunwoo, J.B. CD44+ Cells in Head and Neck Squamous Cell Carcinoma Suppress T-Cell-Mediated Immunity by Selective Constitutive and Inducible Expression of PD-L1. *Clinical Cancer Res.* **2016**, *22*, 3571–3581. [CrossRef] [PubMed]

Publisher's Note: MDPI stays neutral with regard to jurisdictional claims in published maps and institutional affiliations.

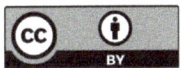

© 2020 by the authors. Licensee MDPI, Basel, Switzerland. This article is an open access article distributed under the terms and conditions of the Creative Commons Attribution (CC BY) license (http://creativecommons.org/licenses/by/4.0/).

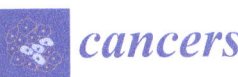

Review

Engineering Metabolism of Chimeric Antigen Receptor (CAR) Cells for Developing Efficient Immunotherapies

Joslyn L. Mangal [1], Jamie L. Handlos [2], Arezoo Esrafili [2], Sahil Inamdar [2], Sidnee Mcmillian [2], Mamta Wankhede [2], Riccardo Gottardi [3,4] and Abhinav P. Acharya [1,2,5,6,*]

1. Biological Design Graduate Program, School for Biological and Health Systems Engineering, Arizona State University, Tempe, AZ 85281, USA; jmangal@asu.edu
2. Department of Chemical Engineering, School for the Engineering of Matter, Transport, and Energy, Arizona State University, Tempe, AZ 85281, USA; jhandlos@asu.edu (J.L.H.); aesrafil@asu.edu (A.E.); sahil.inamdar@asu.edu (S.I.); smcmill4@asu.edu (S.M.); mamta.wankhede@asu.edu (M.W.)
3. Department of Pediatrics, Division of Pulmonary Medicine, Perelman School of Medicine, University of Pennsylvania, Philadelphia, PA 19104, USA; GOTTARDIR@email.chop.edu
4. Fondazione Ri.MED, 90133 Palermo, Italy
5. Department of Materials Science and Engineering, School for the Engineering of Matter, Transport, and Energy, Arizona State University, Tempe, AZ 85281, USA
6. Biodesign Center for Immunotherapy, Vaccines and Virotherapy, Tempe, AZ 85281, USA
* Correspondence: abhi.acharya@asu.edu

Simple Summary: This review paper here describes the recent progress that has been made in chimeric antigen receptor (CAR) -based therapies for treatment of tumors and the role of metabolism in the tumor microenvironment in relation to these therapies. Moreover, this manuscript also discusses role of different CAR-based cells for treatment of solid tumors, which is a major challenge in the CAR immunotherapy field.

Abstract: Chimeric antigen receptor (CAR) T cell-based therapies have shown tremendous advancement in clinical and pre-clinical studies for the treatment of hematological malignancies, such as the refractory of pre-B cell acute lymphoblastic leukemia (B-ALL), chronic lymphocytic leukemia (CLL), and large B cell lymphoma (LBCL). However, CAR T cell therapy for solid tumors has not been successful clinically. Although, some research efforts, such as combining CARs with immune checkpoint inhibitor-based therapy, have been used to expand the application of CAR T cells for the treatment of solid tumors. Importantly, further understanding of the coordination of nutrient and energy supplies needed for CAR T cell expansion and function, especially in the tumor microenvironment (TME), is greatly needed. In addition to CAR T cells, there is great interest in utilizing other types of CAR immune cells, such as CAR NK and CAR macrophages that can infiltrate solid tumors. However, the metabolic competition in the TME between cancer cells and immune cells remains a challenge. Bioengineering technologies, such as metabolic engineering, can make a substantial contribution when developing CAR cells to have an ability to overcome nutrient-paucity in the solid TME. This review introduces technologies that have been used to generate metabolically fit CAR-immune cells as a treatment for hematological malignancies and solid tumors, and briefly discusses the challenges to treat solid tumors with CAR-immune cells.

Keywords: CAR macrophage; CAR T cell; immunotherapy; solid tumors; immunometabolism; tumor microenvironment

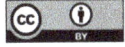

1. Introduction

Adoptive cell transfer (ACT) strategies including tumor-infiltration lymphocytes (TILs), T cell receptor (TCR) engineered T cells, and CAR T cells have been highly efficacious cancer immunotherapies in clinic. CAR T cells are a type of cell-based therapy where autologous T lymphocytes are genetically engineered to express the binding site of specific antibodies for the ability to target tumor-associated antigens (TAAs) [1]. There have been three generations of CAR T cells to date. In the first generation of CARs, the T-cell signaling domain was fused with an intracellular portion of a TCR CD3ζ subunit [2]. However, their poor performance in vivo, due to lack of co-stimulation, led to the development of second-generation CAR T cells where two types of T-cell signaling domains, a co-stimulatory domain, either CD28 or 4-1BB, and a T-cell activation domain were incorporated into the construct. Both of these generations expressed a single chain variable fragment (scFv) against CD19, which is expressed at a high-level on B cell malignancies. However, the second generation of CARs was more efficacious in showing antitumor effects in patients. The later generation of CAR T cells incorporated two co-stimulatory domains derived from different co-stimulatory domains [2], for purposes of enhancing the activation and proliferation of these cells upon interaction with their target antigen [3]. There have been more than 370 clinical trials on CAR T cells to date worldwide (clinicaltrials.gov, accessed on 29 June 2020) [4] and, although there are risks associated with CAR T cells, such as neurotoxicity and cytokine release syndrome (CRS), CAR T cells are the first case of cellular gene therapy to be commercially approved by the U.S. FDA. Figure 1 shows the general methodology of generating CAR expressing cells. Specifically, as the first step, leukocytes are extracted from the patient's blood or donor's body, and T cells are purified. Next, these T cells are genetically modified to express CAR using lentivirus (Kymriah™) or retrovirus (Yescarta™). After T cells are differentiated into their CD4 or CD8 T cells subsets, activation of the T cells is needed. $CD8^+$ T cells can be activated with cytokines, such as IL-2 [5]. Interestingly, in addition to activation and proliferation of CAR $CD8^+$ T cells, IL-2 has also been used clinically as a monotherapy to induce cancer regression in patients [6]. Importantly, the CARs are encoded with viral vectors, which integrate into the genome of the patient T cells, thus allowing them to bind directly to TAA, such as CD19, independent of HLA. However, the efficacy of CAR-T cell therapy is challenged by the nutrient depleted and immunosuppressive TME ensued by tumor cells. The high metabolic demand required for tumor cell proliferation and metastasis, as well as the increased ability for tumor cells to internalize nutrients, leaves the TME nutrient depleted [7,8]. Thereby starving effector T cells and preventing their anti-tumor cytotoxic effects [8]. This increased uptake of nutrients by tumor cells can lead to an increased accumulation of metabolic by-products, such as lactic acid and CO_2, in the TME which in turn has been found to prevent effector T cell activity [9,10]. Additionally, tumor cells can evade the immune system via immunosuppressive mediators, such as immunosuppressive enzyme (Indoleamine-2,3-dioxygenase (IDO) or arginase) [6,11] or cytokine (Interleukin 10 (IL-10) or Transforming growth factor beta (TGFβ) [12,13] production for the induction of T cell suppression or tolerance. This here demonstrates the need to engineer highly resilient and metabolically fit CAR-T cells with capabilities of enduring the nutrient depleted and immunosuppressive TME.

In addition to CAR-T cells, bioengineering technologies have enabled great progress in developing other immune cell types such as CAR-NK cells, CAR-macrophages (CAR-M), and CAR-γδ T cells, which can provide effective responses in persistent solid tumors [14,15]. The following sections will discuss several bioengineering strategies that have led to the development of effective CAR T cell therapies, as well as the metabolic demand of anti-tumor CAR immune cells and an introduction to different types of non-T cell-based CAR therapies.

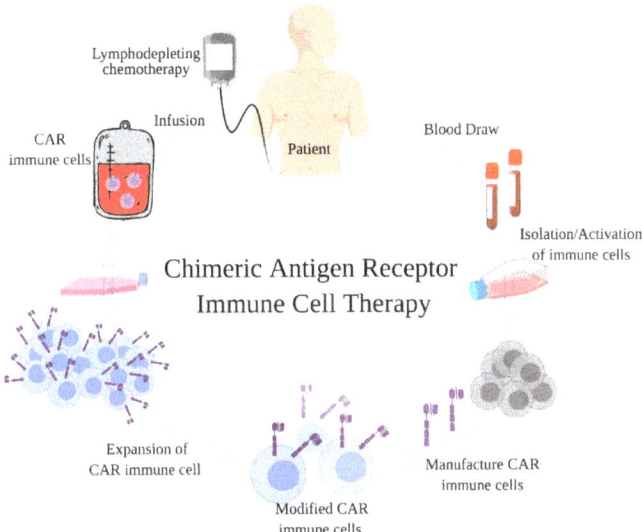

Figure 1. Treatment of patients with CAR immune cells. In the first step, immune cells are isolated from the patient's blood by leukapheresis. These autologous immune cells are then manufactured off-site and genetically modified to target and kill antigen carrying cancer cells. The treatment is initiated by intravenous infusion of CAR immune cells into the patient.

2. Challenges of CAR T Cell Therapy

Although, CAR T cells provide tremendous advantages in killing cancer cells, they also have drawbacks and mechanisms of resistance related to off-targeting effects and antigen loss of cancer cells. Antigen loss in certain cancers is likely contributed to antigen escape or lineage switch [16]. Antigen escape, which is occurs when there is a loss or downregulation of the target antigen, may take place when a patient relapses with a phenotypically similar cancer but lacks the expression of the previously targeted antigen [17]. For example, CAR T therapy can successfully kill one type of cancerous cell, but the patient may relapse if the tumor reforms with a different population of cancerous cells [18,19]. Monitoring CAR T cell efficacy for antigen loss may be essential for relapse prediction and prevention. In contrast, lineage switch can occur when a patient develops a genetically similar tumor with differences in phenotypic expressions [17].

In addition to antigen escape and lineage switch, unforeseen toxicities are another common limitation associated with CAR T cell therapies. The toxicity associated with T cell therapies may be related to incorrect dosages, off targeting effects, and incorrect timing of T cell activity. Specifically, CAR T cells can target healthy B cells in non-tumor tissues, and this can lead to "on-target, off-tumor" toxic responses. Additional mechanisms of resistance to CAR T cell therapy is the inability to harvest enough autologous T cells for CAR engineering, the inability to generate effective CAR technologies from patients who have previously been exposed to chemotherapy, and the inherent tumor heterogeneity being an obstacle in recognizing the most optimal target [20–22] Therefore, in order to overcome the drawbacks of CAR T cell therapies, further research needs to be done to identify multiple tumor-specific antigens, signaling domains, and optimizing and development of safe, reliable CARs, based on the specific type of tumor.

Notably, some of these challenges have been addressed pre-clinically using recent strategies of suicide genes, inhibitory CAR, dual-antigen receptors, or the use of exogenous molecules to help control CAR T cell function [23]. The implementation of these strategies have led to the development of more effective CAR T cell therapies [23]. Despite the deficiencies associated with CAR T cells, studies have clearly shown that CAR-based T-cell therapies can control tumor progression in patients that do not respond to conventional treatments [24,25].

Furthermore, three additional important parameters that should be considered when engineering CAR in T cells include (i) identifying the most relevant T cell subset to induce the most robust antitumor response, (ii) finding the best ex vivo T cell processing procedure to ensure that the most fit T cells are generated, and (iii) determining whether or not additional T cell engineering is required for the most optimal in vivo performance [26]. Each of these aspects require additional study for the further development of effective CAR cells that have a higher capability in targeting and killing cancerous cells within heterogeneous tumor complexes. Moreover, additional research on the manufacturing process of CAR cells can also decrease costs and increase the number of centers that specialize in engineering CAR constructs.

3. CAR T Cell Immunotherapy for Solid Tumors

Despite extensive efforts in pre-clinical studies, CAR T cell therapy has not been successful in treating solid tumors in clinic. There are several limitations to current CAR T cell technologies that need to be addressed in order to have a more efficacious construct when treating solid tumors. Namely, one of the limitations being the physical nature of solid tumors itself. The solid feature of the tumor creates a physical barrier, in turn preventing CAR T cells from successfully infiltrating the tumor. Consequently, this affects the CAR T cells' ability to locate the ideal target antigen as compared to hematological diffused tumors [27]. Moreover, as observed in human tumor cultures, in order to access tumor sites and exert antitumor effects, CAR T cells must be able to degrade heparan sulphate proteoglycans (HSPGs) by releasing specific enzymes, such as heparanase (HPSE) in the TME to reach their target [28,29]. Notably, in solid tumors, chemokine-receptor mismatch, cancer associated fibroblasts (CAFs), physical barriers represented by the extracellular matrix (ECM) and stroma, and abnormal vasculature at tumor sites are also some of the limitations to CAR T cell infiltration [27]. In contrast to hematological cancers, where CAR T cells can circulate the bloodstream to eventually reach the targeted cancer cells without having to overcome physical barriers. Additionally, solid tumors promote infiltrating myeloid cells to produce immunosuppressive signals and molecules within the TME for the inhibition of T effector cell infiltration and activity [30]. Interestingly, a strategy of photothermal therapy has been shown to promote direct tumor cell killing, partial disruption of the ECM, and enhanced tumor infiltration and activation of CAR T cells in mice bearing human melanoma tumors [31]. Additionally, clinical studies have shown that CAR T cell infiltration within solid tumors can be enhanced when targeting a tissue-specific antigen, such as prostate-specific membrane antigen (PSMA), which can be found on malignant prostate cells [32]. However, the selective targeting of conventional CAR T cells is reliant on identifying specific TAAs of interest. Therefore, universal CAR-T cells have become a popular area of study and can promote the selective targeting of various antigens without prior TAA identification. For instance, given that CD16-CAR T cells are capable of identifying the FC-region of monoclonal antibodies, the combinatorial delivery of CD16-CAR T cells and monoclonal antibodies can promote the selective targeting of multiple antigens, and in turn avert the antigen loss, downregulation or mutation limitation that is associated with conventional CAR cell therapy [33–36].

In addition to trafficking and infiltration, multiple challenges in the hostile solid TME can affect the efficacy and function of CAR T cells. For example, nutritional depletion, acidic pH, oxidative stress, and hypoxia that are rendered by the metabolism of tumor cells, can also inhibit CAR T cell function [32,37]. Something that is also important to note when generating effective CAR T cells is to consider the reduction in memory and effector T cell activity in the TME due to (1) the clonal deletion of self/tumor-specific T cells leads to a decreased number in tumor-specific TCRs, (2) poor activation of innate immune cells and antigen-presenting cells (APCs) in the TME, and (3) formation of an overall immunosuppressive TME [38]. Interestingly, these challenges have inspired the development in CAR T cell-based treatments that partially overcome each of these three obstacles. However, the efficacy of CAR T cell therapy is influenced by multiple challenges generated by stromal cells, such as cancer associated fibroblast, and suppressive immune cells, tumor associated macrophages, tumor associated neutrophils, and Tregs. Other factors, such as immunosuppressive cells, the presence of inhibitory soluble factors, and cytokines are also responsible for hindering the ability of CAR T cells to target the solid tumors effectively.

The following sections discuss a few of these issues that are involved in reducing the efficiency of CAR T cells within solid tumors and the TME, as well as how metabolism plays a role in CAR T cell efficacy.

3.1. Impact of TME on T Cell Metabolism

Over the past few decades, the role of immune cell metabolism is being recognized as a major hurdle in limiting the function and efficacy of antitumor T cells for cancer therapy. The metabolic pathways within immune cells, in particular T cells, is known to control T cell activation, proliferation, differentiation, migration and function [39]. Therefore, recent efforts identifying that metabolites within the TME can alter T cell function is vital information for the future development of more stable and effective CAR technologies [40]. Additionally, hypoxia associated with the TME in solid tumors is one of the challenges that has been shown to decrease T-bet expression in TILs and reduce lymphocyte's activation [41], and generation of high level of reactive oxygen species (ROS) by tumor cells can cause oxidative stress in mouse melanoma models. Therefore, such a TME can inhibit T cell immune responses, such as activation, proliferation, differentiation and apoptosis [42]. Interestingly, engineered CAR T cells have been generated to secrete an antioxidant enzyme, catalase (CAT), to reduce hydrogen peroxide to water and oxygen. Thus, these CAT-CAR T cells can maintain their anti-tumor function and were shown to have a reduced oxidative state with decreased levels in ROS accumulation in solid human tumor samples [32]. Moreover, since the metabolism of memory T cells relies on oxygen, hypoxic conditions are a major challenge for these cell types in the TME. Additionally, low oxygen concentrations can limit oxidative phosphorylation [27]. Studies have shown that increased levels of hypoxia can lead to an upregulation of PD-L1 and HIF-1a in myeloid-derived suppressor cells (MDSCs) to ultimately lead to T cell exhaustion and Treg generation [43].

Therefore, understanding the metabolic transition of T cells in the TME, and a change in the cellular metabolic reprogramming of cancer cells due to oncogenic mutations can lead to a better understanding of the issues related to the metabolic state in TME [44]. Glycolysis plays a crucial role in the differentiation and expansion of effector T cells. Upon encountering an antigen (such as lymphoma specific CD20) T cells undergo changes in their metabolic activity for their differentiation into effector cell subsets. Indeed, naïve T cells rely on oxidative phosphorylation (OXPHOS) and fatty acid oxidation (FAO) to meet energy demands. However, activated effector T cells rely on aerobic glycolysis to facilitate faster proliferation [44–46]. On the other hand, glycolysis is also a preferred metabolic program of cancer cells. An increased reliance on glycolysis over OXPHOS, known as Warburg effect, generates energy in the form of adenosine triphosphate (ATP) and lactate [44], under hypoxic conditions during the early avascular phase of tumor development [47]. Therefore, glucose availability in the TME is decreased due to the increased uptake by tumor cells, in turn, leading to lowered AKT and mTOR signaling in T cells, which are vital for a greater reliance on anabolic metabolism of T cells and their function. This then leads to a downregulation of glucose transporter (Glut1) and prevention of effector T cell activation and function [27,46]. Consequently, this process further diminishes an effector T cells ability to have an increased reliance on glycolytic metabolism. More recently, it has been shown that a reduction in glucose availability leads to a decrease of phosphoenolpyruvate, a glycolysis metabolite, which is necessary to sustain TCR signaling and antitumor T-cell effector activity [48]. Glucose deprivation can also lead to an increased expression of programmed cell death protein 1 (PD-1) on

T cells [49], however the inhibition of programmed cell death ligand 1 (PD-L1) on solid tumor cells, to prevent tumor-mediated T cell death, can drive tumor cells to rely more on OXPHOS. This in vivo data, within a sarcoma mouse model, suggested that this increased tumor reliance on OXPHOS may lead to an increase in glucose availability in the TME for effector T cell function and survival [49,50].

Interestingly, lactate, as a major byproduct of aerobic glycolysis is generated in large amounts in the TME and can hinder cytotoxic T lymphocyte activity and disturb T-cell metabolism [30,45,51]. Increased extracellular levels of lactate has shown to decrease the intracellular pH of T cells and inhibit T cell glycolysis, via direct inhibition of hexokinase 2 (HK) and 6-phosphofructo-2-kinase (PFK) [52,53]. Blocking acidification prior to anti-PD-1 or anti-CTLA-4 may lead to efficient anti-tumor responses [52]. Generation of lactate, and factors like vascular endothelial growth factor (VEGF), IDO, Prostaglandin E_2 (PGE2), and adenosine are active players that contribute to the suppression of T cell immune responses within the TME. Moreover, low level of amino acids such as cysteine, arginine, tryptophan, and lysine within the TME can cause malfunctions in protein translation or can induce autophagy responses in effector T cells as well [37,54]. Low levels of arginine can alter T cell responsiveness due to the decreased expression of the CD3ζ chain. However, providing T cells with arginine has demonstrated an increase in pro-inflammatory cytokine production and an increase antitumor T cell responses in vitro [55,56]. Therefore, supplementing CAR-T cells with amino acids, such as cysteine or arginine, may lead to an increase in antitumor CAR T cell activity.

Notably, metabolic adaptation of cancer cells extends beyond ATP production. For example, cellular metabolism of several tumors can be modified by loss of tumor suppressors, such as P53, or activation of oncoproteins, such as phosphoinositide 3-kinase (PI3K). In fact, balance between energy production and macromolecular biosynthesis and redox status are key requirements of metabolic adaptation of tumor cells [44,47]. These factors lead to the immunosuppressive TME and low immunogenicity of cancer cells, which are ultimately responsible for restricting the therapeutic efficacy of CAR T cells in solid tumors. Thus, TME metabolism and immunometabolism is an active area of research to substantially improve clinical outcomes of CAR T immunotherapy for treating solid tumors. For example, to improve cell-based cancer immunotherapy, research has been performed on immune cell metabolism (e.g., T cells, dendritic cells, [57] macrophages) to understand how it is affected by the TME, and how it can be manipulated specifically in adoptive transfer therapies like CAR T immunotherapy [58–61].

Interestingly, studies suggest that cancer cells outcompete T cells for glucose in vivo in cancerous mouse models, therefore preventing the cytokine production that is required for T cells to mount a cellular response against the tumor (Figure 2A) [50,62]. Although further studies are required to understand if this phenomenon is also consistent in human studies. However, it is observed that checkpoint inhibitor therapies (e.g., anti-CTLA-4) combined with other therapies are effective, and it is known that these checkpoint inhibitors accelerate glycolysis in TILs [63,64]. Therefore, this suggests that the ineffectiveness of antitumor T cells may be due to them being deprived of glucose in the TME. Notably, metabolic pathways diverge and converge at many different levels, and therefore, cells have to choose the most optimal path to achieve their metabolic goals to further determine their fate and function [65]. Overall, different metabolic pathway choices affect the function and fate of immune cells. Thus, metabolic commitment to a pathway is influenced by both signaling pathways and substrate availability in the microenvironment. These concepts have been applied to CAR T cell therapies for making these cells more effective in killing cancer cells in the solid TME (Figure 2B). For instance, inhibition of IDO because of increased tryptophan has shown promise for greater success in cancer treatment [66]. Similarly, checkpoint blockade therapy (anti-PD-1, anti-PD-L1, anti-CTLA-4) corrects nutrient restriction experienced by T cells in a progressing tumor by upregulating CD28 mediated glycolysis (Figure 2C) [50]. These elegant studies clearly demonstrate that metabolic regulation affects both the function of T cells and their response to low nutrient microenvironments [67].

These data also suggest that T cell function and cellular metabolism can be modified to treat different types of tumors in vivo [68]. Table 1 demonstrates how the TME modulates immunometabolism and potential strategies to overcome the induced metabolic impairments.

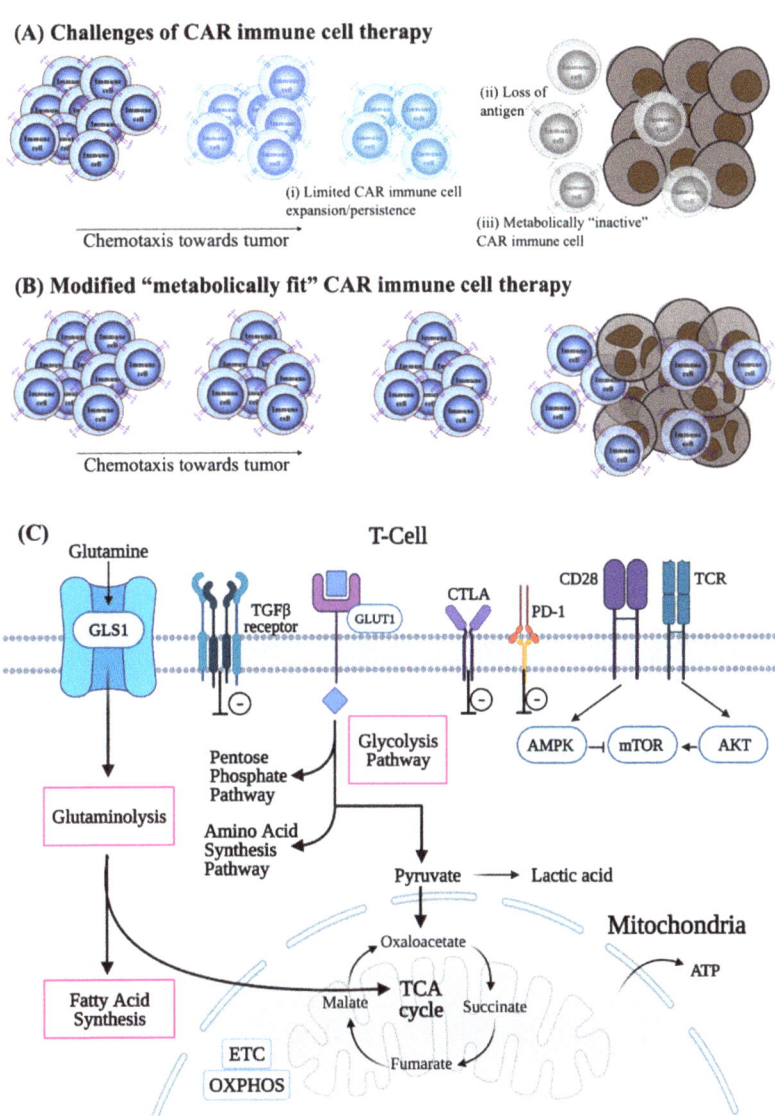

Figure 2. Metabolically fit chimeric antigen receptor (CAR) cells need to be generated for effective CAR immunotherapy. (A) When CAR immune cells reach their target, due to the paucity of nutrients, these cells can become exhausted. This prevents the CAR immune cells from functioning and allows for tumor growth. (B) Metabolically fit CAR immune cells can be generated by modifying the metabolic pathways that endow these immune cells to out-compete cancer cells for nutrients and thus remain active even in the TME for the eradication of cancer cells. (C) Metabolic pathways that are disrupted and can be modified to generate metabolically fit CAR-immune cells.

Table 1. Summary of TME mediated modulation of immunometabolism.

TME Factors Affecting Immune Cell Metabolism	Direct and Indirect Metabolic Impairment of Immune Cells in TME	Strategy to Overcome Induced Metabolic Impairment	References
Increased hypoxia	Increases HIF1-α and PD-L1 on MDSCs for T cell exhaustion and Treg generation	Anti-PD-L1 and HIF inhibitors	[43,69,70]
Increased reactive oxygen species	Oxidative stress-mediated inhibition of NF-kB or mTOR for the prevention of T cell activation	Catalase, an antioxidant enzyme	[32,42]
Decreased glucose availability	Reduced AKT, mTOR, GLUT1, phosphoenolpyruvate, and increased PD-1 expression in T cells	anti-PD-1, anti-PD-L1, anti-CTLA-4	[27,46,48–50]
Increased lactate	Inhibition of T cell glycolysis and function	Blocking acidification prior to anti-PD-1 or anti-CTLA-4 administration	[52]
Low levels of arginine	Reduced responsiveness of T cells due to decreased expression of CD3ζ chain	Administering arginine	[55,56]

Nonetheless, the strategic selection of which co-stimulatory molecule is expressed by a CAR T construct can influence CAR T cell function and fate within the challenging TME. Several examples of T cell co-stimulatory molecules are CD28, ICOS (inducible T cell co-stimulator (CD278)), 4-1BB (CD137), OX40 (CD134), and CD27. The expression of a 4-1BB domain by a CAR T construct has previously demonstrated the induction of CD8+ central memory T cells with increased respiratory capacity and heightened mitochondrial biogenesis. In contrast, the incorporation of a CD28 domain has shown to stimulate effector memory T cell phenotypes with a gene signature signifying glycolytic metabolism [71,72]. Notably, a sustained activation, proliferation, and effector function in resting T cells, via the activation of NFκB, has been observed when combining a CD28 and OX40 domain to a CD3 ζ chain (CD28-OX40-CD3ζ) [73]. Nonetheless, ICOS can activate the PI3K-AKT signaling more effectively than CD28, which may elucidate a mechanism behind the increased T cell persistence within ICOS-based CAR T cells [74]. Furthermore, the incorporation of the CD27 domain, as a CAR co-stimulatory molecule, has exhibited a decrease in apoptotic pathways with an upregulation of B-cell lymphoma-extra large (BCL-(X) L), which is known to modulate metabolic functions of mitochondrial multiprotein complexes [71,75]. Therefore, the incorporation or combination of various intracellular signaling domains can alter the outcome of the CAR construct within the TME.

Among different approaches, one of the most promising approaches to modifying the TME in solid and hematological malignancies may be the combined delivery of CAR T therapies with existing protein therapies for an improvement of CAR T cell function. An example of such as approach is the constitutive expression of IL-12 by CAR T cells for an increased ability to eliminate cancer cells more effectively, which in turn leads to overcoming the immunosuppressive TME [76]. Therefore, generation modified CAR T cell immunotherapy, based on combinatorial engineering and treatments to reprogram T cell properties and the TME, can be unprecedented hope of therapeutic interventions for solid and hematological tumors.

3.2. Metabolic Engineering of CAR Cells

Metabolic engineering of CAR cells has a great potential to develop highly potent CAR T cells. For example, gene engineering approaches, such as overexpression of intercellular metabolic enzymes, [30] can improve CAR T cell activity in solid tumors. Overexpression of PPAR-gamma coactivator 1-α (PGC1-α), which programs mitochondrial biogenesis is one approach to potentially engineering the metabolism of CAR T cells. A defect in PPAR-gamma coactivator 1-α, due to chronic protein kinase B (Akt) signaling inhibiting Foxo transcription factor activity and consequent PGC1-α repression, can lead to loss of mitochondrial function in tumor-reactive T cells in the TME. Therefore, PGC1-α overexpressing T cells significantly increases mitochondrial mass, resulting in greater metabolic efficiency of T cells in the TME [77]. However, studies have not yet implemented this approach in CAR T cell therapies, indicating that further studies are required. Interestingly, another study showed that co-inhibitory factor gene editing, such as the combination of PD-1 blockade in CAR T cells [78] can also enhance CAR T cell function. Specifically, cancer cells often upregulate ligands, such as PD-L1, that bind to inhibitory receptors on T cells and limit the capacity of CAR T cells to combat solid tumors. Using clustered regularly interspaced short palindromic repeats (CRISPR)/Cas9 system to knockout PD-1 has been shown to augment the function of CAR T cells in vitro and in vivo. Indeed, CRISPR/Cas9 system can disrupt PD-1 gene locus in human primary T cells, which leads to reduction of PD-1^{HI} population. Notably, this reduction does not have a significant effect on CAR T cell proliferation. Besides the boosting of CAR T cell cytokine production, a combination of CAR T cells with CRISPR/Cas9-mediated PD-1 genome can enhance the ability of CAR T cells to recognize antigens and target antigen-expressing tumors [78]. Furthermore, the inhibition of PD-1 in T cells, is shown to lead to metabolic changes where T cells transition from glycolysis toward the Krebs cycle with an increased rate of FAO. This alteration in T cell metabolism using PD-1 inhibitors demonstrated an increase in T cell survival, function, and terminal differentiation by relying on a fat-based metabolism and in turn mimicking functions similar to memory T cells. PD-1 ligation has also been shown to enhance the PPAR/PPARγ PGC1-α axis when administering bezafibrate (a pan-PPAR agonist) for the prevention of T cell death and for the initiation of a long-lived T cell phenotype under PD-1 blockade [79–81]. Therefore, utilizing PD-1 therapies in conjunction with CAR T cell therapies may be a feasible approach to altering the metabolic profile of T cells as a strategy to maintain CAR T cell function in a nutrient depleted environment.

Adoptive cell therapy, such as TIL therapy, has also shown success and is a current clinical approach to treating cancer. In comparison to CAR-T cell therapy where circulating T cells from the blood are extracted and engineered to bind to specific proteins expressed by cancer cells, TILs are found and extracted from the tumor. TILs that recognize the tumor cells are then expanded and infused back into the patient. Although TIL therapy does not require engineering of T cells, TIL therapy is a more invasive approach and requires identifying TIL-rich tumor samples which may not exist or may be challenging to acquire [82]. Additionally, TILs have dysregulated metabolism due to the nature of the TME, which has shown to increase exhaustion and deplete effector T cell function [83]. Therefore, acquiring metabolically stable T cells from the periphery for CAR therapy may be an advantage in comparison to expanding metabolically dysregulated TILs for the treatment of cancer.

4. Other Potent CAR Immune Cells

The idea of generating metabolically fit immune cells can also be extended to other CAR immune cells such as NK cells, macrophages, and dendritic cells [84–88]. In fact, recent research is beginning to explore specific metabolic enzymes in these immune cell types, which can be manipulated to make these cells more metabolically fit. The metabolic reprogramming of macrophages and dendritic cells [89] has led to the discovery of metabolic processes, such as glycolysis, the Krebs cycle, and fatty acid metabolism, having significant effects on their cellular function [90]. For example, macrophages undergo metabolic reprogramming in response to environmental cues, danger signals, and cytokines. Macrophage function is also affected by certain metabolites such as succinate and citrate [90]. Overall, the immune system can regulate metabolic pathways to change cell function and fate, thus modulating these pathways in immune cells could generate a metabolically fit CAR-based immunotherapy.

4.1. NK Cell CAR Therapies

CAR NK cells have shown promising results for tumor suppression in pre-clinical testing. Successful pre-clinical tests of anti-CD19 CAR T cell therapy and remission of B cell malignancies has led to further investigations in CAR NK cells and its clinical applications (Figure 3) [87]. The inspiration for generating anti-CD19 CAR NK cells was to overcome the complexity in manufacturing CAR T cells and circumvent their associated toxicities [91]. About 73% of CD19-positive lymphoid tumor patients, who were treated with CAR NK therapy responded to treatment and approximately 88% of those patients had reached complete remission [91]. Additionally, patients had shown a response to the treatment within 30 days of the infusion, regardless of the dosage. Furthermore, CAR NK cells were active for at least 12 months in patients who received low doses [91]. CAR NK cells have also shown success in targeting solid tumors expressing antigens such as HER2, PSMA, mesothelin, ROBO1, or MUC1[92]. Importantly, a majority of the patients receiving CAR NK therapy had a positive response to the treatment, and CAR NK cells were not associated with any toxicity such as cytokine release syndrome, neurotoxicity, or graft-versus-host disease. Therefore, CAR NK cell immunotherapy presents an allogenic therapy that can be readily available for instant use [93,94]. Moreover, CAR NK cells are able to exert anti-tumor effects in addition to the CAR function since they also obtain their native receptors, therefore averting any relapse or resistance associated with antigen loss and CAR therapy [93,95,96]. Additionally, unlike CAR T cells, CAR NK cells can target tumor cells without the requirement of specific TAA recognition and despite the down-regulation of MHC class I on tumor cells [94,97]. This demonstrates the potential of CAR NK cells as universal CAR cells [93,98].

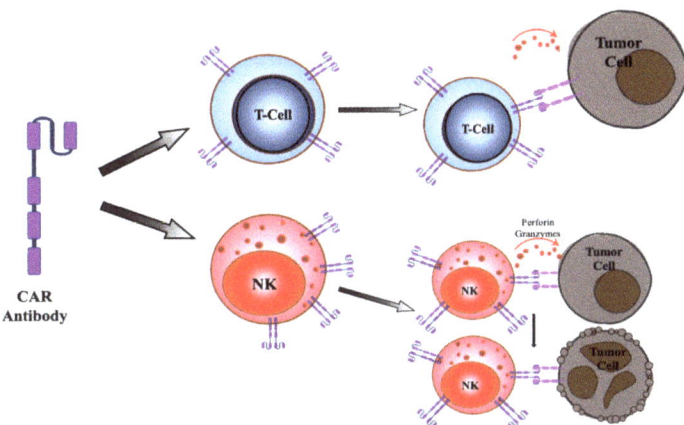

Figure 3. Targeting of tumor cells by T cells and NK cells. T cells and Natural Killer (NK) cells expressing a chimeric antigen receptor (CAR) recognize the antigens present on the tumor cells, bind them and release perforin and granzymes to directly initiate tumor cell death.

Although NK cells are effective phagocytic lymphocytes with high tumor suppressing activity, NK cells are functionally exhausted in the TME [99]. This is likely due to the nutrient and oxygen deprived TME that also consists of high levels of metabolic by-products, such as lactic acid. A reduction in IL-2-induced mitochondrial metabolism, such as OXPHOS and maximal respiration has been observed in human NK cells within the TME [100]. Nonetheless, the hypoxic environment can be used as an advantage when constructing NK cells. Juillerat et al. demonstrated that the incorporation of the oxygen-sensitive domain, HIF-1a, can generate a construct where the expression of CAR is reliant on low oxygen concentrations [101,102]. Additionally, CRISPR/Cas9 can be utilized to alter pathways that are involved in NK exhaustion or function [103]. For instance, CRISPR/Cas9 can successfully express the NKG2D ligand, major histocompatibility complex class I polypeptide-related sequence A (MICA), which may promote NK-mediated anti-tumor effects [104]. It is also important to note that tumor cells in the TME evade NK cell function via TGF-b, metabolic disturbances, and checkpoints among many other immunosuppressive mechanisms [96]. However, NK cells with a chimeric receptor consisting of the activating receptor, NKG2D, along with the cytotoxic ζ-chain of a TCR can overcome the immunosuppressive TME while promoting inflammatory responses within the TME [97,105]. Furthermore, transduction of NK cells with activating cytokines, such as IL-2, IL-12, IL-15, IL-18, and IL-21, can promote the proliferation and function of NK cells [106]. For example, NK cells co-expressing CAR and IL-15 were more potent than unmodified NK cells with and had shown to increase proliferative rates and selective cell-killing activity in breast carcinoma [107]. Furthermore, CAR NK persistence and function can be achieved when engineering memory-like NK cells with CAR [108].

Although CAR NKs have shown some success in recent clinical trials, there are still challenges associated with this treatment option. For example, CAR NK cells have low ex vivo expansion as well as low transduction efficiency and lifespan, which limits their use and warrants further research [94,109]. However, electroporation pulse codes and buffer optimization for protein uptake can improve NK transduction rates [103]. Nonetheless, CAR NK cells may have several advantages over CAR T cells including safer clinical uses, more advanced mechanisms of cancer cell recognition, and an increased abundance of NK cells in clinical samples for the generation of CAR NK cells [109].

4.2. CAR Macrophages

Due to the success of CAR T cell and CAR NK cell therapies in the clinic, further research has been carried out to engineer other potent CAR immune cells in pre-clinical animal models. Among those, a promising cell type, that is gaining traction in CAR-based immunotherapy, is CAR macrophages. Engineering CAR macrophages is a relatively new avenue for CAR research which attempts to overcome some of the previously mentioned limitations associated with CAR T therapies.

Macrophages are known to naturally traffic into solid tumors and may result in a targeted cancer cell treatment that leaves healthy cells unaffected. Interestingly, a family of engineered chimeric antigen receptors for phagocytosis (CAR-Ps) has recently been generated and might direct macrophages towards the desired cancerous cells targets [88]. CAR-P macrophages have shown specificity toward targets as they have been shown to recognize and attack beads coated with the CD19 protein [88]. Furthermore, CAR-P macrophages have been able to phagocytose cancer cells and debris in vitro as well.

In another interesting development, human epidermal growth factor receptor 2 (HER2) targeting-CAR-Ms were developed with the capacity to phagocytose HER2 antigen expressing ovarian cancer cells [14]. Moreover, it was found that a one-time combined treatment of CAR-Ms and T cells decreased tumor burden in a xenograft mouse models. Interestingly, the infusion of CAR-Ms in mice converted the M2 (immunosuppressive macrophage phenotype) type of macrophages in the tumor to M1 (pro-inflammatory macrophage phenotype) [14] and induced antigen specific T cell responses against the tumors. Interestingly, in 2018, Carisma Therapeutics was successful in raising funds for developing CAR macrophage immunotherapies. In addition to CAR-macrophages, the precursor of macrophages, monocytes can also have antitumor activity. The advantage of using monocytes as oppose to macrophages can be that it reduces the time between retrieval and infusion from seven days to one day.

Overall, CAR monocytes/macrophages are a promising avenue of CAR cell-based immunotherapy and has the potential to overcome the shortcomings of CAR T cell-based immunotherapies, especially in targeting solid tumors.

5. Summary

In summary, cellular metabolism plays a crucial role in the immune response and based on different stages of immune cell phenotype (naive, effector, memory, regulatory T cells; M1; M2) and their activation state, the metabolic properties of these cells will change. Additionally, other factors, such as nutrients, cytokines, and growth factors, can affect effector T cell metabolism. Moreover, the high glycolytic metabolism of tumor cells creates a microenvironment that is low in vital nutrients, in turn making it highly hypoxic and acidic, which then leads to the metabolic inhibition of immune cells, poor inflammatory cell trafficking to the tumor, the production of immunosuppressive cytokines, and expression of co-inhibitory ligands. These suppressive influences render significant challenges for CAR cell therapies. Moreover, although several strategies have been tested to tackle solid tumor barriers, such as the use of alternative cytoplasmic activation domains and the use of CRISPR-Cas9 as gene-editing techniques, these need to be validated in clinic. Notably, combination therapy with checkpoint inhibitors and armed CARs has been used to improve the function of CAR T cells in solid tumors and are being tested in clinical trials. Importantly, new strategies are required to improve the metabolic fitness of CAR T cells within the TME and strategies are also required to improve the safety of CAR cells, particularly as they move into clinic. Indeed, CAR cells can be optimally designed based on the metabolic properties of the tumor being targeted, and cultured to promote a less differentiated, long-lived phenotype that can efficiently self-renew and differentiate in vivo into potent effector cells. Next-generation CAR cell immunotherapy based on combinatorial engineering and treatments to reprogram immune cell properties and the TME offer unprecedented hope of therapeutic interventions for solid tumors.

6. Future Directions

Generating highly pure and metabolically fit CAR immune cells is a major challenge, and precision genetic modulation of metabolic pathways may improve efficacy toward treating solid tumors. Moreover, pharmaceutical modification of CAR immune cells can also be utilized to modify these energy metabolic pathways to drive the activation of CAR immune cells, specifically for the treatment of solid tumors. These strategies may pave the way to more efficient CAR therapies against solid tumors.

A major issue that needs to be addressed for CAR therapy is the costs associated with manufacturing. Engineering strategies of non-viral vectors, developing protocols for in-hospital CAR therapy generation and generating CAR expression in non-T cells are some of the approaches that may lead to a decrease in these costs. Furthermore, a significant investment in engineering principles and omics approaches are needed to improve cellular manufacturing and the quality control and assurance of CAR therapies. The next stages in developing CAR immune cells will require marrying the fields of engineering and gene therapy for increasing the efficacy of treatment of solid tumors with low toxicity.

Author Contributions: Conceptualization, A.P.A., R.G. and M.W.; methodology, J.L.M., A.E., J.L.H., S.I., S.M.; Writing—Original draft preparation, J.L.M., A.E., J.L.H., S.I., S.M.; Writing—Review and editing, A.P.A., R.G., and M.W. All authors have read and agreed to the published version of the manuscript.

Funding: This research received no external funding.

Institutional Review Board Statement: Not applicable.

Informed Consent Statement: Not applicable.

Data Availability Statement: Not applicable.

Acknowledgments: This work was supported in part by Ri.MED Foundation (Italy), the Children's Hospital of Philadelphia Research Institute, and the Frontier Program in Airway Disorders of the Children's Hospital of Philadelphia to RLG. This work was also supported by start-up funds from Arizona State University to APA.

Conflicts of Interest: The authors declare no conflict of interest.

Abbreviations

ACT	Adoptive cell transfer
AKT	protein kinase B
APCs	Antigen presenting cells
ATP	Adenosine triphosphate
B-ALL	B cell acute lymphoblastic leukemia
Bcl-X(L)	B-cell lymphoma-extra large
CAFs	Cancer-associated fibroblasts
CAR	Chimeric antigen receptor
CAR-M	Chimeric antigen receptor macrophage
CAR-Ps	Chimeric antigen receptors for phagocytosis
CAT	Catalase
CCR	Chimeric costimulatory receptor
CLL	Chronic lymphocytic leukemia
CRISPR	Clustered Regularly Interspaced Short Palindromic Repeats
CRS	Cytokine release syndrome
ECM	Extracellular matrix
ETBR	Endothelin B receptor
FAO	Fatty acid oxidation

GLUT1	Glucose transporter 1
HER2	Human epidermal growth factor receptor 2
HK	Hexokinase 2
HPSE	Heparinase
HSPG	Heparan sulphate proteoglycans
ICOS	Inducible T cell co-stimulator
IDO	Indoleamine-2,3-dioxygenase
IL-10	Interleukin 10
LBCL	Large B cell lymphoma
MDSC	Myeloid-derived suppressor cells
MICA	Major histocompatibility complex class I polypeptide-related sequence A
NK	Natural killer
OXPHOS	Oxidative phosphorylation
PD-1	Programmed cell death protein 1
PD-L1	Programmed cell death ligand 1
PFK-6	phosphofructo-2-kinase
PGC1-α	PPAR-gamma coactivator 1-α
PGE2	Prostaglandin E2
PI3K	Phosphoinositide 3-kinase
PSMA	Prostate-specific membrane
ROS	Reactive oxygen species
ScFv	Single chain variable fragment
TAA	Tumor-associated antigens
TCR	T cell receptor
TGFβ	Transforming growth factor beta
TILs	Tumor-infiltration lymphocytes
TME	Tumor microenvironment
VEGF	Vascular endothelial growth factor

References

1. Batlevi, C.L.; Matsuki, E.; Brentjens, R.J.; Younes, A. Novel immunotherapies in lymphoid malignancies. *Nat. Rev. Clin. Oncol.* **2016**, *13*, 25–40. [CrossRef] [PubMed]
2. Brudno, J.N.; Kochenderfer, J.N. Chimeric antigen receptor T-cell therapies for lymphoma. *Nat. Rev. Clin. Oncol.* **2018**, *15*, 31–46. [CrossRef]
3. June, C.H.; O'Connor, R.S.; Kawalekar, O.U.; Ghassemi, S.; Milone, M.C. CAR T cell immunotherapy for human cancer. *Science* **2018**, *359*, 1361–1365. [CrossRef]
4. Available online: https://clinicaltrials.gov/ct2/results/details?cond=CAR+T+cells (accessed on 29 June 2020).
5. Zhang, C.; Liu, J.; Zhong, J.F.; Zhang, X. Engineering CAR-T cells. *Biomark. Res.* **2017**, *5*, 22. [CrossRef] [PubMed]
6. Hinrichs, C.S.; Spolski, R.; Paulos, C.M.; Gattinoni, L.; Kerstann, K.W.; Palmer, D.C.; Klebanoff, C.A.; Rosenberg, S.A.; Leonard, W.J.; Restifo, N.P. IL-2 and IL-21 confer opposing differentiation programs to CD8+ T cells for adoptive immunotherapy. *Blood* **2008**, *111*, 5326–5333. [CrossRef] [PubMed]
7. Pavlova, N.N.; Thompson, C.B. The Emerging Hallmarks of Cancer Metabolism. *Cell Metab.* **2016**, *23*, 27–47. [CrossRef] [PubMed]
8. Finicle, B.T.; Jayashankar, V.; Edinger, A.L. Nutrient scavenging in cancer. *Nat. Rev. Cancer* **2018**, *18*, 619–633. [CrossRef] [PubMed]
9. Dietl, K.; Renner, K.; Dettmer, K.; Timischl, B.; Eberhart, K.; Dorn, C.; Hellerbrand, C.; Kastenberger, M.; Kunz-Schughart, L.A.; Oefner, P.J.; et al. Lactic Acid and Acidification Inhibit TNF Secretion and Glycolysis of Human Monocytes. *J. Immunol.* **2009**, *184*, 1200–1209. [CrossRef] [PubMed]
10. Fischer, K.; Hoffmann, P.; Voelkl, S.; Meidenbauer, N.; Ammer, J.; Edinger, M.; Gottfried, E.; Schwarz, S.; Rothe, G.; Hoves, S.; et al. Inhibitory effect of tumor cell-derived lactic acid on human T cells. *Blood* **2007**, *109*, 3812–3819. [CrossRef] [PubMed]
11. Muller, A.J.; Prendergast, G.C. Marrying immunotherapy with chemotherapy: Why say IDO? *Cancer Res.* **2005**. [CrossRef]
12. Itakura, E.; Huang, R.R.; Wen, D.R.; Paul, E.; Wünsch, P.H.; Cochran, A.J. IL-10 expression by primary tumor cells correlates with melanoma progression from radial to vertical growth phase and development of metastatic competence. *Mod. Pathol.* **2011**, *24*, 801–809. [CrossRef] [PubMed]
13. Massagué, J. TGFβ in Cancer. *Cell* **2008**, *134*, 215–230. [CrossRef] [PubMed]
14. Klichinsky, M.; Ruella, M.; Shestova, O.; Lu, X.M.; Best, A.; Zeeman, M.; Schmierer, M.; Gabrusiewicz, K.; Anderson, N.R.; Petty, N.E.; et al. Human chimeric antigen receptor macrophages for cancer immunotherapy. *Nat. Biotechnol.* **2020**, *38*, 947–953. [CrossRef] [PubMed]
15. Patel, S.; Burga, R.A.; Powell, A.B.; Chorvinsky, E.A.; Hoq, N.; McCormack, S.E.; Van Pelt, S.N.; Hanley, P.J.; Cruz, C.R. Beyond CAR T Cells: Other Cell-Based Immunotherapeutic Strategies Against Cancer. *Front. Oncol.* **2019**. [CrossRef]

16. Majzner, R.G.; Heitzeneder, S.; Mackall, C.L. Harnessing the Immunotherapy Revolution for the Treatment of Childhood Cancers. *Cancer Cell.* **2017**, *31*, 476–485. [CrossRef]
17. Majzner, R.G.; Mackall, C.L. Tumor antigen escape from car t-cell therapy. *Cancer Discov.* **2018**, *8*, 1219–1226. [CrossRef] [PubMed]
18. Zah, E.; Lin, M.-Y.; Silva-Benedict, A.; Jensen, M.C.; Chen, Y.Y. T Cells Expressing CD19/CD20 Bispecific Chimeric Antigen Receptors Prevent Antigen Escape by Malignant B Cells. *Cancer Immunol. Res.* **2016**, *4*, 498–508. [CrossRef]
19. Sadelain, M. CAR therapy: The CD19 paradigm. *J. Clin. Investig.* **2015**, *125*, 3392–3400. [CrossRef] [PubMed]
20. Das, R.K.; Storm, J.; Barrett, D.M. Abstract 1631: T cell dysfunction in pediatric cancer patients at diagnosis and after chemotherapy can limit chimeric antigen receptor potential. *Cancer Res.* **2018**. [CrossRef]
21. Heinmöller, P.; Gross, C.; Beyser, K.; Schmidtgen, C.; Maass, G.; Pedrocchi, M.; Rüschoff, J. HER2 Status in Non-Small Cell Lung Cancer: Results from Patient Screening for Enrollment to a Phase II Study of Herceptin. *Clin Cancer Res.* **2003**, *9*, 5238–5243. [CrossRef]
22. Shah, N.N.; Fry, T.J. Mechanisms of resistance to CAR T cell therapy. *Nat. Rev. Clin. Oncol.* **2019**, *16*, 1–385. [CrossRef] [PubMed]
23. Zhang, E.; Xu, H. A new insight in chimeric antigen receptor-engineered T cells for cancer immunotherapy. *J. Hematol. Oncol.* **2017**, *10*, 1. [CrossRef] [PubMed]
24. Frey, N.V.; Porter, D.L. CAR T-cells merge into the fast lane of cancer care. *Am. J. Hematol.* **2016**, *91*, 146–150. [CrossRef] [PubMed]
25. Jena, B.; Moyes, J.S.; Huls, H.; Cooper, L.J.N. Driving CAR-Based T-Cell Therapy to Success. *Curr. Hematol. Malig Rep.* **2014**, *9*, 50–56. [CrossRef] [PubMed]
26. Gilham, D.E.; Debets, R.; Pule, M.; Hawkins, R.E.; Abken, H. CAR–T cells and solid tumors: Tuning T cells to challenge an inveterate foe. *Trends Mol. Med.* **2012**, *18*, 377–384. [CrossRef]
27. Martinez, M.; Moon, E.K. CAR T cells for solid tumors: New strategies for finding, infiltrating, and surviving in the tumor microenvironment. *Front. Immunol.* **2019**, *10*, 1–21. [CrossRef]
28. Caruana, I.; Savoldo, B.; Hoyos, V.; Weber, G.; Liu, H.; Kim, E.S.; Ittmann, M.M.; Marchetti, D.; Dotti, G. Heparanase promotes tumor infiltration and antitumor activity of CAR-redirected T lymphocytes. *Nat. Med.* **2015**, *21*, 524–529. [CrossRef]
29. D'Aloia, M.M.; Zizzari, I.G.; Sacchetti, B.; Pierelli, L.; Alimandi, M. CAR-T cells: The long and winding road to solid tumors review-article. *Cell Death Dis.* **2018**. [CrossRef]
30. Irving, M.; de Silly, R.V.; Scholten, K.; Dilek, N.; Coukos, G. Engineering chimeric antigen receptor T-cells for racing in solid tumors: Don't forget the fuel. *Front. Immunol.* **2017**, *8*, 1–19. [CrossRef]
31. Chen, Q.; Hu, Q.; Dukhovlinova, E.; Chen, G.; Ahn, S.; Wang, C.; Ogunnaike, E.A.; Ligler, F.S.; Dotti, G.; Gu, Z. Photothermal Therapy Promotes Tumor Infiltration and Antitumor Activity of CAR T Cells. *Adv. Mater.* **2019**, *31*, 1900192. [CrossRef]
32. Yong, C.S.M.; Dardalhon, V.; Devaud, C.; Taylor, N.; Darcy, P.K.; Kershaw, M.H. CAR T-cell therapy of solid tumors. *Immunol. Cell Biol.* **2017**, *95*, 356–363. [CrossRef] [PubMed]
33. Rataj, F.; Jacobi, S.J.; Stoiber, S.; Asang, F.; Ogonek, J.; Tokarew, N.; Cadilha, B.L.; Puijenbroek, E.V.; Heise, C.; Duewell, P.; et al. High-affinity CD16-polymorphism and Fc-engineered antibodies enable activity of CD16-chimeric antigen receptor-modified T cells for cancer therapy. *Br. J. Cancer* **2019**, *120*, 79–87. [CrossRef]
34. Clémenceau, B.; Congy-Jolivet, N.; Gallot, G.; Vivien, R.; Gaschet, J.; Thibault, G.; Vié, H. Antibody-dependent cellular cytotoxicity (ADCC) is mediated by genetically modified antigen-specific human T lymphocytes. *Blood* **2006**, *107*, 4669–4677. [CrossRef] [PubMed]
35. Kudo, K.; Imai, C.; Lorenzini, P.; Kamiya, T.; Kono, K.; Davidoff, A.M.; Chng, W.J.; Campana, D. T lymphocytes expressing a CD16 signaling receptor exert antibody-dependent cancer cell killing. *Cancer Res.* **2014**, *74*, 93–103. [CrossRef]
36. Ochi, F.; Fujiwara, H.; Tanimoto, K.; Asai, H.; Miyazaki, Y.; Okamoto, S.; Mineno, J.; Kuzushima, K.; Shiku, H.; Barrett, J.; et al. Gene-modified human α/β-T cells expressing a chimeric CD16-CD3ζ receptor as adoptively transferable effector cells for anticancer monoclonal antibody therapy. *Cancer Immunol. Res.* **2014**. [CrossRef]
37. Newick, K.; O'Brien, S.; Moon, E.; Albelda, S.M. CAR T Cell Therapy for Solid Tumors. *Annu. Rev. Med.* **2017**, *68*, 139–152. [CrossRef] [PubMed]
38. Baitsch, L.; Fuertes-Marraco, S.A.; Legat, A.; Meyer, C.; Speiser, D.E. The three main stumbling blocks for anticancer T cells. *Trends Immunol.* **2012**, *33*, 364–372. [CrossRef] [PubMed]
39. Almeida, L.; Lochner, M.; Berod, L.; Sparwasser, T. Metabolic pathways in T cell activation and lineage differentiation. *Semin. Immunol.* **2016**, *28*, 514–524. [CrossRef]
40. Kouidhi, S.; Elgaaied, A.B.; Chouaib, S. Impact of metabolism on T-cell differentiation and function and cross talk with tumor microenvironment. *Front. Immunol.* **2017**, *8*, 270. [CrossRef] [PubMed]
41. Zhang, Y.; Kurupati, R.; Liu, L.; Zhou, X.Y.; Zhang, G.; Hudaihed, A.; Filisio, F.; Giles-Davis, W.; Xu, X.; Karakousis, G.C.; et al. Enhancing CD8+ T Cell Fatty Acid Catabolism within a Metabolically Challenging Tumor Microenvironment Increases the Efficacy of Melanoma Immunotherapy. *Cancer Cell.* **2017**, *32*, 377–391. [CrossRef]
42. Chen, X.; Song, M.; Zhang, B.; Zhang, Y. Reactive Oxygen Species Regulate T Cell Immune Response in the Tumor Microenvironment. *Oxid. Med. Cell. Longev.* **2016**. [CrossRef]
43. Lim, A.R.; Rathmell, W.K.; Rathmell, J.C. The tumor microenvironment as a metabolic barrier to effector T cells and immunotherapy. *eLife* **2020**, *9*. [CrossRef]
44. Herbel, C.; Patsoukis, N.; Bardhan, K.; Seth, P.; Weaver, J.D.; Boussiotis, V.A. Clinical significance of T cell metabolic reprogramming in cancer. *Clin. Transl. Med.* **2016**, *5*, 29. [CrossRef]

45. Ho, P.C.; Liu, P.S. Metabolic communication in tumors: A new layer of immunoregulation for immune evasion. *J. Immunother. Cancer* **2016**, *4*, 4. [CrossRef] [PubMed]
46. Patsoukis, N.; Weaver, J.D.; Strauss, L.; Herbel, C.; Seth, P.; Boussiotis, V.A. Immunometabolic regulations mediated by coinhibitory receptors and their impact on T cell immune responses. *Front. Immunol.* **2017**, *8*, 1–19. [CrossRef] [PubMed]
47. Cairns, R.A.; Harris, I.S.; Mak, T.W. Regulation of cancer cell metabolism. *Nat. Rev. Cancer.* **2011**, *11*, 85–95. [CrossRef] [PubMed]
48. Ho, P.C.; Bihuniak, J.D.; MacIntyre, A.N.; Staron, M.; Liu, X.; Amezquita, R.; Tsui, Y.; Cui, G.; Micevic, G.; Perales, J.C.; et al. Phosphoenolpyruvate Is a Metabolic Checkpoint of Anti-tumor T Cell Responses. *Cell* **2015**, *162*, 1217–1228. [CrossRef] [PubMed]
49. Chang, C.-H.; Curtis, J.D.; Maggi, L.B.; Faubert, B.; Villarino, A.V.; O'Sullivan, D.; Huang, S.C.-C.; Van Der Windt, G.J.; Blagih, J.; Qiu, J.; et al. Posttranscriptional Control of T Cell Effector Function by Aerobic Glycolysis. *Cell* **2013**, *153*, 1239–1251. [CrossRef]
50. Chang, C.-H.; Qiu, J.; O'Sullivan, D.; Buck, M.D.; Noguchi, T.; Curtis, J.D.; Chen, Q.; Gindin, M.; Gubin, M.M.; Van Der Windt, G.J.; et al. Metabolic Competition in the Tumor Microenvironment Is a Driver of Cancer Progression. *Cell* **2015**, *162*, 1229–1241. [CrossRef] [PubMed]
51. Hope, H.C.; Salmond, R.J. Targeting the tumor microenvironment and T cell metabolism for effective cancer immunotherapy. *Eur. J. Immunol.* **2019**, *49*, 1147–1152. [CrossRef]
52. Brand, A.; Singer, K.; Koehl, G.E.; Kolitzus, M.; Schoenhammer, G.; Thiel, A.; Matos, C.; Bruss, C.; Klobuch, S.; Peter, K.; et al. LDHA-Associated Lactic Acid Production Blunts Tumor Immunosurveillance by T and NK Cells. *Cell Metab.* **2016**, *24*, 657–671. [CrossRef]
53. Haas, R.; Smith, J.; Rocher-Ros, V.; Nadkarni, S.; Montero-Melendez, T.; D'Acquisto, F.; Bland, E.J.; Bombardieri, M.; Pitzalis, C.; Perretti, M.; et al. Lactate regulates metabolic and proinflammatory circuits in control of T cell migration and effector functions. *PLoS Biol.* **2015**. [CrossRef]
54. Srivastava, M.K.; Sinha, P.; Clements, V.K.; Rodriguez, P.; Ostrand-Rosenberg, S. Myeloid-Derived Suppressor Cells Inhibit T-Cell Activation by Depleting Cystine and Cysteine. *Cancer Res.* **2010**, *70*, 68–77. [CrossRef]
55. Lind, D.S. Arginine and cancer. *J. Nutr.* **2004**. [CrossRef] [PubMed]
56. Geiger, R.; Rieckmann, J.C.; Wolf, T.; Basso, C.; Feng, Y.; Fuhrer, T.; Kogadeeva, M.; Picotti, P.; Meissner, F.; Mann, M.; et al. L-Arginine Modulates T Cell Metabolism and Enhances Survival and Anti-tumor Activity. *Cell* **2016**, *167*, 829–842. [CrossRef]
57. Acharya, A.P.; Sinha, M.; Ratay, M.L.; Ding, X.; Balmert, S.C.; Workman, C.J.; Wang, Y.; Vignali, D.A.A.; Little, S.R. Localized Multi-Component Delivery Platform Generates Local and Systemic Anti-Tumor Immunity. *Adv. Funct. Mater.* **2017**, *27*. [CrossRef]
58. Pearce, E.L.; Poffenberger, M.C.; Chang, C.-H.; Jones, R.G. Fueling Immunity: Insights into Metabolism and Lymphocyte Function. *Science* **2013**, *342*, 1242454. [CrossRef] [PubMed]
59. Frauwirth, K.A.; Riley, J.L.; Harris, M.H.; Parry, R.V.; Rathmell, J.C.; Plas, D.R.; Elstrom, R.L.; June, C.H.; Thompson, C.B. The CD28 Signaling Pathway Regulates Glucose Metabolism. *Immunity* **2002**, *16*, 769–777. [CrossRef]
60. Kolev, M.; Dimeloe, S.; Le Friec, G.; Navarini, A.; Arbore, G.; Povoleri, G.A.; Fischer, M.; Belle, R.; Loeliger, J.; Develioglu, L.; et al. Complement Regulates Nutrient Influx and Metabolic Reprogramming during Th1 Cell Responses. *Immunity* **2015**, *42*, 1033–1047. [CrossRef]
61. Delgoffe, G.M.; Pollizzi, K.N.; Waickman, A.T.; Heikamp, E.; Meyers, D.J.; Horton, M.R.; Xiao, B.; Worley, P.F.; Powell, J.D. The kinase mTOR regulates the differentiation of helper T cells through the selective activation of signaling by mTORC1 and mTORC. *Nat. Immunol.* **2011**, *12*, 295–303. [CrossRef]
62. Cham, C.M.; Driessens, G.; O'Keefe, J.P.; Gajewski, T.F. Glucose deprivation inhibits multiple key gene expression events and effector functions in CD8+ T cells. *Eur. J. Immunol.* **2008**, *38*, 2438–2450. [CrossRef] [PubMed]
63. Hamid, O.; Robert, C.; Daud, A.; Hodi, F.S.; Hwu, W.-J.; Kefford, R.; Wolchok, J.D.; Hersey, P.; Joseph, R.W.; Weber, J.S.; et al. Safety and Tumor Responses with Lambrolizumab (Anti–PD-1) in Melanoma. *N. Engl. J. Med.* **2013**, *369*, 134–144. [CrossRef] [PubMed]
64. Wolchok, J.D.; Kluger, H.; Callahan, M.K.; Postow, M.A.; Rizvi, N.A.; Lesokhin, A.M.; Segal, N.H.; Ariyan, C.E.; Gordon, R.-A.; Reed, K.; et al. Nivolumab plus Ipilimumab in Advanced Melanoma. *N. Engl. J. Med.* **2013**, *369*, 122–133. [CrossRef] [PubMed]
65. Pearce, E.L.; Pearce, E.J. Metabolic Pathways in Immune Cell Activation and Quiescence. *Immunity Cell Press* **2013**, *38*, 633–643. [CrossRef]
66. Liu, X.; Shin, N.; Koblish, H.K.; Yang, G.; Wang, Q.; Wang, K.; Leffet, L.; Hansbury, M.J.; Thomas, B.; Rupar, M.; et al. Selective inhibition of IDO1 effectively regulates mediators of antitumor immunity. *Blood* **2010**, *115*, 3520–3530. [CrossRef] [PubMed]
67. Buck, M.D.; O'Sullivan, D.; Pearce, E.L. T cell metabolism drives immunity. *J. Exp. Med.* **2015**, *212*, 1345–1360. [CrossRef]
68. O'Sullivan, D.; Pearce, E.L. Targeting T cell metabolism for therapy. *Trends Immunol.* **2015**, *36*, 71–80. [CrossRef]
69. Noman, M.Z.; DeSantis, G.; Janji, B.; Hasmim, M.; Karray, S.; Dessen, P.; Bronte, V.; Chouaib, S. PD-L1 is a novel direct target of HIF-1α, and its blockade under hypoxia enhanced MDSC-mediated T cell activation. *J. Exp. Med.* **2014**, *211*, 781–790. [CrossRef]
70. Fallah, J.; Rini, B.I. HIF Inhibitors: Status of Current Clinical Development. *Curr. Oncol. Rep.* **2019**. [CrossRef] [PubMed]
71. Weinkove, R.; George, P.; Dasyam, N.; McLellan, A.D. Selecting costimulatory domains for chimeric antigen receptors: Functional and clinical considerations. *Clin. Transl. Immunol.* **2019**, *8*, e1049. [CrossRef]
72. Kawalekar, O.U.; O'Connor, R.S.; Fraietta, J.A.; Guo, L.; McGettigan, S.E.; Posey, A.D.; Patel, P.R.; Guedan, S.; Scholler, J.; Keith, B.; et al. Distinct Signaling of Coreceptors Regulates Specific Metabolism Pathways and Impacts Memory Development in CAR T Cells. *Immunity* **2016**, *44*, 380–390. [CrossRef] [PubMed]

73. Pulè, M.A.; Straathof, K.C.; Dotti, G.; Heslop, H.E.; Rooney, C.M.; Brenner, M.K. A chimeric T cell antigen receptor that augments cytokine release and supports clonal expansion of primary human T cells. *Mol. Ther.* **2005**, *12*, 933–941. [CrossRef] [PubMed]
74. Guedan, S.; Posey, A.D.; Shaw, C.; Wing, A.; Da, T.; Patel, P.R.; Mcgettigan, S.E.; Casado-Medrano, V.; Kawalekar, O.U.; Uribe-Herranz, M.; et al. Enhancing CAR T cell persistence through ICOS and 4-1BB costimulation. *JCI Insight* **2018**, *3*. [CrossRef] [PubMed]
75. Michels, J.; Keep, O.; Senovilla, L.; Lissa, D.; Castedo, M.; Kroemer, G.; Galluzzi, L. Functions of BCL-XL at the interface between cell death and metabolism. *Int. J. Cell Biol.* **2013**. [CrossRef]
76. Abate-Daga, D.; Davila, M.L. CAR models: Next-generation CAR modifications for enhanced T-cell function. *Mol. Ther. Oncolytics* **2016**, *3*, 16014. [CrossRef]
77. Scharping, N.E.; Menk, A.V.; Moreci, R.S.; Whetstone, R.D.; Dadey, R.E.; Watkins, S.C.; Ferris, R.L.; Delgoffe, G.M. The Tumor Microenvironment Represses T Cell Mitochondrial Biogenesis to Drive Intratumoral T Cell Metabolic Insufficiency and Dysfunction. *Immunity* **2016**, *45*, 374–388. [CrossRef] [PubMed]
78. Hu, W.; Zi, Z.; Jin, Y.; Li, G.; Shao, K.; Cai, Q.; Ma, X.; Wei, F. CRISPR/Cas9-mediated PD-1 disruption enhances human mesothelin-targeted CAR T cell effector functions. *Cancer Immunol. Immunother.* **2019**, *68*, 365–377. [CrossRef]
79. Kumar, A.; Chamoto, K. Immune metabolism in PD-1 blockade-based cancer immunotherapy. *Int. Immunol.* **2021**, *33*, 17–26. [CrossRef]
80. Patsoukis, N.; Bardhan, K.; Chatterjee, P.; Sari, D.; Liu, B.; Bell, L.N.; Karoly, E.D.; Freeman, G.J.; Petkova, V.; Seth, P.; et al. PD-1 alters T-cell metabolic reprogramming by inhibiting glycolysis and promoting lipolysis and fatty acid oxidation. *Nat. Commun.* **2015**, *6*, 6692. [CrossRef]
81. Wan, H.; Xu, B.; Zhu, N.; Ren, B. PGC-1α activator–induced fatty acid oxidation in tumor-infiltrating CTLs enhances effects of PD-1 blockade therapy in lung cancer. *Tumori* **2020**. [CrossRef]
82. Yee, C. Adoptive T cell therapy: Points to consider. *Curr. Opin. Immunol.* **2018**, *51*, 197–203. [CrossRef]
83. Le Bourgeois, T.; Strauss, L.; Aksoylar, H.I.; Daneshmandi, S.; Seth, P.; Patsoukis, N.; Boussiotis, V.A. Targeting T cell metabolism for improvement of cancer immunotherapy. *Front. Oncol.* **2018**. [CrossRef] [PubMed]
84. Acharya, A.P.; Dolgova, N.V.; Clare-Salzler, M.J.; Keselowsky, B.G. Adhesive substrate-modulation of adaptive immune responses. *Biomaterials* **2008**, *29*, 4736–4750. [CrossRef] [PubMed]
85. Acharya, A.P.; Carstens, M.R.; Lewis, J.S.; Dolgova, N.; Xia, C.Q.; Clare-Salzler, M.J.; Keselowsky, B.G. A cell-based microarray to investigate combinatorial effects of microparticle-encapsulated adjuvants on dendritic cell activation. *J. Mater. Chem.* **2016**, *4*, 1672–1685. [CrossRef] [PubMed]
86. Acharya, A.P.; Clare-Salzler, M.J.; Keselowsky, B.G. A high-throughput microparticle microarray platform for dendritic cell-targeting vaccines. *Biomaterials* **2009**, *30*, 4168–4177. [CrossRef] [PubMed]
87. Liu, E.; Tong, Y.; Dotti, G.; Shaim, H.; Savoldo, B.; Mukherjee, M.; Orange, J.; Wan, X.; Lu, X.; Reynolds, A.; et al. Cord blood NK cells engineered to express IL-15 and a CD19-targeted CAR show long-term persistence and potent antitumor activity. *Leukemia* **2018**, *32*, 520–531. [CrossRef]
88. A Morrissey, M.; Williamson, A.P.; Steinbach, A.M.; Roberts, E.W.; Kern, N.; Headley, M.B.; Vale, R.D. Chimeric antigen receptors that trigger phagocytosis. *eLife* **2018**, *7*, e36688. [CrossRef]
89. Mangal, J.L.; Inamdar, S.; Yang, Y.; Dutta, S.; Wankhede, M.; Shi, X.; Gu, H.; Green, M.D.; Rege, K.; Curtis, M.; et al. Metabolite releasing polymers control dendritic cell function by modulating their energy metabolism. *J. Mater. Chem. B* **2020**, *8*, 5195–5203. [CrossRef]
90. O'Neill, L.A.J.; Pearce, E.J. Immunometabolism governs dendritic cell and macrophage function. *J. Exp. Med.* **2016**, *213*, 15–23. [CrossRef]
91. Liu, E.; Marin, D.; Banerjee, P.; Macapinlac, H.A.; Thompson, P.; Basar, R.; Kerbauy, L.N.; Overman, B.; Thall, P.; Kaplan, M.; et al. Use of CAR-Transduced Natural Killer Cells in CD19-Positive Lymphoid Tumors. *N. Engl. J. Med.* **2020**, *382*, 545–553. [CrossRef]
92. Xie, G.; Dong, H.; Liang, Y.; Ham, J.D.; Rizwan, R.; Chen, J. CAR-NK cells: A promising cellular immunotherapy for cancer. *EBioMedicine* **2020**, *59*, 102975. [CrossRef]
93. Rezvani, K.; Rouce, R.; Liu, E.; Shpall, E. Engineering Natural Killer Cells for Cancer Immunotherapy. *Mol. Ther.* **2017**, *25*, 1769–1781. [CrossRef]
94. Basar, R.; Daher, M.; Rezvani, K. Next-generation cell therapies: The emerging role of CAR-NK cells. *Blood Adv.* **2020**. [CrossRef]
95. Sotillo, E.; Barrett, D.M.; Black, K.L.; Bagashev, A.A.; Oldridge, D.; Wu, G.; Sussman, R.T.; LaNauze, C.; Ruella, M.; Gazzara, M.R.; et al. Convergence of Acquired Mutations and Alternative Splicing of CD19 Enables Resistance to CART-19 Immunotherapy. *Cancer Discov.* **2015**, *5*, 1282–1295. [CrossRef] [PubMed]
96. Yilmaz, A.; Cui, H.; Caligiuri, M.A.; Yu, J. Chimeric antigen receptor-engineered natural killer cells for cancer immunotherapy. *J. Hematol. Oncol.* **2020**, *13*, 1–22. [CrossRef]
97. Lin, C.-Y.; Gobius, I.; Souza-Fonseca-Guimaraes, F. Natural killer cell engineering—A new hope for cancer immunotherapy. *Semin. Hematol.* **2020**, *57*, 194–200. [CrossRef] [PubMed]
98. Caratelli, S.; Arriga, R.; Sconocchia, T.; Ottaviani, A.; Lanzilli, G.; Pastore, D.; Cenciarelli, C.; Venditti, A.; Del Principe, M.I.; Lauro, D.; et al. In vitro elimination of epidermal growth factor receptor-overexpressing cancer cells by CD32A-chimeric receptor T cells in combination with cetuximab or panitumumab. *Int. J. Cancer* **2020**, *146*, 236–247. [CrossRef] [PubMed]

99. Afolabi, L.O.; Adeshakin, A.O.; Sani, M.M.; Bi, J.; Wan, X. Genetic reprogramming for NK cell cancer immunotherapy with CRISPR/Cas9. *Immunology* **2019**, *158*, 63–69. [CrossRef]
100. Terrén, I.; Orrantia, A.; Vitallé, J.; Zenarruzabeitia, O.; Borrego, F. NK Cell Metabolism and Tumor Microenvironment. *Front. Immunol.* **2019**, *10*. [CrossRef]
101. Juillerat, A.; Marechal, A.; Filhol, J.M.; Valogne, Y.; Valton, J.; Duclert, A.; Duchateau, P.; Poirot, L. An oxygen sensitive self-decision making engineered CAR T-cell. *Sci. Rep.* **2017**, *7*, srep39833. [CrossRef]
102. Navin, I.; Lam, M.T.; Parihar, R. Design and Implementation of NK Cell-Based Immunotherapy to Overcome the Solid Tumor Microenvironment. *Cancers* **2020**, *12*, 3871. [CrossRef]
103. Rautela, J.; Surgenor, E.; Huntington, N.D. Efficient genome editing of human natural killer cells by CRISPR RNP. *bioRxiv* **2018**. [CrossRef]
104. Sekiba, K.; Yamagami, M.; Otsuka, M.; Suzuki, T.; Kishikawa, T.; Ishibashi, R.; Ohno, M.; Sato, M.; Koike, K. Transcriptional activation of the MICA gene with an engineered CRISPR-Cas9 system. *Biochem. Biophys. Res. Commun.* **2017**, *486*, 521–525. [CrossRef]
105. Parihar, R.; Rivas, C.H.; Huynh, M.; Omer, B.; Lapteva, N.; Metelitsa, L.S.; Gottschalk, S.M.; Rooney, C.M. NK Cells Expressing a Chimeric Activating Receptor Eliminate MDSCs and Rescue Impaired CAR-T Cell Activity against Solid Tumors. *Cancer Immunol. Res.* **2019**, *7*, 363–375. [CrossRef]
106. Fang, F.; Xiao, W.; Tian, Z. NK cell-based immunotherapy for cancer. *Semin. Immunol.* **2017**, *31*, 37–54. [CrossRef] [PubMed]
107. Sahm, C.; Schönfeld, K.; Wels, W.S. Expression of IL-15 in NK cells results in rapid enrichment and selective cytotoxicity of gene-modiWed eVectors that carry a tumor-speciWc antigen receptor. *Cancer Immunol. Immunother.* **2012**, *61*, 1451–1461. [CrossRef] [PubMed]
108. Gang, M.; Marin, N.D.; Wong, P.; Neal, C.C.; Marsala, L.; Foster, M.; Schappe, T.; Meng, W.; Tran, J.; Schaettler, M.; et al. CAR-modified memory-like NK cells exhibit potent responses to NK-resistant lymphomas. *Blood* **2020**, *136*, 2308–2318. [CrossRef]
109. Hu, Y.; Tian, Z.-G.; Zhang, C. Chimeric antigen receptor (CAR)-transduced natural killer cells in tumor immunotherapy. *Acta Pharmacol. Sin.* **2017**, *39*, 167–176. [CrossRef]

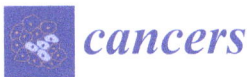

Article

Arming T Cells with a gp100-Specific TCR and a CSPG4-Specific CAR Using Combined DNA- and RNA-Based Receptor Transfer

Bianca Simon [1,2], Dennis C. Harrer [1], Beatrice Schuler-Thurner [1], Gerold Schuler [1] and Ugur Uslu [1,*]

1. Department of Dermatology, Friedrich-Alexander-Universität Erlangen-Nürnberg (FAU), Universitätsklinikum Erlangen, 91054 Erlangen, Germany; bianca.simon@uk-erlangen.de (B.S.); dennis.harrer@uk-erlangen.de (D.C.H.); beatrice.schuler-thurner@uk-erlangen.de (B.S.-T.); gerold.schuler@uk-erlangen.de (G.S.)
2. Division of Genetics, Department of Biology, Friedrich-Alexander-Universität Erlangen-Nürnberg (FAU), 91058 Erlangen, Germany
* Correspondence: ugur.uslu@uk-erlangen.de

Received: 17 April 2019; Accepted: 16 May 2019; Published: 20 May 2019

Abstract: Tumor cells can develop immune escape mechanisms to bypass T cell recognition, e.g., antigen loss or downregulation of the antigen presenting machinery, which represents a major challenge in adoptive T cell therapy. To counteract these mechanisms, we transferred not only one, but two receptors into the same T cell to generate T cells expressing two additional receptors (TETARs). We generated these TETARs by lentiviral transduction of a gp100-specific T cell receptor (TCR) and subsequent electroporation of mRNA encoding a second-generation CSPG4-specific chimeric antigen receptor (CAR). Following pilot experiments to optimize the combined DNA- and RNA-based receptor transfer, the functionality of TETARs was compared to T cells either transfected with the TCR only or the CAR only. After transfection, TETARs clearly expressed both introduced receptors on their cell surface. When stimulated with tumor cells expressing either one of the antigens or both, TETARs were able to secrete cytokines and showed cytotoxicity. The confirmation that two antigen-specific receptors can be functionally combined using two different methods to introduce each receptor into the same T cell opens new possibilities and opportunities in cancer immunotherapy. For further evaluation, the use of these TETARs in appropriate animal models will be the next step towards a potential clinical use in cancer patients.

Keywords: cancer; melanoma; immune escape; antigen loss; immunotherapy; chimeric antigen receptor; electroporation; lentivirus; lentiviral transduction

---

1. Introduction

Adoptive transfer of T cells transfected with tumor-specific T cell receptors (TCRs) or chimeric antigen receptors (CARs) has already been successfully used in clinical trials treating patients suffering from several types of solid and hematologic malignancies [1–5]. Especially for therapy-refractory B-cell acute lymphoblastic leukemia (ALL) and diffuse large B-cell lymphoma, CD19-directed CAR T cell therapy revealed impressive response rates in clinical trials [5–8]. This has resulted in the recent approval of two CD19 CAR T cell constructs in the United States and the European Union [5–8].

However, a major hurdle in the use of adoptively transferred T cells, especially for the use in solid tumors, is posed by mechanisms of tumor cells that enable them to escape T cell recognition [9–11]. Occurrences of, e.g., tumor antigen loss, downregulation of the antigen presenting machinery, or defects in antigen processing are collectively known as "immune escape mechanisms" and give rise to disease progression after an initial response [9–11]. Thus, new strategies to improve the adoptive transfer of engineered T cells are required [12–14]. A possible approach is the introduction of not only one but two tumor-specific receptors into the same T cell in order to generate T cells expressing not only one, but two additional tumor antigen-specific receptors. This would reduce the risk of immune escape, as it is less likely that both tumor antigens recognized by the same T cell will be lost or downregulated by the same tumor cell at the same time. Additionally, a multi-hit therapy by attacking tumor cells via more than one target antigen simultaneously may result in a more efficient tumor cell killing.

In our previous studies, we have already generated so called "T cells expressing two additional receptors" (TETARs) with two TCRs specific for human immunodeficiency virus (HIV)-epitopes [15] or melanoma antigens [16] using co-electroporation of receptor-encoding mRNAs. These TETARs equivalently responded to both epitopes with regard to cytokine secretion and cytotoxic function [15,16]. However, by equipping the same T cells simultaneously with two TCRs, tumor cells could still escape immune recognition by defects in antigen processing or loss of human leukocyte antigen (HLA) expression. This could be circumvented by, e.g., co-transfection of the T cells with a CAR and a TCR: While TCRs recognize intracellular tumor antigens that are presented on the cell surface by major histocompatibility complex (MHC) molecules [17], CARs bind to unprocessed tumor surface antigens independent of MHC restriction and antigen processing [18,19]. Thus, we generated TETARs by simultaneous transfection of a second-generation CAR and a conventional TCR using again co-electroporation of receptor-encoding mRNAs [20]. We could confirm that a CAR and a TCR can be functionally combined, as these TETARs produced cytokines and were cytotoxic upon recognition of each of their cognate antigens, while no reciprocal inhibition of the receptors occurred [20].

Using only transient RNA-based transfection to introduce the two receptors into the same T cells to generate TETARs represents a safer method, as potential side effects will be transient as well. At the same time, a clinical application would require repetitive infusions and thus, a higher amount of engineered T cells [21–23]. The use of only DNA-based receptor transfer to introduce both receptors stably—and not transiently—into the same T cell, however, would most likely result in higher rates of severe side effects [24], complicating its clinical application as well. Thus, the logical strategy would be to stably transfer receptors which have already proven to be effective and safe, and to transiently transfer receptors into the same T cell which are likely potent, but potentially more dangerous regarding on-target off-tumor toxicities. Thus, an effective strategy could be to stably transfer receptors which have already proven to be effective and safe, and to transiently transfer receptors into the same T cells which have been shown to be potent, but potentially more dangerous regarding side effects. In this context, the receptor, which is virally transduced into the T cell using receptor-encoding DNA, should have a strong and permanent anti-tumor effect, whereas the receptor, which is transfected into the same T cell using receptor-encoding RNA, should have an additional "boost" effect at the beginning of the therapy. This initial "boost" effect could massively increase the pressure on the tumor by enhanced induction of direct tumor-cell killing and rapid on-site T cell expansion and could be an effective and fast way to eradicate large quantities of tumor cells.

The CSPG4 antigen (chondroitin sulfate proteoglycan 4, also known as melanoma-associated chondroitin sulfate proteoglycan, MCSP, or high molecular weight melanoma-associated antigen, HMW-MAA) is expressed in 90% of melanoma lesions [25] and other malignancies, e.g., gliomas and sarcomas [26,27]. It is a major driver of melanoma progression by influencing adhesion/spreading, migration, invasion, and metastasis [25]. It is also expressed on healthy tissue, e.g., precursor cells of hair follicle and epidermal cells, as well as on endothelial cells and on activated pericytes [28,29]. The gp100 antigen (also known as premelanosome protein, PMEL) is an intracellular transmembrane glycoprotein enriched in melanosomes, which is involved in the synthesis of melanin [30]. Thus, both antigens, CSPG4 and gp100, may represent effective target antigens for the use in adoptive T cell transfer.

The aim of this study was to simultaneously transfer two receptors into the same T cell to generate TETARs by combining stable DNA- and transient RNA-based receptor transfer. Since the gp100 antigen has been previously used as a target antigen in adoptive T cell therapy and has proven to be an effective as well as a safe target antigen [1,31], we decided to stably introduce a gp100-specific TCR into the T cells via lentiviral transduction. Due to the more distributed expression pattern of CSPG4 in malignant as well as healthy tissue, we additionally introduced a CSPG4-specific second-generation CAR transiently into the same T cell via electroporation of receptor-encoding RNA. Following pilot experiments to optimize the combined DNA- and RNA-based receptor transfer, we examined the functional activity, i.e., cytokine production and cytotoxicity, of TETARs and compared them to T cells either transfected with the TCR only or the CAR alone to provide a proof of principle of this novel approach.

2. Results

2.1. Generation of TETARs

At the beginning of experimental procedures, healthy donor T cells were extracted from peripheral blood mononuclear cells (PBMCs) via magnetic-activated cell sorting (MACS) and short-time activated with the anti-CD3 antibody OKT-3, IL-2, and αCD28 (Figure 1). At day two, T cells were lentivirally transduced with a gp100-specific TCR. Non-transduced cells served as a negative control. In order to directly expand transduced cells, antigen-specific stimulation was performed with A375M melanoma cells pulsed with the HLA-A2-restricted peptide gp100$_{280-288}$ for one week (Figure 1). This antigen-specific stimulation of cells was performed twice consecutively, adding IL-2 and fresh medium at day four after each stimulation. At the same time, non-transduced cells were again activated with OKT-3, IL-2, and αCD28. On day 20, half of the transduced cells as well as non-transduced cells were electroporated with a CSPG4-specific CAR leading to the following T cell conditions: non-transduced cells (mock), CSPG4 CAR-transfected cells (CAR T cells; CAR only), gp100 TCR-transduced T cells (TCR T cells; TCR only), and TCR-transduced plus CAR-transfected T cells (TETARs). After T cell engineering, cells were examined for their receptor expression levels. In the next step, functionality of these TETARs, i.e., cytokine production and cytotoxicity, was analyzed and compared to CAR T cells and TCR T cells (Figure 1).

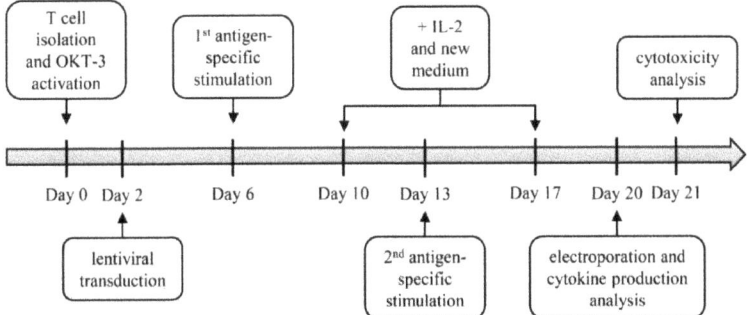

Figure 1. Experimental procedure for the generation of T cells expressing two additional receptors (TETARs). CD8$^+$ T cells were first isolated from peripheral blood mononuclear cells (PBMCs) and subsequently activated with OKT-3, CD28 antibody, and IL-2 (T cell isolation and activation). After two days, T cells were lentivirally transduced with the gp100 TCR virus (lentiviral transduction). On day 6 and 13, antigen-specific stimulation of transduced T cells with gp100 peptide-loaded A375M melanoma cells was performed (antigen-specific stimulation). New medium and IL-2 was added to the cells on day 10 and 17 (+ IL-2 and new medium). Transduced T cells were then electroporated with mRNA encoding the CSPG4-specific chimeric antigen receptor (CAR), and functionality assays, i.e., analysis of cytokine secretion and cytotoxicity, were conducted at day of or one day after electroporation. In addition, a receptor expression analysis was performed in a time-course experiment.

2.2. Gp100-Specific TCR T Cells Can Be Efficiently Transfected with a CSPG4-Specific CAR Using mRNA Electroporation

In order to determine whether the lentivirally transduced T cells can be additionally transfected with mRNA coding for a tumor-specific CAR, the surface expression of the gp100-specific TCR and the CSPG4-specific CAR were examined following RNA electroporation. The expression of the gp100-specific TCR was confirmed using an MHC-Dextramer (HLA-A*0201/YLEPGPVTV), whereas successful CAR transfection was detected via an anti-IgG1 antibody. Successive TCR and CAR stainings were performed in a time-course experiment at 4, 8, and 24 h after CAR transfection.

Mock-transfected cells showed no or only few unspecific TCR- or CAR-positive cell populations (Figure 2A,B). The gp100-specific TCR was constantly expressed on lentivirally transduced cells indicated by the similar expression pattern exhibited by TCR T cells and TETARs (Figure 2A and Figure S1). Regarding transient CAR expression, an increase from 4 to 8 h after RNA-electroporation was observed in both CAR T cells and TETARs, with a subsequent decrease of receptor expression at 24 h after transfection (Figure 2A and Figure S1). TETARs revealed expression of both receptors on the cell surface, indicated by a single double-positive population as seen in the dot plots (Figure 2B). Further analysis of transfection efficacy displayed no significant differences in CAR-positive cells when cells engineered with the CAR only were compared to TETARs (Figure 2C and Table S1).

Taken together, these results demonstrate that it is feasible to generate TETARs through additional mRNA-transfection of already lentivirally transduced T cells. In addition, TETARs showed an equal transfection efficacy in comparison to CAR T cells and TCR T cells.

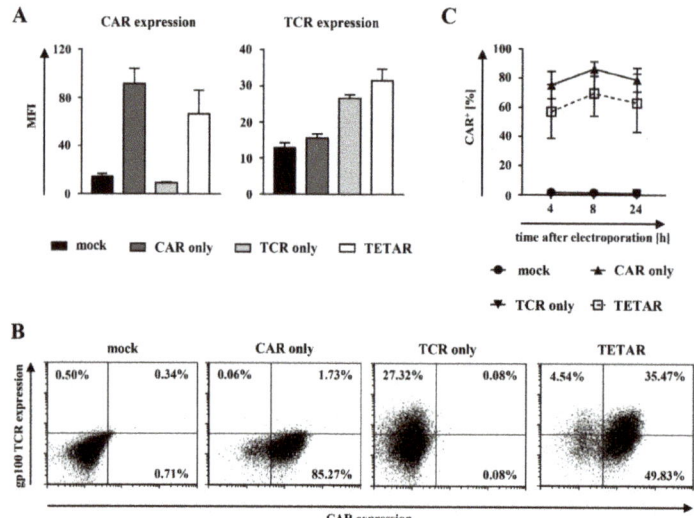

Figure 2. Gp100-specific T cell receptor (TCR) T cells can be additionally equipped with a CSPG4-specific CAR via mRNA electroporation. (**A–C**) CD8$^+$ T cells were lentivirally transduced with a gp100-specific TCR (TCR only) and electroporated with mRNA coding for the CSPG4-specific CAR (TETARs), as indicated. Non-transduced T cells were either transfected without mRNA (mock) or with CSPG4-specific CAR mRNA (CAR only). Mock-transfected cells served as a negative control. (**A,B**) The surface expression of the gp100-specific TCR and the CSPG4-specific CAR at eight hours after electroporation are shown. (**A**) Average geometric mean values of three independent experiments with SEM and (**B**) dot plots of one representative out of three independent experiments are depicted. (**C**) Mean percentages of CAR-positive cells of three independent experiments ± SEM are shown. The *p*-values were calculated by unpaired Student's *t*-test and are listed in Table S1.

2.3. TETARs Antigen-Specifically Secrete Cytokines

In the next step, antigen-specific cytokine production of engineered T cells in response to tumor cells, expressing either one of the antigens or both, was examined. Lentivirally transduced T cells were subsequently electroporated either without mRNA (TCR T cells; TCR only) or with mRNA coding for the CSPG4-specific CAR (TETARs). Non-transduced cells were either transfected without mRNA as a control (mock) or with the CSPG4 CAR mRNA (CAR T cells; CAR only). As target cells, either the human TxB cell hybridoma T2.A1 (HLA-A2$^+$, CSPG4$^-$, gp100$^-$) or the human melanoma cell line A375M (HLA-A2$^+$, CSPG4$^+$, gp100$^-$), both either unpulsed or pulsed with the HLA-A2-restricted peptide gp100$_{280-288}$, were used. At 4 h after electroporation, T cells were co-incubated with target cells to assess cytokine production profiles. The specific tumor necrosis factor (TNF) and interferon-gamma (IFNγ) secretion were calculated by subtracting the number of cytokines produced after stimulation with T2.A1, which served as a negative control target cell line (Figure 3).

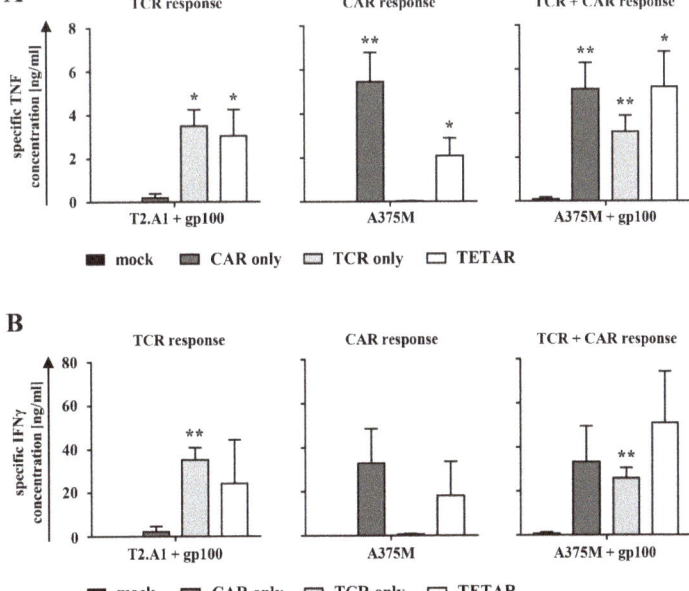

Figure 3. TETARs specifically produced cytokines after antigen encounter. (**A,B**) CD8$^+$ T cells were lentivirally transduced with a gp100-specific TCR (TCR only) and electroporated with mRNA coding for the CSPG4-specific CAR (TETARs). Non-transduced T cells were either transfected without mRNA (mock) or with CSPG4-specific CAR mRNA (CAR only). Mock-transfected cells were used as a negative control. Following overnight stimulation of T cells with either gp100 peptide-loaded or unpulsed T2.A1 (HLA-A2$^+$, CSPG4$^-$, gp100$^-$) and A375M (HLA-A2$^+$, CSPG4$^+$, gp100$^-$) tumor cells, the production of cytokines was measured in a cytometric bead array (CBA). (**A**) Specific secretion of tumor necrosis factor (TNF) and (**B**) interferon-gamma (IFNγ) were calculated by subtracting the number of produced cytokines after co-incubation with unpulsed T2.A1 target cells, which served as a negative control. (**A,B**) Mean values of four independent experiments with SEM are shown. The p-values were calculated by unpaired Student's t-test and are listed in Table S2. ** $p \leq 0.01$, * $p \leq 0.05$.

Mock-electroporated T cells, which served as a negative control, showed no specific TNF or IFNγ secretion following incubation with any of the abovementioned tumor cells (Figure 3). Stimulation with gp100 peptide-loaded T2.A1 cells (expected TCR response only) revealed significantly higher production of TNF by TCR T cells and TETARs compared to mock-transfected cells, whereas no or only little unspecific cytokine expression was observed in CAR T cells (Figure 3A and Table S2). CAR T cells and TETARs exhibited a significant TNF secretion after co-incubation with unpulsed A375M melanoma cells (expected CAR response only) in comparison to mock-electroporated cells, while no cytokine secretion was observed in TCR T cells (Figure 3A and Table S2). Following stimulation with gp100-pulsed A375M cells (expected TCR and CAR response), CAR T cells, TCR T cells, as well as TETARs showed a significant TNF production when compared to mock-transfected cells (Figure 3A and Table S2). IFNγ secretion patterns were similar to that of TNF (Figure 3B and Table S2). Compared to the T cells transfected with only one receptor, TETARs secreted in general lower quantities of cytokines when stimulated with only one of the two antigens (Figure 3). Of note is, however, that TETARs stimulated with both cognate antigens showed at least the same amount of cytokine secretion (TNF) or a trend towards higher secretion (IFNγ) in comparison to T cells engineered with the CAR only or the TCR alone, indicating an additive effect through recognition of both target antigens by the same T cell (Figure 3).

Analysis of the anti-inflammatory cytokine interleukin-4 (IL-4) showed only very low production levels with values below 100 pg/mL in all T cell conditions (Figure S2).

In summary, these results display that TETARs produce significant amounts of pro-inflammatory cytokines after stimulation with target cells expressing either one of the targeted tumor antigens or both.

2.4. TETARs Antigen-Specifically Eliminate Tumor Cells

An important characteristic of tumor-specific T cells is their ability to lyse antigen-positive tumor cells. Thus, for cytotoxicity testing, $CD8^+$ T cells were lentivirally transduced with the gp100-specific TCR and subsequently electroporated either without mRNA (TCR T cells; TCR only) or with mRNA encoding the CSPG4-specific CAR (TETARs). Non-transduced cells were either mock-transfected (mock) and used as a control or electroporated with the CSPG4 CAR mRNA (CAR T cells; CAR only). Receptor-transfected T cells were then analyzed in a standard ^{51}chromium-release assay for their antigen-specific cytotoxicity after incubation with the abovementioned target cells at following effector-to-target cell ratios (E:T): 60:1, 20:1, 6:1, and 2:1.

With decreasing effector-to-target cell ratios, a decline in lysis of target cells was observed, as expected (Figure 4 and Figure S3). All T cell conditions showed no or only little unspecific response after incubation with unpulsed T2.A1 cells, which served as negative control target cells (Figure 4 and Figure S3). Stimulation with gp100-loaded T2.A1 cells (expected TCR response only) revealed a significant lysis by TCR T cells and TETARs, while no or only little unspecific background effect was observed in mock or CAR T cells (Figure 4 and Table S3). Lysis of peptide-pulsed T2.A1 cells by TETARs was, however, in general lower when compared to TCR T cells (Figure 4). Following co-incubation with A375M melanoma cells (expected CAR response only), CAR T cells and TETARs exhibited significant cytolytic capacity after antigen encounter at a 60:1 ratio, whereas only few unspecific effects were observed in the case of mock and TCR T cells (Figure 4 and Table S3). In addition, CAR T cells, TCR T cells, and TETARs showed a significantly higher killing of gp100-pulsed A375M melanoma cells (expected TCR and CAR response) at a 60:1 and 20:1 ratio in comparison to mock-electroporated cells, while cytotoxicity of TETARs was in general lower when compared to TCR T cells (Figure 4 and Table S3).

Altogether, these results show that TETARs specifically kill tumor cells expressing either one of the targeted antigens or both through the equipment with a gp100-specific TCR and a CSPG4-specific CAR.

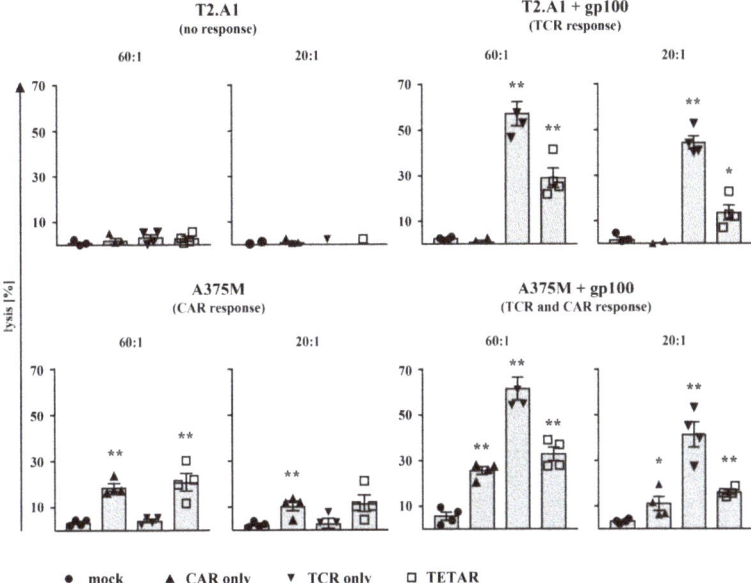

Figure 4. TETARs lyse tumor cells in an antigen-specific manner. CD8$^+$ T cells were lentivirally transduced with a gp100-specific TCR (TCR only) and electroporated with mRNA coding for the CSPG4-specific CAR (TETARs), as indicated. Non-transduced T cells were either transfected without mRNA (mock) or with CSPG4-specific CAR mRNA (CAR only). Mock-transfected cells served as a negative control. One day after electroporation, T cells were co-incubated for 4–6 h with the target cell lines T2.A1 (HLA-A2$^+$, CSPG4$^-$, gp100$^-$) and A375M (HLA-A2$^+$, CSPG4$^+$, gp100$^-$), which were either used unpulsed or loaded with gp100 peptide beforehand. Cytotoxicity of T cells was assessed in a ^{51}chromium-release assay, and the percentages of lysed cells were determined at the effector-to-target ratios (E:T) of 60:1 and 20:1. Average values of four independent experiments, each additionally depicted as an individual symbol, ± SEM are shown. The p-values were calculated by unpaired Student's t-test and are listed in Table S3. ** $p \leq 0.01$, * $p \leq 0.05$.

3. Discussion

To transfer not only one, but simultaneously two different antigen-specific receptors into the same T cell represents a logical consequence to counteract possible immune escape mechanisms, which may be developed by tumor cells under adoptive T cell therapy. TCRs of CD8$^+$ T cells bind to intracellular tumor antigens which upon antigen processing are presented on the cell surface by MHC molecules [17]. In addition, a TCR can also recognize target antigens, which are cross-presented by tumor stromal cells, leading to a more efficient tumor regression [32]. The repertoire of available tumor-specific TCRs has increased in the last decades, as many tumor antigens are expressed intracellularly, and more epitopes have been discovered for the use in adoptive transfer of receptor-transfected cells, especially for the use in solid tumors [33]. CARs consist of an antibody-derived single chain variable fragment (scFv) fused to intracellular domains to provide T cell stimulation [34,35]. A major advantage presented by the use of CARs is their ability to recognize an unprocessed tumor surface antigen independent of MHC restriction and antigen processing [18,19]. The combination of the best of both worlds, the expression of a TCR and a CAR within the same T cell, as well as the combination of stable DNA-based receptor transfer (for receptors which are known to be potent but comparably safe at the same time) and transient RNA-based receptor transfer (for receptors, which are known to be potent, but possibly more dangerous regarding side effects) to generate TETARs, will represent in this context a novel approach in the immunotherapy of cancer, which has yet to be explored.

In our study, it was possible to introduce a gp100-specific TCR into T cells using stable lentiviral transduction, and in addition a second-generation CSPG4-specific CAR into the same T cells by subsequent transient RNA-electroporation. These TETARs were able to secrete cytokines and showed cytotoxicity after stimulation with one of the targeted antigens or both. However, the lytic capacity of TETARs was not as high as that of T cells transfected with the TCR only and unlike in previously reported studies [20,35], no or only little additive or enhanced effect was observed after stimulation with target cells which expressed both target antigens. For further evaluation of a potential benefit of these TETARs, their use in appropriate animal models will be the next important step towards a clinical use in cancer patients.

The approved CD19-directed CAR T cell therapy represents a milestone in cancer immunotherapy for the treatment of therapy-refractory B-cell ALL and diffuse large B-cell lymphoma [6,7]. Patients with a previously poor outcome now have a realistic chance to achieve a complete response and long-term disease remission. However, in a significant number of these patients as well as patients suffering from other types of leukemia and solid tumors, tumor cells are able to develop escape mechanisms under adoptive T cell therapy that lead to resistance and relapse [9–11,14,35,36]. For instance, June and colleagues at the University of Pennsylvania observed that up to 60% of B-cell ALL patients may relapse despite CD19-directed CAR T cell persistence [35]. These patients are characterized by the occurrence of CD19-negative leukemia under therapy, most likely due to potent selective pressure by CD19 CAR T cells [35]. Thus, as a potential strategy to counteract the loss of CD19 on leukemia cells, they generated T cells expressing both a CD19-specific CAR and a CD123-specific CAR [35] using stable lentiviral transfection to transfer both receptors into the same T cell. They observed that these engineered T cells prevented antigen loss relapses and revealed higher T cell activation and enhanced anti-tumor efficacy in a mouse model against B-cell ALL compared to T cells expressing CD19 CAR only, CD123 CAR only, or a pooled combination of both CD19 or CD123 CAR T cell populations [35]. In another study, Slaney et al. introduced two receptors, a Her2/ERBB2-specific CAR and additionally a gp100-specific TCR, into the same T cell [37]. They used a regimen of adoptive cell transfer incorporating vaccination (ACTIV) with recombinant vaccinia virus expressing gp100 to treat a range of tumors including breast tumors and large liver tumors and observed a massive infiltration of T cells into the tumor, resulting in durable complete remission of Her2$^+$ tumors in mice [37].

However, a drawback of CAR T cell therapy is the presence of on-target off-tumor toxicities, depending on the used target antigen [24]. In the approved CD19 CAR T cell therapy, loss of healthy CD19$^+$ cells can be compensated by supplementing intravenous immunoglobulins. The CD123 antigen, for instance, which was used in the above discussed study, is known to be also expressed on non-malignant cells [24]. Thus, although anti-CD123 CAR T cell therapy proved to be efficient for the treatment of acute myeloid leukemia (AML) in a preclinical setting [38,39], its clinical use is impeded due to CD123 expression on healthy stem cells [40]. Furthermore, Her2/ERBB2, which was used by Slaney et al. as the target antigen of their CAR construct [37], is known to be expressed on lung epithelial cells, which might cause fatal side effects [24]. For instance, a patient with colon cancer metastatic to the lungs and liver received Her2/ERBB2-specific CAR T cells [41] and within 15 minutes after cell infusion the patient experienced respiratory distress and displayed a dramatic pulmonary infiltrate on a chest X-ray [41]. Despite intensive medical intervention, the patient died 5 days after treatment [41]. The administered cells most likely localized to the lungs immediately following infusion and were triggered to release cytokines by the recognition of low levels of ERBB2 on lung epithelial cells, which then caused the fatal side effects [41].

A possible strategy to bypass these hurdles and still use the dual-CAR or TCR+CAR expressing T cells by Ruella et al. and Slaney et al. for further clinical development could be the combined DNA- and RNA-based receptor transfer [35,37]. In this context the "safer" receptor, which is lentivirally transduced into the T cells using receptor-encoding DNA (e.g., the CD19 CAR or the gp100 TCR) should have a strong and permanent anti-tumor effect, whereas the "more dangerous" receptor, that is transfected into the same T cell using receptor-encoding RNA (e.g., the CD123 CAR or Her2/ERBB2

CAR), should have an additional "boost" effect at the beginning of the therapy. This could massively increase the pressure on the tumor by enhanced induction of direct tumor-cell killing and rapid on-site T cell expansion and might be an effective and fast way to eradicate large quantities of tumor cells before tumor cells might escape immune recognition.

4. Materials and Methods

4.1. Cells

Blood was collected from healthy donors after informed consent and approval by the institutional review board of the Friedrich-Alexander-University (FAU) of Erlangen-Nürnberg (Reference Number: 65_16 B) had been obtained. First, peripheral blood mononuclear cells (PBMCs) were extracted using density centrifugation via Lymphoprep reagent (Axis-Shield, Oslo, Norway). $CD8^+$ T cells were then obtained via MACS according to manufacturer's instructions (Miltenyi, Bergisch-Gladbach, Germany). Purified T cells were cultured in X-Vivo 15 medium already containing L-glutamine, gentamycin, and phenol red (Biozym Scientific GmbH, Hessisch Oldendorf, Germany). Target cell lines included the TxB cell hybridoma T2.A1 ($HLA-A2^+$, $CSPG4^-$, $gp100^-$ [20]; kind gift from Prof. Dr. Schulz, Nuremberg, Germany) and the melanoma cell line A375M ($HLA-A2^+$, $CSPG4^+$, $gp100^-$ [20]; kind gift from Dr. Aarnoudse, Leiden, Netherlands; ATCC CRL-3223). Prior to co-incubation with T cells, we cultured the target cells in R10 medium (RPMI 1640 (Lonza, Basel, Switzerland) supplemented with 2 mM L-glutamine (Lonza), 100 IU/mL penicillin (Lonza), 100 mg/ml streptomycin (Lonza), 10% (v/v) heat-inactivated fetal calf serum (PAA, GE healthcare, Piscataway, NY, USA), 2 mM HEPES (PAA, GE healthcare, Little Chalfont, UK), and 2 mM β-mercaptoethanol (Gibco, Life Technologies, Carlsbad, CA, USA)). The above-mentioned target cells were additionally pulsed with HLA-A2-restricted peptide $gp100_{280-288}$ (YLEPGPVTA) as previously described [16], where indicated. Peptide-loading was performed in DC-medium (RPMI 1640 (Lonza) supplemented with 1% heat-inactivated human serum (Sigma-Aldrich, Taufkirchen, Germany), 2 mM L-glutamine (Lonza), and 0.04% of 20 mg/L gentamycin (Lonza)).

4.2. Lentiviral Transduction of T Cells

The gp100 TCR α- and β-chains were encoded in a lentiviral vector (pcLV-EF1a-MCS-WPRE) and expressed under control of an EF1a promotor (designed by and purchased from Sirion Biotech, Planegg-Martinsried, Germany). Lentiviral transduction of T cells was performed as follows: After MACS-isolation, T cells were subsequently stimulated with 0.1 µg/mL anti-CD3 antibody OKT-3 (Orthoclone OKT-3; Janssen-Cilag, Neuss, Germany), 0.25 µg/mL anti-CD28 antibody (BD Biosciences, Franklin Lakes, NJ, USA), and 1000 IU/mL interleukin-2 (IL-2) (Proleukin; Novartis, Nuremberg, Germany). Two days later, T cells were lentivirally transduced with a gp100-specific TCR using a multiplicity of infection (MOI) of 10 and the transduction enhancer LentiBOOST™ (consisting of 1000 µg/mL P338 and 10 µg/mL polybrene, Sirion Biotech, Planegg-Martinsried, Germany) together with 1000 IU/mL IL-2 (Novartis) via spinoculation (800 g for 90 min). As a negative control, only IL-2 was added to the cells prior to spinoculation. On the following day, culture medium of T cells was replaced by fresh X-Vivo 15 medium, and 5 ng/mL IL-7 (PeproTech, Rocky Hill, NJ, USA), 5 ng/mL IL-15 (Miltenyi), and 1000 IU/mL IL-2 (Novartis) were added. After three days, T cells were antigen-specifically stimulated with irradiated (140 gray for 6 min) and gp100 peptide-pulsed A375M target cells for one week and subsequently stimulated for another week. Non-transduced cells were re-stimulated with 0.1 µg/mL OKT-3 (Janssen-Cilag), 0.25 µg/mL anti-CD28 antibody (BD Bisosciences, Franklin Lakes, NJ, USA), and 1000 IU/mL (Novartis). New culture medium and IL-2 was added to the cells at day four after each stimulation.

4.3. RNA Production and Transfection

The mMESSAGE mMACHINE T7 Ultra Transcription Kit (Life Technologies, Carlsbad, CA, USA) was used for the generation of mRNA. The mRNA was further purified with the RNeasy Kit (Qiagen, Hilden, Germany) according to manufacturer's instructions. Then, T cells were electroporated with the generated mRNA encoding a CSPG4-specific CAR (MCSP$_{HL}$ CD28-CD3ζ) [42] by the GenePulser Xcell system (Bio-Rad, Hercules, CA, USA) with the square-wave protocol and 500 V for 5 ms, as previously described [43]. Following electroporation, cells were rapidly transferred to X-Vivo 15 medium.

4.4. Receptor Expression Analysis of Engineered T Cells

The goat-F(ab')2 anti-human IgG antibody (Southern Biotech, Birmingham, AL, USA) directed against the extracellular IgG1 CH2-CH3 CAR domain was used to determine the CAR expression on T cells. TCR expression on the cell surface of T cells was analyzed using an MHC Dextramer (HLA-A*0201/YLEPGPVTV; Immudex, Copenhagen, Denmark) directed against the gp100-specific TCR. In addition, the anti-7-AAD antibody (BD Biosciences) was used to exclude nonviable T cells. The detailed procedure of cell surface staining was previously described [44]. Immunofluorescence was measured via the FACS Calibur (BD Biosciences, Heidelberg, Germany), which was equipped with the CellQuest Pro software (BD Biosciences). Data were analyzed using the FCS Express software, version 5 (DeNovo Software, Glendale, CA, USA).

4.5. Cytokine Secretion Analysis of Engineered T Cells

Cytokine production of T cells was analyzed as previously described [45]. In brief, transfected T cells were co-incubated with target cell lines T2.A1 and A375M (either unpulsed or pulsed with the HLA-A2-restricted peptide gp100$_{280-288}$) overnight at a 1:1 effector-to-target cell ratio. Cytokine concentrations of TNF, IFNγ, and IL-4 in the supernatants were measured utilizing the Th1/Th2 Cytometric Bead Array Kit II (BD Biosciences) according to manufacturer's instructions. Immunofluorescence was detected using the FACSCanto II (BD Biosciences) equipped with FACSDiva software (BD Biosciences). Data were analyzed via FCS Express software, version 5 (DeNovo Software).

4.6. Cytotoxicity Analysis of Engineered T Cells

Cytolytic capacity of transfected T cells was assessed with a standard 4–6 h ^{51}chromium-release assay, as previously described [16]. First, target cell lines T2.A1 and A375M were labelled with 20 µCi of Na$_2$^{51}CrO$_4$/10^6 cells (Perkin Elmer, Waltham, MA, USA) for one hour. Subsequently, half of the target cells were pulsed with the HLA-A2-restricted peptide gp100$_{280-288}$ for one hour. Transfected T cells and target cells were co-incubated to obtain the following effector-to-target cell ratios (E:T): 60:1, 20:1, 6:1, and 2:1. Chromium release in supernatants was analyzed with the Wallac 1450 MicroBeta plus Scintillation Counter (Wallac, Turku, Finland). The percentage of lysis was calculated as follows: [(measured release − background release)/(maximum release − background release)] × 100%.

4.7. Figure Preparation and Statistical Analysis

Graphs were created and statistical analysis was performed using GraphPad Prism, version 7 (GraphPad Software, La Jolla, CA, USA). The p-values were analyzed using the unpaired Student's t-test, assuming a Gaussian distribution. * indicates $p \leq 0.05$ and ** indicates $p \leq 0.01$.

5. Conclusions

We have shown here that it is feasible to co-transfect the same T cells with a TCR specific for gp100 and a CAR specific for CSPG4 using a combined DNA- and RNA-based receptor transfer to generate TETARs for the use in adoptive T cell therapy of cancer. These TETARs proved to be functional regarding cytokine secretion and cytolytic activity upon stimulation with each of their cognate antigens. The confirmation that two antigen-specific receptors can be functionally combined using two different methods to introduce each receptor into the same T cell may open up new possibilities and opportunities in cancer immunotherapy, which should be further evaluated in suitable preclinical models towards a potential use in cancer patients.

Supplementary Materials: The following are available online at http://www.mdpi.com/2072-6694/11/5/696/s1, Figure S1: Gp100 TCR and CSPG4 CAR expression of TETARs, Figure S2: Antigen-specific IL-4 production of TETARs, Figure S3: TETARs show antigen-specific cytotoxicity. Table S1: *p*-values corresponding to Figure 2C, Table S2: *p*-values corresponding to Figure 3, Table S3: *p*-values corresponding to Figure 4 and Figure S3.

Author Contributions: B.S. performed the experiments, analyzed and illustrated the data, and wrote the manuscript. D.C.H. provided valuable technical advice for conducting the experiments and participated in data analysis and interpretation. B.S.-T. and G.S. influenced the outline of the experimental study design and critically revised the manuscript. U.U. masterminded the study, planned the experimental setting, participated in the data analysis and interpretation, and critically revised the manuscript. All authors read and approved the final manuscript.

Funding: This study was funded by the ELAN-fonds ("Erlanger Leistungsbezogene Anschubfinanzierung und Nachwuchsförderung") of the IZKF ("Interdisziplinäres Zentrum für Klinische Forschung"), Friedrich-Alexander-Universität Erlangen-Nürnberg (FAU) (DE-18-03-04-1-Uslu).

Acknowledgments: The authors acknowledge the support by the Deutsche Forschungsgemeinschaft and the Friedrich-Alexander-Universität Erlangen-Nürnberg (FAU) within the funding program 'Open Access Publishing'. We want to thank Christian Thirion, Michael Salomon, and Silke Schrödel (Sirion Biotech GmbH, Martinsried, Germany) for technical support regarding lentiviral transduction. We also wish to acknowledge Matthias Peipp and Georg Fey for preliminary work on the CSPG4-specific single chain variable fragment, Reno Debets for the gp100-specific TCR, Kris Thielemans for providing the pGEM4Z RNA-production vector, and Hinrich Abken for the CAR backbone. Finally, we also express our gratitude to the voluntary blood donors and the medical staff for the acquisition of the blood.

Conflicts of Interest: The authors declare no conflict of interest.

References

1. Morgan, R.A.; Dudley, M.E.; Wunderlich, J.R.; Hughes, M.S.; Yang, J.C.; Sherry, R.M.; Royal, R.E.; Topalian, S.L.; Kammula, U.S.; Restifo, N.P.; et al. Cancer regression in patients after transfer of genetically engineered lymphocytes. *Science* **2006**, *314*, 126–129. [CrossRef] [PubMed]
2. Barrett, D.M.; Grupp, S.A.; June, C.H. Chimeric Antigen Receptor- and TCR-Modified T Cells Enter Main Street and Wall Street. *J. Immunol.* **2015**, *195*, 755–761. [CrossRef] [PubMed]
3. Lu, Y.C.; Parker, L.L.; Lu, T.; Zheng, Z.; Toomey, M.A.; White, D.E.; Yao, X.; Li, Y.F.; Robbins, P.F.; Feldman, S.A.; et al. Treatment of Patients with Metastatic Cancer Using a Major Histocompatibility Complex Class II-Restricted T-Cell Receptor Targeting the Cancer Germline Antigen MAGE-A3. *J. Clin. Oncol.* **2017**, *35*, 3322–3329. [CrossRef]
4. June, C.H.; O'Connor, R.S.; Kawalekar, O.U.; Ghassemi, S.; Milone, M.C. CAR T cell immunotherapy for human cancer. *Science* **2018**, *359*, 1361–1365. [CrossRef] [PubMed]
5. Schuster, S.J.; Svoboda, J.; Chong, E.A.; Nasta, S.D.; Mato, A.R.; Anak, O.; Brogdon, J.L.; Pruteanu-Malinici, I.; Bhoj, V.; Landsburg, D.; et al. Chimeric Antigen Receptor T Cells in Refractory B-Cell Lymphomas. *N. Engl. J. Med.* **2017**, *377*, 2545–2554. [CrossRef] [PubMed]
6. Neelapu, S.S.; Locke, F.L.; Bartlett, N.L.; Lekakis, L.J.; Miklos, D.B.; Jacobson, C.A.; Braunschweig, I.; Oluwole, O.O.; Siddiqi, T.; Lin, Y.; et al. Axicabtagene Ciloleucel CAR T-Cell Therapy in Refractory Large B-Cell Lymphoma. *N. Engl. J. Med.* **2017**, *377*, 2531–2544. [CrossRef]
7. Maude, S.L.; Laetsch, T.W.; Buechner, J.; Rives, S.; Boyer, M.; Bittencourt, H.; Bader, P.; Verneris, M.R.; Stefanski, H.E.; Myers, G.D.; et al. Tisagenlecleucel in Children and Young Adults with B-Cell Lymphoblastic Leukemia. *N. Engl. J. Med.* **2018**, *378*, 439–448. [CrossRef]
8. Park, J.H.; Riviere, I.; Gonen, M.; Wang, X.; Senechal, B.; Curran, K.J.; Sauter, C.; Wang, Y.; Santomasso, B.; Mead, E.; et al. Long-Term Follow-up of CD19 CAR Therapy in Acute Lymphoblastic Leukemia. *N. Engl. J. Med.* **2018**, *378*, 449–459. [CrossRef]
9. Olson, B.M.; McNeel, D.G. Antigen loss and tumor-mediated immunosuppression facilitate tumor recurrence. *Expert Rev. Vaccines* **2012**, *11*, 1315–1317. [CrossRef]
10. Poggi, A.; Musso, A.; Dapino, I.; Zocchi, M.R. Mechanisms of tumor escape from immune system: Role of mesenchymal stromal cells. *Immunol. Lett.* **2014**, *159*, 55–72. [CrossRef] [PubMed]

11. Guedan, S.; Ruella, M.; June, C.H. Emerging Cellular Therapies for Cancer. *Annu. Rev. Immunol.* **2018**. [CrossRef]
12. Hammerl, D.; Rieder, D.; Martens, J.W.M.; Trajanoski, Z.; Debets, R. Adoptive T Cell Therapy: New Avenues Leading to Safe Targets and Powerful Allies. *Trends Immunol.* **2018**, *39*, 921–936. [CrossRef]
13. Castellarin, M.; Watanabe, K.; June, C.H.; Kloss, C.C.; Posey, A.D., Jr. Driving cars to the clinic for solid tumors. *Gene Ther.* **2018**. [CrossRef]
14. Simon, B.; Uslu, U. CAR-T cell therapy in melanoma: A future success story? *Exp. Dermatol.* **2018**, *27*, 1315–1321. [CrossRef] [PubMed]
15. Hofmann, C.; Hofflin, S.; Huckelhoven, A.; Bergmann, S.; Harrer, E.; Schuler, G.; Dorrie, J.; Schaft, N.; Harrer, T. Human T cells expressing two additional receptors (TETARs) specific for HIV-1 recognize both epitopes. *Blood* **2011**, *118*, 5174–5177. [CrossRef] [PubMed]
16. Hofflin, S.; Prommersberger, S.; Uslu, U.; Schuler, G.; Schmidt, C.W.; Lennerz, V.; Dorrie, J.; Schaft, N. Generation of CD8(+) T cells expressing two additional T-cell receptors (TETARs) for personalised melanoma therapy. *Cancer Biol. Ther.* **2015**, *16*, 1323–1331. [CrossRef] [PubMed]
17. Davis, M.M.; Bjorkman, P.J. T-cell antigen receptor genes and T-cell recognition. *Nature* **1988**, *334*, 395–402. [CrossRef] [PubMed]
18. Gross, G.; Waks, T.; Eshhar, Z. Expression of immunoglobulin-T-cell receptor chimeric molecules as functional receptors with antibody-type specificity. *Proc. Natl. Acad. Sci. USA* **1989**, *86*, 10024–10028. [CrossRef]
19. Hombach, A.; Sent, D.; Schneider, C.; Heuser, C.; Koch, D.; Pohl, C.; Seliger, B.; Abken, H. T-cell activation by recombinant receptors: CD28 costimulation is required for interleukin 2 secretion and receptor-mediated T-cell proliferation but does not affect receptor-mediated target cell lysis. *Cancer Res.* **2001**, *61*, 1976–1982. [PubMed]
20. Uslu, U.; Schuler, G.; Dorrie, J.; Schaft, N. Combining a chimeric antigen receptor and a conventional T-cell receptor to generate T cells expressing two additional receptors (TETARs) for a multi-hit immunotherapy of melanoma. *Exp. Dermatol.* **2016**, *25*, 872–879. [CrossRef]
21. Schaft, N.; Dorrie, J.; Muller, I.; Beck, V.; Baumann, S.; Schunder, T.; Kampgen, E.; Schuler, G. A new way to generate cytolytic tumor-specific T cells: Electroporation of RNA coding for a T cell receptor into T lymphocytes. *Cancer Immunol. Immunother.* **2006**, *55*, 1132–1141. [CrossRef] [PubMed]
22. Zhao, Y.; Moon, E.; Carpenito, C.; Paulos, C.M.; Liu, X.; Brennan, A.L.; Chew, A.; Carroll, R.G.; Scholler, J.; Levine, B.L.; et al. Multiple injections of electroporated autologous T cells expressing a chimeric antigen receptor mediate regression of human disseminated tumor. *Cancer Res.* **2010**, *70*, 9053–9061. [CrossRef]
23. Riet, T.; Holzinger, A.; Dorrie, J.; Schaft, N.; Schuler, G.; Abken, H. Nonviral RNA transfection to transiently modify T cells with chimeric antigen receptors for adoptive therapy. *Methods Mol. Biol.* **2013**, *969*, 187–201. [PubMed]
24. Bedoya, F.; Frigault, M.J.; Maus, M.V. The Flipside of the Power of Engineered T Cells: Observed and Potential Toxicities of Genetically Modified T Cells as Therapy. *Mol. Ther.* **2017**, *25*, 314–320. [CrossRef] [PubMed]
25. Campoli, M.R.; Chang, C.C.; Kageshita, T.; Wang, X.; McCarthy, J.B.; Ferrone, S. Human high molecular weight-melanoma-associated antigen (HMW-MAA): A melanoma cell surface chondroitin sulfate proteoglycan (MSCP) with biological and clinical significance. *Crit. Rev. Immunol.* **2004**, *24*, 267–296. [CrossRef]
26. Chekenya, M.; Rooprai, H.K.; Davies, D.; Levine, J.M.; Butt, A.M.; Pilkington, G.J. The NG2 chondroitin sulfate proteoglycan: Role in malignant progression of human brain tumours. *Int. J. Dev. Neurosci.* **1999**, *17*, 421–435. [CrossRef]
27. Godal, A.; Bruland, O.; Haug, E.; Aas, M.; Fodstad, O. Unexpected expression of the 250 kD melanoma-associated antigen in human sarcoma cells. *Br. J. Cancer* **1986**, *53*, 839–841. [CrossRef]
28. Ferrone, S.; Chen, Z.J.; Liu, C.C.; Hirai, S.; Kageshita, T.; Mittelman, A. Human high molecular weight-melanoma associated antigen mimicry by mouse anti-idiotypic monoclonal antibodies MK2-23. Experimental studies and clinical trials in patients with malignant melanoma. *Pharmacol. Ther.* **1993**, *57*, 259–290. [CrossRef]
29. Schlingemann, R.O.; Rietveld, F.J.; de Waal, R.M.; Ferrone, S.; Ruiter, D.J. Expression of the high molecular weight melanoma-associated antigen by pericytes during angiogenesis in tumors and in healing wounds. *Am. J. Pathol.* **1990**, *136*, 1393–1405. [PubMed]
30. Watt, B.; van Niel, G.; Raposo, G.; Marks, M.S. PMEL: A pigment cell-specific model for functional amyloid formation. *Pigment Cell Melanoma Res.* **2013**, *26*, 300–315. [CrossRef]

31. Johnson, L.A.; Morgan, R.A.; Dudley, M.E.; Cassard, L.; Yang, J.C.; Hughes, M.S.; Kammula, U.S.; Royal, R.E.; Sherry, R.M.; Wunderlich, J.R.; et al. Gene therapy with human and mouse T-cell receptors mediates cancer regression and targets normal tissues expressing cognate antigen. *Blood* **2009**, *114*, 535–546. [CrossRef]
32. Spiotto, M.T.; Yu, P.; Rowley, D.A.; Nishimura, M.I.; Meredith, S.C.; Gajewski, T.F.; Fu, Y.X.; Schreiber, H. Increasing tumor antigen expression overcomes "ignorance" to solid tumors via crosspresentation by bone marrow-derived stromal cells. *Immunity* **2002**, *17*, 737–747. [CrossRef]
33. June, C.H.; Maus, M.V.; Plesa, G.; Johnson, L.A.; Zhao, Y.; Levine, B.L.; Grupp, S.A.; Porter, D.L. Engineered T cells for cancer therapy. *Cancer Immunol. Immunother.* **2014**, *63*, 969–975. [CrossRef]
34. Boyiadzis, M.M.; Dhodapkar, M.V.; Brentjens, R.J.; Kochenderfer, J.N.; Neelapu, S.S.; Maus, M.V.; Porter, D.L.; Maloney, D.G.; Grupp, S.A.; Mackall, C.L.; et al. Chimeric antigen receptor (CAR) T therapies for the treatment of hematologic malignancies: Clinical perspective and significance. *J. Immunother. Cancer* **2018**, *6*, 137. [CrossRef] [PubMed]
35. Ruella, M.; Barrett, D.M.; Kenderian, S.S.; Shestova, O.; Hofmann, T.J.; Perazzelli, J.; Klichinsky, M.; Aikawa, V.; Nazimuddin, F.; Kozlowski, M.; et al. Dual CD19 and CD123 targeting prevents antigen-loss relapses after CD19-directed immunotherapies. *J. Clin. Investig.* **2016**, *126*, 3814–3826. [CrossRef] [PubMed]
36. Hegde, M.; Corder, A.; Chow, K.K.; Mukherjee, M.; Ashoori, A.; Kew, Y.; Zhang, Y.J.; Baskin, D.S.; Merchant, F.A.; Brawley, V.S.; et al. Combinational targeting offsets antigen escape and enhances effector functions of adoptively transferred T cells in glioblastoma. *Mol. Ther.* **2013**, *21*, 2087–2101. [CrossRef]
37. Slaney, C.Y.; von Scheidt, B.; Davenport, A.J.; Beavis, P.A.; Westwood, J.A.; Mardiana, S.; Tscharke, D.C.; Ellis, S.; Prince, H.M.; Trapani, J.A.; et al. Dual-specific Chimeric Antigen Receptor T Cells and an Indirect Vaccine Eradicate a Variety of Large Solid Tumors in an Immunocompetent, Self-antigen Setting. *Clin. Cancer Res.* **2017**, *23*, 2478–2490. [CrossRef]
38. Gill, S.; Tasian, S.K.; Ruella, M.; Shestova, O.; Li, Y.; Porter, D.L.; Carroll, M.; Danet-Desnoyers, G.; Scholler, J.; Grupp, S.A.; et al. Preclinical targeting of human acute myeloid leukemia and myeloablation using chimeric antigen receptor-modified T cells. *Blood* **2014**, *123*, 2343–2354. [CrossRef] [PubMed]
39. Tasian, S.K.; Kenderian, S.S.; Shen, F.; Ruella, M.; Shestova, O.; Kozlowski, M.; Li, Y.; Schrank-Hacker, A.; Morrissette, J.J.D.; Carroll, M.; et al. Optimized depletion of chimeric antigen receptor T cells in murine xenograft models of human acute myeloid leukemia. *Blood* **2017**, *129*, 2395–2407. [CrossRef]
40. Taussig, D.C.; Pearce, D.J.; Simpson, C.; Rohatiner, A.Z.; Lister, T.A.; Kelly, G.; Luongo, J.L.; Danet-Desnoyers, G.A.; Bonnet, D. Hematopoietic stem cells express multiple myeloid markers: Implications for the origin and targeted therapy of acute myeloid leukemia. *Blood* **2005**, *106*, 4086–4092. [CrossRef] [PubMed]
41. Morgan, R.A.; Yang, J.C.; Kitano, M.; Dudley, M.E.; Laurencot, C.M.; Rosenberg, S.A. Case report of a serious adverse event following the administration of T cells transduced with a chimeric antigen receptor recognizing ERBB2. *Mol. Ther.* **2010**, *18*, 843–851. [CrossRef] [PubMed]
42. Krug, C.; Birkholz, K.; Paulus, A.; Schwenkert, M.; Schmidt, P.; Hoffmann, N.; Hombach, A.; Fey, G.; Abken, H.; Schuler, G.; et al. Stability and activity of MCSP-specific chimeric antigen receptors (CARs) depend on the scFv antigen-binding domain and the protein backbone. *Cancer Immunol. Immunother.* **2015**, *64*, 1623–1635. [CrossRef] [PubMed]
43. Simon, B.; Harrer, D.C.; Schuler-Thurner, B.; Schaft, N.; Schuler, G.; Dorrie, J.; Uslu, U. The siRNA-mediated downregulation of PD-1 alone or simultaneously with CTLA-4 shows enhanced in-vitro CAR-T cell functionality for further clinical development towards the potential use in immunotherapy of melanoma. *Exp. Dermatol.* **2018**, *27*, 769–778. [CrossRef] [PubMed]
44. Schaft, N.; Dorrie, J.; Thumann, P.; Beck, V.E.; Muller, I.; Schultz, E.S.; Kampgen, E.; Dieckmann, D.; Schuler, G. Generation of an optimized polyvalent monocyte-derived dendritic cell vaccine by transfecting defined RNAs after rather than before maturation. *J. Immunol.* **2005**, *174*, 3087–3097. [CrossRef] [PubMed]
45. Simon, B.; Wiesinger, M.; Marz, J.; Wistuba-Hamprecht, K.; Weide, B.; Schuler-Thurner, B.; Schuler, G.; Dorrie, J.; Uslu, U. The Generation of CAR-Transfected Natural Killer T Cells for the Immunotherapy of Melanoma. *Int. J. Mol. Sci.* **2018**, *19*, 2365. [CrossRef] [PubMed]

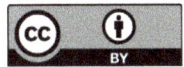

© 2019 by the authors. Licensee MDPI, Basel, Switzerland. This article is an open access article distributed under the terms and conditions of the Creative Commons Attribution (CC BY) license (http://creativecommons.org/licenses/by/4.0/).

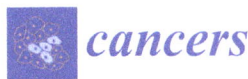

Article

Hypoxia Selectively Impairs CAR-T Cells In Vitro

Robert Berahovich [1], Xianghong Liu [1], Hua Zhou [1], Elias Tsadik [1], Shirley Xu [1], Vita Golubovskaya [1,2,*] and Lijun Wu [1,*]

1. ProMab Biotechnologies, 2600 Hilltop Drive, Richmond, CA 94806, USA; robert.berahovich@promab.com (R.B.); Xianghong.liu@promab.com (X.L.); hua.zhou@promab.com (H.Z.); elias.tsadik@promab.com (E.T.); shirley.xu@promab.com (S.X.)
2. Department of Medicine, University of Oklahoma, Health Sciences Center, Oklahoma City, OK 73104, USA
* Correspondence: vita.gol@promab.com (V.G.); john@promab.com (L.W.); Tel.: +1-510-974-0687 (V.G.); +1-866-339-0871 (L.W.)

Received: 4 March 2019; Accepted: 26 April 2019; Published: 30 April 2019

Abstract: Hypoxia is a major characteristic of the solid tumor microenvironment. To understand how chimeric antigen receptor-T cells (CAR-T cells) function in hypoxic conditions, we characterized CD19-specific and BCMA-specific human CAR-T cells generated in atmospheric (18% oxygen) and hypoxic (1% oxygen) culture for expansion, differentiation status, and CD4:CD8 ratio. CAR-T cells expanded to a much lower extent in 1% oxygen than in 18% oxygen. Hypoxic CAR-T cells also had a less differentiated phenotype and a higher CD4:CD8 ratio than atmospheric CAR-T cells. CAR-T cells were then added to antigen-positive and antigen-negative tumor cell lines at the same or lower oxygen level and characterized for cytotoxicity, cytokine and granzyme B secretion, and PD-1 upregulation. Atmospheric and hypoxic CAR-T cells exhibited comparable cytolytic activity and PD-1 upregulation; however, cytokine production and granzyme B release were greatly decreased in 1% oxygen, even when the CAR-T cells were generated in atmospheric culture. Together, these data show that at solid tumor oxygen levels, CAR-T cells are impaired in expansion, differentiation and cytokine production. These effects may contribute to the inability of CAR-T cells to eradicate solid tumors seen in many patients.

Keywords: CAR-T; hypoxia; tumor; microenvironment; CD19; BCMA; immunotherapy

1. Introduction

Autologous chimeric antigen receptor (CAR) T cells specific for CD19 provide a substantial therapeutic benefit for a large percentage of patients with B cell leukemias and lymphomas [1–3]. Two types of CD19-specific CAR-T cells, tisagenlecleucel (Kymriah) and axicabtagene ciloleucel (Yescarta), have been approved for clinical use by the FDA [4]. Unlike B cell-specific CAR-T cells, CAR-T cells specific for antigens on solid tumors have to overcome multiple immunosuppressive mechanisms intrinsic to the tumor microenvironment [5–8]. Solid tumors are hypoxic (1% oxygen or less), contain high levels of soluble factors like TGF-β that directly inhibit T cell function [9,10], contain immunosuppressive myeloid cells and regulatory T cells [11,12], and express ligands for checkpoint proteins like PD-1 that down-regulate T cell function [13,14]. Each of these mechanisms have been studied using tumor-specific T cells, but little is known about how these mechanisms affect CAR-T cells.

Hypoxia is also present in bone marrow hematopoietic niches where B lineage cells reside [15]. Therefore, in this study, we analyzed the effects of hypoxia on CD19 CAR-T cells [16,17] and B cell maturation antigen (BCMA) CAR-T cells in vitro [18]. We generated CD19 and BCMA CAR-T cells at atmospheric (18%) and hypoxic (1%) oxygen levels, and characterized the cells for expansion, CAR expression, CD4:CD8 ratio and differentiation status. We then cultured the CAR-T cells with antigen-positive and antigen-negative tumor cells at the same or lower oxygen level, and measured

CAR-T cell cytotoxicity, cytokine production and PD-1 upregulation. The data show that both CD19 and BCMA CAR-T cells are not impaired by hypoxia with regards to CAR expression, cytotoxicity or PD-1 expression. However, hypoxia reduces CAR-T cell expansion and differentiation, increases the CD4:CD8 ratio, and substantially reduces cytokine and granzyme B production. These data are critical for the development of next-generation CAR-T cells against tumors with hypoxic microenvironments.

2. Results

2.1. Hypoxia Greatly Decreases CAR-T Cell Expansion

To determine the effects of hypoxia on CAR-T cell expansion, CD19 CAR-T cells and BCMA CAR-T cells were transferred into a chamber continually maintaining an oxygen level of 1% on day 5 of the expansion period. The hypoxia chamber was placed inside a tissue culture incubator (humidified, with 5% carbon dioxide), and cell expansion was monitored for another eight days. As shown in Figure 1, hypoxia greatly diminished the expansion of both CAR-T cells and control (non-transduced) T cells.

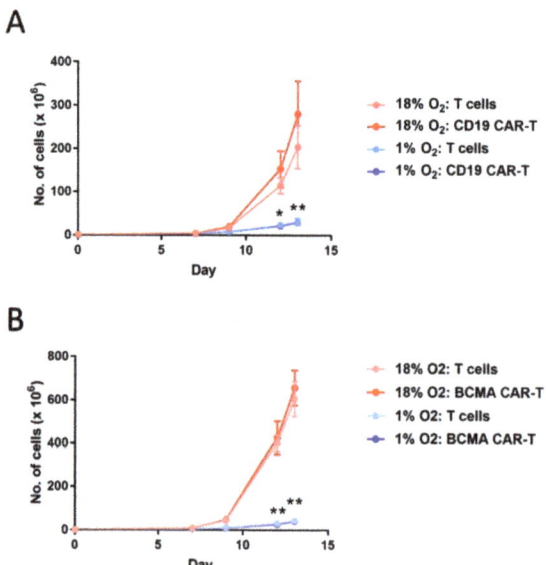

Figure 1. Hypoxia decreases chimeric antigen receptor-T cell (CAR-T cell) expansion. CD19 CAR-T cells (**A**) and B cell maturation antigen (BCMA) CAR-T cells (**B**), along with control T cells, were cultured in an 18% oxygen incubator for the entire 13-day expansion period (red lines), or were cultured in the 18% oxygen incubator for the first 5 days and then in a hypoxia chamber for the remaining 8 days (blue lines). Data-points represent the average and standard error of 4 separate experiments. * $p = 0.02$ (day 12) and ** $p < 0.001$ (day 13) for hypoxic vs. atmospheric CD19 CAR-T cells. ** $p < 0.001$ for hypoxic vs. atmospheric BCMA CAR-T cells.

2.2. Hypoxia Does Not Affect CAR-T Cell Frequency

The cells were analyzed by flow cytometry on days 8 and 13 of the expansion period for CAR expression. CD19 CAR-T cells were detected with an anti-FLAG antibody, whereas BCMA CAR-T cells were detected with BCMA protein. As shown in Figure 2, hypoxia did not affect the percentage of cells that expressed the CAR (i.e., the CAR-T cell frequency).

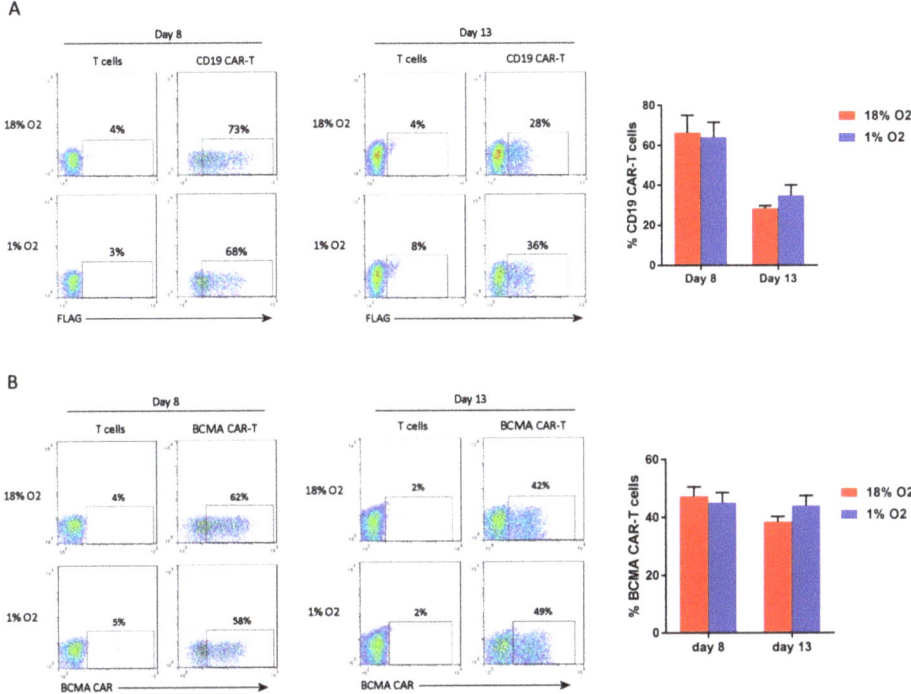

Figure 2. Hypoxia does not affect CAR-T cell frequency. CD19 CAR-T cells (**A**) and BCMA CAR-T cells (**B**) were stained with an anti-FLAG antibody or BCMA protein, respectively. Representative flow cytometry plots showing CAR expression on the X-axis (the Y-axis is an empty channel) are on the left. Charts showing the average and standard error of 4 separate experiments are shown on the right.

2.3. Hypoxia Inhibits CAR-T Cell Differentiation

The cells were analyzed by flow cytometry on day 13 of the expansion period for T cell differentiation subsets. Antibodies specific for CD27 and CD45RO were used, as they discriminate the 4 primary subsets (from least to most differentiated): naïve T cells (Tn, CD27$^+$CD45RO$^-$), central memory T cells (Tcm, CD27$^+$CD45RO$^+$), effector memory T cells (Tem, CD27$^-$CD45RO$^+$), and effector T cells (Teff, CD27$^-$CD45RO$^-$). The FLAG antibody or BCMA protein was included, to identify the CD19 CAR-T cells or BCMA CAR-T cells, respectively (see Figure S1 for the gating strategy). As shown in Figure 3, all of the CAR-T cells and control T cells, in both the 18% oxygen culture and 1% oxygen culture, were memory T cells (CD45RO$^+$). Hypoxia caused an increase in the frequency of central memory cells (CD27$^+$) in the control T cell cultures and the BCMA CAR-T cell culture, and showed a trend towards doing the same in the CD19 CAR-T cell culture (Figure 3). Hence, the differentiation of Tcm cells into Tem cells was largely impaired in the hypoxic cultures.

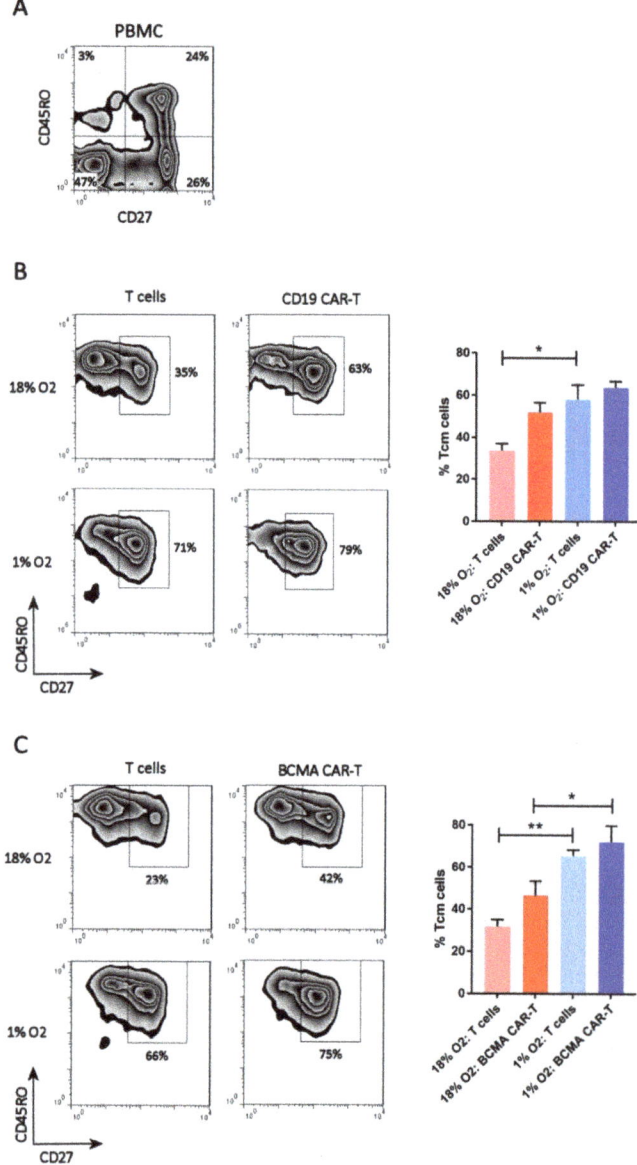

Figure 3. Hypoxia inhibits CAR-T cell differentiation. PBMC (**A**), CD19 CAR-T cells (**B**) and BCMA CAR-T cells (**C**) were stained with antibodies for CD27 and CD45RO. CAR-T cells were first gated using the anti-FLAG antibody or BCMA protein. Representative flow cytometry plots showing CD27 and CD45RO expression are on the left; the CAR-T plots show only the gated CAR-T cells. Charts showing the average and standard error of 4 separate experiments are shown on the right. * $p < 0.05$ and ** $p < 0.005$.

2.4. Hypoxia Increases the CAR-T Cell CD4:CD8 Ratio

The cells were analyzed on day 13 for the ratio of CD4 T cells to CD8 T cells. In normal human PBMC, this ratio is typically 2:1. The FLAG antibody or BCMA protein was included in the staining, to gate on the CD19 CAR-T cells or BCMA CAR-T cells, respectively. As shown in Figure 4, the CD4:CD8 ratio of atmospheric T cells was approximately 2.5:1, whereas the CD4:CD8 ratio of atmospheric CAR-T cells was approximately 5:1. In contrast, the CD4:CD8 ratio of hypoxic T cells was 5:1 and the CD4:CD8 ratio of hypoxic CAR-T cells was 8.6:1 (BCMA CAR-T cells) or 11:1 (CD19 CAR-T cells). Hence, hypoxia increased the CD4:CD8 ratio of both CD19 and BCMA CAR-T cells, and the CAR-T cells themselves had a higher CD4:CD8 ratio than non-transduced T cells.

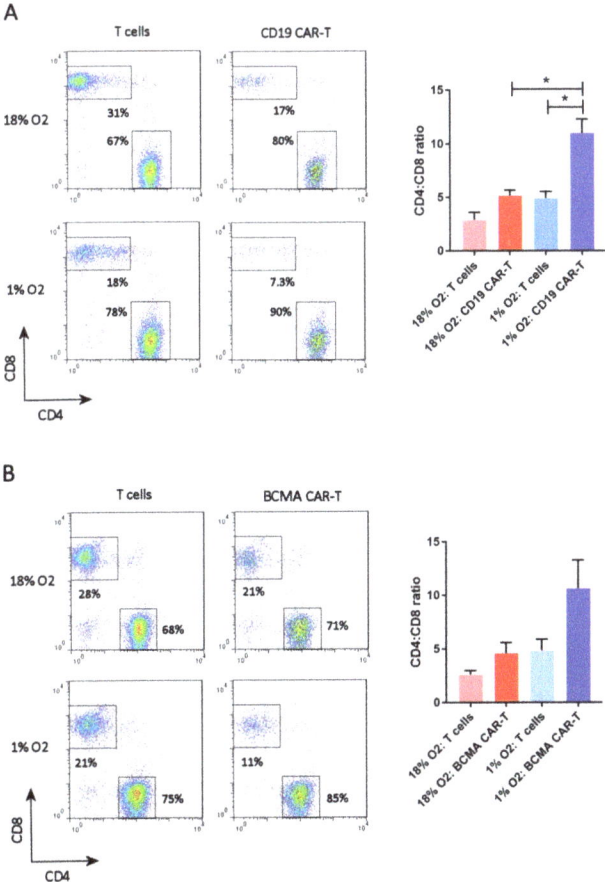

Figure 4. Hypoxia increases the CD4:CD8 ratio. CD19 CAR-T cells (**A**) and BCMA CAR-T cells (**B**) were stained with antibodies for CD27 and CD45RO, along with the anti-FLAG antibody or BCMA protein. Representative flow cytometry plots showing CD27 and CD45RO expression are on the left; the CAR-T plots show only the gated CAR-T cells. Charts showing the average and standard error of 4 separate experiments are shown on the right. * $p = < 0.05$.

2.5. Hypoxia Does Not Affect CAR-T Cell Cytotoxicity

The cytolytic activity of the cells was evaluated on day 13 using a real-time cellular analysis (RTCA) assay. In this assay, the effector cells (CAR-T cells or control T cells) are added to a monolayer of antigen-positive or antigen-negative target cells and the integrity of the monolayer—determined by its impedance in an electrical field—is monitored over time. If the effector cells kill the target cells, the impedance of the monolayer decreases. As shown in Figure 5, both CD19 CAR-T cells and BCMA CAR-T cells killed cell lines stably expressing CD19 and BCMA, respectively, to a significantly greater extent than the control T cells. In the parental cell lines, the CAR-T cells exhibited cytotoxicity comparable to the control T cells. This CAR-independent cytotoxicity is likely an allogeneic phenomenon, since the effector cells and target cells are not HLA-matched, and does not produce cytokines like IFNγ and IL-2. CAR-mediated cytotoxicity did not differ significantly between the three conditions tested: (1) Atmospheric CAR-T cells mixed with atmospheric target cells, (2) atmospheric CAR-T cells mixed with hypoxic target cells in the hypoxia chamber, and (3) hypoxic CAR-T cells mixed with hypoxic target cells in the hypoxia chamber (Figure 5).

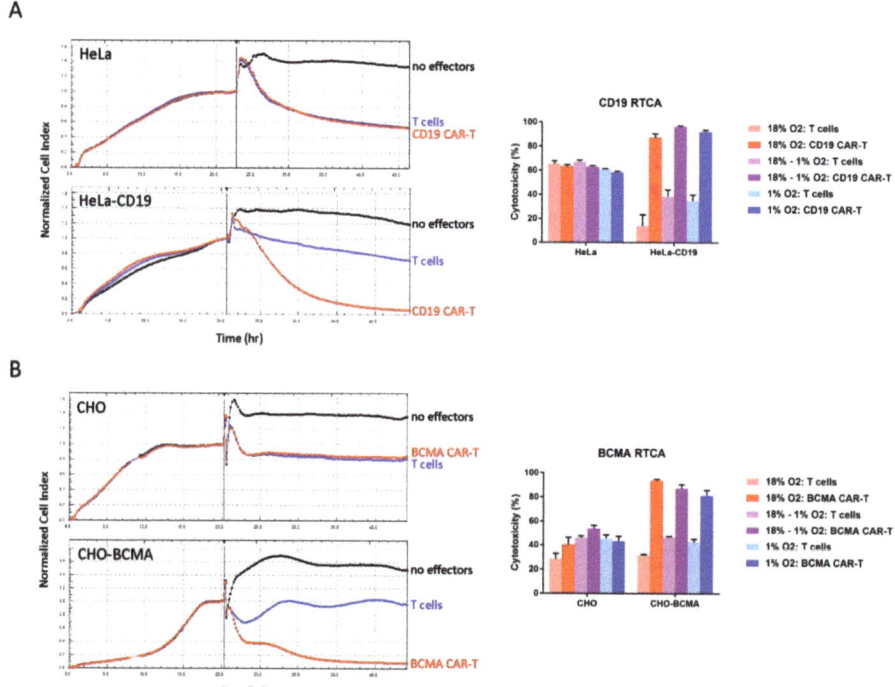

Figure 5. Hypoxia does not affect CAR-T cell cytotoxicity. (**A**) CD19 CAR-T cell RTCA assay. (**B**) BCMA CAR-T cell RTCA assay. Left: HeLa, HeLa-CD19, CHO, and CHO-BCMA cells were monitored overnight as they adhered to the plate and formed a monolayer. The next day, atmospheric CD19 CAR-T cells, BCMA CAR-T cells or control T cells were added to the monolayers at an E:T ratio of 10:1 (vertical bars). The cultures were monitored for approximately 24 more hours. Traces show the average of 3 wells. Right: Cytotoxicity in the RTCA assays was calculated at the end of the assays. Data-points represent the average and standard error of 4 separate experiments.

2.6. Hypoxia Decreases CAR-T Cell Granzyme B and Cytokine Production in Response to Transfected Cell Lines

The cell culture media from the RTCA assays was analyzed for the levels of the serine protease granzyme B and the cytokines IFN-γ, IL-2 and IL-6. In most cases, the levels of all 4 analytes were substantially decreased when the RTCA assay was performed in 1% oxygen compared to 18% oxygen, regardless of whether the CAR-T cells were originally expanded in 18% oxygen or 1% oxygen (Figure 6). BCMA CAR-T cell production of IL-2 did not follow this pattern, as atmospheric cells cultured in either

18% oxygen or 1% oxygen produced low IL-2 levels and hypoxic cells produced 2.5-fold higher levels. BCMA CAR-T cells produced extremely low levels of IL-6 regardless of oxygen level.

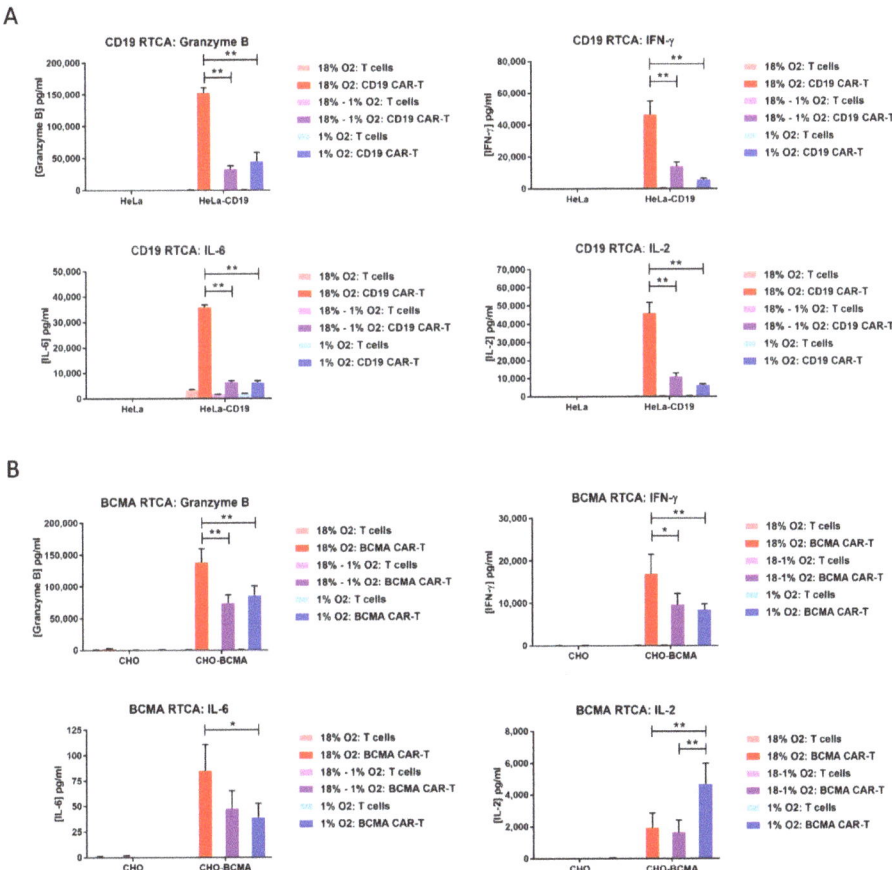

Figure 6. Hypoxia decreases CAR-T cell granzyme B and cytokine production. The media from the CD19 RTCA assay (**A**) and BCMA RTCA assay (**B**) was analyzed by ELISA for the levels of granzyme B, IFN-γ, IL-2 and IL-6. Data-points represent the average and standard error of 2–4 separate experiments. * $p < 0.05$ and ** $p < 0.005$.

2.7. Hypoxia Decreases CAR-T Cell Granzyme B and Cytokine Production in Response to Tumor Cells

On day 12 of the expansion period, the CAR-T cells or control T cells were co-cultured overnight at a 10:1 E:T ratio with hematopoietic cell lines endogenously expressing or lacking CD19 or BCMA. CD19 CAR-T cells were cultured with B lymphoma Raji cells, which express CD19, or with myelogenous leukemia K562 cells, which do not express CD19. BCMA CAR-T cells were cultured with multiple myeloma RPMI8226 cells or MM1S cells, both of which express BCMA, or with K562 cells, which do not express BCMA. As before, three conditions were tested: (1) Atmospheric CAR-T cells mixed with atmospheric tumor cells in the normal incubator, (2) atmospheric CAR-T cells mixed with hypoxic tumor cells in the hypoxia chamber, and (3) hypoxic CAR-T cells mixed with hypoxic tumor cells in the hypoxia chamber. The next day, the medium in the co-cultures was assayed for the levels of granzyme B, IFN-γ, IL-2, and IL-6. For both CD19 CAR-T cells and BCMA CAR-T cells, the levels of granzyme B, IFN-γ and IL-6 were lower in the co-cultures incubated at 1% oxygen than the co-cultures incubated at

18% oxygen, regardless of whether the CAR-T cells were originally atmospheric or hypoxic (Figure 7). This was also true for IL-2 production by CD19 CAR-T cells, but not BCMA CAR-T cells. Hypoxic BCMA CAR-T cells produced low levels of IL-2, whereas atmospheric BCMA CAR-T cells produced very low levels of IL-2. Both CD19 CAR-T cells and BCMA CAR-T cells produced very low levels of IL-6.

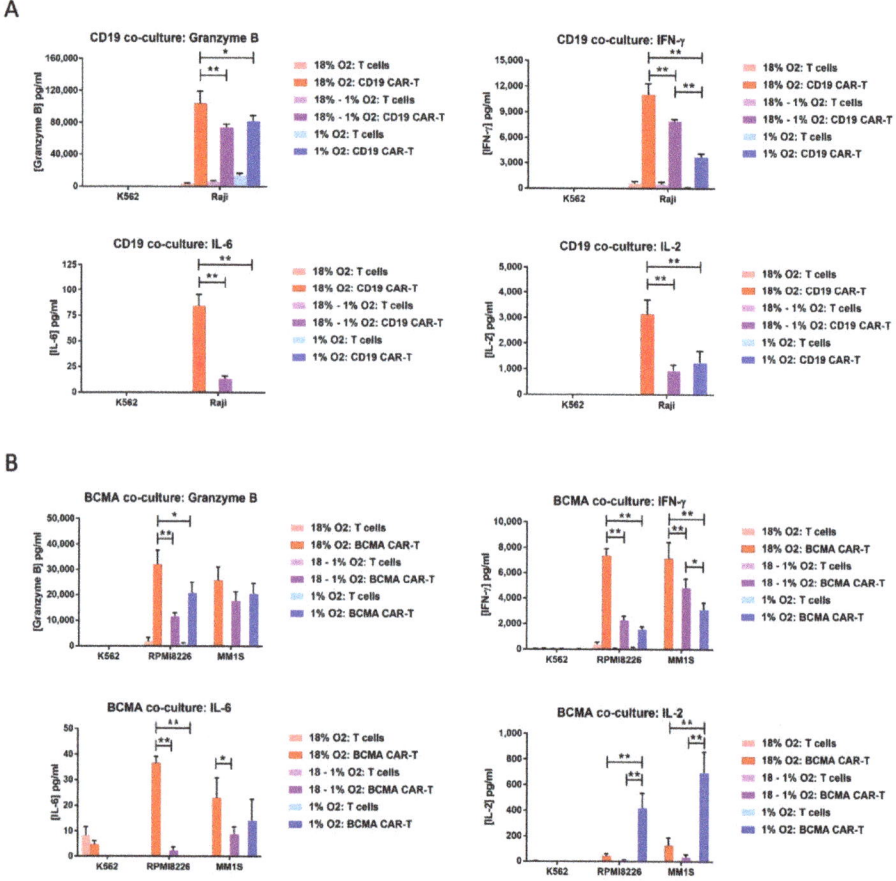

Figure 7. Hypoxia decreases CAR-T cell granzyme B and cytokine production in response to tumor cells. CD19 CAR-T cells or control T cells (**A**) were co-cultured with CD19$^+$ Raji cells or CD19$^-$ K562 cells. BCMA CAR-T cells or control T cells (**B**) were cultured with BCMA$^+$ RPMI8226 cells, BCMA$^+$ MM1S cells or BCMA$^-$ K562 cells. The medium from the co-cultures was analyzed by ELISA for the levels of granzyme B, IFN-γ, IL-2, and IL-6. Data-points represent the average and standard error of 2-4 separate experiments. * $p < 0.05$ and ** $p < 0.005$.

2.8. Hypoxia Does Not Affect CAR-T Cell PD-1 Upregulation

Since T cells upregulate PD-1 upon tumor cell recognition, we wanted to know whether PD-1 upregulation is altered in hypoxic settings; if hypoxia amplifies PD-1 upregulation, higher levels of checkpoint protein inhibitors like Kymriah might be required for activity in solid tumors. Therefore, the cells from the co-cultures were analyzed by flow cytometry for expression of PD-1. The FLAG antibody or BCMA protein was included in the staining, to gate on the CD19 CAR-T cells or BCMA CAR-T cells, respectively. As shown in Figure 8, PD-1 was expressed on a significantly higher percentage of

CAR-T cells than control T cells when the cells were co-cultured with antigen-positive tumor cells (Raji, MM1S or RPMI8226). In contrast, PD-1 expression was comparable between CAR-T cells and control T cells when the cells were cultured with antigen-negative K562 cells. Importantly, the frequency of antigen-mediated PD-1 upregulation on CAR-T cells was not affected by the level of oxygen during the expansion period or during the co-culture.

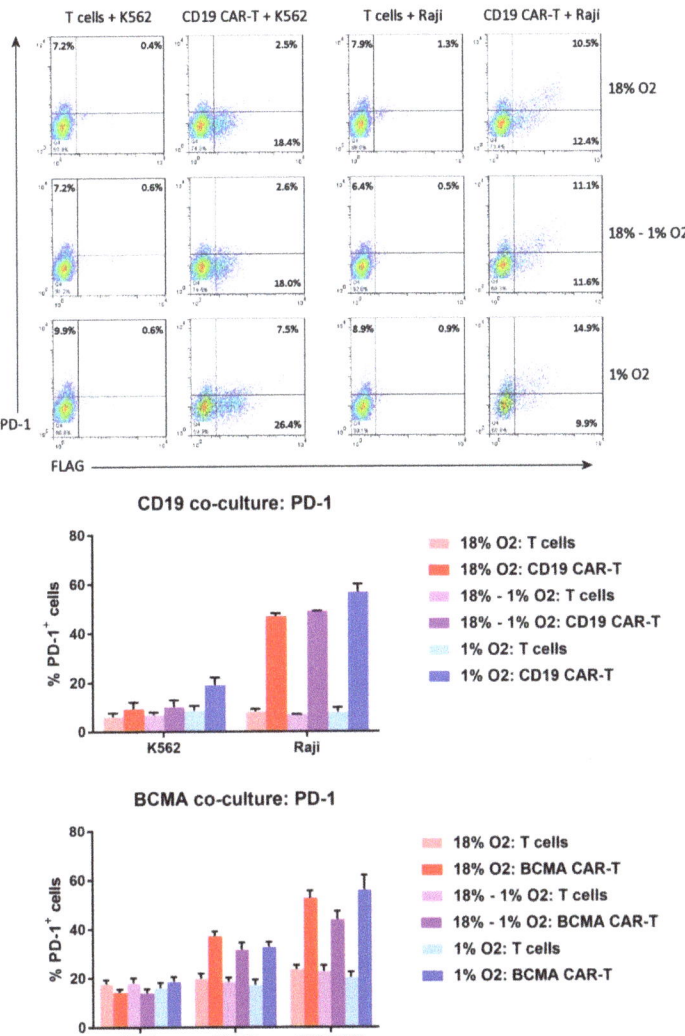

Figure 8. Hypoxia does not affect CAR-T cell PD-1 upregulation. Top: the cells from the CD19 CAR-T cell co-cultures were analyzed by flow cytometry for FLAG staining (i.e., CD19 CAR expression) vs. PD-1 expression. Bottom: the percentages of CD19 CAR-T cells, BCMA CAR-T cells, or control T cells expressing PD-1 were plotted; data-points represent the average and standard error of 2–4 separate experiments.

2.9. CAR-T Cell Expansion in 5% Oxygen Results in Greater Cytotoxicity and Decreased IFN-γ/IL-2 Production

Since hematological cancers reside partly in the bloodstream, which is more oxygenated than solid tumors, we tested the effect of 5% oxygen on CD19 CAR-T cell expansion, differentiation, cytotoxicity and cytokine production. Unlike 1% oxygen, 5% oxygen did not impair CAR-T cell expansion or CAR-T cell differentiation (Figure 9). Interestingly, CAR-T cells expanded in 5% oxygen were actually more cytotoxic against HeLa-CD19 target cells than were CAR-T cells expanded in 18% oxygen, even if the latter cells were assayed in 5% oxygen. Despite the increased cytotoxicity, CAR-T expanded and assayed in 5% oxygen produced lower levels of IFN-γ and IL-2 than CAR-T cells expanded and assayed in 18% oxygen. In addition, CAR-T cells expanded in 18% oxygen produced less IFN-γ and IL-2 when assayed in 5% oxygen—similar to when the cells were assayed in 1% oxygen (Figures 6 and 7). In contrast to IFN-γ and IL-2, IL-6 levels were not decreased by expanding or assaying the CD19 CAR-T cells in 5% oxygen. These data show that 1% oxygen has much stronger effect on CAR-T cell functions than 5% oxygen.

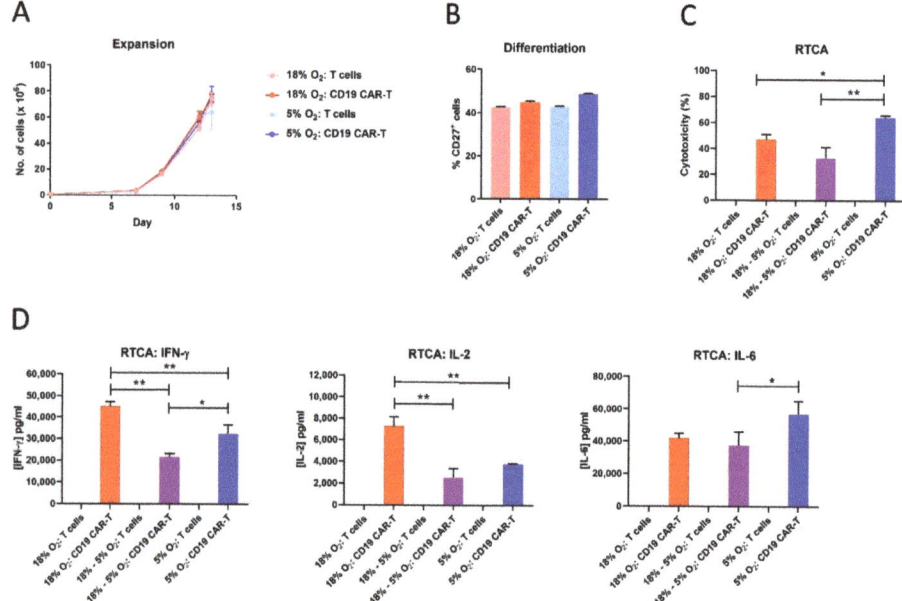

Figure 9. CAR-T cell expansion in 5% oxygen results in greater cytotoxicity and decreased IFN-γ/IL-2 production. CD19 CAR-T cells and control T cells expanded in 18% oxygen or 5% oxygen were analyzed for cell expansion (**A**), differentiation (**B**), cytotoxicity (**C**), and cytokine production during the RTCA assay (**D**). Data points indicate averages of 2–3 replicates; * $p < 0.05$ and ** $p < 0.005$.

3. Discussion

In this study we compared CAR-T cells expanded under atmospheric (18%) oxygen levels to CAR-T cells expanded under hypoxic (1%) oxygen levels. Expansion of hypoxic CD19 CAR-T cells and BCMA CAR-T cells, as well as control T cells, was impaired 10–20-fold over the eight-day expansion period. The impairment was not due to altered T cell activation or lentiviral transduction, since these events occurred in the 5-day period before expansion, when all cultures were kept in atmospheric oxygen. Previous studies of non-CAR-T cells found that hypoxia reduced proliferation rates and increased apoptosis rates [19–24]. However, the mechanisms by which hypoxia affects proliferation and apoptosis are not clear. Prior studies have indicated that hypoxia is associated with alterations in Kv1.3 potassium channel activity that impair CD3ζ-mediated Ca^{2+} signaling [25], and that IL-2 signaling might also be impaired [26]. Hypoxia inducible factor 1α may be involved, as it can interact with MCM replication proteins to regulate cell cycle progression [27]. Clearly, this is an important area requiring a future detailed, comprehensive analysis.

Although hypoxia inhibited CAR-T cell expansion, the frequency of CAR-T cells in the cultures was not affected by hypoxia. This suggests that hypoxia affects the expansion of CAR-T cells and non-transduced T cells equally, and does not cause CAR down-regulation. Hypoxia did impair the differentiation of central memory BCMA CAR-T cells into effector memory BCMA CAR-T cells, and showed a trend towards doing the same to CD19 CAR-T cells. This suggests that differentiation of CAR-T cells is oxygen-dependent, which is consistent with prior studies on non-CAR-T cells [19,21–23]. The impaired differentiation of CAR-Tcm cells into CAR-Tem cells might actually be favorable therapeutically, since Tcm cells exhibit enhanced persistence after adoptive transfer [28]. Since culture of CD19 CAR-T cells in 5% oxygen did not affect their expansion or differentiation, oxygen levels below 5% are required for the reduction in differentiation. In addition, initial experiments indicate that hypoxia skews the balance of CAR-T cell functional subsets from a Th1/Tc1-dominated composition to a Treg-dominated composition.

Hypoxia also increased the CD4:CD8 ratio of the CAR-T cells, suggesting that $CD4^+$ CAR-T cell expansion is less oxygen-dependent than $CD8^+$ CAR-T cell expansion. Previous studies of non-CAR-T cells also found hypoxia-mediated increases in the CD4:CD8 ratio [19]. In fact, it is possible that the hypoxia-mediated increased CD4:CD8 ratio and decreased differentiation we observed might be related; perhaps $CD4^+$ CAR-T cells differentiate more slowly than $CD8^+$ CAR-T cells in culture. In addition, we observed that, in both atmospheric and hypoxic cultures, both CD19 CAR-T cells and BCMA CAR-T cells had a higher CD4:CD8 ratio than control T cells. This suggests either that $CD4^+$ T cells are transduced by the CAR lentivirus more readily than $CD8^+$ T cells, or that CAR expression impacts $CD4^+$ T cell expansion less than $CD8^+$ T cell expansion. These important questions should be answered in our next study, when we analyze CAR-T cells generated from isolated $CD4^+$ T cells and $CD8^+$ T cells.

Functionally, CAR-T cells expanded under hypoxia were not impaired in their ability to kill cells transfected to stably express the target antigen, consistent with prior studies on non-CAR-T cells [19,24,29]. The equivalent cytotoxicity coupled with the increased CD4:CD8 ratio indicates that $CD4^+$ CAR-T cells are cytotoxic in vitro [30]. In the clinic, a 1:1 mixture of separate $CD4^+$ CAR-T cells and $CD8^+$ CAR-T cells was found to be highly efficacious in adult B-ALL patients [31]. However, several recent studies indicate that a CD4:CD8 ratio greater than 1:1 might be beneficial, especially in solid tumors. Wang et al found that IL-13 receptor α2-specific $CD4^+$ CAR-T cells exhibited long-term cytotoxicity against primary glioblastoma cells, whereas $CD8^+$ CAR-T cells exhibited short-term cytotoxicity but became exhausted, permitting tumor relapse [32]. The $CD4^+$ CAR-T cells had significant upregulation of genes responsible for stem cell renewal and memory function such as WNT9B, WNT9A, AXIN2, LEF, TWIST1, ALDH1A3 and EGFR [32]; perhaps these genes helped $CD4^+$ CAR-T cells overcome the hypoxia-mediated inhibition of expansion we observed, increasing the CD4:CD8 ratio. Analysis of CAR-T cell products from GBM patients indicated that the products with decreased CD4:CD8 ratios demonstrated decreased cytotoxicity [32]. In multiple myeloma, Cohen et al showed that a higher CD4:CD8 T cell ratio in the leukapheresis product was associated with greater CAR-T cell expansion in the patient and with a greater therapeutic response [33]. Interestingly, since the CAR-T cells we expanded in 5% oxygen were more cytotoxic than the CAR-T cells expanded in 18% oxygen, it is possible that the clinical efficacy of CAR-T cells could be improved by expanding them in 5% oxygen.

Despite their high cytolytic activity, hypoxic CAR-T cells produced relatively low levels of granzyme B, IFN-γ, IL-2, and IL-6 in response to transfected cells and tumor cell lines endogenously expressing the target antigen. This is consistent with prior studies on non-CAR-T cells [19,23,24]. Interestingly, this effect also occurred when atmospheric CAR-T cells were cultured with hypoxic target cells. The decreased levels were not due to decreased target expression on the transfected cells and tumor cells; flow cytometric analysis indicated that CD19 and BCMA expression levels on the target cells were not altered in 1% oxygen. Thus, decreased granzyme B and cytokine production occurs in the hypoxic setting, even if the CAR-T cells are expanded in atmospheric oxygen. This is the case in vivo, where CAR-T cells in the bloodstream move out of the capillaries and into the hypoxic tumor or bone marrow. Next-generation CAR-T cells with increased production of cytokines might be needed to overcome this hypoxia-mediated effect.

Lastly, hypoxia did not affect checkpoint protein PD-1 upregulation. Hence, PD-1 blocking antibodies should be as active in solid tumors as the antibodies are in non-hypoxic settings. In fact, next-generation CAR-T cells with down-regulation of the PD-1 pathway exhibit enhanced activity in solid tumors [7,34,35]. CRISPR/Cas9-mediated disruption of the PD-1 pathway was actually more effective than adding a PD-1 neutralizing antibody in enhancing CAR-T cytotoxicity against solid tumors [35].

In summary, this is the first report to describe the effects of hypoxia on CAR-T cells. The effects we observed were consistent between CD19 CAR-T cells and BCMA CAR-T cells, indicating that the effects are CAR-independent and likely to apply to other targets. These data are critical for clinical studies because the success of CAR-T cell therapy depends on multiple parameters affected by hypoxia, including CAR-T cell expansion, CAR-T cell functional activity, and CAR-T cell differentiation/maturation status [36,37]. In particular, the less differentiated phenotype of CAR-T cells was found to preferable for expansion and persistence in patients, and adequate number of $CD4^+$ CAR-T cells and $CD8^+$ CAR T cells in the manufactured CAR-T product was obtained without pre-selection of T cell subsets [36]. Our experiments also provide baseline data important for the design of hypoxia-resistant next-generation CAR-T cells. Analyzing the other aspects of the solid tumor microenvironment on CAR-T cell expansion, differentiation, cytotoxicity, cytokine production, and checkpoint protein expression will be critical for developing successful CAR-T cell therapies against solid tumors in the future.

4. Materials and Methods

4.1. Cells

HeLa cells were purchased from the ATCC (Manassas, VA, USA) and cultured in DMEM (GE Healthcare, Chicago, IL, USA) containing 10% FBS (Lonza, Walkersville, MD, USA). K562, Raji, MM1S and RPMI8226 cells were purchased from the ATCC and cultured in RPMI-1640 medium (Thermo Fisher, Waltham, MA, USA) containing 10% FBS. CHO-CD22 and CHO-BCMA cells were purchased from BPS Bioscience (San Diego, CA, USA) and cultured in Ham's F-12K medium (Thermo Fisher) containing 10% FBS and 1 mg/mL geneticin (Thermo Fisher). HeLa-CD19 cells were generated in our laboratory [16] and cultured in DMEM containing 10% FBS and 1 uM puromycin (Thermo Fisher). Human peripheral blood mononuclear cells (PBMC) were isolated from LRS chambers (Stanford Blood Center, Palo Alto, CA, USA) by density sedimentation over Ficoll-Paque (GE Healthcare). HEK293FT cells were a gift from AlStem (Richmond, CA, USA) and were cultured in DMEM containing 10% FBS.

4.2. Generation of CAR-Encoding Lentivirus

Ten million growth-arrested HEK293FT cells were seeded into T75 flasks and cultured overnight, then transfected with the pPACKH1 Lentivector Packaging mix (System Biosciences, Palo Alto, CA, USA) and 10 µg of either the CD19-FLAG [16] or BCMA 4C8A [18] lentiviral vector using the CalPhos Transfection Kit (Takara, Mountain View, CA, USA). The next day the medium was replaced with fresh medium, and 48 h later the lentivirus-containing medium was collected. The medium was cleared of cell debris by centrifugation at 2100× g for 30 min. The virus particles were collected by centrifugation at 110,000× g for 100 min, suspended in AIM V medium (Thermo Fisher), aliquoted and frozen at −80 °C, as described [16,37–39].

4.3. Generation and Expansion of CAR-T Cells

Treated 24-well plates were incubated at 37 °C for 2 hours with PBS containing 0.1 µg/mL anti-CD3 clone OKT3 (Biolegend, San Diego, CA, USA) and 0.1 µg/mL anti-CD28 clone CD28.2 (Thermo Fisher). PBMC were suspended at 1×10^6 cells/mL in AIM V medium containing 10% FBS and 10 ng/ml of IL-2 (Thermo Fisher). The wells were rinsed with PBS, then 0.5 mL of PBMC were added per well. The next day, 20 uL of lentivirus was added to the cells, along with 5 µg/mL of DEAE-dextran (Sigma, St. Louis, MO, USA). The day after that (day 2), another 20 ul of lentivirus was added to the cells. Three days later, half of the cells were transferred into a humidified C chamber (Biospherix, Parish, NY, USA) set to 5% carbon dioxide and either 5% oxygen or 1% oxygen. As the T cells proliferated over the next 8 days, the cells in the normal incubator and hypoxia chamber were counted every 2–3 days and fresh medium (equilibrated overnight in the hypoxia chamber for the hypoxic cultures) with IL-2 was added to the cultures to maintain the proper cell density.

4.4. Flow Cytometry

To measure CAR expression, cells were first suspended in 100 µL of cold buffer (PBS containing 0.5% BSA and 2 mM EDTA) supplemented with 2 µg of goat IgG (Jackson Immunoresearch, West Grove, PA, USA) and incubated on ice. CD19-FLAG CAR-T cells were stained with 2 µL of PE- or Alexa Fluor 488-conjugated anti-FLAG (Biolegend), whereas BCMA CAR-T cells were first stained with 0.4 µg of BCMA-huFc protein (Acro Biosystems, Newark, DE, USA) and then stained with 1 µL of PE- or Alexa Fluor 488-conjugated goat anti-human IgG (Jackson Immunoresearch). Cells were co-stained with either FITC-conjugated anti-CD4 and APC-conjugated anti-CD8; PE-conjugated anti-CD27 and APC-conjugated CD45RO; or APC-conjugated anti-PD-1 (all from Biolegend). Dead cells were identified with 7-aminoactinomycin D (7-AAD, BioLegend). The cells were rinsed with 3 mL of buffer, then suspended in buffer and acquired on a FACSCalibur (BD Biosciences, San Jose, CA, USA). Gating strategies are shown in Supplemental Figure S1.

4.5. Cytotoxicity Assay

Adherent target cells were seeded into 96-well E-plates (Acea Biosciences, San Diego, CA) at 1.5×10^4 cells per well (HeLa-CD19), 3×10^4 cells per well (HeLa), or 4×10^4 cells per well (CHO-CD22, CHO-BCMA), and monitored in the normal incubator or hypoxia chamber overnight with the xCELLigence impedance-based RTCA system (Acea Biosciences). The next day, the medium was removed and replaced with normal or equilibrated RPMI-1640 medium containing 10% FBS ± CAR-T cells or non-transduced T cells at an E:T ratio of 10:1, in triplicate. The cells in the E-plates were monitored for another 20–24 h with the RTCA system, and impedance (normalized to the time of effector cell addition) was plotted over time. Cytotoxicity was calculated as the percentage $(X - Y) \times 100/X$, where X = normalized impedance of target cells without effector cells and Y = normalized impedance of target cells with effector cells. For hypoxic RTCA assays, target cells were cultured in the hypoxia chamber for three days before use.

4.6. Cytokine and PD-1 Induction Assay

Effector cells (CAR-T cells or non-transduced T cells) were co-cultured overnight with target cells (Raji, K562, MM1S or RPMI8226 cells) at a 10:1 E:T ratio in normal or equilibrated RPMI-1640 medium containing 10% FBS, in duplicate or triplicate. The next day, the cultures were centrifuged at 300 g, the supernatants were transferred to new tubes and frozen, and the cells were suspended in FACS buffer and analyzed by flow cytometry for expression of the CAR and PD-1. Culture supernatants were later thawed and analyzed by ELISA for the levels of IFN-γ, IL-2, IL-6, and Granzyme B according to the manufacturer's protocols (R&D Systems, Minneapolis, MN, USA). For hypoxic co-cultures, tumor cells were cultured in the hypoxia chamber for three days before use.

4.7. Statistical Analysis

Data were analyzed and plotted with Prism software v8.1.1 (GraphPad, San Diego, CA, USA). Comparisons between two groups were performed by unpaired Student's *t* test, and comparisons between three or more groups were performed by one-way or two-way ANOVA with Tukey's post-hoc test.

5. Conclusions

CD19-specifc CAR-T cells and BCMA-specific CAR-T cells were selectively affected by exposure to hypoxia (1% oxygen). CAR expression, CAR-T cell cytolytic activity and target antigen-induced PD-1 upregulation were not affected by hypoxia. However, CAR-T cell expansion, differentiation, CD8:CD4 ratio, and production of granzyme B and cytokines IFN-γ, IL-2, and IL-6 were all significantly decreased by hypoxia. These effects may underlie the failure of CAR-T cells to eradicate solid tumors in some patients and point to areas in which CAR-T cells may be modified for future clinical studies.

Supplementary Materials: The following are available online at http://www.mdpi.com/2072-6694/11/5/602/s1, Figure S1: Gating strategies used to identify cells by flow cytometry.

Author Contributions: Conceptualization, R.B., V.G. and L.W.; Investigation, R.B., X.L., H.Z., E.T. and S.X.; Data Curation, R.B.; Writing—Original Draft Preparation, R.B.; Writing—Review & Editing, R.B. and V.G.

Funding: This research was funded by the Science and Technology Department, China [grant number 2016SK2071].

Acknowledgments: The authors would like to thank Alicia Henn and Ray Gould of Biospherix for providing the hypoxia chamber and scientific advice. We would like to thank Martyn Lewis and Brandon Lamarche of Acea Biosciences for installation and technical advice.

Conflicts of Interest: Robert Berahovich, Xianghong Liu, Hua Zhou, Elias Tsadik, Shirley Xu, Vita Golubovskaya and Lijun Wu are employees of Promab Biotechnologies. Other authors declare no conflict of interest.

References

1. Maus, M.V.; June, C.H. Making better chimeric antigen receptors for adoptive T-cell therapy. *Clin. Cancer Res.* **2016**, *22*, 1875–1884. [CrossRef] [PubMed]
2. Porter, D.L.; Levine, B.L.; Kalos, M.; Bagg, A.; June, C.H. Chimeric antigen receptor-modified T cells in chronic lymphoid leukemia. *N. Engl. J. Med.* **2011**, *365*, 725–733. [CrossRef]
3. Grupp, S.A.; Kalos, M.; Barrett, D.; Aplenc, R.; Porter, D.L.; Rheingold, S.R.; Teachey, D.T.; Chew, A.; Hauck, B.; Wright, J.F.; et al. Chimeric antigen receptor-modified T cells for acute lymphoid leukemia. *N. Engl. J. Med.* **2013**, *368*, 1509–1518. [CrossRef] [PubMed]
4. Feins, S.; Kong, W.; Williams, E.F.; Milone, M.C.; Fraietta, J.A. An introduction to chimeric antigen receptor (CAR) T cell immunotherapy for human cancer. *Am. J. Hematol.* **2019**, *94*, S3–S9. [CrossRef] [PubMed]
5. Abken, H. Adoptive therapy with CAR redirected T cells: The challenges in targeting solid tumors. *Immunotherapy* **2015**, *7*, 535–544. [CrossRef]
6. Beatty, G.L.; Moon, E.K. Chimeric antigen receptor T cells are vulnerable to immunosuppressive mechanisms present within the tumor microenvironment. *Oncoimmunology* **2014**, *3*, e970027. [CrossRef] [PubMed]
7. Guedan, S.; Calderon, H.; Posey, A.D.J.; Maus, M.V. Engineering and design of chimeric antigen receptors. *Mol. Ther. Methods Clin. Dev.* **2019**, *12*, 145–156. [CrossRef] [PubMed]
8. Eshhar, Z.; Waks, T.; Gross, G. The emergence of T-bodies/CAR T cells. *Cancer J.* **2014**, *20*, 123–126. [CrossRef]
9. Becker, A.; Stadler, P.; Krause, U.; Utzig, D.; Hansgen, G.; Lautenschlager, C.; Rath, F.W.; Molls, M.; Dunst, J. Association between elevated serum VEGF and polarographically measured tumor hypoxia in head and neck carcinomas. *Strahlenther. Onkol.* **2001**, *177*, 182–188. [CrossRef]
10. Dunst, J.; Stadler, P.; Becker, A.; Kuhnt, T.; Lautenschlager, C.; Molls, M.; Haensgen, G. Tumor hypoxia and systemic levels of vascular endothelial growth factor (VEGF) in head and neck cancers. *Strahlenther. Onkol.* **2001**, *177*, 469–473. [CrossRef]
11. Bollinger, T.; Gies, S.; Naujoks, J.; Feldhoff, L.; Bollinger, A.; Solbach, W.; Rupp, J. HIF-1alpha- and hypoxia-dependent immune responses in human $CD4^+CD25^{high}$ T cells and T helper 17 cells. *J. Leukoc. Biol.* **2014**, *96*, 305–312. [CrossRef] [PubMed]

12. Kumar, V.; Gabrilovich, D.I. Hypoxia-inducible factors in regulation of immune responses in tumour microenvironment. *Immunology* **2014**, *143*, 512–519. [CrossRef] [PubMed]
13. Badoual, C.; Combe, P.; Gey, A.; Granier, C.; Roussel, H.; De Guillebon, E.; Oudard, S.; Tartour, E. PD-1 and PDL-1 expression in cancer: Significance and prognostic value. *Med. Sci. (Paris)* **2013**, *29*, 570–572. [CrossRef]
14. Denis, H.; Davoine, C.; Bermudez, E.; Grosjean, G.; Schwager, M.; Ifrah, N.; Dahan, M.; Negellen, S. Specific immunotherapies in the treatment of cancers. *Bull. Cancer* **2019**, *106*, 37–47. [CrossRef] [PubMed]
15. Irigoyen, M.; Garcia-Ruiz, J.C.; Berra, E. The hypoxia signalling pathway in haematological malignancies. *Oncotarget* **2017**, *8*, 36832–36844. [CrossRef]
16. Berahovich, R.; Xu, S.; Zhou, H.; Harto, H.; Xu, Q.; Garcia, A.; Liu, F.; Golubovskaya, V.M.; Wu, L. FLAG-tagged CD19-specific CAR-T cells eliminate CD19-bearing solid tumor cells in vitro and in vivo. *Front. Biosci. (Landmark Ed.)* **2017**, *22*, 1644–1654.
17. Davila, M.L.; Bouhassira, D.C.; Park, J.H.; Curran, K.J.; Smith, E.L.; Pegram, H.J.; Brentjens, R. Chimeric antigen receptors for the adoptive T cell therapy of hematologic malignancies. *Int. J. Hematol.* **2014**, *99*, 361–371. [CrossRef]
18. Berahovich, R.; Zhou, H.; Xu, S.; Wei, Y.; Guan, J.; Guan, J.; Harto, H.; Fu, S.; Yang, K.; Zhu, S.; et al. CAR-T cells based on novel BCMA monoclonal antibody block multiple myeloma cell growth. *Cancers (Basel)* **2018**, *10*, 323. [CrossRef]
19. Caldwell, C.C.; Kojima, H.; Lukashev, D.; Armstrong, J.; Farber, M.; Apasov, S.G.; Sitkovsky, M.V. Differential effects of physiologically relevant hypoxic conditions on T lymphocyte development and effector functions. *J. Immunol.* **2001**, *167*, 6140–6149. [CrossRef]
20. Atkuri, K.R.; Herzenberg, L.A.; Herzenberg, L.A. Culturing at atmospheric oxygen levels impacts lymphocyte function. *Proc. Natl. Acad. Sci. USA* **2005**, *102*, 3756–3759. [CrossRef]
21. Larbi, A.; Zelba, H.; Goldeck, D.; Pawelec, G. Induction of HIF-1alpha and the glycolytic pathway alters apoptotic and differentiation profiles of activated human T cells. *J. Leukoc. Biol.* **2010**, *87*, 265–273. [CrossRef]
22. Ikejiri, A.; Nagai, S.; Goda, N.; Kurebayashi, Y.; Osada-Oka, M.; Takubo, K.; Suda, T.; Koyasu, S. Dynamic regulation of Th17 differentiation by oxygen concentrations. *Int. Immunol.* **2012**, *24*, 137–146. [CrossRef]
23. Westendorf, A.M.; Skibbe, K.; Adamczyk, A.; Buer, J.; Geffers, R.; Hansen, W.; Pastille, E.; Jendrossek, V. Hypoxia enhances immunosuppression by inhibiting CD4$^+$ effector T cell function and promoting Treg activity. *Cell. Physiol. Biochem.* **2017**, *41*, 1271–1284. [CrossRef] [PubMed]
24. Vuillefroy de Silly, R.; Ducimetiere, L.; Yacoub Maroun, C.; Dietrich, P.Y.; Derouazi, M.; Walker, P.R. Phenotypic switch of CD8($^+$) T cells reactivated under hypoxia toward IL-10 secreting, poorly proliferative effector cells. *Eur. J. Immunol.* **2015**, *45*, 2263–2275. [CrossRef]
25. Robbins, J.R.; Lee, S.M.; Filipovich, A.H.; Szigligeti, P.; Neumeier, L.; Petrovic, M.; Conforti, L. Hypoxia modulates early events in t cell receptor-mediated activation in human t lymphocytes via kv1.3 channels. *J. Physiol.* **2005**, *564*, 131–143. [CrossRef]
26. Gaber, T.; Tran, C.L.; Schellmann, S.; Hahne, M.; Strehl, C.; Hoff, P.; Radbruch, A.; Burmester, G.R.; Buttgereit, F. Pathophysiological hypoxia affects the redox state and il-2 signalling of human cd4+ t cells and concomitantly impairs survival and proliferation. *Eur. J. Immunol.* **2013**, *43*, 1588–1597. [CrossRef]
27. Hubbi, M.E.; Luo, W.; Baek, J.H.; Semenza, G.L. Mcm proteins are negative regulators of hypoxia-inducible factor 1. *Mol. Cell* **2011**, *42*, 700–712. [CrossRef]
28. Berger, C.; Jensen, M.C.; Lansdorp, P.M.; Gough, M.; Elliott, C.; Riddell, S.R. Adoptive transfer of effector cd8+ t cells derived from central memory cells establishes persistent t cell memory in primates. *J. Clin. Investig.* **2008**, *118*, 294–305. [CrossRef] [PubMed]
29. Nakagawa, Y.; Negishi, Y.; Shimizu, M.; Takahashi, M.; Ichikawa, M.; Takahashi, H. Effects of extracellular pH and hypoxia on the function and development of antigen-specific cytotoxic T lymphocytes. *Immunol. Lett.* **2015**, *167*, 72–86. [CrossRef] [PubMed]
30. Hombach, A.A.; Abken, H. Most do, but some do not: CD4($^+$)CD25(-) T cells, but not CD4($^+$)CD25($^+$) Treg cells, are cytolytic when redirected by a chimeric antigen receptor (CAR). *Cancers (Basel)* **2017**, *9*, 112. [CrossRef] [PubMed]
31. Turtle, C.J.; Hanafi, L.A.; Berger, C.; Hudecek, M.; Pender, B.; Robinson, E.; Hawkins, R.; Chaney, C.; Cherian, S.; Chen, X.; et al. Immunotherapy of non-hodgkin's lymphoma with a defined ratio of cd8+ and cd4+ cd19-specific chimeric antigen receptor-modified t cells. *Sci. Transl. Med.* **2016**, *8*, 355ra116. [CrossRef]

32. Wang, D.; Aguilar, B.; Starr, R.; Alizadeh, D.; Brito, A.; Sarkissian, A.; Ostberg, J.R.; Forman, S.J.; Brown, C.E. Glioblastoma-targeted CD4$^+$ CAR T cells mediate superior antitumor activity. *JCI Insight* **2018**, *3*, 99048. [CrossRef]
33. Cohen, A.D.; Garfall, A.L.; Stadtmauer, E.A.; Melenhorst, J.J.; Lacey, S.F.; Lancaster, E.; Vogl, D.T.; Weiss, B.M.; Dengel, K.; Nelson, A.; et al. B cell maturation antigen-specific car t cells are clinically active in multiple myeloma. *J. Clin. Investig.* **2019**, *130*, 126397. [CrossRef] [PubMed]
34. Hu, W.; Zi, Z.; Jin, Y.; Li, G.; Shao, K.; Cai, Q.; Ma, X.; Wei, F. CRISPR/Cas9-mediated PD-1 disruption enhances human mesothelin-targeted CAR T cell effector functions. *Cancer Immunol. Immunother.* **2019**, *68*, 365–377. [CrossRef] [PubMed]
35. Chen, N.; Morello, A.; Tano, Z.; Adusumilli, P.S. CAR T-cell intrinsic PD-1 checkpoint blockade: A two-in-one approach for solid tumor immunotherapy. *Oncoimmunology* **2017**, *6*, e1273302. [CrossRef] [PubMed]
36. Locke, F.L.; Neelapu, S.S.; Bartlett, N.L.; Siddiqi, T.; Chavez, J.C.; Hosing, C.M.; Ghobadi, A.; Budde, L.E.; Bot, A.; Rossi, J.M.; et al. Phase 1 results of zuma-1: A multicenter study of kte-c19 anti-cd19 car t cell therapy in refractory aggressive lymphoma. *Mol. Ther.* **2017**, *25*, 285–295. [CrossRef]
37. Locke, F.L.; Ghobadi, A.; Jacobson, C.A.; Miklos, D.B.; Lekakis, L.J.; Oluwole, O.O.; Lin, Y.; Braunschweig, I.; Hill, B.T.; Timmerman, J.M.; et al. Long-term safety and activity of axicabtagene ciloleucel in refractory large b-cell lymphoma (zuma-1): A single-arm, multicentre, phase 1-2 trial. *Lancet Oncol.* **2019**, *20*, 31–42. [CrossRef]
38. Xu, Q.; Harto, H.; Berahovich, R.; Xu, S.; Zhou, H.; Golubovskaya, V.; Wu, L. Generation of CAR-T cells for cancer immunotherapy. *Methods Mol. Biol.* **2019**, *1884*, 349–360.
39. Golubovskaya, V.; Berahovich, R.; Zhou, H.; Xu, S.; Harto, H.; Li, L.; Chao, C.C.; Mao, M.M.; Wu, L. CD47-CAR-T cells effectively kill target cancer cells and block pancreatic tumor growth. *Cancers (Basel)* **2017**, *9*, 139. [CrossRef] [PubMed]

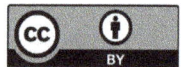

© 2019 by the authors. Licensee MDPI, Basel, Switzerland. This article is an open access article distributed under the terms and conditions of the Creative Commons Attribution (CC BY) license (http://creativecommons.org/licenses/by/4.0/).

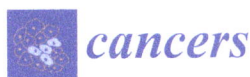

Article

Targeted Killing of Monocytes/Macrophages and Myeloid Leukemia Cells with Pro-Apoptotic Peptides

Mouldy Sioud [1,*], Solveig Pettersen [1], Ieva Ailte [1] and Yngvar Fløisand [2]

[1] Department of Cancer Immunology, Institute for Cancer Research, Oslo University Hospital-Radiumhospitalet, Ullernchausseen 70, N0379 Oslo, Norway
[2] Department of Haematology, Oslo University Hospital-Rikshospitalet, Sognsvannvien 20, N0372 Oslo, Norway
* Correspondence: Mouldy.Sioud@rr-research.no or mosioud@ous-hf.no; Tel.: +47-22-78-14-14

Received: 18 April 2019; Accepted: 26 July 2019; Published: 31 July 2019

Abstract: Several cells of myeloid origin, such as monocytes and macrophages are involved in various human disorders, including cancer and inflammatory diseases. Hence, they represent attractive therapeutic targets. Here we developed three lytic hybrid peptides, by fusing a monocyte- and macrophage-binding peptide to pro-apoptotic peptides, and investigated their killing potency on blood monocytes, macrophages, and leukemia cells. We first showed that the targeting NW peptide is effective for depleting monocytes from whole peripheral blood mononuclear cells (PBMCs). Incubating the cells with biotin-conjugated NW peptide, and the subsequent capture on streptavidin-conjugated magnetic beads, depleted monocytes from the PBMCs. The NW peptide also depleted myeloid leukemia blasts from patient PBMCs. The treatment of the PBMCs with the lytic hybrid NW-KLA peptide killed monocytes, but not lymphocytes and primary mammary epithelial cells. Additionally, the fusion peptide exhibited a potent toxicity against macrophages and leukemia cells. The free lytic KLA peptide did not affect cells. Similarly, a second lytic hybrid peptide killed macrophages, leukemia cell lines, and blood leukemia blasts from patients with acute and chronic myeloid leukemia. The IC_{50} towards target cells were in the low macromolar range (4–12 µM). Overall, the data indicate that the NW peptide could be a potential drug delivery agent for monocytes, macrophages, and leukemia cells. Moreover, the engineered lytic hybrid peptides acting alone, or in combination with other therapeutic agents, might benefit many cancer patients and overcome drug resistance.

Keywords: tumor microenvironment; macrophages; leukemia cells; lytic peptides; targeted therapy; immunotherapy; cancer

1. Introduction

Circulating blood monocytes extravasate into tissues, where they differentiate into M1 or M2 macrophages, controlled by local environmental signals, such as colony-stimulating factor-1 (CSF-1) [1,2]. Under normal conditions, macrophages protect the host against infection and injury and facilitate tissue remodeling [2]. However, in most solid tumors, high macrophage infiltration into tumor tissues has been associated with poor clinical outcome [2–9]. These tumor associated macrophages (TAMs) promote numerous important features of tumor progression, including angiogenesis, motility, metastasis, and inhibition of T cell function [3]. Additionally, TAMs are known to suppress responses to standard-of-care-therapeutics, including chemotherapy, irradiation and angiogenic inhibitors [7–9]. In cancer, both the resident and the infiltrating macrophages have the pro-tumorigenic M2 phenotype [4]. Similarly, some studies suggested that elevated number of circulating blood monocytes was associated with poor prognosis in patients with various cancer types [5,7]. In addition to malignancies, macrophages are associated with the progression of a number of other diseases, such as asthma, allergic inflammation, and rheumatic inflammatory diseases [10–13]. In rheumatoid arthritis (RA), M1 macrophages secrete pro-inflammatory cytokines, such as tumor necrosis factor- (TNF-α) and interleukin-1. The role of these cytokines in RA pathogenesis is well documented by several experimental and clinical findings [11,12]. Hence, therapeutic strategies that either target TAM recruitment from inflammatory monocytes, or deplete TAMs will benefit patients with cancer or inflammatory diseases.

To therapeutically target TAMs, several pharmacological and immunological strategies have been used. Trabecdedin is a synthetic tetrahydroisoquinoline drug originally isolated from the marine Caribbean tunicate *Ecteinascidia turbinate*, approved for the treatment of sarcoma and ovarian carcinoma [14]. In sarcoma patients, trabectedin reduced the density of TAMs and improved patient outcome [15]. Clodronate is a bisphosphonate-family compound found to deplete macrophages, and is currently used to prevent or block the development of bone metastases, as well as to treat inflammatory diseases [16]. In animal models, an antibody targeting the CSF-1 receptor (R) reduced TAMs [17]. Treatment of patients with diffuse-type giant cell tumor with this antibody resulted in clinical benefit that correlated with reduction of TAMs and blood circulating monocytes. Similarly, CSF-1 inhibition by antisense oligonucleotides or small interfering RNAs (siRNAs) suppressed tumor growth in mice xenografted with human cancer cells as a result of macrophages reduction in tumor tissues [18]. Despite these advances, the current therapeutic strategies are not monocyte- and/or TAM-specific, and can thus have substantial side effects over time. Moreover, there is a need for the development of new therapeutic agents to treat drug-resistant cancers.

In recent years, antimicrobial peptides have attracted interest as potential anti-cancer drugs [19–23]. Usually these peptides do not bind to mammalian cell membrane, however, they can kill the cells if internalized via targeting moieties, such as antibodies and peptides [22,23]. Within the cytosol, they selectively disrupt mitochondrial membranes, leading to cell death by apoptosis [20]. Since their killing activity is not dependent on cell proliferation, they do not have many of the undesirable toxic effects of other chemo drugs. In the present study, we evaluated the effects of lytic peptides fused to a targeting peptide on blood monocytes, M1 and M2 macrophages, and leukemia cell lines. In addition, we included blood leukemia blasts from patients with myeloid leukemia, a disease that remains incurable, despite improvement in treatment options. The targeting peptide was identified using phage display libraries [24,25]. Two of the engineered lytic hydrid peptides killed monocytes, macrophages, and leukemia cells in vitro at low peptide concentrations, supporting their further clinical development.

2. Materials and Methods

2.1. Peptides

The following peptides were purchased from Biosynthesis (Lewisville, TX, USA). Italic letters indicate the pro-apoptotic domains.

NW peptide: NWYLPWLGTNDW-NH$_2$
NW peptide-biotin: NWYLPWLGTNDW-GGK-biotin
Control peptide: MEWSLEKGYTIK-GGK-biotin
KLA peptide: *KLAKLAKKLAKLAK*-NH$_2$
KLL peptide: *KLLLKLLKKLLKLLKKK*-NH$_2$
QLG peptide: *QLGKKKHRRRPSKKRHW*-NH$_2$

Fusion lytic peptides:

NW-KLA: NWYLPWLGTNDWGGG*KLAKLAKKLAKLAK*-NH$_2$
NW-KLL: NWYLPWLGTNDWGGG*KLLLKLLKKLLKLLKKK*-NH$_2$
NW-QLG: NWYLPWLGTNDWGGG*QLGKKKHRRRPSKKRHW*-NH$_2$

All peptides were dissolved in sterile water at 600 µM and aliquots and stored at −80 °C until use. Biotin-conjugated NW peptide and control peptide were dissolved in DMSO and stored at −80 °C. A flexible short glycine linker (GGG) was placed between the NW peptide and the lytic domain to minimize potential steric hindrance which may block the binding to target cells.

2.2. Antibodies and Cytokines

Cell staining was performed using fluorescein isothiocyanate (FITC), phycoerythrin (PE), allophycocyanin (APC), or pacific blue (PB)-conjugated mouse monoclonal antibodies against CD80, CD86, CD83, CD14, and CD163 (all purchased from BD Biosciences, San Jose, CA, USA). Fluorochrome conjugated antibodies against CD8, CD4, CD56, and CD19 were purchased from BioLegends (Nordic BioSite AS, Kristiansand, Norway). The following cytokines were used: Interleukin-4 (IL-4), granulocyte-colony stimulating factor (GM-CSF), monocyte-colony stimulating factor (M-CSF), tumor necrosis factor-α (TNF-α), interleukin-10 (IL-10), and interferon-γ (IFN-γ; all purchased from R&D Systems (Minneapolis, MN, USA).

2.3. Cell Lines and Peripheral Blood Mononuclear Cells

Leukemia cell lines MV-4-11 and U937 were purchased from the American Type Culture Collection (ATCC, Rockville, MD, USA). Cells were cultured in RPMI medium-1640 supplemented with 10% fetal calf serum (FCS) and antibiotics (complete medium). Primary human mammary epithelial cells were purchased from ATCC. Peripheral blood mononuclear cells (PBMCs) were obtained from buffy coats of healthy individuals and isolated by density gradient centrifugation (Lymphoprep; Nycomed Pharm, Oslo, Norway). Monocytes were prepared using plastic adherence. Briefly, PBMCs were plated into T-75 flasks (3×10^6/mL) in complete RPMI medium and incubated at 37 °C for 1–2 h. Non-adherent cells were removed, and adherent monocytes were harvested by gentle scraping with a plastic cell scraper. CD4+ and CD8+ T cells were isolated using Dynabeads' positive selection kits (Invitrogen Dynal AS, Oslo, Norway), following the manufacturer's instructions. CD19+ B cells were isolated by positive selection using CD19 MicroBeads, following the manufacturer's instructions, using manual labeling and automated separation on autoMACS™ Pro Separator (Miltenyi Biotec, Lund, Sweden). Natural Killer (NK) cells were isolated by negative selection using the NK Cell Isolation Kit (Miltenyi Biotec Norden AB, Lund, Sweden), following the manufacturer's instructions, in combination with automated separation using autoMACS™ Pro Separator (Miltenyi Biotec Norden AB, Lund, Sweden). The purity of the cells was verified using antibody staining and analysis by flow cytometry.

2.4. Primary Leukemia Cells

A single sample of 10 mL of peripheral blood was obtained from each patient with leukemia at Oslo University Hospital. Cells were isolated by density gradient centrifugation as indicated above. All cells were re-suspended in the growth medium, counted, frozen down, or freshly used in downstream experiments. The collection of patient blood samples was approved by the Regional Committees for Medical and Health Research Ethics (REK = 2017/1596). The study was conducted in accordance with the declaration of Helsinki.

2.5. Generation of Immature Human Dendritic Cells

Blood monocytes were cultured in complete medium supplemented with IL-4 (100 ng/mL) and GM-CSF (50 ng/mL) for 6 days. Under these conditions, immature DCs are in the supernatant while macrophages stick well to the culture flask. We verified the floating cells to be DCs using flow cytometry detection of CD80, CD86 and CD83. Adherent macrophages are positive for CD14.

2.6. Generation of M1 and M2 Macrophages

To generate macrophages, blood monocytes were cultured in X-vivo 15 medium, supplemented with 50 ng/mL GM-CSF (M1) or 50 ng/mL M-CSF (M2), followed by additional two days of culture in the presence of 50 ng/mL LPS and 100 U/mL IFN-γ (M1), or 50 ng/mL IL-4 and 1 ng/mL IL-10 (M2). Under these conditions, the cells showed the morphological characteristic features of M1 or M2 macrophages.

2.7. Flow Cytometry

Flow cytometry was performed to analyze the expression of certain surface markers and peptide binding to tested human cells. Conjugated antibodies specific for cell surface markers were incubated with the cells (1–2 × 10^5 cells/100 µL/sample) in PBS buffer containing 1% FCS or BSA (staining buffer) for 30–60 min at 4 °C. After washing, the cells were re-suspended in 300 µL staining buffer before being analyzed on BD FACS Canto II Flow cytometer, using BD FACSDiva™ software (BD Biosciences, San Jose, CA, USA). Similarly, cells were incubated with biotinylated NW peptide or control peptide (5 µg/mL each) in staining buffer at 4 °C for 40 min. After washing, the cells were incubated with phycoethrin (PE)-conjugated streptavidin, and then processed as indicated above. All data were analyzed by FlowJo software (FlowJo LLC, Ashland, OR, USA).

2.8. Depletion of Monocytes and Blast Cells from Peripheral Blood Mononuclear Cells

Peripheral blood mononuclear cells (10^6 cells) were incubated with biotin-conjugated NW peptide (20 µg/mL) for 40 min at 4 °C with gentle rotation. After washing, streptavidin-magnetic beads were added at a concentration of 4 beads per target cell, and incubation continued for 20 min at 4 °C. The samples were placed on a magnet for 5 min, and non-attached cells were carefully removed and analyzed by flow cytometry to check for the removal of the peptide-binding cells.

2.9. Cell Viability Assays

Leukemia cell lines MV-4-11 and U937 were seeded at 10^5 cells/100 µL complete medium and incubated for 1 h at 37 °C. Cells were subsequently incubated with various concentrations of the different peptides for 1 h at 37 °C. Cell viability was then assessed using CellTiter 96® AQueous One Solution Reagent (Promega, Madison, WI, USA) according to the manufacturer's instructions. Optical densities were measured at 492 nm. For the M1 and M2 macrophages, monocytes were initially seeded in a 96-well plate (1.5 × 10^5/100 µL complete medium) and differentiated into M1 or M2 macrophages as described above. After, the culture medium was replaced to remove dead cells and viable adherent cells were treated with various peptide concentrations and processed as above. The effects of the engineered lytic peptides on monocytes and primary leukemia cell viability were measured using propidium iodide (PI) uptake.

2.10. Apoptosis Assay

The induction of apoptosis subsequent to peptide treatment was measured using the annexin V/PI staining dual assay, combined with flow cytometry analysis as described previously [22]. Cells stained with annexin alone (green fluorescence) were considered apoptotic, whereas those stained both green and red were considered necrotic.

2.11. Uptake of the NW-Peptide Streptavidin-PE-Complexes by Macrophages

Streptavidin-PE conjugates (10 µg/mL) were incubated with biotinylated NW peptide or control peptide (10 µg/mL) for 30 min at room temperature in PBS buffer supplemented with 1% FCS. Then the mixtures were added to macrophages growing in Lab-Tek chamber slides (Nalge Nunc International, Naperville, IL, USA). After incubation for 30 min at 4 °C, the cells were washed 3 times with culture medium and incubated at 37 °C for 60 min to allow internalization of the bound peptide-streptavidin-PE complexes. To visualize the nuclei, Hoechst 33342 (Invitrogen Dynal AS, Oslo, Norway) was added to the cells for 5 min. Subsequently, the cells were washed 3 times with PBS buffer, fixed with 4% paraformaldehyde for 20 min at 4 °C, washed, and then slides were covered with Dako fluorescent mounting medium before analysis by a Zeiss LSM 510 confocal laser scanning microscope (Carl Zeiss, Olympus, Tokyo, Japan). MV-4-11 leukemia cells were analyzed by Zeiss LSM 880 confocal microscope.

2.12. Statistical Analysis

All experiments were performed at least three times, except if otherwise indicated. Differences between control and treated cells were measured by the standard student's t test. For multiple comparisons, a two-way ANOVA analysis was used. p values < 0.05 were considered significant.

3. Results

3.1. The NW Peptide Displays Strong Binding to Human Monocytes

Unlike standard cancer treatments, targeted therapies are gaining importance, due to their specificity towards cancer cells. Over the last few years, we have developed a panel of peptides that can guide therapeutics to either cancer cells or immune cells [25]. With respect to the latter, we recently identified a peptide (named NW peptide) which binds to monocytes, macrophages and dendritic cells [24]. Figure 1A shows the binding to blood monocyte (gate R2) and lymphocyte (gate R1) populations. The mean fluorescence intensity (MFI) of the peptide binding to monocytes was 38-fold higher than that of the control peptide. By contrast to monocytes, the NW peptide showed no significant binding to the lymphocyte population (T, B, and NK cells).

To further evaluate the specificity of the NW peptide towards blood cells, we analyzed its binding to purified CD14+ monocytes, CD4+ T cells, CD8+ T cells, CD19 B cells, and CD56+ NK cells. The cells were co-stained with the biotinylated NW peptide in combination with cell-lineage specific antibodies (Figure 1B). Under our experimental conditions, only monocytes bound to the NW peptides (first panel). This means that the receptor of the NW peptide is not expressed by cells of lymphoid origin. Immature DCs and macrophages also showed a significant binding to the NW peptide (Figure 1C,D). The binding to macrophages and iDCs had 24 (±2) and 11 (±3) -fold increases over those of the control peptide ($p < 0.0001$ and $p < 0.001$, respectively). Hence, the receptor of the NW peptide seems to be preferentially expressed by monocytes followed by macrophages, and then iDCs.

Most peptides isolated from phage display libraries have affinities unsuitable for clinical use when synthesized as monomers [25,26]. On the phage, peptides are displayed on the pIII coat protein in five copies at the tip of the filamentous phage particle. As such, peptides selected may bind the cell surface in a multivalent manner [25]. However, the NW peptide exhibited a strong binding to monocytes, even at low peptide concentrations (Figure 2A). This strength of peptide binding is comparable to that of monoclonal antibodies.

Given the high affinity of the NW peptide towards blood monocytes, we next investigated its use in magnetic cell separation protocols. In the majority of such separation techniques, target cells are labeled with magnetic beads that are conjugated to specific antibodies [27]. When different cell populations are placed in a magnetic field, those cells that express the antibody receptor and bind to the beads will be attracted to the magnet, and therefore separated from non-targetted cells. Peripheral blood mononuclear cells were incubated with biotin-conjugated NW peptide for 40 min at 4 °C. After addition of streptavidin-conjugated Dynabeads and magnetic separation, non-attached cells were carefully aspirated off and analyzed by flow cytometry to verify the removal of the monocytes (Figure 2B). The data show that most, if not all, monocytes were depleted from blood PBMCs. Although further optimization is required, recovery of the monocytes from the beads can be done by adding larger excess of competing peptide, thus supporting the use of the NW peptide and derivatives in magnetic separation techniques.

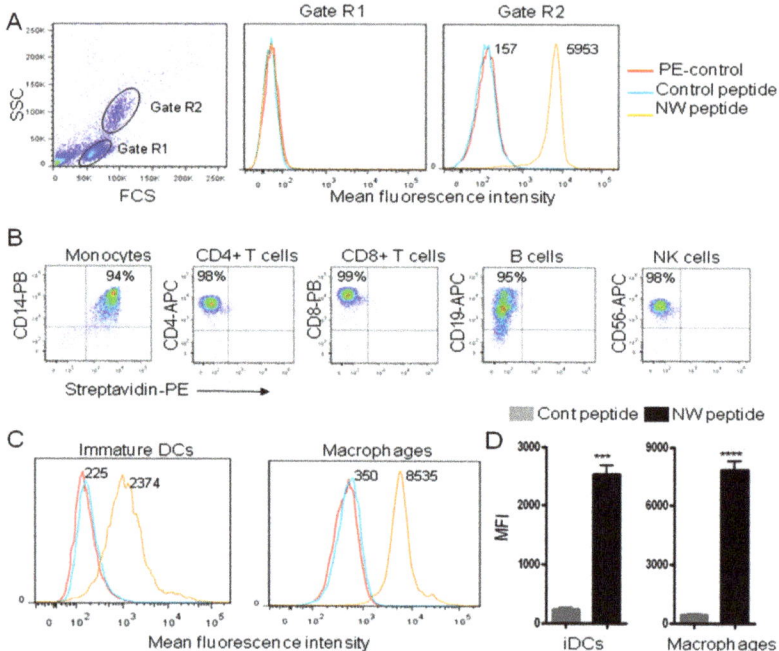

Figure 1. Binding of the NW peptide to blood cells. (**A**) Peripheral blood mononuclear cells (PBMCs) were incubated with the biotinylated W peptide or control peptide (5 μg/mL each) for 40 min at 4 °C. After washing, they were incubated with phycoerythrin (PE)-conjugated streptavidin before analysis by flow cytometry. Gated cells are indicated. The numbers indicate the mean fluorescence intensities (MFI) of the peptide binding. (**B**) Purified blood cell populations were stained with the biotinylated NW peptide in combination with fluorochrome conjugated antibodies specific for CD14, CD4, CD8, CD19, or CD56 cell surface marker, and then analyzed by flow cytometry. The percentages of positive cells are indicated. (**C**) Representative flow cytometry histograms showing the binding of the NW peptide to immature (i) DCs or macrophages. Experimental conditions are as in (**A**). Quantitative data from three independent experiments are shown in (**D**). *** $p < 0.001$, **** $p < 0.0001$.

3.2. Specific Killing of Monocytes by a Lytic Hybrid Peptide

Since the NW peptide efficiently depleted monocytes from PBMCs, we generated a peptide fusion with a pro-apoptotic peptide, and investigated the killing potency of the lytic hybrid peptide. For the pro-apoptotic domain, we first selected the cationic -helix peptide (KLAKLAK)$_2$ (named KLA peptide), a mitochondrial membrane disrupting agent that has been extensively characterized with respect to structure and killing mechanism [20]. PBMCs were incubated with either NW peptide, KLA peptide, or NW-KLA fusion peptide for 15 min at 4 °C, washed to remove excess of peptides and then incubated at 37 °C for 60 min to allow cell killing. Flow cytometry analysis of cells is shown in Figure 3A. The hybrid lytic peptide killed monocytes, but not lymphocytes, indicating that the killing is specific for monocytes. When the cells were incubated with propidium iodide (PI), only dead monocytes (gate R2) incorporated the dye (Figure 3A, last panel, red histogram). Under the same experimental conditions, the lymphocytes were not killed (gate R1, blue histogram).

We next compared the cytotoxic effect of the NW-KLA peptide to a second lytic hybrid peptide (named NW-QLG) that has been found to possess a potent cytotoxic effect against breast cancer cell lines, when internalized via a targeting moiety [28]. Unlike the NW-KLA, the NW-QLG peptide did not induce a significant cell killing at lower peptide concentrations (Figure 3B). The IC$_{50}$ values for the two peptides were 9 M and >30 M, respectively. As shown in Figure 3C, exposing monocytes to the NW-KLA fusion peptide resulted in time-dependent loss of cell viability. Most of the cells were killed within a 10–15 min incubation time. Purified T cells were used as a control, as they did not bind to the NW peptide. Under the same experimental conditions, T cells were not killed (Figure 3C).

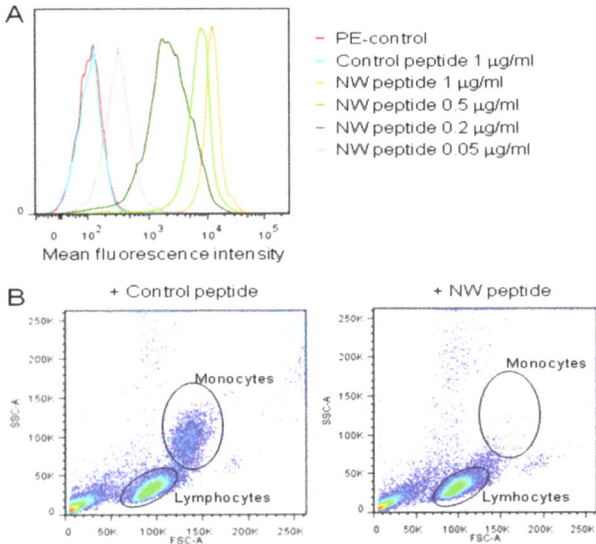

Figure 2. Binding and depletion of blood monocytes. (**A**) Representative flow cytometry histograms showing the peptide binding to purified blood monocytes. Cells were incubated with various concentrations of the biotinylated NW peptide, followed by streptavidin-conjugate PE and analysis by flow cytometry. (**B**) Monocyte depletion. PBMCs were incubated with the biotinylated NW peptide or control peptide (20 µg/mL each), and then processed as described in Material and Methods. The cells were analyzed by flow cytometry to check for monocyte depletion after peptide addition and capture on streptavidin beads. The data are representative of four independent experiments.

Usually, cells expose on their surface phosphatidylserine (PS) when they undergo apoptosis [29]. Annexin V binds to PS and therefore can be used to monitor this early event in apoptosis process. Hence, we performed a flow cytometry analysis to determine the death pathway of the targeted lytic peptide using a Dead Cell Apoptosis Kit with Annexin V-FITC and PI. In these experiments, purified monocytes were used. Treatment of the cells with the NW-KLA peptide caused an increase in annexin V positive cells (Figure 3D, a representative example). More than half of the cells (52.8%, ± 10%, $p < 0.01$) were at late apoptosis/secondary necrosis phases (Annexin V+ and PI+) (Figure 3E). Although PS may be exposed under a variety of circumstances and could be a general indicator of membrane instability [30–32], the data suggest that monocytes undergo both apoptosis and necrosis pathways after treatment with the NW-KLA peptide. Again, the KLA peptide showed no significant effect as compared to untreated cells.

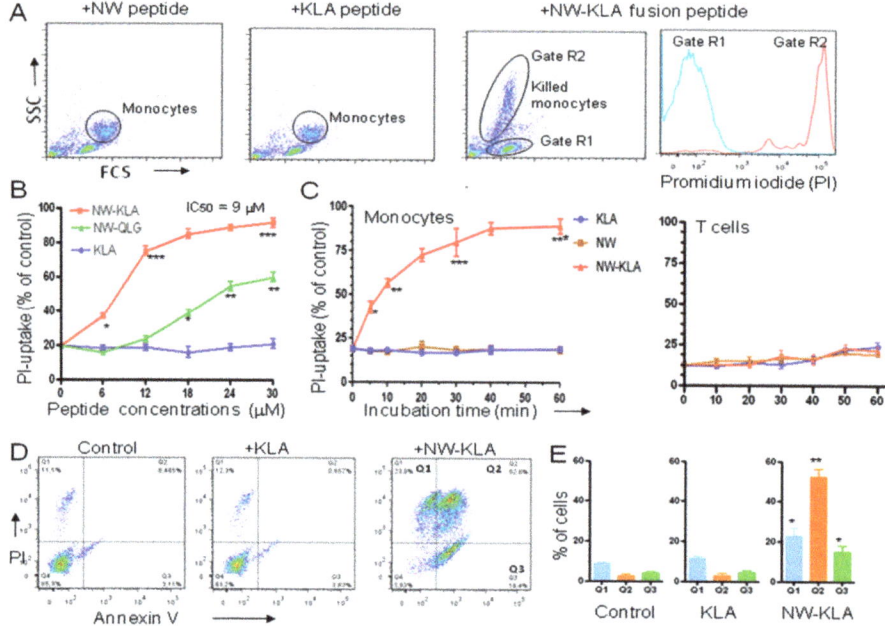

Figure 3. Effects of the fusion peptides on monocyte viability. (**A**) Selective killing of monocytes. Peripheral blood mononuclear cells were incubated with the indicated peptides as described in the text, and then they were analyzed by flow cytometry. Cells were also incubated with propidium iodide (PI) to check for membrane integrity. Data are representative of at least three independent experiments. (**B**) Cytotoxic effects of the fusion peptides. Purified monocytes were cultured in complete medium and then treated for 60 min with various peptide concentrations, incubated with PI and then analyzed by flow cytometry. Data are from three independent experiments. (**C**) Killing kinetics. Purified CD14+ monocytes or CD4+ T cells were incubated with the tested peptides (10 µM each) and then analyzed by flow cytometry at various time points after PI incubation. Data are from three independent experiments. (**D**) Induction of apoptosis. After incubation with the peptides for 60 min at 37 °C, monocytes were analyzed by dual-color flow cytometry for annexin V and PI staining. Quantitative data from three independent experiments are shown in (**E**). * $p < 0.05$, ** $p < 0.01$, *** $p < 0.001$.

3.3. Effects of the Fusion Lytic Peptides on M1 and M2 Macrophages

One strategy to deplete TAMs is to cut off their replenishment, by circulating inflammatory monocytes. Hence, the killing of blood monocytes, as demonstrated in Figure 3, should result in reduced numbers of TAMs in primary and metastatic sites. As M2 TAMs promote cancer progression and resistance to therapy, we investigated whether the engineered targeted lytic peptides could preferentially kill M2 or M1 macrophages. Monocyte polarization into M1 or M2 macrophages was induced in vitro as described in Materials and Methods. In accordance to previous studies [33], M1 and M2 cells presented either an elongated (M1) or round (M2) morphology, respectively (Figure 4A). The M2 phenotype was further characterized by analyzing the expression of the specific marker CD163. At day eight after differentiation, the expression of CD163 by M2 was significantly increased when compared to M1 macrophages (Figure 4B,C, $p < 0.001$). In contrast to M2, M1 macrophages are characterized by the expression of CD80 and the absence of CD163 [34]. In this respect, the expression of CD80 on M1 macrophages was significantly upregulated, as compared to M2 macrophages (Figure 4B,C, $p < 0.01$). As expected, both cell populations expressed the CD14 marker.

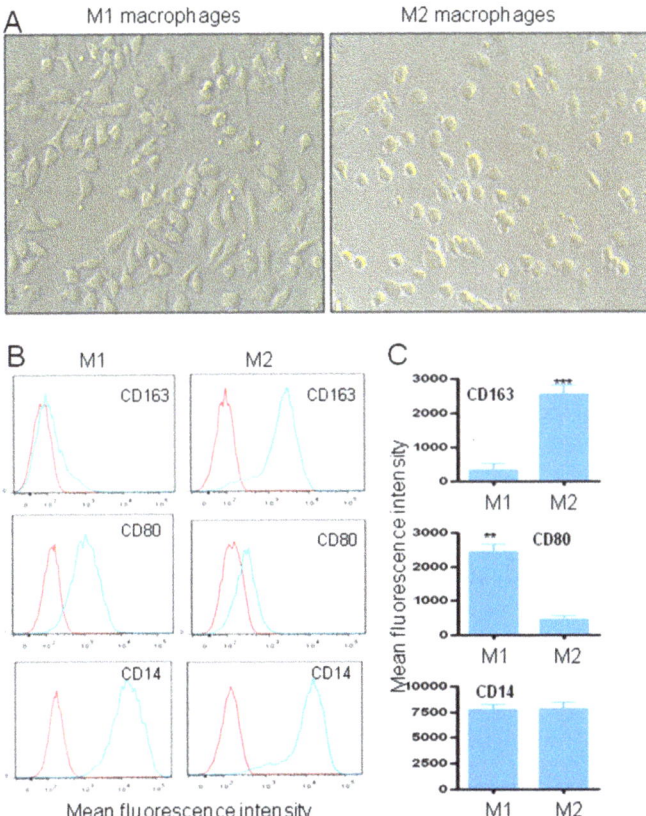

Figure 4. Monocyte-derived M1 and M2 macrophages. (**A**) Morphology of monocyte-derived M1 or M2 macrophages in X-vivo 15 medium. Original magnification, x20. (**B**) Phenotypic characterization of M1 and M2 macrophages. Cell surface expression of CD163, CD80 and CD14 markers by M1 and M2 macrophages. (**C**) Quantitative data from three independent experiments are presented as a mean ± SD. ** $p < 0.01$, *** $p < 0.001$.

Having confirmed the polarization status of the cells, we next tested their binding to the NW peptide (Figure 5A). The peptide bound to both M1 and M2 macrophages. The MFIs of the NW peptide binding to M1 and M2 macrophages were, respectively, 27 and 15 fold higher than those of the control peptide. In most experiments, a small population of M1 macrophages showed a strong binding to the NW peptide. Such binding may contribute to the overall MFI increase.

The potential of using the NW peptide to deliver polypeptides/proteins to macrophages was investigated by examining its ability to promote the internalization of streptavidin-PE conjugates. The cells were pre-incubated for 30 min at 4 °C with preformed biotin-peptide/streptavidin-PE complexes, washed, and subsequently transferred to 37 °C to allow peptide internalization. Since active endocytosis occurs in cells at 37 °C, but not at 4 °C, the complexes can be internalized only after specific binding of the NW peptide to macrophages. Whereas macrophages incubated with the control peptide-PE complexes showed no red fluorescence, those incubated with the NW-peptide-PE-complexes showed intensive cytoplasmic fluorescence resulting from peptide internalization (Figure 5B). It should be noted that streptavidin-PE conjugates did not bind to macrophages (Figure 5A).

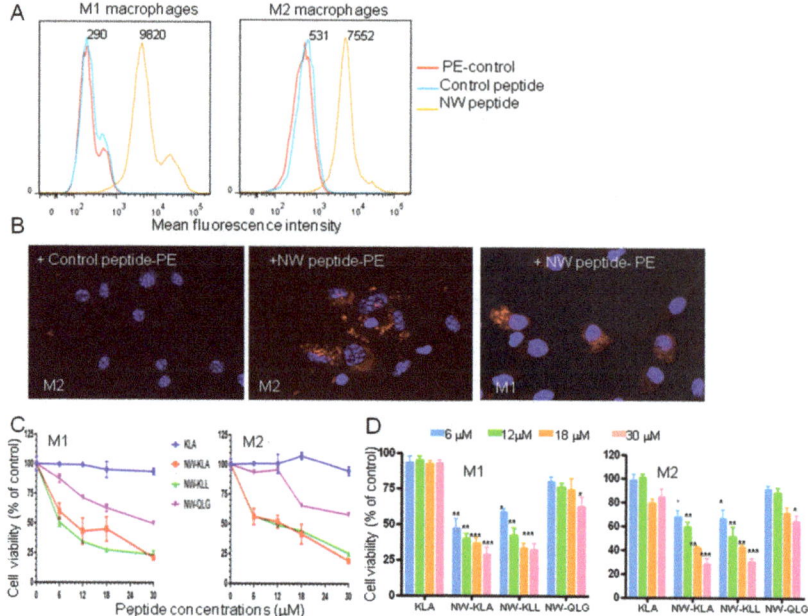

Figure 5. Effects of the fusion lytic peptides on M1 and M2 macrophages. (**A**) Representative flow cytometry histograms showing the binding of the NW peptide to M1 and M2 macrophages. The numbers indicate the mean fluorescence intensities of the peptide binding. (**B**) Internalization of the NW-peptide-streptavidin-PE complexes by M2 and M1 macrophages. Biotinylated NW peptide- or control peptide-streptavidin-PE complexes were added to M2 macrophages and incubated for 40 min at 4 °C. After washing, the cells were incubated at 37 °C for 60 min, further washed, fixed, and then confocal microscopy images were taken. Original magnification, x40. The uptake of the NW peptide-PE complexes by M1 is also shown. (**C**) Cell viability. The cells were incubated with various concentrations of the tested peptides for 60 min at 37 °C, and cell viability was determined using the CellTiter 96R Aqueous One Solution reagent. The results are represented as mean ± SD of triplicate determination. Quantitative data (mean ± SD) from three independent experiments are shown in (**D**). ** $p < 0.01$, *** $p < 0.001$.

In the next experiments, we evaluated the cytotoxic effects of the lytic fusion peptides on macrophages. We included a third lytic domain containing several leucine residues (KLL; KLLLKLLKKLLKLLKKKK) that was shown to induce apoptosis in cancer cells [35]. Although the NW peptide bound better to M1 macrophages when compared to their M2 counterparts, the killing effects of the lytic peptides were comparable (Figure 5C,D). Cells treated with either NW-KLA or NW-KLL lytic peptide were killed effectively when compared to those treated with the other peptides. The IC_{50} values for NW-KLA, NW-KLL and NW-QLG peptides were around 10 ± 2, 6 ± 1, 30 ± 3 µM, for M1 macrophages, and 9 ± 1.5, 9 ± 1.4, >30 µM, for M2 macrophages, respectively. When tested at higher concentrations, the IC_{50} values for the NW-QLG peptide were found to be around 40 µM for M1 and 70 µM for M2 macrophages.

3.4. Effects of the Fusion Lytic Peptides on Leukemia Cell Lines

Although many advances have occurred in the treatment of blood malignancies, the treatment of relapsed/refractory acute myeloid leukemia (AML) remains one of the most challenging tasks in oncology today [36,37]. Hence, novel treatment strategies are needed. We first tested the binding of the NW peptide to MV-4-11, a human acute myeloid leukemia cell line, and to U937, a pro-monocytic human myeloid leukemia cell line. As shown in Figure 6A, the NW peptide bound to both cell lines. Cells incubated with the lytic hybrid NW-KLA or the NW-KLL peptide showed significant toxicity when compared to those incubated with free KLA or NW-QLG peptide (Figure 6B). In the case of U937 cells, both NW-KLA and NW-KLL peptides had comparable IC_{50} values (5–8 µM). MV-4-11 cells seem to be more sensitive to the NW-KLA peptide (IC_{50} = 4 µM) than the NW-KLL peptide (IC_{50} = 12 µM). Again, the pro-apoptosis QLG domain did not induce killing of leukemia cell lines at lower concentrations (<12 µM). At higher concentrations, the NW-QLG IC_{50} values for MV4 and U937 were around 60 and 90 µM, respectively.

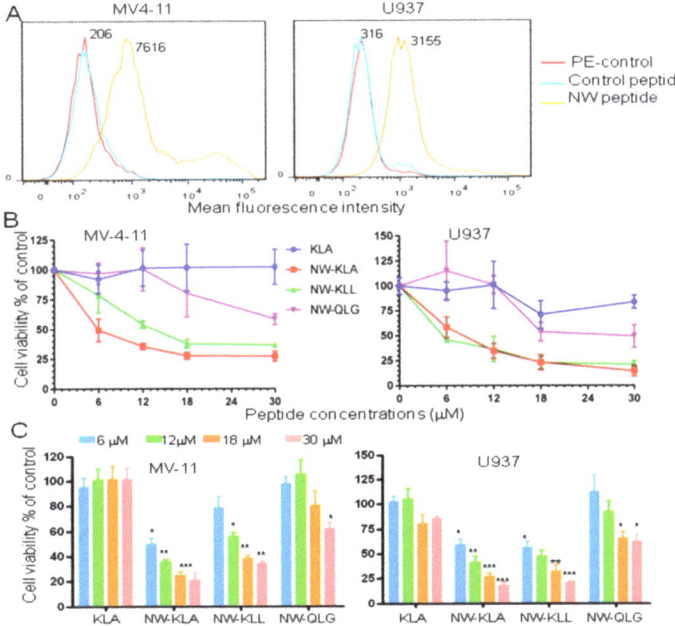

Figure 6. Effects of the fusion lytic peptides on human leukemia cell lines. (**A**) Representative flow cytometry histograms showing the binding of the NW peptide to MV-4-11 and U937 leukemia cells. The numbers indicate the mean fluorescence intensities of the peptide binding. (**B**) Cell viability in response to the peptides. The cells were incubated with various peptide concentrations for 60 min at 37 °C, and then cell viability was determined using the CellTiter 96R Aqueous One Solution reagent. The results are represented as mean ± SD of triplicate determination. Quantitative data (mean ± SD) from three independent experiments are shown in (**C**). * $p < 0.05$, ** $p < 0.01$, *** $p < 0.001$.

We next evaluated the permeability of MV-4-11 cells to promidium iodide (PI) after peptide treatment. PI does not stain live cells, due to the presence of an intact plasma membrane. As indicated by the forward scatter (Figure 7A), cells treated with the NW-KLA peptide for 20 min showed a smaller size and most cells were porous to PI (Figure 7B, last panel), indicating that they were killed. In contrast, cells treated with the control peptides remained unchanged compared to untreated cells. In accordance with the flow data, confocal microscopy images showed that the cells treated with the NW-KLA peptide were permeable to PI, making them become red.

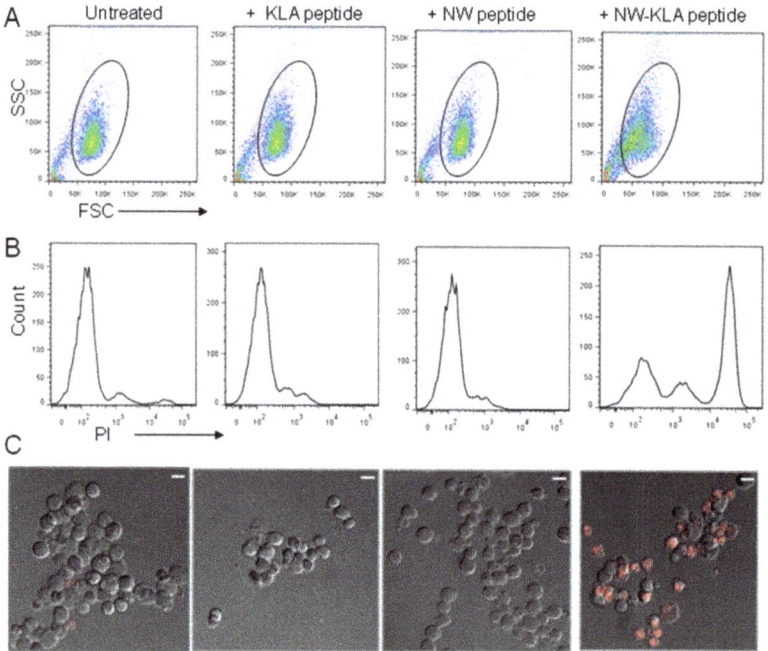

Figure 7. Permeability of MV-4-11 cells after treatment with the NW-KLA peptide. (**A,B**) MV-4-11 cells were treated with the test peptides (6 µM each) for 20 min at 37 °C, incubated with PI and then analyzed by flow cytometry. (**C**) Confocal microscopy images. After incubation with PI, the cells were washed and resuspended in 100 µL PBS buffer. One drop of each cell suspension was spotted onto microscope glass slips and processed for confocal microscopy. Images are of single sections through the middle of cells. Scale bar represents 10 µm. The same samples shown in A were analyzed in B and C.

3.5. Effects of the Lytic Peptides on Primary Leukemia Cells

Although the life expectancy of patients with acute myeloid leukemia (AML) or chronic myeloid leukemia (CML) has improved in recent years, treatment resistant and refractory leukemia are still a major problem [36,37]. Hence, novel approaches to treatment are urgently needed to further improve the prognosis of these diseases. Prompted by the strong cytotoxic effects of the engineered lytic hybrid peptides on leukemia cell lines, we investigated next, whether the NW-KLA peptide would kill primary leukemia cells. Figure 8 shows the binding of the NW peptide and control peptide to freshly isolated blood AML (Figure 7A) and CML (Figure 7B) blasts. By contrast to the control peptide, the NW peptide showed a very strong binding to both blast types, indicating that the peptide receptor is overexpressed in primary leukemia cells when compared to leukemia cell lines and macrophages. In the case of the CML, the lymphocyte population (gate R1) did not bind to the NW peptide, again arguing that the peptide binds to a receptor that is expressed by cells of myeloid, but not lymphoid origin. Treatment with the NW-KLA peptide induced cell death in a dose-dependent manner (Figure 8C). When tested at 10 µM for 2 h, the lytic hybrid peptides showed significant cytotoxic effects on blast cells (Figure 9). The average decrease in viability of freshly isolated AML blasts due to the treatment with the NW-KLA and NW-KLL lytic peptides were 88 ± 5% ($p < 0.001$), 75 ± 6% ($p < 0.001$), respectively. Similarly, these two lytic peptides induced around 74 ± 7% of cell death in CML blasts ($p < 0.001$). There was no significant difference in viability between untreated cells and those treated with the control peptides. Comparable results were obtained with additional three patients with AML and four patients with CML.

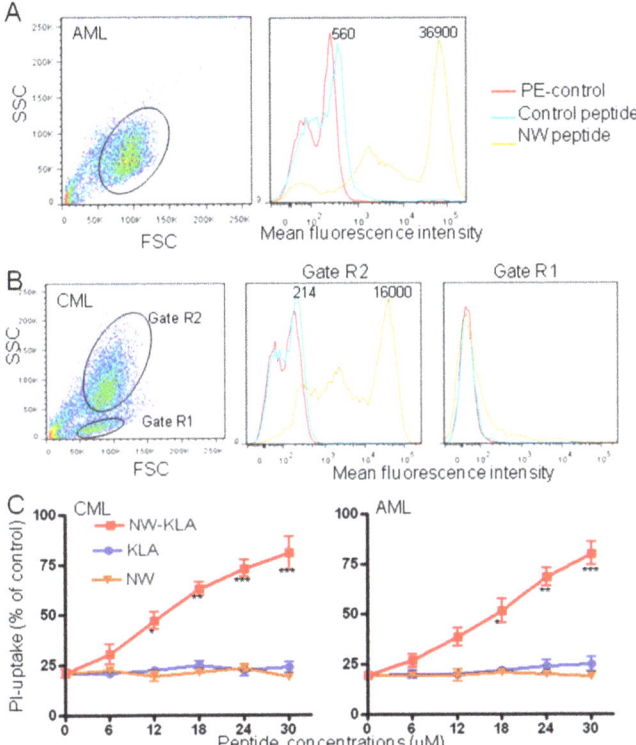

Figure 8. Effects of the targeted lytic peptides on human primary leukemia cells. Representative flow cytometry histograms showing the binding of the NW peptide to primary leukemia cells from a patient with acute myeloid leukemia (AML) (**A**) or from a patient with chronic myeloid leukemia CML (**B**). Gated cells are indicated. The numbers indicate the mean fluorescence intensities of the peptide binding (**C**). Cell viability in response to the peptide treatment. The cells were incubated with various concentrations of the tested peptides for 60 min at 37 °C, and then cell viability was determined using flow cytometry subsequent to PI incubation. The results are represented as mean ± SD of three independent experiments. * $p < 0.05$, ** $p < 0.01$, *** $p < 0.001$.

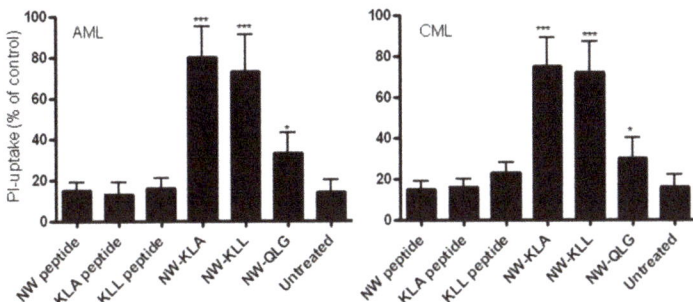

Figure 9. Cytotoxic effects of the fusion peptides on primary leukemia cells. Cells were incubated with the indicated test peptides (12 μM each) for 120 min at 37 °C followed with PI staining and analysis by flow cytometry. The data are from three independent experiments and are presented as mean ± SD. * $p < 0.05$, *** $p < 0.001$.

3.6. Depletion of Blood Blast Cells

A number of methods have been used to remove leukemia cells from blood or bone marrow aspirates [38]. In such techniques, the specificity of magnetic affinity separation is based on the selectivity of monoclonal antibody binding to target cells. Given the strong binding of the NW peptide to primary leukemia cells, we investigated whether it can be used to deplete or reduce blast cells from PBMCs. Peptide mediated blast depletion in each PBMC sample was determined by flow cytometry by counting the cells in blast population (gate R2) vs those in lymphocyte population (gate R1) and by relating the ratios with those of the corresponding untreated sample (Figure 10 as a representative example). For both samples, fifteen thousand ungated events were collected. The NW peptide depleted most blood leukemia blasts (9.5% vs. 52%). Notably, the lymphocyte population was significantly enriched (7.2% vs. 51.1%). Thus, the NW peptide can be used to remove blast cells and enrich for other cell types, such as lymphocytes.

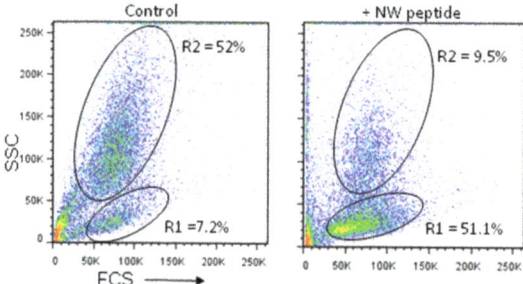

Figure 10. Depletion of blast cells from whole PBMCs. PBMCs from a patient with CML were incubated or not with the biotinylated NW peptide (10 µg/mL), followed by streptavidin-conjugated magnetic beads, as described in Materials and Methods. After magnetic separation, non-binding cells were analyzed by flow cytometry to verify blast depletion. 15,000 events were recorded for each sample.

3.7. Effects of the NW-KLA Peptide on Primary Mammary Epithelial Cells

Having demonstrated that the lytic hybrid peptides can kill monocytes, macrophages, and leukemia cells, we investigated their cytotoxic effects on primary human mammary epithelial cells (HMECs). We first analyzed the binding of the NW peptide to the cells (Figure 11A). No significant binding was detected, suggesting that the peptide receptor is not expressed by non-hematopoietic cells. Treatment of HMECs by the lytic fusion peptides did not result in significant cytotoxic effects (Figure 11B). Thus, the expression of the peptide receptor on target cells is indispensable for the cytotoxicity of the engineered fusion lytic peptides.

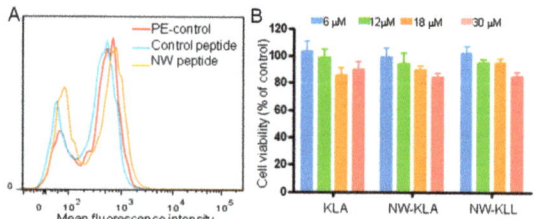

Figure 11. Effects of the fusion lytic peptides on normal mammary epithelial cells. (**A**) Representative flow cytometry histograms showing the binding of the NW peptide to primary human mammary epithelial cells. (**B**) Cell viability. The cells were incubated with various concentrations of the tested peptides for 60 min at 37 °C and cell viability was determined using the CellTiter 96R Aqueous One Solution reagent. The results are represented as mean ± SD of three independent experiments.

4. Discussion

Although abnormalities of cancer genes are essential contributors to cancer, cells within the tumor microenvironment, such as macrophages, myeloid-derived suppressor cells, and T regulatory cells play an important part in the initiation and progression of solid tumors [18,39]. Additionally, host macrophages can promote lymphoma and leukemia cell survival in vitro and in vivo [40–42]. By coupling pro-apoptotic peptides to the NW peptide, we engineered new targeted lytic peptides that killed monocytes and macrophages. At the concentrations used, the lytic hybrid peptides did not kill blood lymphocytes. Monocytes and macrophages are widely acknowledged as one of the central suppressive populations within solid tumors, and depleting these cells should benefit patients with solid and blood malignancies. Therapies that deplete TAMs and/or cut off their replenishment by circulating inflammatory monocytes would also benefit patients with various inflammatory diseases.

In several types of cancers, including ovarian, pancreatic, breast, and brain cancers, most, if not all, TAMs express the M2 phenotype [4,5]. In these cancers, specific therapy targeting M1 or M2 macrophages may not be required. Indeed, untargeted depletion of monocytes and macrophages in experimental settings has been successful in inhibiting tumor growth and enhancing responses to standard chemo and anti-angiogenic therapies [43,44]. Recently, Galletti et al. showed that eliminating TAMs along with neutrophils, sensitizes mammary tumors to chemotherapy, resulting in tumor eradication in mice [42]. The authors used a monoclonal antibody to block CSF-1R signaling, required for macrophage development and infiltration into tumor tissues. Similarly, the use of small molecule inhibitors or antisense RNA strategies to inhibit CSF-1R signaling, also inhibited tumor growth in both xenograft and genetically engineered mouse models [45–47]. Our current targeting strategy would preferentially eliminate both circulating monocytes and macrophages, and might be better than previously tested strategies. Unlike tissue resident macrophages, which are derived largely from the yolk sac in embryogenesis, TAMs derive from circulating blood monocytes [3]. Using phage display, Cieslewicz et al. selected a peptide specific for murine macrophages [48]. When fused to a pro-apoptotic peptide, the fusion peptide inhibited tumor growth in a subcutaneous tumor model [48]. Unfortunately, the selected peptide showed no significant binding to human M1 and M2 macrophages [48].

With respect to blood malignancies, adults with AML have some of the highest unmet treatment needs of all cancer patients. The outcomes for patients with relapsed or refractory AML are poor, with overall survival estimated at no more than 10% at 3 years [49,50]. In addition to cell lines, the killing potency of the NW-KLA and the NW-KLL fusion peptides was confirmed in leukemia patient samples at low concentrations. In all experiments, the NW-QKG fusion peptide killed leukemia cells only at higher concentrations. Early reports from Ghosh's group showed that the leucine residues were essential for peptide structure and cytotoxic effect [51]. Most anti-cancer peptides, natural and synthetic, contain several leucine residues. By contrast, the lytic QLG domain contains only one leucine residue, which may explain its weak cytotoxic effects at lower concentrations. Interestingly, the NW-QLG fusion peptide preferentially killed M1 rather than M2 macrophages at high peptide concentrations.

Although promising agents such as Bcr-Abl tyrosine kinase inhibitors have shown a significant therapeutic efficacy in patients with CML [52], the search for innovative therapeutic alternatives in this disease is also essential, due to the emergence of primary or secondary resistance to treatment. Moreover, there is a need in improving the management of CML in blast crisis. A large number of patients with hyperleucytosis can develop leukostasis, a life-threatening situation where leukemia cells are thought to cause organ dysfunction [53]. The lytic hybrid NW-KLA and NW-KLL peptides showed a strong cytotoxic effect against CML blasts. Moreover, we demonstrated that the targeting NW peptide can selectively deplete blast cells from PBMCs. Although in vivo work is needed, the data would support the development of the engineered lytic hybrid peptides as a myeloid cytoreduction therapy.

In addition to solid tumors, macrophages have recently been reported to be involved in tumor progression in several hematological malignancies, such as CML, AML, and B-cell lymphomas [40–42,54]. TAMs are highly present in relapsed and refractory lymphomas, most likely playing an important role in multiple types of drug resistance [50]. Recently, Al-Matary et al. showed that myeloid leukemia-associated macrophages can support the progression of AML [40]. The authors showed a significant increase in M2 macrophages in the bone marrow of AML patients when compared to healthy volunteers. These M2 macrophages supported the growth of both human and murine AML cells in vitro. Targeting macrophages using anti-CSF-1R antibody or clodrolip (clodronate encapsulated liposomes) also impaired chronic lymphocytic leukemia cell engraftment. Macrophage depletion sensitized leukemia cells to apoptosis via induction of TNF-α signaling, and leukemia cells were killed through a TNF-α-dependent mechanism [39]. The NW-KLA peptide, unlike other targeted cytotoxins, offers the possibility of targeting monocytes, macrophages, and leukemia cells.

With respect to chemotherapy, cancer cells become resistant to a variety of structurally different drugs, even after treatment with only one single drug [55]. By contrast, lytic peptides, when delivered via a targeting moiety, damage cell membranes within minutes which would hinder formation of resistance. Most lytic peptides killed both drug-sensitive and drug-resistant cancer cells [19,22]. Notably, the tumor selectivity of lytic peptides was considerably enhanced after the fusion to tumor targeting domains, such as antibodies and peptides [20,56]. Moreover, a variety of nanoparticles were also applied for the delivery of lytic peptides, resulting in reduced side effects, and an increase in targeted accumulation in tumor tissues [57,58]. Under our experimental conditions, the KLA peptide did not kill target cells, whereas the hybrid peptides did. Thus, the killing activity requires the presence of the targeting NW domain. Out of the three designed peptides, the NW-KLA and NW-KLL peptides showed the strongest lytic activity. It should be noted that the NW peptide has no effect on cell viability, even at high concentrations.

With respect to peptide selection, a primary advantage of the phage display technology is that affinity-based interactions are detected in native biological systems. The screening on intact cells preserves the original conformation of cell surface proteins and protein-protein interactions that could be relevant in vivo. While a number of selected peptides from phage display libraries have been used as tumor imaging agents, or disease biomarkers without knowledge of their binding receptors [25,59], the clinical use of such peptides will be further facilitated better by the characterization of their binding partners. Moreover, once the partner is known, certain amino acid chains of the peptide can be modified to improve its binding affinity and specificity. Unfortunately, immunoprecipitation experiments with the biotinylated NW peptide failed to identify potential partners. This is most likely due to the intrinsic nature of membrane proteins. They are present in low abundance, and their solubility in most buffers is a major issue. The selection of detergents suitable for the solubilization and purification of a specific membrane protein is critical for the outcome of the experiments. A combination of proteomic and genomic approaches will be needed to tackle this challenging task that is under investigation.

5. Conclusions

Macrophages are among the most abundant normal cells in the tumor microenvironment, and usually play a pro-tumoral role. Additionally, they support the proliferation and survival of leukemia and lymphoma cells. By fusing a targeting peptide to pro-apoptotic peptides, we engineered new lytic hybrid peptides that killed monocytes, macrophages and leukemia cells. Killing leukemia cells and macrophages with one single agent, such as the lytic fusion NW-KLA peptide should benefit patients with blood malignancies. In addition to therapy, the NW peptide could be a good candidate for cell depletion from blood and/or bone marrow aspirates.

Author Contributions: M.S. designed the study, supervised the project, performed some of the experiments shown in Figures 1–11, and analyzed the data. S.P. performed some of the experiments shown in Figures 3–6, and analyzed the data. I.A. performed the experiment shown in Figure 7C (confocal imaging), and analyzed the data. Y.F. provided patient blood samples, analyzed the data, and discussed the project plans. M.S. wrote the manuscript. All authors edited the final version of the manuscript.

Funding: This work was supported by the Norwegian Cancer Society (Grant No. 182593).

Acknowledgments: We are thankful to Linn A. Rosenberg and Anne Mobergslien for excellent technical assistance with the project.

Conflicts of Interest: The authors declare no conflict of interest.

References

1. Sica, A.; Mantovani, A. Macrophage plasticity and polarization: In vivo veritas. *J. Clin. Investig.* **2012**, *122*, 787–795. [CrossRef] [PubMed]
2. Murray, P.J.; Wynn, T.A. Protective and pathogenic functions of macrophage subsets. *Nat. Rev. Immunol.* **2011**, *11*, 723–737. [CrossRef] [PubMed]
3. Brown, J.M.; Recht, L.; Strober, S. The promise of targeting Macrophages in Cancer Therapy. *Clin. Cancer Res.* **2017**, *23*, 3241–3250. [CrossRef] [PubMed]
4. Mantovani, A.; Sozzani, S.; Locati, M.; Allavena, P.; Sica, A. Macrophage polarization: Tumor-associated macrophages as a paradigm for polarized M2 mononuclear phagocytes. *Trends Immunol.* **2002**, *23*, 549–555. [CrossRef]
5. Pollard, J.W. Tumour-educated macrophages promote tumour progression and metastasis. *Nat. Rev. Cancer* **2004**, *4*, 71–78. [CrossRef] [PubMed]
6. Qian, B.Z.; Li, J.; Zhang, H.; Kitamura, T.; Zhang, J.; Campion, L.R.; Kaiser, E.A.; Snyder, L.A.; Pollard, J.W. CCL2 recruits inflammatory monocytes to facilitate breast-tumour metastasis. *Nature* **2011**, *475*, 222–225. [CrossRef] [PubMed]
7. Qian, B.Z.; Pollard, J.W. Macrophage diversity enhances tumor progression and metastasis. *Cell* **2010**, *141*, 39–51. [CrossRef] [PubMed]
8. Steidl, C.; Lee, T.; Shah, S.P.; Farinha, P.; Han, G.; Nayar, T.; Delaney, A.; Jones, S.J.; Iqbal, J.; Weisenburger, D.D.; et al. Tumor-associated macrophages and survival in classic Hodgkin's lymphoma. *N. Engl. J. Med.* **2010**, *362*, 875–885. [CrossRef]
9. Gupta, V.; Yull, F.; Khabele, D. Bipolar Tumor-associated macrophages in ovarian cancer as targets for therapy. *Cancers* **2018**, *10*, 366. [CrossRef]
10. Davignon, J.L.; Hayder, M.; Baron, M.; Boyer, J.F.; Constantin, A.; Apparailly, F.; Poupot, R.; Cantagrel, A. Targeting monocytes/macrophages in the treatment of rheumatoid arthritis. *Reumatology* **2013**, *52*, 590–598. [CrossRef]
11. Roberts, C.A.; Dickinson, A.K.; Taams, L.S. The Interplay Between Monocytes/Macrophages and CD4$^+$ T Cell Subsets in Rheumatoid Arthritis. *Front Immunol.* **2015**, *6*, 571. [CrossRef] [PubMed]
12. Rana, A.K.; Li, Y.; Dang, Q.; Yang, F. Monocytes in rheumatoid arthritis: Circulating precursors of macrophages and osteoclasts and, their heterogeneity and plasticity role in RA pathogenesis. *Int. Immunopharmacol.* **2018**, *65*, 348–359. [CrossRef] [PubMed]
13. Balhara, J.; Gounni, A.S. The alveolar macrophages in asthma: A double-edged sword. *Mucosal Immunol.* **2012**, *5*, 605–609. [CrossRef] [PubMed]
14. Carter, N.J.; Keam, S.J. Trabectedin: A review of its use in soft tissue sarcoma and ovarian cancer. *Drugs* **2010**, *70*, 355–376. [CrossRef] [PubMed]
15. Germano, G.; Frapolli, R.; Belgiovine, C.; Anselmo, A.; Pesce, S.; Liguori, M.; Erba, E.; Uboldi, S.; Zucchetti, M.; Pasqualini, F.; et al. Role of Macrophage Targeting in the Antitumor Activity of Trabectedin. *Cancer Cell* **2013**, *23*, 249–262. [CrossRef]
16. Roelofs, A.J.; Thompson, K.; Ebetino, F.H.; Rogers, M.J.; Coxon, F.P. Bisphosphonates: Molecular mechanisms of action and effects on bone cells, monocytes and macrophages. *Curr. Pharm. Des.* **2010**, *16*, 2950–2960. [CrossRef] [PubMed]
17. Ries, C.H.; Cannarile, M.A.; Hoves, S.; Benz, J.; Wartha, K.; Runza, V.; Rey-Giraud, F.; Pradel, L.P.; Feuerhake, F.; Klaman, I.; et al. Targeting tumor-associated macrophages with anti-CSF-1R antibody reveals a strategy for cancer therapy. *Cancer Cell* **2014**, *25*, 846–859. [CrossRef]
18. Zins, K.; Sioud, M.; Aharinejad, S.; Lucas, T.; Abraham, D. Modulating the tumor microenvironment with RNA interference as a cancer treatment strategy. *Methods Mol. Biol.* **2015**, *1218*, 143–161.
19. Papo, N.; Shai, Y. Host defence peptides as new weapons in cancer treatment. *Cell. Mol. Life Sci.* **2005**, *62*, 785–790. [CrossRef]
20. Leuschner, C.; Hansel, W. Membrane disrupting lytic peptides for cancer treatments. *Curr. Pharm. Des.* **2004**, *10*, 2299–2310. [CrossRef]

21. Barua, S.; Linton, R.S.; Gamboa, J.; Banerjee, I.; Yarmush, M.L.; Rege, K. Lytic peptide-mediated sensitization of TRAIL-resistant prostate cancer cells to death receptor agonists. *Cancer Lett.* **2010**, *293*, 240–253. [CrossRef] [PubMed]
22. Sioud, M.; Mobergslien, A. Selective killing of cancer cells by peptide-targeted elivery of an anti-microbial peptide. *Biochem. Pharm.* **2012**, *84*, 1123–1132. [CrossRef] [PubMed]
23. Rege, K.; Patel, S.J.; Megeed, Z.; Yarmush, M.L. Amphipathic peptide-based fusion peptides and immunoconjugates for the targeted ablation of prostate cancer cells. *Cancer Res.* **2007**, *67*, 785–790. [CrossRef] [PubMed]
24. Sioud, M.; Skorstad, G.; Mobergslien, A.; Sæbøe-Larssen, S. A novel peptide carrier for efficient targeting of antigens and nucleic acids to dendritic cells. *FASEB J.* **2013**, *27*, 3272–3283. [CrossRef] [PubMed]
25. Sioud, M. Phage Display Libraries: From binders to targeted drug delivery and human therapeutics. *Mol. Biotechnol.* **2019**, *61*, 286–303. [CrossRef] [PubMed]
26. Galán, A.; Comor, L.; Horvatić, A.; Kuleš, J.; Guillemin, N.; Mrljak, V.; Bhide, M. Library-based display technologies: Where do we stand? *Mol. Biosyst.* **2016**, *12*, 2342–2358. [CrossRef] [PubMed]
27. Jain, R.; Gray, D.H. Isolation of thymic epithelial cells and analysis by flow cytometry. *Curr. Protoc. Immunol.* **2014**, *107*, 3–26. [PubMed]
28. Neo, S.H.; Lew, Q.J.; Koh, S.M.; Zheng, L.; Bi, X.; Chao, S.H. Use of a novel cytotoxic HEXIM1 peptide in the directed breast cancer therapy. *Oncotarget* **2015**, *7*, 5483–5494. [CrossRef]
29. Vermes, I.; Haanen, C.; Steffens-Nakken, H.; Reutelingsperger, C. A novel assay for apoptosis. Flow cytometric detection of phosphatidylserine expression on early apoptotic cells using fluorescein labelled Annexin V. *J. Immunol. Methods* **1995**, *184*, 39–51. [CrossRef]
30. Arakawa, S.; Nakanomyo, I.; Kudo-Sakamoto, Y.; Akazawa, H.; Komuro, I.; Shimizu, S. Identification of a novel compound that inhibits both mitochondria-mediated necrosis and apoptosis. *Biochem. Biophys. Res. Commun.* **2015**, *467*, 1006–1011. [CrossRef]
31. Lecoeur, H.; Prévost, M.C.; Gougeon, M.L. Oncosis is associated with exposure of phosphatidylserine residues on the outside layer of the plasma membrane: A reconsideration of the specificity of the annexin V/propidium iodide assay. *Cytometry* **2001**, *44*, 65–72. [CrossRef]
32. Zargarian, S.; Shlomovitz, I.; Erlich, Z.; Hourizadeh, A.; Ofir-Birin, Y.; Croker, B.A.; Regev-Rudzki, N.; Edry-Botzer, L.; Gerlic, M. Phosphatidylserine externalization, "necroptotic bodies" release, and phagocytosis during necroptosis. *PLoS Biol.* **2017**, *15*, e2002711. [CrossRef] [PubMed]
33. Rey-Giraud, F.; Hafner, M.; Ries, C.H. In vitro generation of monocyte-derived macrophages under serum-free conditions improves their tumor promoting functions. *PLoS ONE* **2012**, *7*, e42656. [CrossRef] [PubMed]
34. Martinez, F.O.; Scia, A.; Mantovani, A.; Locati, M. Macrohagae activation and polarization. *Front. Biosci.* **2008**, *13*, 453–461. [CrossRef] [PubMed]
35. Kohno, M.; Horibe, T.; Haramoto, M.; Yano, Y.; Ohara, K.; Nakajima, O.; Matsuzaki, K.; Kawakami, K. A novel hybrid peptide targeting EGFR-expressing cancers. *Eur. J. Cancer* **2011**, *47*, 773–783. [CrossRef] [PubMed]
36. Bose, P.; Vachhani, P.; Cortes, J.E. Treatment of relapsed/refractory acute myeloid leukemia. *Curr. Treat. Opt. Oncol.* **2017**, *18*, 17. [CrossRef] [PubMed]
37. Guinn, B.A.; Mohamedali, A.; Thomas, N.S.B.; Mills, K.I. Immunotherapy of myeloid leukaemia. *Cancer Immunol. Immunother.* **2007**, *56*, 943–957. [CrossRef]
38. Canals, C.; Torrico, C.; Picón, M.; Amill, B.; Cancelas, J.A.; Fraga, G.; Badell, I.; Cubells, J.; Olivé, T.; Ortega, J.; et al. Immunomagnetic bone marrow purging in children with acute lymphoblastic leukemia. *J. Hematother.* **1997**, *6*, 261–268. [CrossRef]
39. Engblom, C.; Pfirschke, C.; Pittet, M.J. The role of myeoloid cells in cancer therapies. *Nat. Rev. Cancer* **2016**, *16*, 447–462. [CrossRef]
40. Al-Matary, Y.; Botezatu, L.; Opalka, B.; Hones, J.M.; Lames, R.F.; Thivakaran, A.; Schutte, J.; Köster, R.; Lennartz, K.; Schroeder, T.; et al. Acute meyeloid leukemia cells polarize macrophages towards a leukemia supporting state in a growth factor independence 1 dependent manner. *Haematologica* **2016**, *101*, 1216–1227. [CrossRef]
41. Van Attekum, M.; Terpstra, S.; Reinen, E.; Kater, A.; Eldering, E. Macrophage-mediated chronic lymphocytic leukemia cell survival is independent of APRIL signaling. *Cell Death Discov.* **2016**, *2*, 16020. [CrossRef] [PubMed]

42. Galletti, G.; Scielzo, C.; Barbaglio, F.; Rodriguez, T.V.; Riba, M.; Lazarevic, D.; Cittaro, D.; Simonetti, G.; Ranghetti, P.; Scarfò, L.; et al. Targeting macrophages sensitizes chronic lymphocytic leukemia to apoptosis and inhbit disease progression. *Cell Rep.* **1016**, *14*, 1748–1760. [CrossRef] [PubMed]
43. Ruffell, B.; Coussens, L.M. Macrophages and therapeutic resistance in cancer. *Cancer Cell* **2015**, *27*, 462–472. [CrossRef] [PubMed]
44. Noy, R.; Pollard, J.W. Tumor-associated macrophages: From mechanisms to therapy. *Immunity* **2014**, *41*, 49–61. [CrossRef] [PubMed]
45. Aharinejad, S.; Paulus, P.; Sioud, M.; Hofmann, M.; Zins, K.; Schäfer, R.; Stanley, E.R.; Abraham, D. Colony-stimulating factor-1 blockade by antisense oligonucleotides and small interfering RNAs suppresses growth of human mammary tumor xenografts in mice. *Cancer Res.* **2004**, *64*, 5378–5384. [CrossRef]
46. Cannarile, M.A.; Weisser, M.; Jacob, W.; Jegg, A.M.; Ries, C.H.; Rüttinger, D. Colony-stimulating factor 1 receptor (CSF1R) inhibitors in cancer therapy. *J. Immunother. Cancer* **2017**, *5*, 53. [CrossRef]
47. Quail, D.F.; Joyce, J.A. Microenvironmental regulation of tumor progression and metastasis. *Nat. Med.* **2013**, *19*, 1423–1437. [CrossRef]
48. Cieslewicz, M.; Tang, J.; Yu, J.L.; Cao, H.; Zavaljevski, M.; Motoyama, K.; Lieber, A.; Raines, E.W.; Pun, S.H. Targeted delivery of proapoptotic peptides to tumor associated macrophages improves survival. *Proc. Natl. Acad. Sci. USA* **2013**, *110*, 15919–15924. [CrossRef]
49. Dohner, H.; Weisdorf, D.J.; Bloomfield, C.D. Acute myeloid leukemia. *N. Engl. J. Med.* **2015**, *373*, 1136–1152. [CrossRef]
50. Rowe, J.M.; Tallman, M.S. How I treat acute myeloid leukemia. *Blood* **2010**, *116*, 3147–3156. [CrossRef]
51. Pandey, K.B.; Srivastava, S.; Singh, M.; Ghosh, J.K. Inducing toxicity by introducing a leucine-Zipper-like motif in from antimicrobial peptides, magainin 2. *Biochem. J.* **2011**, *436*, 609–620. [CrossRef] [PubMed]
52. Soverini, S.; De Benedittis, C.; Mancini, M.; Martinelli, G. Best practices in chronic myeloid leukemia monitoring and managment. *Oncologist* **2016**, *21*, 626–633. [CrossRef] [PubMed]
53. Saubele, S.; Silver, R.T. Management of chronic myeloid leukemia in blast crisis. *Ann. Hematol.* **2015**, *94*, S159–S165.
54. Pham, L.V.; Pogue, E.; Ford, R.J. The role of macrophage/B cell interactions in the pathophysiology of B cell lymphomas. *Front. Oncol.* **2018**, *8*, 147. [CrossRef] [PubMed]
55. Yuan, R.; Hou, Y.; Sun, W.; Yu, J.; Liu, X.; Niu, Y.; Lu, J.J.; Chen, X. Natural products to prevent drug resistance in cancer chemotherapy: A review. *Ann. N. Y. Acad. Sci.* **2017**, *1401*, 19–27. [CrossRef] [PubMed]
56. Marks, A.J.; Cooper, M.S.; Anderson, R.J.; Orchard, K.H.; Hale, G.; North, J.M.; Ganeshaguru, K.; Steele, A.J.; Mehta, A.B.; Lowdell, M.W.; et al. Selective apoptotic killing of malignant hemopoietic cells by antibody-targeted delivery of an amphipathic peptide. *Cancer Res.* **2005**, *65*, 2373–2377. [CrossRef] [PubMed]
57. Aronson, M.R.; Simonson, A.W.; Orchard, L.M.; Llinás, M.; Medina, S.H. Lipopeptisomes: Anticancer peptide-assembled particles for fusolytic oncotherapy. *Acta Biomater.* **2018**, *80*, 269–277. [CrossRef]
58. Gonzalez-Horta, A.; Matamoros-Acosta, A.; Chavez-Montes, A.; Castro-Rios, R.; Lara-Arias, J. Biodegradable nanoparticles loaded with tetrameric melittin: Preparation and membrane disruption evaluation. *Gen. Physiol. Biophys.* **2017**, *36*, 373–381. [CrossRef]
59. Dybwad, A.; Førre, O.; Natvig, J.B.; Sioud, M. Structural characterization of peptides that bind synovial fluid antibodies from RA patients: A novel strategy for identification of disease-related epitopes using a random peptide library. *Clin. Immunol. Immunopathol.* **1995**, *75*, 45–50. [CrossRef]

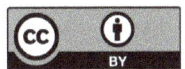

© 2019 by the authors. Licensee MDPI, Basel, Switzerland. This article is an open access article distributed under the terms and conditions of the Creative Commons Attribution (CC BY) license (http://creativecommons.org/licenses/by/4.0/).

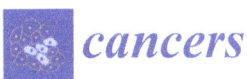

Article

Sequential Blockade of PD-1 and PD-L1 Causes Fulminant Cardiotoxicity—From Case Report to Mouse Model Validation

Shin-Yi Liu [1,†], Wen-Chien Huang [2,†], Hung-I Yeh [3], Chun-Chuan Ko [3], Hui-Ru Shieh [1], Chung-Lieh Hung [3], Tung-Ying Chen [4] and Yu-Jen Chen [1,5,6,*]

1. Department of Medical Research, MacKay Memorial Hospital, New Taipei City 25160, Taiwan; syliu0830@gmail.com (S.-Y.L.); ru123@mmh.org.tw (H.-R.S.)
2. Department of Thoracic Surgery, MacKay Memorial Hospital, Taipei 10449, Taiwan; wjhuang0@yahoo.com.tw
3. Department of Internal Medicine, MacKay Memorial Hospital, Taipei 10449, Taiwan; yehmmc@mmc.edu.tw (H.-I.Y.); kochunchuan1113@gmail.com (C.-C.K.); jotaro3791@gmail.com (C.-L.H.)
4. Department of Pathology, MacKay Memorial Hospital, Taipei 10449, Taiwan; wax921@gmail.com
5. Department of Radiation Oncology, MacKay Memorial Hospital, Taipei 10449, Taiwan
6. Department of Chinese Medicine, China Medical University Hospital, Taichung 40402, Taiwan
* Correspondence: chenmdphd@gmail.com or oncoman@mmh.org.tw; Tel.: +886-2-2543-3535
† These authors contributed equally to this work.

Received: 25 March 2019; Accepted: 22 April 2019; Published: 24 April 2019

Abstract: The combined administration of programmed cell death 1 (PD-1) and programmed cell death ligand 1 (PD-L1) inhibitors might be considered as a treatment for poorly responsive cancer. We report a patient with brain metastatic lung adenocarcinoma in whom fatal myocarditis developed after sequential use of PD-1 and PD-L1 inhibitors. This finding was validated in syngeneic tumor-bearing mice. The mice bearing lung metastases of CT26 colon cancer cells treated with PD-1 and/or PD-L1 inhibitors showed that the combination of anti-PD-1 and anti-PD-L1, either sequentially or simultaneously administered, caused myocarditis lesions with myocyte injury and patchy mononuclear infiltrates in the myocardium. A significant increase of infiltrating neutrophils in myocytes was noted only in mice with sequential blockade, implying a role for the pathogenesis of myocarditis. Among circulating leukocytes, concurrent and subsequent treatment of PD-1 and PD-L1 inhibitors led to sustained suppression of neutrophils. Among tumor-infiltrating leukocytes, combinatorial blockade increased CD8[+] T cells and NKG2D[+] T cells, and reduced tumor-associated macrophages, neutrophils, and natural killer (NK) cells in the lung metastatic microenvironment. The combinatorial treatments exhibited better control and anti-PD-L1 followed by anti-PD-1 was the most effective. In conclusion, the combinatory use of PD-1 and PD-L1 blockade, either sequentially or concurrently, may cause fulminant cardiotoxicity, although it gives better tumor control, and such usage should be cautionary.

Keywords: check point inhibitors; programmed cell death protein 1; programmed cell death 1 ligand 1; cardiotoxicity; lung metastasis

1. Introduction

The efficacy of immunotherapies that use antibodies to block programmed cell death 1 (PD-1) or its ligand 1 (PD-L1) have been extensively investigated for a variety of cancer types [1]. These types of immunotherapy, immune checkpoint inhibitors (ICIs), have been proved effective in advanced/metastatic non-small cell lung cancer (NSCLC) [2], colorectal cancer with high mismatch repair deficiency or microsatellite instability [3], and others [4,5]. In clinical practice, sequential shifting from a PD-1 inhibitor to its ligand, a PD-L1 inhibitor, or re-treatment with immunotherapy due to ineffectiveness or toxicity, is becoming more common to prolong survival in terminally ill patients [6].

The benefits of ICIs can be offset by the serious immune-related adverse events (irAEs), which mostly involve damage to the dermatologic, gastrointestinal, endocrine, respiratory, hepatic, and musculoskeletal systems [7,8]. So far, irAEs are reported and often encountered in patients treated with ipilimumab, an anti-CTLA-4 (cytotoxic T-lymphocyte–associated antigen 4) therapy [9,10], and are less frequent in patients treated with anti-PD-1 agents [11,12] or anti-PD-L1 antibodies [13,14]. A combination of ICIs has demonstrated a significant benefit to overall survival compared to monotherapy [15,16]. However, unexpected toxicities mediated by irAEs are also significantly higher using a combined ICI strategy [17,18], and require early detection and appropriate management [19]. Cardiotoxicity is regarded as a rare event of irAEs after ICI treatment [20–22]; nevertheless, recent reports indicate that immune-related myocarditis might be a serious and underestimated complication of immunotherapy [23–25]. Inflammation-mediated cardiotoxic effects can include myocarditis, pericarditis, perimyocarditis, left ventricular dysfunction without myocarditis, Takotsubo syndrome, and others [26]. The diagnosis of immune-related myocarditis should exclude viral and autoimmune myocarditis, coronary artery disease, and pulmonary embolism. Cardiac magnetic resonance imaging (MRI) to detect myocardial edema and late gadolinium enhancement is important, but sensitivity is currently inadequate [27,28]. Endomyocardial biopsy could be considered for tissue proof in clinical practice.

Here, we report a patient in whom fatal myocarditis developed after sequential use of PD-1 and PD-L1 inhibitors. To validate this finding, an immune competent tumor-bearing mouse model was used for the evaluation of myocarditis and immune responses.

2. Experimental Section

2.1. Patient Record

Study of the patient's medical records was approved by the Institute Review Board of Mackay Memorial Hospital, Taipei, Taiwan. Treatment courses and clinical features of this patient were collected.

2.2. Cell Culture

The mouse colorectal adenocarcinoma cell line CT26 was purchased from the American Type Culture Collection (Manassas, VA, USA) and maintained in Roswell Park Memorial Institute (RPMI)-1640 medium supplemented with 10% heat-inactivated fetal calf serum (FCS, Hyclone, Logan, UT, USA) and L-glutamine (200 mM). Stable clones expressing luciferase (CT26-Luc cells) were established by transducing lentivirus containing the North American Firefly Luciferase gene under the control of the SV40 promoter. CT26-Luc cells were maintained in the above medium containing G418 (500 µg/mL; Sigma-Aldrich, St. Louis, MO, USA).

2.3. Experimental Animal Model for ICI Treatment

Four-week-old male BALB/c mice were purchased from the Animal Resource Center of the National Science Council of Taiwan (Taipei, Taiwan). All animal experiments were approved by the Animal Ethics Committee of Mackay Memorial Hospital (Taipei, Taiwan). Approval was received on 24 January 2019 and the IRB approval number is 19MMHIS008e. CT26-Luc cells (1×10^6) were injected into tail veins of Balb/c mice to establish lung metastasis. The IVIS 200 imaging system (Xenogen Biosciences, Cranbury, NJ, USA) was used to estimate lung metastatic burden. After lung metastasis was established, the anti-mouse PD-1 monoclonal antibody (200 µg per mouse, RMP1-14, BioXcell, Lebanon, NH, USA), anti-mouse PD-L1 monoclonal antibody (150 µg per mouse, 10F.9G2, BioXcell, Lebanon, NH, USA), or their isotype control mAbs (rat IgG2a or rat IgG2b) were intraperitoneally administered. For concurrent combination, the anti-PD-1 and anti-PD-L1 mAbs were injected on the same days (days 0, 2, and 4). For subsequent combination, the second mAb was administered on days 6, 8, and 10. Mice were sacrificed on day 11 or day 17 for tumor microenvironment assessment as described in the text.

2.4. Immunohistochemistry (IHC) and Grading of Myocarditis

Sections of formalin-fixed and paraffin-embedded mouse hearts were treated with heat-induced antigen retrieval in sodium citrate buffer (10 mM sodium citrate, 0.05% Tween 20, pH 6.0) at 95–100 °C for 15 min, followed with 3% H_2O_2 at room temperature for 10 min. Blocking was performed with BlockPROTM Protein Blocking Buffer (Visual Protein Biotech., Taipei, Taiwan) at room temperature for 1 h. Sections were incubated with primary antibodies against Ly6C (1:200; Abcam, Cambridge, UK) and Ly6G (1:100; Abcam, Cambridge, UK) at room temperature for 1 h, with secondary antibodies of SignalStain® Boost IHC Detection Reagent and Rabbit Anti-Rat IgG (1:200; Abcam, Cambridge, UK) at room temperature for 1 h, and developed for 5–10 min with DAB (3,3'-Diaminobenzidine) chromogen kit (EnVision™+ Dual Link System-HRP, DAKO, Carpinteria, CA, USA) before counterstaining with hematoxylin (Merck, Darmstadt, Germany). The proportion of cells with Ly6C and Ly6G staining were calculated from a high-power field for 10 different portions by microscopy. Sections with 4 μm thickness were stained with hematoxylin and eosin (H&E). Myocarditis was graded as previously described [29] by examination of H&E-stained specimens at mid-ventricular cross sections. The grading using a 0–4 scale was recorded as follows: Grade 0, no inflammation; Grade 1, one to five distinct inflammatory foci with total involvement of 5% or less of the cross-sectional area; Grade 2, more than five distinct inflammatory foci, or involvement of more than 5% but less than 20% of the cross-sectional area; Grade 3, diffuse inflammation involving 20–50% of the area; Grade 4, diffuse inflammation involving more than 50% of the area.

2.5. Hemogram and Biochemistry

White blood cell (WBC) counts of the blood samples were analyzed by an automatic Coulter counter (HEMAVET HV950; Drew Scientific, Inc., Dallas, TX, USA). The plasma levels of alanine aminotransferase (ALT), creatinine (CRE), and creatine kinase (CK) were measured with the colorimetric method (Fuji Dri-Chem Slide, Fuji, Japan), according to instructions given by the manufacturer.

2.6. Flow Cytometry Analysis

Lung metastatic colon cancer-bearing mice were euthanized by intramuscular injection of a mixture of ketamine (100 mg/kg) and xylazine (10 mg/kg). The whole spleen, lung, and heart tissues were removed en bloc, and digested with solution containing collagenase A (1.5 mg/mL) and DNase I (0.4 mg/mL) at 37 °C for 30 min [30]. Cells were mashed through a 70 μm cell strainer to obtain single-cell suspensions, and further incubated with ACK (Ammonium-Chloride-Potassium) solution to lyse red blood cells. Before staining with cell surface markers, cells were incubated with an Fc receptor block (1 μg/1 × 10^6 cells; BD Bioscience, San Diego, CA, USA) to reduce non-specific binding. Then, cells (1 × 10^6 cells/mL for spleen, 1 × 10^7 cells/mL for heart and lung) were stained with antibodies conjugated with the indicated fluorochromes for 20 min on ice, including anti-CD3-Alexa488, anti-NKG2D-PE, anti-PD-L1-PE/Dazzle 594, anti-Ly6G-PE/Cy7, anti-PD-1-APC, anti-F4/80-APC/Cy7, anti-Ly6C-BV421, anti-CD45-BV510, anti-CD11b-BV605, anti-CD4-BV650, and anti-CD8-BV785 antibodies (BioLegend, San Diego, CA, USA). After washing, cells were immediately analyzed on the CytoFLEX 13-color cytometer (Beckman Coulter, Brea, CA, USA) and quantified using CytExpert analysis software (Beckman Coulter, Brea, CA, USA). Immune cell populations were defined as the following: T cells ($CD3^+/CD11b^-$), $CD8^+$ T cells ($CD3^+/CD11b^-/CD8^+$), $CD4^+$ T cells ($CD3^+/CD11b^-/CD4^+$), $NKG2D^+$ T cells ($CD3^+/CD11b^-/NKG2D^+$), neutrophils ($CD11b^+/Ly6G^+$), macrophages ($CD3^-/CD11b^+/Ly6C^+/F4/80^+$), NK cells ($CD3^-/Ly6G^-/CD11b^-/NKG2D^+$), and inflammation monocytes ($CD11b^+/Ly6C^{++}$).

2.7. Statistical Analysis

Results were expressed as mean ± standard error of the mean (SEM). Statistical comparison in each experiment was performed using Student's *t*-test or one-way analysis of variance (ANOVA). The difference was considered significant at $p < 0.05$. We used SigmaPlot version 8.0 (IBM SPSS, Armonk, NY, USA) with written syntax.

3. Results

3.1. Patient and Treatment

A 61-year-old woman with lung adenocarcinoma was sent to the emergency department with dyspnea and fatigue, three days after receiving her first dose of atezolizumab (1000 mg). Ten weeks before atezolizumab administration, she received five biweekly doses of nivolumab (3 mg/kg) with whole brain radiotherapy (RT) (30 Gy in 10 fractions) for brain metastasis, delivered after the first dose of nivolumab. Due to enlargement of lung nodules, shifting anti-PD-1 nivolumab to anti-PD-L1 atezolizumab was discussed in an oncology team meeting (Figure 1A). At day 3 of atezolizumab administration, the chest X-ray revealed right lung consolidation without fever and choking, which was not evident before atezolizumab administration (Figure 1B). Under the impression of pneumonitis, the dyspnea and lung consolidation subsided one week after treatment, which included high-dose methylprednisolone (5 mg/kg/day). However, the chest tightness and dyspnea developed four weeks later (day 40 of atezolizumab administration). The workup revealed sinus tachycardia by electrocardiography (Figure 1C), a normal troponin I level (<0.01 ng/mL, normal level <0.1), an elevated creatine kinase-myocardial band (CK-MB) level (10 ng/mL, normal level <7.2 ng/mL), and an elevated N-terminal pro-brain natriuretic peptide (NT-proBNP) level (2960 ng/mL, normal level <300 ng/mL) (Table 1). An echocardiogram revealed normal cardiac size and preserved global contractility of the left ventricle with an ejection fraction of 66.3% and no regional wall motion abnormality. Under a highly suspected diagnosis of myocarditis, she was treated with intravenous methylprednisolone at 5 mg/kg/day, and oral mycophenolate mofetil at 1000 mg/day. The progressive clinical deterioration was noted with serial elevation of troponin I, CK-MB, and NT-proBNP levels up to 1.3 ng/mL, 24 ng/mL, and 15,738 ng/mL, respectively. A subsequent echocardiogram revealed a non-significant decline of the ejection fraction to 59.2%. Cardiac arrest was noted at day 68 of atezolizumab administration, the 28th day after the development of cardiac symptoms.

Table 1. Data from echocardiogram and serum cardiac enzyme levels.

Cardiac Function Parameters	d40 of Atezo	d45 of Atezo	d55 of Atezo
LV ejection fraction	66.3%	N.A.	59.2%
Troponin I (ng/mL)	<0.01	0.3	1.3
CK-MB (ng/mL)	10	27	24
NT-proBNP (ng/mL)	2960	8668	15,738

d = day; LV = left ventricular; CK-MB = creatine kinase-myocardial band; NT-proBNP = N-terminal pro-brain natriuretic peptide.

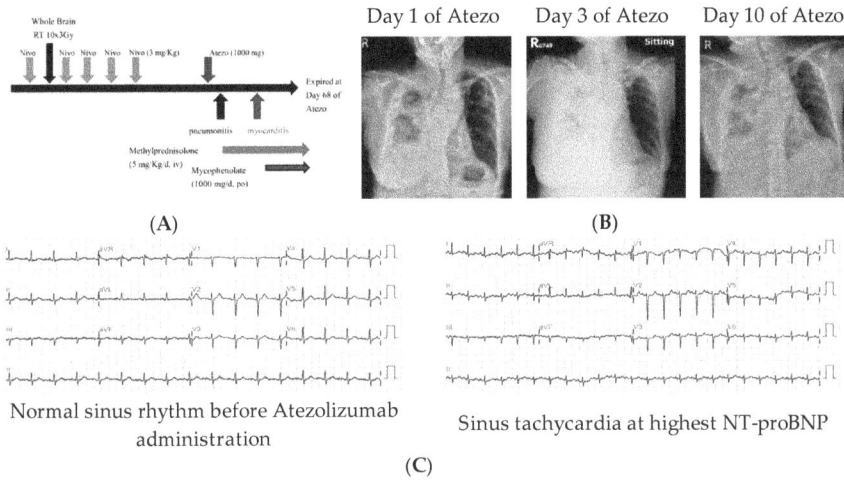

Figure 1. Clinical course of the presented patient. (A) Scheme of immune checkpoint inhibitor treatment course for the patient with brain metastatic lung adenocarcinoma. (B) Chest X-ray films demonstrated Atezolizumab (Atezo)-associated pneumonitis. (C) Electrocardiography of the patient before and after Atezolizumab administration. Nivo = nivolumab; RT = radiotherapy; NT-proBNP = N-terminal pro-brain natriuretic peptide.

3.2. Assessment of Cardiotoxicity after Combined ICI Therapies in Lung Metastasis Animal Model

To reveal the cardiotoxicity risk arising from ICI treatment, lung metastatic colon cancer-bearing mice were established using the intravenous injection method and were treated with the scheme simulating the treatment course of the aforementioned patient (Figure 2A). After three administrations of anti-PD-1/anti-PD-L1 antibodies, with either simultaneous or sequential treatment, heart tissues were collected for pathology and flow cytometry analysis. Hematoxylin and eosin staining showed no myocarditis lesions were observed in mice treated with anti-PD-1 or anti-PD-L1 alone (Figure 2B). However, in mice with the combination of anti-PD-1 and anti-PD-L1, either sequentially or simultaneously administered, myocarditis lesions equal or greater than grade 3 were noted. The characteristic features included extensive myocyte injury and patchy mononuclear infiltrates in the myocardium (Figure 2B, upper panel). Heart size in all groups had no marked alteration. Immunohistochemistry analysis showed Ly6C-positive staining was higher in the groups of PD-L1 inhibitor alone and concurrent PD-1 and PD-L1 blockade, whereas a Ly6G-positive signal appeared in the groups of blockade of PD-L1 alone, PD-1 plus PD-L1, and PD-1 followed with PD-L1 (Figure 2B, lower panel). Plasma levels of creatine kinase (CK) on 5 days, 10 days and 15 days post-treatment were further detected after ICI treatment. On day 10 post-treatment, plasma CK levels were statistically higher in the group of PD-L1 alone, concurrent and sequential treatment of PD-1 and PD-L1 inhibitors. On day 15 post-treatment, treatment with sequential blockade of PD-1 and PD-L1 caused a higher level of plasma CK but this was not statistically significant (Figure 2C). An abnormal infiltration of leukocytes within hearts were further examined by flow cytometry, and a higher level of inflammatory monocytes (CD11b$^+$/Ly6C^{++}) were detected in the hearts of mice treated with anti-PD-1 plus anti-PD-L1 antibody (12.85% ± 3.38%) than those of control group mice (2.80% ± 0.36%) (Figure 2D,E). Sequential administration of PD-1 and PD-L1 inhibitors in lung metastasis mice showed an increase of neutrophils (17.01% ± 0.12%) rather than inflammatory monocytes, as compared to control mice (4.49% ± 2.43%). Besides, macrophages in the heart also decreased after sequential treatment of PD-1 and PD-L1 inhibitors (51.42% ± 3.25%) than untreated mice (59.67% ± 2.69%). Intriguingly, when treatment with the PD-L1 inhibitor was followed with a PD-1 blocker (α-PD-L1, α-PD-1), accumulation of inflammatory monocytes or neutrophils was not observed in murine heart tissues (Figure 2D,E). Other immune cells in the hearts did not show significant changes after combined ICI treatment, including T cells, dendritic cells (DCs), and NK cells.

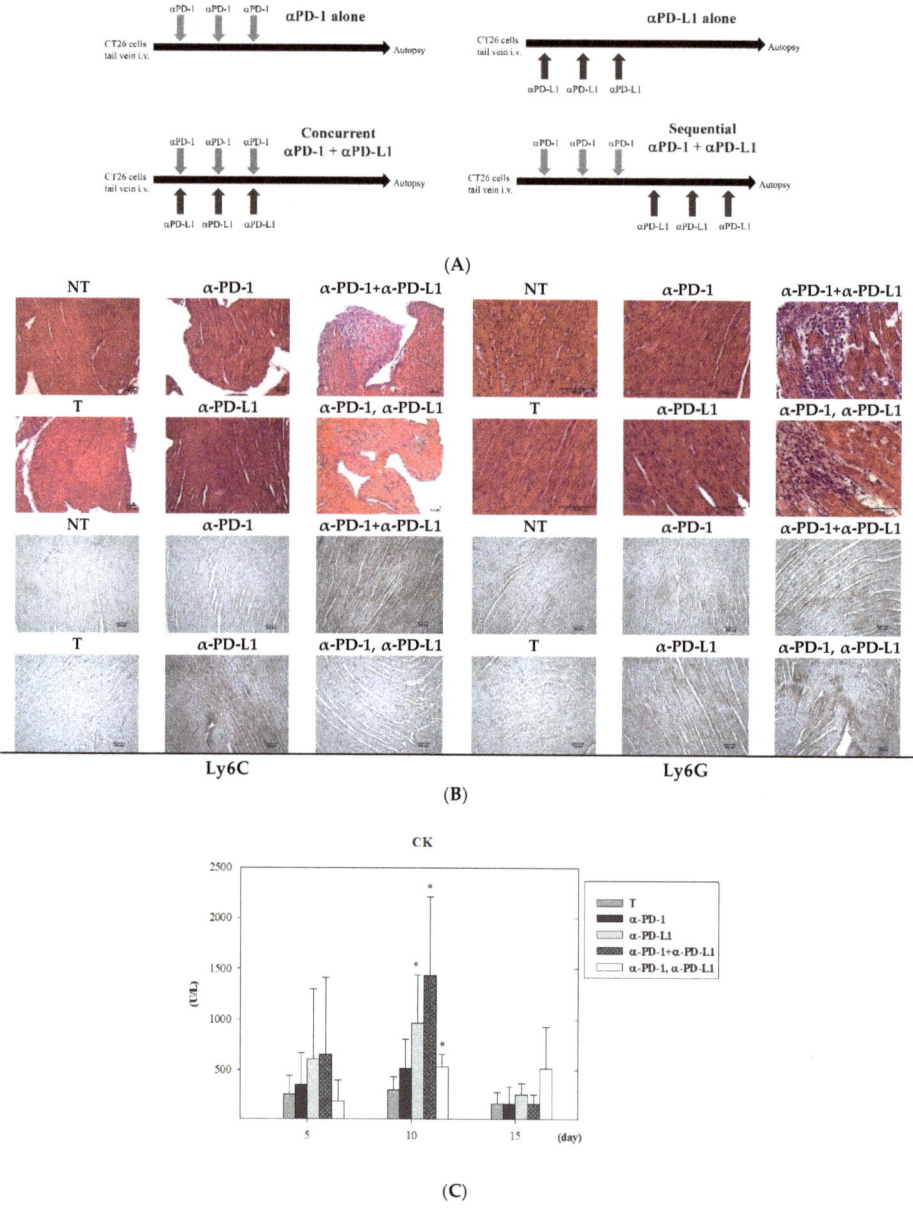

Figure 2. Cont.

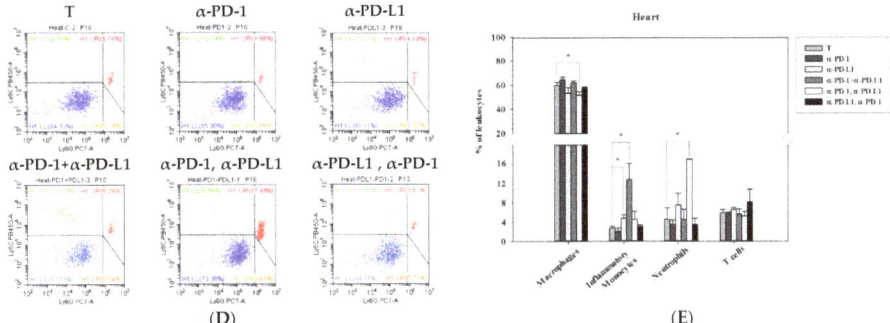

Figure 2. Combination treatment of programmed cell death 1/programmed cell death ligand 1 (PD-1/PD-L1) blockade induced myocarditis in a lung metastatic colon cancer mouse model. (**A**) Scheme of experimental design. Balb/c mice were intravenously (i.v.) injected with CT26-luciferase expressing cells. Single and combined treatment of anti-PD-1 and anti-PD-L1 were administered intraperitoneally (i.p.) on days 0, 2, and 4. Sequential treatments were administered on days 0, 2, and 4, followed by another antibody on days 6, 8, and 10. Mice were sacrificed for analysis on day 11. (**B**) Representative hematoxylin and eosin-stained (H&E) slides of heart tissues from each group (left panel: 200×; right panel: 400×). Lower panel shows the immunohistochemistry (IHC) stain of Ly6C and Ly6G expression in heart sections at 100× magnification. Scale bars indicate 100 µm. (**C**) Plasma levels of creatine kinase (CK) on 5 days, 10 days and 15 days post-treatment after immune checkpoint inhibitor (ICI) therapies. (**D**) Flow cytometric analysis of immune cell profiles from heart tissues revealed an increase of inflammatory monocytes (Ly6C^{++}) and neutrophils (Ly6G$^+$) in lung metastatic mice treated with concurrent and sequential PD-1/PD-L1 inhibitors, respectively. (**E**) Quantification results from flow cytometric data indicated that administration of anti-PD-1 followed with anti-PD-L1 antibodies led to the accumulation of neutrophils in the hearts of lung metastatic mice. NT and T indicate the no tumor and tumor group, respectively. In ICI-treated groups, statistical analysis was performed with the tumor (T) group (* $p < 0.05$). Total leukocytes (CD45$^+$) = 100%. $n = 3$ for each group.

3.3. Assessment of Tumor Control after Combined ICI Therapies in Lung Metastasis Animal Model

In order to determine whether different courses of ICI treatment can lead to different adverse effects and tumor control, biological toxicity and survival analyses were performed. IVIS images showed that combinatorial treatments exhibited better tumor control than monotherapy of anti-PD-1 or anti-PD-L1 in lung metastatic colon cancer-bearing mice (Figure 3A). Among combinatorial treatments, lung metastatic mice treated with anti-PD-L1 following anti-PD-1 presented the lowest signal of IVIS images, indicating tumor growth was successfully attenuated with sequential treatment of anti-PD-L1 and anti-PD-1 therapy (Figure 3A). No significant changes in body weight and renal function were noted within 15 days post-treatment in any mouse group (Figure 3B,E). Consistent and significant suppression of white blood cells were observed on day 5 and day 10 in all ICI therapies (Figure 3C). Among the combined ICI treatment groups, only sequential administration of PD-1 and PD-L1 inhibitors generated a transient increase of alanine aminotransferase (ALT), an indicator of liver function, on day 10 post-treatment ($p = 0.09$, 3/6 mice showed abnormal ALT). Survival analysis was revealed, and ICI treatment was started on day 7 of the designed scheme to make sure that the lung metastatic tumor cells were undergoing exponential growth. Among all treatment groups, the anti-PD-L1 followed by anti-PD-1 was the most effective combination protocol to control lung metastasis from CT26 colon cancer cells ($p = 0.03$) (Figure 3F). Monotherapy of anti-PD-L1 also showed improvement of overall survival compared to control mice ($p = 0.05$), even though tumor volumes were big. These data indicate that in the lung metastatic mouse model, ICI-mediated infiltration of immune cells into the myocardium did not cause severe lethality but showed better survival benefit.

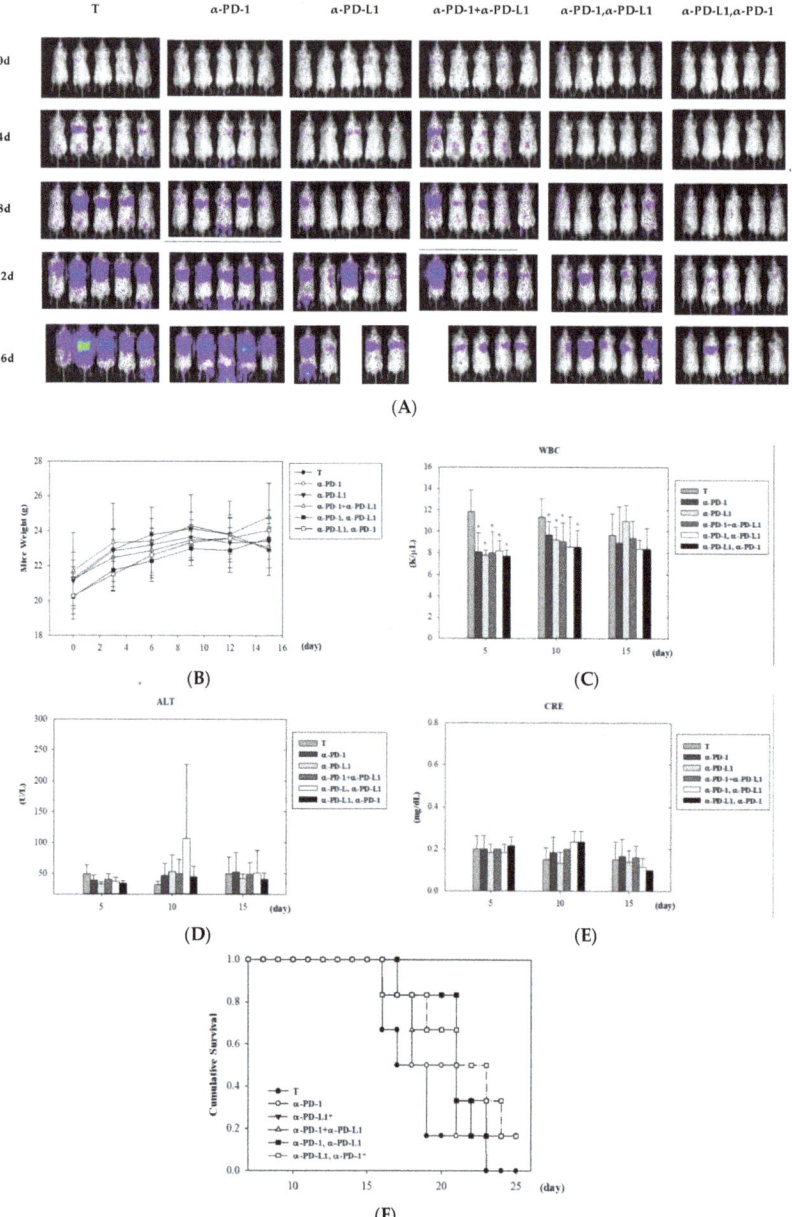

Figure 3. Therapeutic effects and toxicity in a lung metastatic animal model of monotherapy and various combination treatments of anti-PD-1 and anti-PD-L1. (**A**) Tumor growth of lung metastatic colon cancer-bearing mice after mono-, combined, and sequential treatment of PD-1 and PD-L1 antibodies. After seven days of intravenous cell injection (day 0), mice were treated with the indicated ICI therapies. Tumor growth of lung metastatic colon cancer was monitored using the IVIS imaging system at four-day intervals. General toxicities were examined by mouse weight (**B**), white blood cells (**C**), liver function with ALT (**D**), and renal function with CRE (**E**) within 15 days post-treatment. (**F**) Survival analysis was assessed in lung metastatic mice with visible tumor burden in the lung. In ICI-treated groups, statistical analysis was performed with the tumor (T) group (* $p < 0.05$). $n = 6$ for each group. ALT = alanine aminotransferase; CRE = creatinine.

3.4. Alternation of Circulating Immune Cells in Lung Metastatic Mice after Combined ICI Therapies

First, the effectiveness of ICI treatment on the expression of PD-1 and PD-L1 in a lung metastatic colon cancer mouse model was revealed on day 10 by flow cytometric analysis. Our data indicated that PD-1 blockade caused prolonged and effective inhibition of PD-1 expression in both leukocytes and non-leukocytes (including tumor cells) in the lung (Figure 4A). In contrast, PD-L1 blockade presented with a more transient suppression of PD-L1, as the level of PD-L1 was lower in the group of anti-PD-1 followed with anti-PD-L1 inhibitors, but recovered to normal levels in the anti-PD-L1 alone group (Figure 4A). Combinatorial blockade exhibited various effects on PD-1 and PD-L1 expression in lung metastatic mice. Intriguingly, only the sequential combination of anti-PD-L1 followed by anti-PD-1 (the most effective regimen for controlling lung metastasis) universally inhibited the up-regulated expression of both PD-1 and PD-L1 in lung metastasis (Figure 4A). It was worth noting that both anti-PD-1 and anti-PD-L1 monotherapy resulted in the elevation of PD-L1 expression in the tumor microenvironment seven days post-treatment. Besides, the expression of PD-1 and PD-L1 on immune cells in the spleen made them more susceptible to treatment with the anti-PD-L1 inhibitor (Figure 4A). Circulating immune cells such as neutrophils, inflammatory monocytes, macrophages, NK cells, and DCs were further examined in lung metastatic mice in response to ICI therapies. Lung metastasis of colon cancer led to increased neutrophils and decreased T cells in the spleen, and combinatorial and sequential treatments of PD-1/PD-L1 inhibitors reversed these alternations (Figure 4B). A consistent suppression of neutrophils was observed on day 17 post-treatment (Figure 4C). Macrophages in the spleen were significantly increased on day 17 after monotherapy and various combination treatments of PD-1 and PD-L1 inhibitors (Figure 4C).

3.5. Alternations of Local Immune Cells in Lung Metastatic Mice after Combined ICI Therapy

The immune cell profiles at the tumor site were assessed on day 17 post-treatment in lung metastatic colon cancer-bearing mice with or without ICI treatment. Flow cytometric analysis showed the alternation of T cells and neutrophils (Figure 5A) and the changes of monocytes and macrophage populations (Figure 5B) in response to ICI treatment. Compared to lung metastatic mice and normal mice, tumor cells that metastasized to the lungs caused a decrease in T cells, including $CD8^+$ T cells and $CD4^+$ T cells. This decrease in number was restored by a combination of PD-1 and PD-L1 inhibitors (both sequential and simultaneous), but not by each inhibitor alone (Figure 5E). Lung metastasis increased the numbers of local immune cells such as tumor associated-neutrophils, macrophages, and NK cells. Combination blockade (both sequential and simultaneous) subverted the increase in numbers to an extent greater than each inhibitor alone (Figure 5E). In addition to the comprehensive profile of immune cells, tumor-infiltrating leukocytes expressing PD-1 or PD-L1 were simultaneously examined. Among T cells in the tumor microenvironment, $CD8^+$ T cells and $NKG2D^+$ T cells were the major cells expressing PD-1 (Figure 5C) and PD-L1 (Figure 5D), respectively. Quantification analysis summarized that up-regulated expression of PD-1 in $CD8^+$ T cells, NK cells, and macrophages—as well as PD-L1 in $NKG2D^+$ T cells, macrophages, and neutrophils—was noted in lung metastatic mice compared to normal mice (Figure 5F,G). Combination blockade inhibited the expression of PD-1 in $CD8^+$ T cells, NK cells, macrophages, and that of PD-L1 in $NKG2D^+$ T cells, macrophages, and neutrophils (Figure 5F,G).

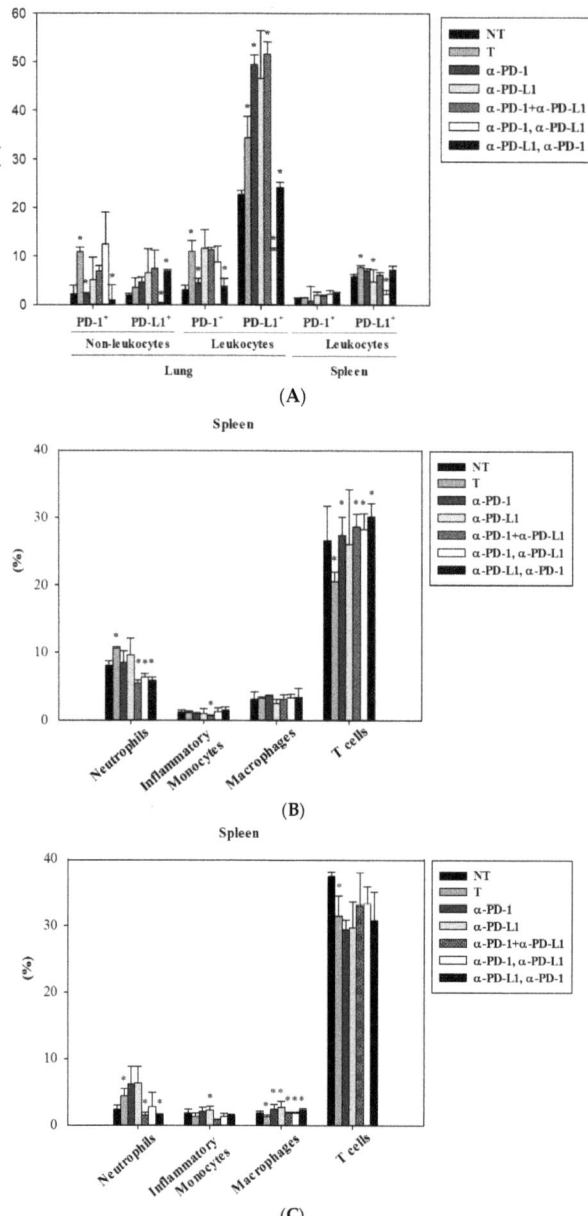

Figure 4. Alterations of circulating immune cells in a lung metastatic animal model after monotherapy and various combination treatments of anti-PD-1 and anti-PD-L1. (**A**) Flow cytometric analysis for expression of PD-1 and PD-L1 on leukocytes (CD45$^+$) and non-leukocytes (CD45$^−$) in the lung and spleen on day 11 post-treatment. (**B**) Immune cell composition in the spleen on day 11 post-treatment in lung metastasis mice. (**C**) Immune cell composition in the spleen on day 17 post-treatment in lung metastasis mice. The tumor (T) group from lung metastatic mice was compared with the no tumor (NT) group from normal mice. In ICI-treated groups, statistical analysis was performed with the tumor (T) group (* $p < 0.05$). Total leukocytes (CD45$^+$) = 100%. Immune cells were defined as follows: neutrophils (CD11b$^+$/Ly6G$^+$), inflammatory monocytes (CD11b$^+$/Ly6C^{++}), macrophages (CD3$^−$/CD11b$^+$/Ly6C$^+$/F4/80$^+$), T cells (CD3$^+$/CD11b$^−$). $n = 3$ for each group.

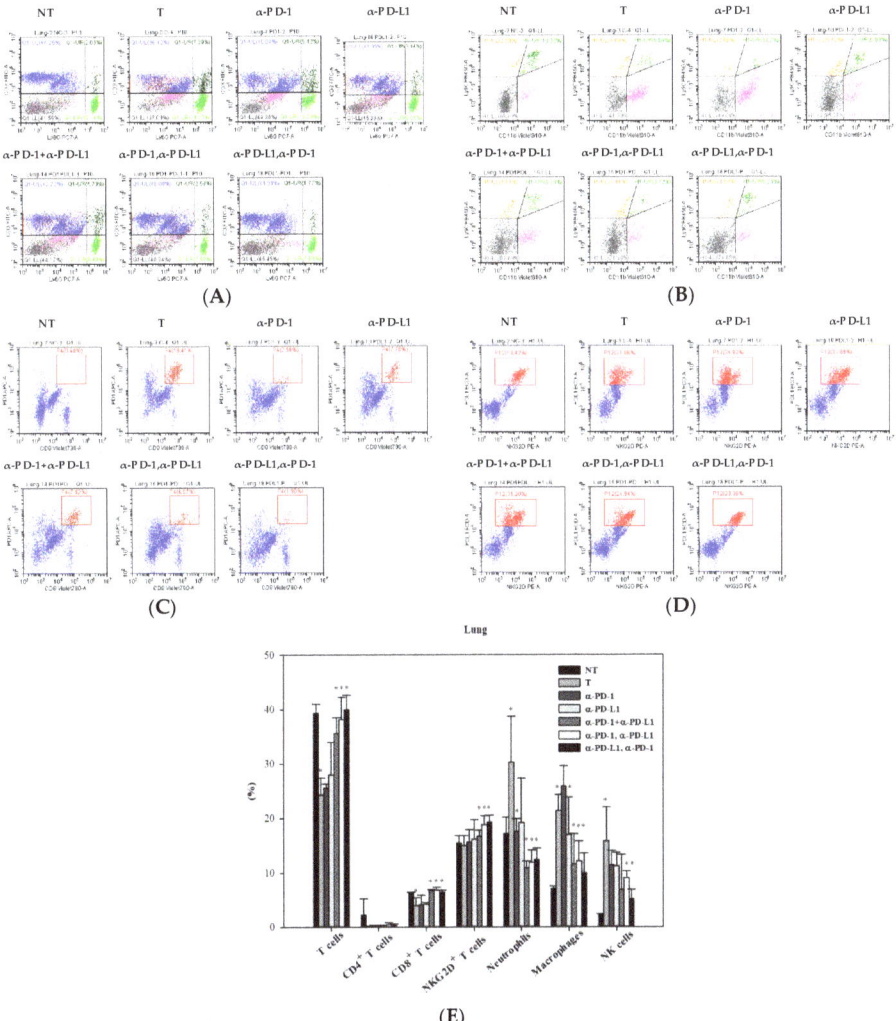

Figure 5. *Cont.*

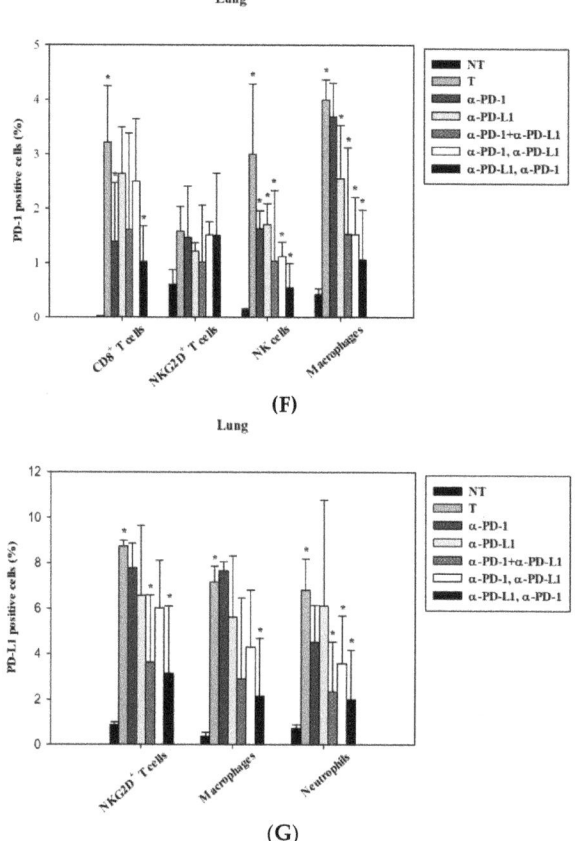

Figure 5. Alterations of local immune cells in a lung metastatic animal model after monotherapy and various combination treatments of anti-PD-1 and anti-PD-L1. (**A**) Dot plots of flow cytometric analysis revealed the alteration of T cells (upper left region in blue) and neutrophils (upper and lower right region in green) on day 17 post-treatment. (**B**) Other immune cells with double negative CD3 and Ly6G (lower left region of **A**) were further gated and analyzed to distinguish macrophages/monocytes/DCs (lower right, pink color) and inflammatory monocytes (upper right, dark green color) by Ly6C and CD11b staining. (**C**) The proportion of PD-1-positive cells in $CD8^+$ T cells in response to ICI therapies. (**D**) The proportion of PD-L1 positive cells in $NKG2D^+$ T cells in response to ICI treatment. (**E**) Quantification of the immune cell profile in the lung on day 17 post-treatment in lung metastasis mice. (**F**) Quantification of major immune cells expressing PD-1 in lung metastases on day 17 post-treatment. (**G**) Quantification of major immune cells expressing PD-L1 in lung metastases on day 17 post-treatment. The tumor (T) group from lung metastatic mice was compared with the no tumor (NT) group from normal mice. In ICI-treated groups, statistical analysis was performed with the tumor (T) group (* $p < 0.05$). Total leukocytes ($CD45^+$) = 100%. Immune cells were defined as follows: T cells ($CD3^+/CD11b^-$), $CD8^+$ T cells ($CD3^+/CD11b^-/CD8^+$), $CD4^+$ T cells ($CD3^+/CD11b^-/CD4^+$), $NKG2D^+$ T cells ($CD3^+/CD11b^-/NKG2D^+$), neutrophils ($CD11b^+/Ly6G^+$), macrophages ($CD3^-/CD11b^+/Ly6C^+/F4/80^+$), NK cells ($CD3^-/Ly6G^-/CD11b^-/NKG2D^+$). $n = 3$ for each group.

4. Discussion

Cardiotoxicity induced by ICI therapy is an underestimated and emerging issue in clinical trials, especially for those with a combination design of ICIs. Myocarditis is life-threatening and difficult to detect early. So far, the pathogenesis of immune-related myocarditis remains unclear. For validating the finding from a lung adenocarcinoma patient, we applied a colon CT26 cancer with lung metastases model to test the effect of dual blockade in mice. The main reason for choosing this model is that it has been widely used in immune checkpoint blockade studies, including for the blockade for PD-1 and PD-L1 independently, with a more comprehensive understanding of dynamic alterations in immune profiles. After this proof-of-concept study, further investigations using various types of cancers are warranted. In our animal model, concurrent and sequential treatment of PD-1 and PD-L1-blocking antibodies resulted in infiltrating leukocyte accumulation in the heart, an abnormality that was not observed in mono-therapy groups. Intriguingly, the administration of the PD-L1 inhibitor prior to the PD-1 inhibitor did not cause leukocytic infiltration of the myocardium. PD-1 is a co-inhibitory molecule of the B7/CD28 superfamily, which can bind PD-L1 and PD-L2 to negatively regulate responses of immune cells including T cells, B cells, macrophages, and dendritic cells [31]. Genetic deletion of PD-1 has been reported to cause autoimmune myocarditis with dilated cardiomyopathy in mice [32]. This implies that PD-1 may play a role in myocardial immune responses and may protect against inflammation and myocyte damage in T-cell-mediated myocarditis. Tarrio et al. revealed transfer of ovalbumin-specific CD8$^+$ T cells into cMyc-mOVA (cMyc oncogene and membrane-bound form of ovalbumin) mice resulted in enhanced immunization accompanied with more myocardial inflammation in recipients receiving PD-1 null T cells [33]. They concluded that PD-1 deficient T cells are more efficient killers of target cells and induce more inflammation, as evident with the increase of CD8$^+$ T cells, neutrophils, and macrophages in murine myocardium. In our case, there is no significant induction of CD8$^+$ T cells in the heart, and inflammatory monocytes (Ly6C^{++}), but not macrophages (Ly6C$^+$) are significantly increased on day 11 post-treatment of PD-1 plus PD-L1 blockade in the lung metastasis mouse model. Another case report that resembled our clinical case mentioned that PD-1 blockade-induced myocarditis was identified in a patient with lung squamous cell carcinoma who received simultaneous whole brain radiotherapy [34]. In our case, myocarditis suddenly appeared on day 3 post-treatment of PD-L1 blockade but not in the therapeutic period of the PD-1 inhibitor combined with radiotherapy, implying that the combinatorial use of PD-1 and PD-L1 inhibitors may lead to a substantial increase of immunotherapy-induced cardiomyopathy.

In the inflamed myocardia of patients with fatal myocarditis after a combination of CTLA-4 and PD-1 blockade, PD-L1 was expressed on the membranous surface of injured cardiac myocytes and on infiltrating CD8$^+$ T cells and histiocytes of the inflamed myocardium, but not skeletal muscles. The mRNA expression data from another ICI-induced myocarditis patient showed 10-fold more abundant expression of PD-L1 in affected cardiac tissue, which was five-fold higher than in affected skeletal muscle [23]. Given that human and murine myocytes constitutively express PD-1 and PD-L1, and expression of PD-L1 is up-regulated in injured myocytes [35,36], the PD-1 blockade-injured myocytes may cause secondary PD-L1 up-regulation, aiming to attenuate pro-inflammatory reactions. This raises the possibility that concurrent or subsequent blockade of PD-L1 added to PD-1 treatment may block the salvage mechanism of anti-PD-1-injured myocytes, leading to the development of fulminant myocarditis. In our animal model, the level of PD-L1 in the myocardium is susceptible to anti-PD-L1 blockade treatment. Besides, a higher dosage (over 200 µg/mice per treatment) of anti-PD-L1 antibody led to significant lethality in our animal system, implying that the toxicity of anti-PD-L1 in vivo should be carefully manipulated while changing the dosage. A recent study reported synergistic toxicities (pneumonitis and colitis) were found only in patients treated with sequential PD-(L)1 blockade and an EGFR (epidermal growth factor receptor) tyrosine kinase inhibitor, osimertinib [37]. Based on their observation, receptor occupancy of the anti-PD-(L)1 antibody is longer than that of osimertinib; thus, there was evident toxicity in lung metastatic mice treated with PD-1 followed by PD-L1 inhibitors. Furthermore, myocarditis was also reported in a patient with multiple myeloma who was treated with an immunomodulatory drug (lenalidomide-dexamethasone) combined with an anti-PD-1 inhibitor (pembrolizumab) [38]. Autopsy revealed the increase of infiltrating macrophages, CD8$^+$ T cells and focal fibrosis in the myocardium after combination therapy. A better understanding of the mechanism of this ICI-induced cardiac toxicity may provide insight into the development of preventive or therapeutic agents for immune-related cardiotoxicity.

The infiltrating CD68$^+$ macrophages in ICI-induced myocarditis were noted in a patient with fatal myocarditis after a combination of CTLA-4 and PD-1 blockade. PD-1 expression in M2 macrophages in tumors is reported to be associated with disease progression and impaired phagocytotic potency against tumors in the same animal model used in this study [39]. In our animal system, combination blockade of PD-1 and PD-L1 reduced the expression of PD-1 and PD-L1 in macrophages, which may imply the validation of the blockade effect but, on the other hand, may represent the relative activation of macrophage function. Besides, transient elevation of neutrophils in the heart and abnormal liver function were only observed on day 10 of the sequential treatment of PD-1 and PD-L1 blockade, indicating the ability of animals to recover differs with clinical results in response to ICI therapy. Moreover, macrophages and neutrophils are the major immune cells expressing PD-L1 in the tumor microenvironment; thus, the inhibition of PD-L1 may influence the activities and functions of tumor-associated macrophages and neutrophils. It is worth noting that a subset of T cells, NKG2D$^+$ T cells, also expressed PD-L1. The NKG2D receptor has received great attention in the development of novel therapeutic agents, and was found to be expressed on NK cells and T cells in both humans and mice [40,41]. For T cells, both NKG2D and CD28 function as costimulatory receptors for CD8$^+$ T cell memory formation, and the ligands of NKG2D are broadly expressed in many cell types upon stress stimuli [42]. Our data indicate that combination blockade could reverse the tumor-associated alterations in immune cell lineages, including the increase of CD8$^+$ T cells and NKG2D$^+$ T cells. Whether this immunomodulatory effect is correlated to toxicity and greater tumor control by combination blockade remains to be elucidated.

5. Conclusions

The combinatory use of PD-1 and PD-L1 blockade, either sequentially or concurrently, may cause fulminant cardiotoxicity, and such usage should be cautionary. The combinatorial treatment of anti-PD-L1 followed by anti-PD-1 is more effective than other mono- or combined strategy.

Author Contributions: Y.-J.C. conceived, designed, discussed the experiments and supervised all works; S.-Y.L. performed the experiments, data acquisition and wrote the paper; W.-C.H. provided clinical data; H.-I.Y., C.-C.K., H.-R.S., C.-L.H., T.-Y.C. finalized experimental works, analyzed the data and prepared the final figures and tables. All authors read and approved the final manuscript.

Funding: This study was supported by grants from National Science Council (MOST 106-2314-B-195 -002 -MY3, MOST 107-2623-E-195-001 -NU), and Mackay Memorial Hospital (MMH-E-107-13, MMH-TH-10703), Taiwan.

Conflicts of Interest: The authors declare no conflict of interest.

References

1. Ribas, A.; Wolchok, J.D. Cancer immunotherapy using checkpoint blockade. *Science* **2018**, *359*, 1350–1355. [CrossRef]
2. Sui, H.; Ma, N.; Wang, Y.; Li, H.; Liu, X.; Su, Y.; Yang, J. Anti-PD-1/PD-L1 Therapy for Non-Small-Cell Lung Cancer: Toward Personalized Medicine and Combination Strategies. *J. Immunol. Res.* **2018**, *2018*, 6984948. [CrossRef]
3. Le, D.T.; Hubbard-Lucey, V.M.; Morse, M.A.; Heery, C.R.; Dwyer, A.; Marsilje, T.H.; Brodsky, A.N.; Chan, E.; Deming, D.A.; Diaz, L.A., Jr.; et al. A Blueprint to Advance Colorectal Cancer Immunotherapies. *Cancer Immunol. Res.* **2017**, *5*, 942–949. [CrossRef]
4. Yang, H.; Shen, K.; Zhu, C.; Li, Q.; Zhao, Y.; Ma, X. Safety and efficacy of durvalumab (MEDI4736) in various solid tumors. *Drug Des. Dev. Ther.* **2018**, *12*, 2085–2096. [CrossRef] [PubMed]

5. Li, H.; Yu, J.; Liu, C.; Liu, J.; Subramaniam, S.; Zhao, H.; Blumenthal, G.M.; Turner, D.C.; Li, C.; Ahamadi, M.; et al. Time dependent pharmacokinetics of pembrolizumab in patients with solid tumor and its correlation with best overall response. *J. Pharmacokinet. Pharmacodyn.* **2017**, *44*, 403–414. [CrossRef]
6. Santini, F.C.; Rizvi, H.; Plodkowski, A.J.; Ni, A.; Lacouture, M.E.; Gambarin-Gelwan, M.; Wilkins, O.; Panora, E.; Halpenny, D.F.; Long, N.M.; et al. Safety and Efficacy of Re-treating with Immunotherapy after Immune-Related Adverse Events in Patients with NSCLC. *Cancer Immunol. Res.* **2018**, *6*, 1093–1099. [CrossRef] [PubMed]
7. Postow, M.A.; Sidlow, R.; Hellmann, M.D. Immune-Related Adverse Events Associated with Immune Checkpoint Blockade. *N. Engl. J. Med.* **2018**, *378*, 158–168. [CrossRef]
8. Baxi, S.; Yang, A.; Gennarelli, R.L.; Khan, N.; Wang, Z.; Boyce, L.; Korenstein, D. Immune-related adverse events for anti-PD-1 and anti-PD-L1 drugs: Systematic review and meta-analysis. *BMJ* **2018**, *360*, k793. [CrossRef] [PubMed]
9. Hodi, F.S.; O'Day, S.J.; McDermott, D.F.; Weber, R.W.; Sosman, J.A.; Haanen, J.B.; Gonzalez, R.; Robert, C.; Schadendorf, D.; Hassel, J.C.; et al. Improved survival with ipilimumab in patients with metastatic melanoma. *N. Engl. J. Med.* **2010**, *363*, 711–723. [CrossRef]
10. Ascierto, P.A.; Del Vecchio, M.; Robert, C.; Mackiewicz, A.; Chiarion-Sileni, V.; Arance, A.; Lebbe, C.; Bastholt, L.; Hamid, O.; Rutkowski, P.; et al. Ipilimumab 10 mg/kg versus ipilimumab 3 mg/kg in patients with unresectable or metastatic melanoma: A randomised, double-blind, multicentre, phase 3 trial. *Lancet Oncol.* **2017**, *18*, 611–622. [CrossRef]
11. Reck, M.; Rodriguez-Abreu, D.; Robinson, A.G.; Hui, R.; Csoszi, T.; Fulop, A.; Gottfried, M.; Peled, N.; Tafreshi, A.; Cuffe, S.; et al. Pembrolizumab versus Chemotherapy for PD-L1-Positive Non-Small-Cell Lung Cancer. *N. Engl. J. Med.* **2016**, *375*, 1823–1833. [CrossRef]
12. Weber, J.S.; Hodi, F.S.; Wolchok, J.D.; Topalian, S.L.; Schadendorf, D.; Larkin, J.; Sznol, M.; Long, G.V.; Li, H.; Waxman, I.M.; et al. Safety Profile of Nivolumab Monotherapy: A Pooled Analysis of Patients with Advanced Melanoma. *J. Clin. Oncol.* **2017**, *35*, 785–792. [CrossRef]
13. Rosenberg, J.E.; Hoffman-Censits, J.; Powles, T.; van der Heijden, M.S.; Balar, A.V.; Necchi, A.; Dawson, N.; O'Donnell, P.H.; Balmanoukian, A.; Loriot, Y.; et al. Atezolizumab in patients with locally advanced and metastatic urothelial carcinoma who have progressed following treatment with platinum-based chemotherapy: A single-arm, multicentre, phase 2 trial. *Lancet* **2016**, *387*, 1909–1920. [CrossRef]
14. Antonia, S.J.; Villegas, A.; Daniel, D.; Vicente, D.; Murakami, S.; Hui, R.; Yokoi, T.; Chiappori, A.; Lee, K.H.; de Wit, M.; et al. Durvalumab after Chemoradiotherapy in Stage III Non-Small-Cell Lung Cancer. *N. Engl. J. Med.* **2017**, *377*, 1919–1929. [CrossRef]
15. You, W.; Liu, M.; Miao, J.D.; Liao, Y.Q.; Song, Y.B.; Cai, D.K.; Gao, Y.; Peng, H. A Network Meta-analysis Comparing the Efficacy and Safety of Anti-PD-1 with Anti-PD-L1 in Non-small Cell Lung Cancer. *J. Cancer* **2018**, *9*, 1200–1206. [CrossRef]
16. Hao, C.; Tian, J.; Liu, H.; Li, F.; Niu, H.; Zhu, B. Efficacy and safety of anti-PD-1 and anti-PD-1 combined with anti-CTLA-4 immunotherapy to advanced melanoma: A systematic review and meta-analysis of randomized controlled trials. *Medicine* **2017**, *96*, e7325. [CrossRef]
17. Zhang, B.; Wu, Q.; Zhou, Y.L.; Guo, X.; Ge, J.; Fu, J. Immune-related adverse events from combination immunotherapy in cancer patients: A comprehensive meta-analysis of randomized controlled trials. *Int. Immunopharmacol.* **2018**, *63*, 292–298. [CrossRef]
18. Davies, M.; Duffield, E.A. Safety of checkpoint inhibitors for cancer treatment: Strategies for patient monitoring and management of immune-mediated adverse events. *Immunotargets Ther.* **2017**, *6*, 51–71. [CrossRef]
19. Brahmer, J.R.; Lacchetti, C.; Schneider, B.J.; Atkins, M.B.; Brassil, K.J.; Caterino, J.M.; Chau, I.; Ernstoff, M.S.; Gardner, J.M.; Ginex, P.; et al. Management of Immune-Related Adverse Events in Patients Treated with Immune Checkpoint Inhibitor Therapy: American Society of Clinical Oncology Clinical Practice Guideline. *J. Clin. Oncol.* **2018**, *36*, 1714–1768. [CrossRef]
20. Eigentler, T.K.; Hassel, J.C.; Berking, C.; Aberle, J.; Bachmann, O.; Grunwald, V.; Kahler, K.C.; Loquai, C.; Reinmuth, N.; Steins, M.; et al. Diagnosis, monitoring and management of immune-related adverse drug reactions of anti-PD-1 antibody therapy. *Cancer Treat. Rev.* **2016**, *45*, 7–18. [CrossRef]

21. Boutros, C.; Tarhini, A.; Routier, E.; Lambotte, O.; Ladurie, F.L.; Carbonnel, F.; Izzeddine, H.; Marabelle, A.; Champiat, S.; Berdelou, A.; et al. Safety profiles of anti-CTLA-4 and anti-PD-1 antibodies alone and in combination. *Nat. Rev. Clin. Oncol.* **2016**, *13*, 473–486. [CrossRef]
22. Naidoo, J.; Page, D.B.; Li, B.T.; Connell, L.C.; Schindler, K.; Lacouture, M.E.; Postow, M.A.; Wolchok, J.D. Toxicities of the anti-PD-1 and anti-PD-L1 immune checkpoint antibodies. *Ann. Oncol.* **2016**, *27*, 1362. [CrossRef] [PubMed]
23. Johnson, D.B.; Balko, J.M.; Compton, M.L.; Chalkias, S.; Gorham, J.; Xu, Y.; Hicks, M.; Puzanov, I.; Alexander, M.R.; Bloomer, T.L.; et al. Fulminant Myocarditis with Combination Immune Checkpoint Blockade. *N. Engl. J. Med.* **2016**, *375*, 1749–1755. [CrossRef] [PubMed]
24. Heinzerling, L.; Ott, P.A.; Hodi, F.S.; Husain, A.N.; Tajmir-Riahi, A.; Tawbi, H.; Pauschinger, M.; Gajewski, T.F.; Lipson, E.J.; Luke, J.J. Cardiotoxicity associated with CTLA4 and PD1 blocking immunotherapy. *J. Immunother. Cancer* **2016**, *4*, 50. [CrossRef]
25. Moslehi, J.J.; Salem, J.E.; Sosman, J.A.; Lebrun-Vignes, B.; Johnson, D.B. Increased reporting of fatal immune checkpoint inhibitor-associated myocarditis. *Lancet* **2018**, *391*, 933. [CrossRef]
26. Lyon, A.R.; Yousaf, N.; Battisti, N.M.L.; Moslehi, J.; Larkin, J. Immune checkpoint inhibitors and cardiovascular toxicity. *Lancet Oncol.* **2018**, *19*, e447–e458. [CrossRef]
27. Escudier, M.; Cautela, J.; Malissen, N.; Ancedy, Y.; Orabona, M.; Pinto, J.; Monestier, S.; Grob, J.J.; Scemama, U.; Jacquier, A.; et al. Clinical Features, Management, and Outcomes of Immune Checkpoint Inhibitor-Related Cardiotoxicity. *Circulation* **2017**, *136*, 2085–2087. [CrossRef] [PubMed]
28. Mahmood, S.S.; Fradley, M.G.; Cohen, J.V.; Nohria, A.; Reynolds, K.L.; Heinzerling, L.M.; Sullivan, R.J.; Damrongwatanasuk, R.; Chen, C.L.; Gupta, D.; et al. Myocarditis in Patients Treated with Immune Checkpoint Inhibitors. *J. Am. Coll. Cardiol.* **2018**, *71*, 1755–1764. [CrossRef] [PubMed]
29. Lucas, J.A.; Menke, J.; Rabacal, W.A.; Schoen, F.J.; Sharpe, A.H.; Kelley, V.R. Programmed death ligand 1 regulates a critical checkpoint for autoimmune myocarditis and pneumonitis in MRL mice. *J. Immunol.* **2008**, *181*, 2513–2521. [CrossRef]
30. Yu, Y.R.; O'Koren, E.G.; Hotten, D.F.; Kan, M.J.; Kopin, D.; Nelson, E.R.; Que, L.; Gunn, M.D. A Protocol for the Comprehensive Flow Cytometric Analysis of Immune Cells in Normal and Inflamed Murine Non-Lymphoid Tissues. *PLoS ONE* **2016**, *11*, e0150606. [CrossRef]
31. Francisco, L.M.; Sage, P.T.; Sharpe, A.H. The PD-1 pathway in tolerance and autoimmunity. *Immunol. Rev.* **2010**, *236*, 219–242. [CrossRef] [PubMed]
32. Nishimura, H.; Okazaki, T.; Tanaka, Y.; Nakatani, K.; Hara, M.; Matsumori, A.; Sasayama, S.; Mizoguchi, A.; Hiai, H.; Minato, N.; et al. Autoimmune dilated cardiomyopathy in PD-1 receptor-deficient mice. *Science* **2001**, *291*, 319–322. [CrossRef] [PubMed]
33. Tarrio, M.L.; Grabie, N.; Bu, D.X.; Sharpe, A.H.; Lichtman, A.H. PD-1 protects against inflammation and myocyte damage in T cell-mediated myocarditis. *J. Immunol.* **2012**, *188*, 4876–4884. [CrossRef]
34. Semper, H.; Muehlberg, F.; Schulz-Menger, J.; Allewelt, M.; Grohe, C. Drug-induced myocarditis after nivolumab treatment in a patient with PDL1-negative squamous cell carcinoma of the lung. *Lung Cancer* **2016**, *99*, 117–119. [CrossRef] [PubMed]
35. Baban, B.; Liu, J.Y.; Qin, X.; Weintraub, N.L.; Mozaffari, M.S. Upregulation of Programmed Death-1 and Its Ligand in Cardiac Injury Models: Interaction with GADD153. *PLoS ONE* **2015**, *10*, e0124059. [CrossRef] [PubMed]
36. Freeman, G.J.; Long, A.J.; Iwai, Y.; Bourque, K.; Chernova, T.; Nishimura, H.; Fitz, L.J.; Malenkovich, N.; Okazaki, T.; Byrne, M.C.; et al. Engagement of the PD-1 immunoinhibitory receptor by a novel B7 family member leads to negative regulation of lymphocyte activation. *J. Exp. Med.* **2000**, *192*, 1027–1034. [CrossRef] [PubMed]
37. Schoenfeld, A.J.; Arbour, K.C.; Rizvi, H.; Iqbal, A.N.; Gadgeel, S.M.; Girshman, J.; Kris, M.G.; Riely, G.J.; Yu, H.A.; Hellmann, M.D. Severe immune related adverse events are common with sequential PD-(L)1 blockade and osimertinib. *Ann. Oncol.* **2019**. [CrossRef] [PubMed]
38. Martinez-Calle, N.; Rodriguez-Otero, P.; Villar, S.; Mejias, L.; Melero, I.; Prosper, F.; Marinello, P.; Paiva, B.; Idoate, M.; San-Miguel, J. Anti-PD1 associated fulminant myocarditis after a single pembrolizumab dose: The role of occult pre-existing autoimmunity. *Haematologica* **2018**, *103*, e318–e321. [CrossRef] [PubMed]

39. Gordon, S.R.; Maute, R.L.; Dulken, B.W.; Hutter, G.; George, B.M.; McCracken, M.N.; Gupta, R.; Tsai, J.M.; Sinha, R.; Corey, D.; et al. PD-1 expression by tumour-associated macrophages inhibits phagocytosis and tumour immunity. *Nature* **2017**, *545*, 495–499. [CrossRef] [PubMed]
40. Prajapati, K.; Perez, C.; Rojas, L.B.P.; Burke, B.; Guevara-Patino, J.A. Functions of NKG2D in CD8(+) T cells: An opportunity for immunotherapy. *Cell. Mol. Immunol.* **2018**, *15*, 470–479. [CrossRef]
41. Bauer, S.; Groh, V.; Wu, J.; Steinle, A.; Phillips, J.H.; Lanier, L.L.; Spies, T. Activation of NK cells and T cells by NKG2D, a receptor for stress-inducible MICA. *Science* **1999**, *285*, 727–729. [CrossRef] [PubMed]
42. Markiewicz, M.A.; Carayannopoulos, L.N.; Naidenko, O.V.; Matsui, K.; Burack, W.R.; Wise, E.L.; Fremont, D.H.; Allen, P.M.; Yokoyama, W.M.; Colonna, M.; et al. Costimulation through NKG2D enhances murine CD8+ CTL function: Similarities and differences between NKG2D and CD28 costimulation. *J. Immunol.* **2005**, *175*, 2825–2833. [CrossRef] [PubMed]

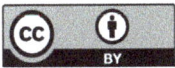

© 2019 by the authors. Licensee MDPI, Basel, Switzerland. This article is an open access article distributed under the terms and conditions of the Creative Commons Attribution (CC BY) license (http://creativecommons.org/licenses/by/4.0/).

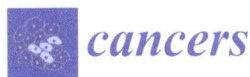

Review

Strategies to Improve Cancer Immune Checkpoint Inhibitors Efficacy, Other Than Abscopal Effect: A Systematic Review

Vito Longo [1,†], Oronzo Brunetti [2,†], Amalia Azzariti [3], Domenico Galetta [1], Patrizia Nardulli [4], Francesco Leonetti [5,‡] and Nicola Silvestris [6,*,‡]

1. Medical Thoracic Oncology Unit, IRCCS Istituto Tumori "Giovanni Paolo II", Viale Orazio Flacco, 65, 70124 Bari, Italy; vito.longo79@tiscali.it (V.L.); galetta@oncologico.bari.it (D.G.)
2. Medical Oncology Unit, Hospital of Barletta, Viale Ippocrate, 15, 70051 Barletta, Italy; dr.oronzo.brunetti@tiscali.it
3. Experimental Pharmacology Laboratory, IRCCS Istituto Tumori "Giovanni Paolo II", Viale Orazio Flacco, 65, 70124 Bari, Italy; a.azzariti@oncologico.bari.it
4. Pharmacy Unit, IRCCS Istituto Tumori "Giovanni Paolo II", Viale Orazio Flacco, 65, 70124 Bari, Italy; p.nardulli@oncologico.bari.it
5. Dipartimento di Farmacia-Scienze del Farmaco, University of Bari, Piazza Umberto I, 1, 70121 Bari, Italy; francesco.leonetti@uniba.it
6. Scientific Guidance, IRCCS Istituto Tumori "Giovanni Paolo II", Viale Orazio Flacco, 65, 70124 Bari, Italy
* Correspondence: n.silvestris@oncologico.bari.it; Tel.: +39-0805-555-419
† These authors contributed equally to this work as the first authors.
‡ These authors contributed equally to this work as the last authors.

Received: 26 March 2019; Accepted: 12 April 2019; Published: 15 April 2019

Abstract: Despite that the impact of immune checkpoint inhibitors on malignancies treatment is unprecedented, a lack of response to these molecules is observed in several cases. Differently from melanoma and non-small cell lung cancer, where the use of immune checkpoint inhibitors results in a high efficacy, the response rate in other tumors, such as gastrointestinal cancers, breast cancer, sarcomas, and part of genitourinary cancers remains low. The first strategy evaluated to improve the response rate to immune checkpoint inhibitors is the use of predictive factors for the response such as PD-L1 expression, tumor mutational burden, and clinical features. In addition to the identification of the patients with a higher expression of immune checkpoint molecules, another approach currently under intensive investigation is the use of therapeutics in a combinatory manner with immune checkpoint inhibitors in order to obtain an enhancement of efficacy through the modification of the tumor immune microenvironment. In addition to the abscopal effect induced by radiotherapy, a lot of studies are evaluating several drugs able to improve the response rate to immune checkpoint inhibitors, including microbiota modifiers, drugs targeting co-inhibitory receptors, anti-angiogenic therapeutics, small molecules, and oncolytic viruses. In view of the rapid and extensive development of this research field, we conducted a systematic review of the literature identifying which of these drugs are closer to achieving validation in the clinical practice.

Keywords: immune checkpoint inhibitors; chemotherapy; tyrosine kinase inhibitors; angiogenesis

---

1. Introduction

Today, immune checkpoint inhibitors (ICIs) represent a gold standard treatment in the first-line setting of several tumors, including non-small cell lung cancer (NSCLC) [1–3], BRAF wild-type (WT) melanoma [4] and metastatic renal cell carcinoma (mRCC) [5]. These molecules are antibodies which block checkpoint molecules such as s cytotoxic T-lymphocyte-associated antigen-4 (CTLA-4) and programmed-death1/programmed death-ligand 1 (PD-1/PD-L1). These interferences reduce the immune suppressive mechanisms increasing the immune responses against cancer and can result in tumor regression in many patients. Over time, the CTLA-4 and PD-1 blockade improved overall survival and the survival rate of many tumors, and have been tested in many others with excellent oncological outcomes. Although these molecules appear to be very promising, there are many limitations such as notable side effects (i.e., endocrine failure, gastrointestinal and pulmonary toxicities). Anyway, one of the biggest disadvantages is that ICIs present a lower activity in several cancers, such as those with low mutational burden. Moreover, even for some pathologies where ICIs have a greater activity, there are some patients that do not show any benefit. However, in some cases there is a lack of response to these molecules [6–8].

Mainly, two strategies are considered to improve the response rate to ICIs. The first is represented by the selection of patients according to specific predictive factors (i.e., PD-L1 expression, tumor mutational burden (TMB), and clinical features). The second strategy has the aim to enhance the efficacy of ICIs, with the abscopal effect induced by radiotherapy representing the most frequently evaluated approach in both pre-clinical and clinical setting [9,10]. However, in the last few years, several studies were focused on the potential role of molecules as it is able to improve the response rate to ICIs by modifying the immune microenvironment of the tumor, increasing the number of activated T cells exerting effector functions, and decreasing the number of immunosuppressive cells thus transforming a cold tumor into a hot one. These drugs include microbiota modifiers, drugs targeting co-inhibitory receptors, anti-angiogenic therapeutics, small molecules, and oncolytic viruses. A systematic review of the literature was conducted, considering only the drug classes which are under evaluation in the clinical setting and as far as they could be considered in the clinical practice in the near future. The research has been conducted considering papers published on PubMed and data presented to the ASCO and ESMO annual meeting. The aim of this systematic review is to evaluate all the drugs, molecules, and viruses which could improve the activity of ICIs. In particular, we evaluate the immunological mechanisms, which lead to enhance ICIs immune anti-cancer.

2. Materials and Methods

2.1. Research Strategy

The research strategy was designed to identify published peer-reviewed studies that research the combination of ICIs and other therapies to improve the anti-tumor immune response. The review covered all countries; no time limit has been set to ensure the identification of a wide range of articles. A web-based search of MEDLINE/PubMed library data published from 2010 to December 2018 was performed. Additional research was performed on ClinicalTrials.gov (Figure 1). Search terms were generated to encapsulate the effect of ICIs on cancer and the increase in the antitumor effect (Table 1).

2.2. Inclusion/Exclusion Criteria

To be eligible, papers had to be written in English, published in a peer-reviewed journal, be original primary research including experimental, observational, and qualitative studies.

The relevant outcomes explored were further investigated as there was a demonstrated role for greater efficacy of the ICI anti-cancer effect when these were administrated in combination with other therapies. The authors excluded the use of ICIs in combination with radiotherapies or other local or regional treatments.

2.3. Study Selection

All studies identified through the search process were exported to EndNoteversion X7(ClarivateAnalytic 22 Thomson Place, 36T3 Boston, MA, USA). Duplicates were removed. Two authors (O.B. and V.L.) have independently doubled the titles, abstracts and keywords with the eligibility criteria. The results were compared and full-text records of potentially relevant publications were obtained and screened using the inclusion criteria for the final selection of studies for systematic review (Figure 1).

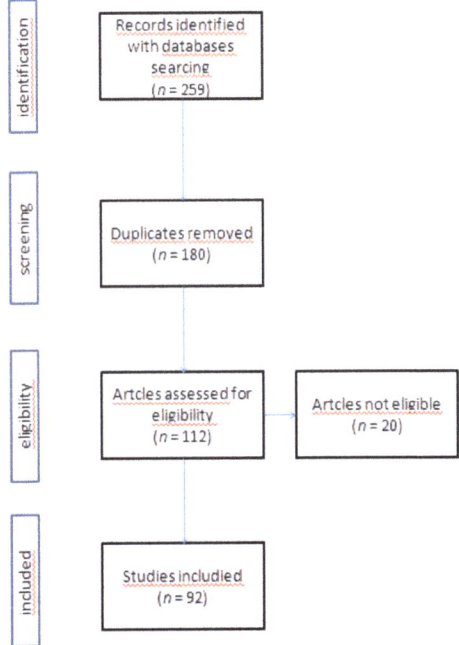

Figure 1. Research strategy with PRISMA flow diagram.

Table 1. Search terms.

Immune Therapy	Enhancer
'immune checkpoint inhibitors', 'anti-PD-(L)1', 'anti-CTLA-4'.	"microbiote" OR "microbiota" OR "gut microbe" OR "bacteria"
'immune checkpoint inhibitors', 'anti-PD-(L)1', 'anti-CTLA-4'.	"chemotherapy" OR "chemotherapeutics" OR "metronomic chemotherapy"
'immune checkpoint inhibitors', 'anti-PD-(L)1', 'anti-CTLA-4'.	"anti-angiogenetic therapies" OR "bevacizumab" OR "nintedanib" OR "Aflibercept" OR "pazopanib" OR "sunitinib"
'immune checkpoint inhibitors', 'anti-PD-(L)1', 'anti-CTLA-4'.	"co-inhibitor receptors" OR "TIGIT" OR "LAG3" OR "TIM-3"
'immune checkpoint inhibitors', 'anti-PD-(L)1', 'anti-CTLA-4'.	"Oncolytic virus" OR "adenovirus" OR "vaccinia viruses" OR "Coxsackieviruses" OR "Reoviruses"
'immune checkpoint inhibitors', 'anti-PD-(L)1', 'anti-CTLA-4'.	"small molecules" OR "tyrosine kinase inhibitor" OR "mTOR inhibitor" OR "cyclin inhibitor"

A group of experts provided additional biological and clinical information, greatly helping to clarify some issues in the absence of clear information from the literature.

The final draft was then submitted to expert evaluation and modified according to their suggestions and comments.

3. Microbiota and ICIs

Microbiota plays a crucial role in the development of host immunity [11]. In several pathologies (i.e., inflammatory bowel disease, diabetes, obesity, atherosclerosis, asthma, and dysmetabolic syndromes) gut commensals resulted in being disrupted in comparison with those of unaffected individuals [12,13].

Regarding the relationship between microbiota and ICIs, the administration of a combination of broad-spectrum antibiotics (i.e., ampicillin plus colistin plus streptomycin) as well as imipenem alone compromised antitumor effects of CTLA-4 monoclonal antibody (mAb) as a consequence of microbiota impairment. Moreover, prescription of antibiotics in patients treated with anti–PD-1/PD-L1 mAb between two months before and two months after the start of immunotherapy resulted in a worse prognosis [14], implying a critical role of microbiota in the modulation of response to ICIs.

In 2015 Vetizou et al. [15] found that antitumor effects of anti-CTLA-4 mAb depended on distinct samples of Bacteroides (B). In particular, the authors demonstrated that the specific T cell response for B. thetaiotaomicron and B. fragilis was associated to the efficacy of anti-CTLA-4 administration in mice inoculated with MCA205 sarcomas, Ret melanoma, and MC38 colon cancer cells. Gut bacterial disruption led to a reduction of anticancer response. This deficiency was overcome by administration of B. fragilis, through immunization with B. fragilis polysaccharides, or by adoptive transfer of B. fragilis-specific T cells. Feces transplantation from patients with metastatic melanoma responsive to anti-CTLA-4 in mice inoculated with cancer cells favored the outcome of these mouse tumor models [15]. In fact, the authors re-colonized both germ-free mice and antibiotics treated with bacterial species, finding that B. fragilis, B. thetaiotaomicron, B. cepacia, or the combination of B. fragilis and B. cepacia could restore the anti-CTLA-4 mAb effects. Oral combination of B. fragilis and Burkholderia cepacia could restore the efficacy of CTLA4 blockade in animals treated with antibiotics, without incurring colitis [15,16]. These data were confirmed in a prospective study considering patients with metastatic melanoma treated with ipilimumab. The intestinal microbiome enriched with B. phylum was correlated with a low incidence of checkpoint-block-induced colitis [17].

In another preclinical study, Sivan et al. [18] compared the growth kinetics of B16.SIY melanoma cells subcutaneously inoculated in two genetically similar C57BL/6 mice from Taconic Farms (TAC) and the Jackson Laboratory (JAX) which contained different intestinal bacterial communities [18]. TAC mice generated more aggressive tumors than JAX mice. On the contrary, tumor-infiltrating specific CD8+ T cells were more evident in JAX mice than in TAC mice. The Bifidobacterium genus was identified as a driver of tumor response in JAX mice. When both mice were co-housed, all animals showed a JAX phenotype, suggesting that an enhanced immune response was potentiated by microbes. Moreover, administration of a mixed Bifidobacterium subspecies altered tumor growth in TAC mice [18].

Patients with baseline bacterial species with a prevalence of the Faecalibacterium genus and other Firmicutes had a significantly longer progression-free survival (PFS) and overall survival (OS) with a more frequent occurrence of colitis than patients with microbiota characterized by the prevalence of B. Moreover, some of these patients reached an OS longer than 18 months [19].

Another study evaluated the therapeutic efficacy of human intestinal microbiota and its metabolites with different ICIs (i.e., ipilimumab, nivolumab, ipilimumab plus nivolumab, or pembrolizumab). The intestinal microbiota of responder patients was enriched by B. caccae with high levels of anacardic acid. In particular, the bacterial microbiome of patients responsive to the combination of nivolumab plus ipilimumab and pembrolizumab was enriched by Faecalibacteriumprausnitzii, B. thetaiotamicron, Holdemaniafiliformis, and Doreaformicogenerans [20].

In 2018, two parallel studies evaluated the role of the microbiome of melanoma patients treated with anti-PD-1. The first analyzed the oral microbiome of 112 patients without significant differences between responders and non-responders, although the fecal microbiota samples of 30 responders to ICI showed a significant presence of Ruminococcaceae bacteria ($p < 0.01$). In the second study 38 and four patients were treated with anti PD1 and anti CTLA4, respectively. A higher presence of Bifidobacterium longum, Collinsellaaerofaciens, Enterococcus faecium, Bifidobacterium adolescentis,

Kleibsiella pneumonia, Veillonellaparvula, Parabacteriodesmerdae, and lactobacillus sp. was observed in the intestines of responders compared to those found in non-responders. Moreover, transplantation of fecal material from responding patients into germ-free mice improved tumor control more effectively than anti-PD-L1 therapy in both studies [21,22].

The microbiome was evaluated in 249 patients with NSCLC, mRCC, and urothelial carcinoma (UC) treated with anti-PD-1 [14]. Genomic analysis of patients' stool samples revealed a significant correlation between response to treatment and high presence of Akkermansia muciniphila. The antitumor effects of the anti PD-1 blockade were improved when the fecal microbiota from patients with a responding tumor were transplanted into germ-free or antibiotic-treated mice. In contrast, fecal transplantation from patients who did not respond to germ-free mice did not achieve any results. Oral supplementation with Akkermansia muciniphila in these latter mice has restored the efficacy of PD-1.

Sivan et al. [18] demonstrated greater expression of the major class I and II histocompatibility complex in dendritic cells (DCs) of JAX mice or Bifidobacterium colonized TAC mice. All the above studies showed an influence of the microbiota on DC maturation and activation (Figure 2). An increase in the rate ofCD8+/Treg was observed in mice transplanted with fecal samples from ICI-sensitive patients. The analysis of tumor infiltrates also revealed the increase of innate effector cells and the reduction of myeloid-derived suppressor cells (MDSCs) [21,22]. Moreover, the administration of Akkermansia muciniphila in germ-free mice treated with anti-PD-1was associated with increased frequency of T helper1 Tregs/tumoral helper1 cells. Finally, the oral administration of A. muciniphila and E. hiraestimulates leads DCs to increase the production of IL-12, a cytokine involved in the inhibition of PD-1 under physiological conditions [14].

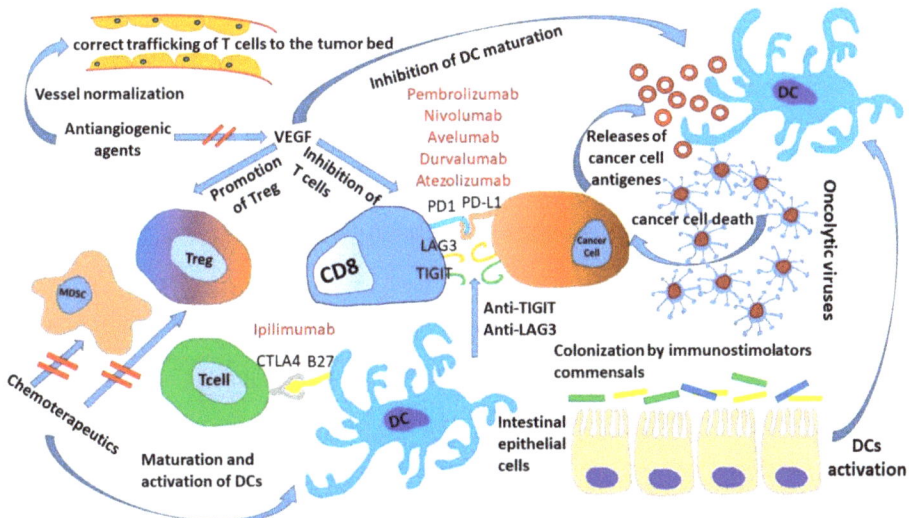

Figure 2. Summarizes the mechanisms implicated in improving the efficacy of immune checkpoint inhibitors (ICIs): The influence of microbiota on dendritic cell (DC) maturation and activation; the correct trafficking of T cells to the tumor bed due to the normalization of endothelium by anti-angiogenic drugs and the VEGF immunosuppressive activity; the impact of chemotherapy on immunosuppressive cells and on DC maturation; release of damaged molecular patterns after oncolytic viruses induce tumor cell lysis.

In conclusion, there is evidence supporting the relationship between some bacterial species and the enhanced response to ICIs (i.e., Ruminococaceae family of the Firmicutes phylum as Firmicutesprausnitzii) [19–21]. Similarly, other intestine microbiome components (i.e., Bacterioides and Firmicutes phylum) have been associated with a lack of response to immune checkpoint blockade [19–21]. Data concerning Firmicutes (Roseburia, Streptococcus) [20,22] and other B. (i.e., Alistipes, Porphyromonaspasteri, and C. aerofaciens) are still not univocal [14,21,22]. It is interesting to note how different bacteria are beneficial in different types of cancer. The differences in the methods used for sample feces and the analysis of the intestinal microbiome, the databases used for analysis, and the populations with both dietary and microbiotic differences are responsible for the ambiguity of these data. These heterogeneous results make it difficult to interpret the reason for such different data. In particular, it is still unclear why different microbiota improve ICI in different types of cancer. Clinical trials are underway to define the possible role of the microbiota in improving the ICI response.

4. Chemotherapeutics Sensitizing Tumor to ICIs

Recently, the combination of immunotherapy and chemotherapy has been approved for the treatment of both metastatic and locally advanced NSCLC [1–3]. Chemotherapy not only achieves an ulterior efficacy to immunotherapy but it also acts in a synergistic manner in two significant ways: (a) Induction of immunogenic cell death as part of its independent therapeutic effects and (b) disruption strategies used by neoplastic cells to evade immune response. The first process involves the release of tumor antigens and the emission of danger-associated molecular patterns within tumor microenvironment during cell death. At the same time, chemotherapy decreases the number of immunosuppressive cells in the microenvironment including Tregs and MDSCs, increases the number of cytotoxic T lymphocytes (CTLs) and promotes maturation and activation of DCs (Figure 2). In addition, chemotherapeutics modifies the levels of several cytokines, down-regulates immune suppressive cytokines (i.e., transforming growth factor-β (TGF β) and IL10), and up-regulates cytokines promoting tumor immunity (i.e., tumor necrosis factor-α (TNF-α), IL-2, and interferon (IFN)–γ) [23].

As far as ICIs are concerned, preclinical models showed that autochthonous tumors that lacked CTLs infiltration were resistant to these agents, while on the contrary the exposure to appropriately selected immunogenic chemotherapeutics induces CTLs tumor infiltration, sensitizing tumor to ICIs. In the mouse model of lung adenocarcinoma, refractory to an anti-PD-1 and anti-CTLA-4 mAb combination therapy, the use of oxaliplatin in combination with a low-dose of cyclophosphamide increased the lung CTLs/Treg cell ratio sensitizing the tumor to ICIs [24]. Similarly, oxaliplatin increased the amounts of CTLs and activated DCs in a murine colorectal cancer, enhancing the efficacy of a PD-L1 trap [25]. A low-dose of cyclophosphamide combined with an anti-PD1 synergistically induced antigen-specific immunity and the infiltration of CD8+ and CD4+FoxP3−T cells as well as it induced the suppression of the CD4+ CD25+ FoxP3+ regulatory T cell function, thus resulting in the increase of tumor-free survival in a model of cervical cancer [26,27]. According to these studies, 5-fluoruracil (5-FU) increased tumor immunity in a mouse model by renal cell xenograft through an increase of CTL infiltration mediated by the High Mobility Group Box 1 (HMGB1). Interestingly, a combined 5-FU and anti-PD-L1 treatment significantly improved the relationship between CTL and MDSCs compared to 5-FU and anti-PD-L1 single treatments with a longer OS [28].

On the other hand, several chemotherapeutics have been shown to induce an up-regulation of PD-L1 expression, as a possible mechanism of chemotherapy immune suppression. However, the increase of PD-L1 expression may support the synergism between chemotherapy and immunotherapy targeting the PD-L1/PD-1 axis. 5-FU demonstrated up-regulation of PD-L1 in two preclinical studies evaluating colorectal cancer patients [25,29]. Similarly, the administration of trabectedin induced the IFN-γ-dependent PD-L1 expression within a tumor in a murine model of ovarian cancer [30]. Others drugs able to up-regulate PD-L1 expression in ovarian cancer models are paclitaxel, carboplatin, cisplatin, gemcitabine, and capecitabine [31].Interestingly, Peng J et al. showed, from a collection of cancer cells from ovarian cancer patients with massive ascites, that the expression of PD-L1 increased 5-fold on day four after combined paclitaxel and carboplatin therapy and decreased to pre-treatment levels on day 11, demonstrating the reversibility of PD-L1 expression induced by chemotherapy [31]. Finally, the evaluation of 150 specimens of patients with ovarian cancer treated with neoadjuvant chemotherapy showed the up-regulation of PD-L1 [32].

Several clinical trials are evaluating the combination of chemotherapy with ICIs, but in the majority of these, chemotherapy and chemotherapeuticsis administered concurrently and at full doses. Only a few trials are focused on the role of chemotherapeutics as sensitizers for immunotherapy, exploring the optimal dose, or the sequence of administration, while preclinical data have shown that these parameters might affect the results.

An open, multi-center, single-arm label, Phase Ib/II, evaluated the daily metronomic dose of 50 mg of cyclophosphamide without interruption of administration, 10 mg/kg of avelumab on day one and every two weeks until progression, and a single fraction of 8Gy radiotherapy in pretreated head and neck cancer patients, showing noun acceptable toxicity [27]. A study concerning metastatic patients with triple negative breast cancer (TNBC) patients investigated induction therapy with various types of chemotherapy [33]. For the induction phase, low doses of chemotherapy were given for two weeks: 50 mg daily cyclophosphamide, twice 40 mg/m^2 cisplatin or twice 15 mg doxorubicin. Response rates with chemotherapy appear higher in the cohorts where low-dose chemotherapy was used as induction, compared with nivolumab alone. Conversely, an immunotherapy induction phase may also be useful. An induction phase with durvalumab followed by combination therapy of nab-paclitaxel weekly for 12 weeks followed by four cycles of combined therapy with epirubicin and cyclophosphamide was evaluated in patients with TNBC, resulting in a higher pathological CR rate when compared with chemotherapy alone (53.4% versus 44.2%, respectively) [34].

Other trials evaluating the combination of metronomic chemotherapy with ICIs [35] or the impact of chemotherapy on TMB [36] are underway. Future studies should evaluate drugs capable of inducing immune cell death and CTLs tumor microenvironment infiltration, optimizing ICI integration with chemotherapy.

5. ICIs and Antiangiogenic Drugs

The vascular network with its specific components (endothelial cells, pericytes, growth factors, and receptors) plays a key role in the regulation of inflammatory response, wound healing, and immune surveillance. Antigen-primed T cells require a healthy endothelium for the trafficking to tissue districts and the cell-to-cell cross-talk during the priming and effector phase of the immune response. The transit of immune cells in the tumor plays a critical role in the outcome of immunotherapeutic strategies, similarly to classical chemotherapeutic drugs. In particular, a normalized endothelium ensures the correct trafficking of T cells to the tumor bed [37]. In fact, tumor angiogenesis contributes to the escape of the immune tumor through the immunosuppressive activity exerted by VEGF, PGE2, IL-10, and tumor hypoxia. In particular, VEGF acts through both the inhibition of lymphocyte adhesion to activated endothelial cells and the systemic effect on immune-regulatory cell function, including the suppression of DCs maturation, the inhibition of T cell development, and the increase of inhibitory immune cells [38] (Figure 2). Therefore, the possibility of administering ICIs during an anti-angiogenic treatment has been studied in different types of cancers according to the hypothesis that anti-angiogenic drug-induced normalization of the vessels may improve immunotherapeutic strategies. On the other hand, ICI activation of Th1 cells blocked vessel normalization, suggesting the existence of a mutually regulatory circuit [39].

In a phase II study, 46 patients with metastatic melanoma were treated in four dosing cohorts of ipilimumab (3 or 10 mg/kg) with four doses at three-week intervals and then every 12 weeks in combination with bevacizumab (7.5 or 15 mg/kg every three weeks). Eight partial responses and 22 stable diseases were observed, with a disease-control rate of 67.4% and a median OS of 25.1 months [40]. Bevacizumab has been evaluated also in combination with ICI targeting the PD-1/PD-L1 axis in a phase II study considering HER2-negative advanced breast cancer patients. The combination of nivolumab, paclitaxel, and bevacizumab showed an overall response rate ORR of 70% [41]. The same combination demonstrated clinical activity in women with recurrent ovarian cancer, which showed a global confirmed response rate of 21% and a median PFS of 9.4 months [42]. In another study patients with pre-treated NSCLC with platinum-based first-line chemotherapy received nivolumab plus bevacizumab as maintenance therapy with 1-yr OS rate of 75% and a manageable toxicity profile [43]. Recently, the phase III IM power 150 trial showed no new safety signals of the combination of atezolizumab plus bevacizumab, carboplatin, and taxol in first-line non-squamous NSCLC patients with a median OS of 20.5 months [2]. Interestingly, the first randomized phase III trial of a PD-L1/PD-1 pathway inhibitor combined with bevacizumab in first-line mRCC showed longer PFS for atezolizumab plus bevacizumab compared to sunitinb in PD-L1+ patients [44]. The safety and efficacy of a combined treatment of bevacizumab with atezolizumab was assessed in pre-treated patients with metastatic colon rectal cancer (MCRC), or in oxaliplatin-naïve patients in conjunction with FOLFOX (fluorouracil, folinic acid, leucovorin, and oxaliplatin), with an ORR of 44% in the combination group. In a phase 1 a/b study [45] concerning patients with gastric or gastroesophageal junction (G/GEJ), NSCLC, UC, or biliary tract cancer (BTC), the combination of ramucirumab (10 mg/kg) with pembrolizumab (200 mg on the first day of q3w) showed a disease control rate DCR of 85% with no relevant toxicity [46]. Regarding antiangiogenic TKIs, the combination of nivolumab and either pazopanib or sunitinib has been evaluated in mRCC pre-treated with at least one previous systemic therapy. An 45% ORR was demonstrated in the nivolumab plus pazopanib arm, compared to 52% in the nivolumab plus sunitinib arm, with a manageable safety profile. These combination approaches might benefit patients with poor prognosis, such as those with a low probability to respond to ICI monotherapy (i.e., refractory to patients on first-line therapy or showing PDL1–negative tumors) [47]. Considering the potential role of antiangiogenenic therapies of changing a cold tumor into a hot one, several trials are currently underway investigating other combinations of antiangiogenic agents and ICIs.

6. Strategies Involving Other Co-Inhibitor Receptors

The encouraging outcome obtained by the co-inhibitory receptors CTLA-4 and PD-1 prompted the research of additional co-inhibitory molecules. T cell immunoglobulin and immune-receptor tyrosine-based inhibitory motif domain (TIGIT) is a newly identified co-inhibitory receptor expressed by Tregs, activated T cells, and natural killer (NK) cells [48]. TIGIT expression is elevated on CD8$^+$TILs and Tregs in a variety of tumors, as well as the expression of its three ligands, namely CD155, CD112, and CD11 3 [49]. Moreover, TIGT and PD-1 are co-expressed and up-regulated on TILs. Dual blockade of two immune checkpoints enhances function of TILs resulting in a significant tumor rejection, as demonstrated by the combination of anti-CTLA-4 with anti-PD-1/PD-L1.Anti-PD-1 and anti-TIGT dual therapy significantly improved survival compared to control and monotherapy in a murine glioblastoma (GBM) model. Clinically, TIGIT expression on tumor-infiltrating lymphocytes was shown to be elevated in GBM samples, suggesting that the TIGIT pathway may be a valuable therapeutic target [50]. A phase II, randomized, blinded, placebo-controlled trial is currently underway that considersMTIG7192A, an anti-TIGIT antibody, in combination with atezolizumab patients with chemotherapy-naïve NSCLC [51].

Lymphocyte activation gene-3 (LAG3), an immune checkpoint up-regulated on activated T cells, Treg, and NK cells in different types of cancer, is required for the maintenance of Treg suppressive function. LAG3 blocks either by soluble LAG3 immunoglobulin or antibodies have shown efficacy in the antitumor response. Similarly, to TIGT, LAG3 coexisted and upregulated with PD-1 on TILs [52]. According to preclinical data showing a significant increase in the activity of dual blockade of LAG3 and PD-1 [53], numerous clinical trials are underway with the aim of translating this combination modality into clinical practice.

An open-label phase 1/2a trial evaluating BMS-986016, an experimentalanti-LAG-3, in combination with nivolumab in patients with advanced melanoma previously treated with anti-PD-1/PD-L1 therapy (n = 55). ORR was 12.5% in evaluable patients (n = 48). The expression of LAG-3in at least 1% (n = 25) of tumor-associated immune cells within the tumor margin was associated with an almost triple improvement in ORRs compared to patients without LAG-3 expression (n = 14) (20% and 7.1%, respectively) [54]. LAG525, a humanized IgG4 mAbs capable of blocking the binding of LAG-3 to class IIMHC, is being studied in a phase I/II study in combination with an anti-PD1 treatment.

Common adverse events (≥10%) were fatigue (10%) for LAG525 alone and fatigue (18%), diarrhea (15%), and nausea (12%) in the combination group. LAG525 plus the anti-PD1 spartalizumab drug led to durable RECIST responses (11 PR, 1 CR) in a variety of solid tumors, including mesothelioma (2/8 pts) and triple-negative breast cancer (TNBC) (2/5 pts). In TNBC tumor biopsies, a tendency to convert immuno-cooled biomarker profiles to immune-activated has been reported [55]. T cell immunoglobulin containing the mucin domain 3 (TIM-3) is widely expressed on helper 1 T cells, CD8+ lymphocytes, Treg, DCs, NK cells, and monocytes. Similarly, to TIGIT and LAG3, the high expression of TIM-3 and PD-1 is observed in the tumor microenvironment, in particular on TIL and Treg, suggesting the possible re-establishing of T cell function through the targeting of TIM-3 and PD-1 [56]. A phase 1 study is evaluating the anti-TIM-3 antibody (T cell immunoglobulin and protein-containing mucin 3) TSR-022 as monotherapy and in combination with an anti-PD-1 antibody, in pre-treated patients with advanced solid tumors [57].

7. Oncolytic Virus and ICIs

The oncolytic virus vectors are designed to have a high tumor tropism, maximize cancer killing effects and minimized a mage to surrounding normal tissue. It is interesting to note that these viruses not only facilitate the lysis of tumor cells, but also cause a strong change in the tumor immune microenvironment. In particular, oncolytic viruses transfer the genes encoding IFN-α, GM-CSF, and others cytokines that induce tumor-specific immunity by promoting DC maturation and function. On the other hand, tumor cell lysis induced by oncolytic viruses determines the release of damage-associated molecular patterns (DAMPS) that include cell surface proteins, membrane proteins, and nucleic acids (Figure 3) [58,59].

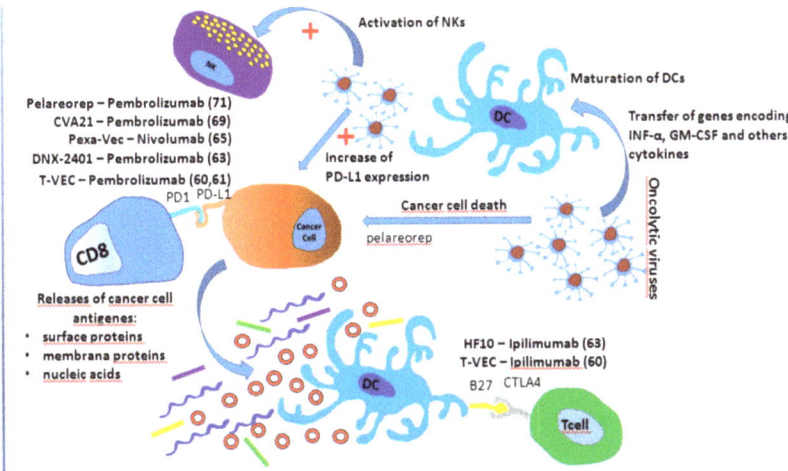

Figure 3. Summary of the mechanisms involved in improving of ICI efficacy by oncolytic viruses: Release of damage-associated molecular patterns after tumor cell lysis, transfer of genes encoding INF-α, GM-CSF and others cytokines, DC maturation and activation, natural killer (NK) cell activation, and increase in PD-L1 expression. The main studies evaluating the combination of oncolytic viruses are also reported.

Talimogene Laherparepvec (T-VEC) replicates within tumors and produces GM-CSF, resulting in a first-rate FDA-approved intralesional oncolytic immune therapy for stage IIIb and IV melanoma. A recent phase II trial comparing ipilimumab plus T-VEC with ipilimumab alone showed that the ORR in the combination arm was significantly higher than in the monotherapy arm (39% vs. 18%; $p < 0.02$) [60]. Distant non-injection sites demonstrated an adjuvant effect with a reduction in visceral lesions size in 52% of patients in the combination arm versus only 2% of the patients in the ipilimumab arm. T-Vec has been also tested in patients with melanoma in combination with pembrolizumab in a phase Ib study. No dose-limiting toxicity was observed with an ORR of 62% and a CRR of 33% [58]. A phase III trial is underway [61]. It is interesting to note that an analysis performed prior to the administration of anti-PD1 antibodies showed that T-VEC increased the PD-L1 expression and inflammation distant from the injection sites. HF 10, another virus included in the HSV family, in combination with ipilimumab showed in a phase II clinical trial regarding stage IIIB/IIIC or IV unresectable melanoma a DCR of 68% without disease limiting toxicity [62]. An oncolytic adenovirus competent for replication with tumor selectivity, namely Tasadenoturev (DNX-2401), was able to overcome the exhaustion of T cells demonstrating a reduction in tumor size in a phase I study for patients with recurrent GBM. A phase II study employing DNX-2401 and pembrolizumab in GBM progressed after initial therapy is currently underway [63]. Another group of oncolytic viruses is represented by vaccinia viruses, members of the Poxviridae family, which are suitable for transgene insertion. Pexa-Vec targeted tumor-associated endothelial cells resulting in vascular disruption and oncolysis [64]. A single dose of Pexa-Vec intravenously demonstrated activation of NK, CD4/CD8 T cells, and antigen presenting cells in surgically treated liver metastases. The combination of Pexa-Vec and nivolumab is under investigation for the treatment of liver tumors [65]. Furthermore, the combination of Pexa-Vec with other ICIs is being evaluated in colorectal cancer and other advanced tumors, respectively [66,67]. When speaking about Coxackieviruses, CVA 21 is able to increase infiltration of immune cells and checkpoint molecules, several clinical trials concerning the combination of CVA 21 with ICIs are ongoing [68]. In particular, in the CAPRA clinical trial, patients who receive multiple intratumoral injections of CVA 21 and pembrolizumab showed an ORR of 73% [69]. Finally, the reoviruses, characterized by icosahedral capsid and double-stranded RNA genomes, have been shown to increase cytotoxic T cells infiltrating the CD8+tumor in an Ib phase concerning GBM patients undergoing debulking neurosurgery [70]. A clinical trial [71] is underway evaluating the use of a reovirus, namely pelareorep in combination with pembrolizumab and chemotherapy in patients with recurrent metastatic pancreatic cancers.

8. Small Molecule Inhibitors and ICIs

Various evidence suggests that small molecule inhibitors could improve host-tumor interactions, improving antigen expression and the immune response against tumor cells [72]. Several small molecules in combination with ICIs have been studied for the treatment of different types of tumor histotypes (Table 2).

The first combination of small molecule inhibitors and ICIs have been evaluated in melanoma. In particular, since the administration of BRAFi/MEKi represents a standard treatment of metastatic BRAF^{V600E} melanoma, the possibility that this association would be improved by ICIs has been evaluated. It has been demonstrated that BRAF inhibition is associated with enhanced melanoma antigen expression [73–75]. Moreover, selective BRAF inhibitors induce marked T cell infiltration in human metastatic melanoma [74], with an up-regulation of PD-L1 in the tumor microenvironment [72,74]. Nevertheless, the benefit of this combination in preclinical models has been modest [76–79]. In particular, in a mouse model of syngeneic BRAF^{V600E} driven melanoma, the combination of dabrafenib and trametinib with pmel-1 adoptive cell transfer showed a complete tumor regression with increased T cell infiltration in tumors and improved in vivo cytotoxicity. Single agent dabrafenib increased the number of tumor-associated macrophages and Tregs in tumors that conversely decreased with the addition of trametinib. The combination of BRAFi/MEKi and ICI induced either an increased expression of the melanosomal antigens and MHC or the global immune-related gene up-regulation. Moreover, a combination of dabrafenib and trametinib with anti-PD1 therapy in SM1 tumors led to a greater anti-tumor effect compared to the results obtained with the only small molecules combination [80].

Table 2. Small Molecule Inhibitors and ICIs.

Small Molecule Enhancer	ICI	Cancer	Study Design	Results/Enhancing	Reference
BRAFi	Not associated	Melanoma	In vitro	BRAF inhibition enhance melanoma antigen expression	Wilmott, 2013. [72]
Selective BRAF inhibitors	Not associated	Melanoma	In vitro	Induction of Tcell infiltration into human metastatic melanoma Up-regulation of PD-L1 in tumor microenvironment	Wilmott, 2012. [74]
Dabrafenib and trametinib	(pmel-1 adoptive cell transfer)	BRAFV600E driven melanoma	In vivo—mouse model	Complete tumor regression with increased T cell infiltration into tumors and improved in vivo cytotoxicity	Cooper, 2014. [79]
Dabrafenib and trametinib	anti-PD1	SM1 tumors (melanoma)	In vivo—mouse model	Superior anti-tumor effect compared to the results obtained with the only small molecules combination	Hu-Lieskovan, 2015. [80]
Vemurafenib	Ipilimumab	Melanoma	Phase 1 trial	Stopped after one month due to liver toxicity	Ribas, 2013. [81]
Dabrafenib, trametinib	Ipilimumab	Melanoma	Phase 1 trial	Stopped due to excessive colon toxicity	Minor, 2015. [82]
Dabrafenib	Ipilimumab	BRAF-mutated melanoma	Phase 1 trial	ORR of 69% Good safety profile	Puzanov, 2014. [83]
Dabrafenib and trametinib	pembrolizumab	BRAF-mutated melanoma	KEYNOTE-022, an ongoing phase I/II trial	ORR of 60% (n = 9 PR, n = 2 SD, n = 3 PD)	NCT02130466, Ribas, 2016. [85]
Vemurafenib (V)	Atezolizumab (A)	Melanoma	Phase Ib trial (V-run in vs. concurrent V-A)	Higher ORR was seen with V run-in than with concurrent A + V start	Sullivan, 2016. [86]
Vemurafenib, and cobimetinib	Atezolizumab	BRAF^{V600}-mutant melanoma	Phase I/II trial	Manageable safety profile and promising antitumor activity	NCT01656642. [84]
imatinib	Not associated	GIST	In vitro study	Reduction of Treg immunosuppressive function	Larmonier, 2008. [87]
Imatinib	Not associated	GIST	In vivo study	PFS correlated with IFN-γ secretion by NK cells	Ménard, 2009. [88]
Imatinib	Not associated	GIST	In vivo—mouse model	Activated CD8+ T cells and induced Treg apoptosis in tumor sample	Balachandran, 2011. [89]
Imatinib	Anti-PD-1 (RMP1-14) or anti-PD-L1 (10F.9G2)	GIST	In vivo—mouse model	Increased antitumor effects by enhancing cytotoxic T cell effector function	Seifert, 2017. [90]
Imatinib	Ipilimumab	GIST and other c-Kit positive solid cancers	Phase 1 trial	Manageable safety profile in multiple tumor types. Low activity with no clear signal for synergy in escalation or GIST expansion cohorts	NCT01738139, Reilley, 2017. [91]
Rapamycin	Not associated	Oral cancer	In vivo—mouse model	Reduction of tumor growth through CD8-activity	Cash, 2015. [93]
Rapamycin	Not associated	Oral cancer	In vivo—mouse model	Enhancing of IFNγ production by peripheral and tumor-infiltrating CD8 T cells	Moore, 2016. [94]
Rapamycin	PD-L1 mAb	Oral cancer	In vivo—mouse model	Activation of CD8 T cells in tumor infiltration increased by the addition of rapamycin	Moore, 2016. [94]
CDK4/6 inhibitor	Not associated	Breast cancer	In vivo—mouse model/blood sample patients	Anti-tumor immunity through proliferation of Tregs	Goel, 2017. [95]
CDK4/6 inhibitor	anti-PD-1	Breast cancer	In vivo—mouse model	Enhancing of tumor regression and dramatically improving of OS	Zhang, 2018. [96]
CDK4/6 inhibitor and PI3K antagonist	Anti PD-1 and anti CTLA-4	Triple negative breast cancer	In vivo—mouse model	Inhibition induced complete and durable regressions (> one year) of breast tumors in in vivo models.	Teo, 2017. [97]

The first phase 1 trial evaluating the role of ipilimumab in combination with vemurafenib was stopped after one month due to liver toxicity [81]. Another phase 1 study evaluated the safety of the combination of dabrafenib, trametinib, and ipilimumab. This study was also stopped due to excessive colon toxicity [82]. A combination of dabrafenib and ipilimumab demonstrated an ORR of 69% in the 26 BRAF-mutated patients with a good safety profile [83]. The KEYNOTE-022, an ongoing phase I/II trial [98], is evaluating the combination of pembrolizumab with dabrafenib and trametinib. Preliminary data on 15 patients enrolled across dose determination and dose confirmation arms showed a safety profile and an ORR of 60% (n = 9 PR, n = 2 SD, n = 3 PD) [85]. A phase Ib study is investigating vemurafenib and atezolizumab combination and comparing this combination concurrently or after a run-in period with vemurafenib alone [99]. It was demonstrated that the vemurafenib run-in showed a higher ORR than concomitant atezolizumab plus the onset of vemurafenib. The combination of atezolizumab, vemurafenib, and cobimetinib in this subgroup of patients is being investigated [84]. Preliminary results confirmed that this combination has a manageable safety profile with a promising antitumor activity in patients with BRAF^{V600}-mutant metastatic melanoma [86].

Also, in gastrointestinal stromal tumors (GIST), preclinical studies demonstrated that imatinib in combination with ICIs should improve the immune response. It is well known that this drug induces NK cells activity through DCs in several cancers [100,101]. Furthermore, in an in vitro study, imatinib reduced the Treg immunosuppressive function and the FoxP3 expression with the inhibition of phosphorylation of both ZAP70 and LAT, impairing their immunosuppressive function [87]. Moreover, PFS correlated with IFN-γ secretion by NK cells in patients affected by GIST treated with imatinib [88]. In a mouse model of spontaneous GIST, Balachandran et al. demonstrated that the immune system substantially contributed to the anti-tumor effects of imatinib. In fact, it activated CD8+ T cells and induced Treg apoptosis in the tumor sample by reducing immunosuppressive enzyme indoleamine 2,3-dioxygenase (IDO) [89]. In a more recent study, PD-1 was expressed more on T cells in imatinib-treated human GISTs as compared to untreated patients. Imatinib inhibited the upregulation of PD-L1 through IFNγ in human GIST cell lines. In a GIST mouse model, imatinib down-regulated IFNγ related genes and reduced the PD-L1 expression on tumor cells. Moreover, PD-1 or PD-L1 blockade without imatinib achieved no response in GIST mouse model. On the contrary, association of ICIs and imatinib increased antitumor effects by enhancing cytotoxic T cell effector function [90].

A current phase I study is evaluating the effect of a combination of ipilimumab and imatinib GIST positive solid cancers and other-Kit [91]. Preliminary results have shown that this combination is safe on most types of tumors. Nevertheless, low activity without a clear synergy signal is observed in GIST expansion or escalation cohorts [92].

It is interesting to note that a combination of small molecules and ICIs have been evaluated in a mouse model of oral cancer. In this neoplasia, both activation of PI3K/mTOR and MEK/ERK pathways promoted the immunosuppressive tumor microenvironment [102]. In an immunogenic model of cancer of the oral cavity, rapamycin reduced tumor growth in a CD8-dependent manner [93]. More recently, Moore et al. [94] demonstrated that rapamycin improved IFNγ production by peripheral and tumor-infiltrating CD8 T cells in a mouse model of oral cancer. Furthermore, antitumor efficacy was enhanced by the CD8 T cell but not by NK cell. Non-inflamed tumor models, which represent the low level of response to immune therapies, did not induce T cell or NK CD8 cell–mediated antitumor immunity when treated with combinations of targeted and ICIs. In other models, antitumor immune responses to PD-L1 mAb treatment were enhanced when treated with mTOR inhibitors. These data suggested that a combination of mTOR and ICIs inhibitors should be evaluated in clinical trials setting.

There are few preclinical studies considering small molecules inhibitors and ICIs combinations in breast cancer patients. In both murine models and breast cancer patients, CDK4/6 inhibition induced anti-tumor immunity through suppression of Tregs and contributing to anticancer effects [95]. Since cyclin D-CDK4 regulated PD-L1 protein expression, inhibition of CDK4/6 in vivo increases PD-L1 protein levels through inhibition of cyclin D-CDK4. Combination of CDK4/6 inhibitor and anti-PD-1 immunotherapy enhanced tumor regression and dramatically improved OS rates in mouse breast cancer models [96]. Teo et al. demonstrated that PI3K antagonist and CDK4/6 inhibition significantly increased tumor immunogenicity through generating immunogenic cell death in triple negative breast cancer model. Moreover, this combination significantly increased tumor-infiltrating T cell activation and cytotoxicity with reduction of immune-suppressive myeloid-derived suppressor cells. Association of immune checkpoints PD-1, CTLA-4 to PI3K antagonist and CDK4/6 inhibition induced complete and durable regressions (> one year) of breast tumors in in vivo models [97].

In the era of precision medicine, several small molecules have been demonstrated to be active in targeting specific pathways leading to apoptosis of cancer cells with impressive results in anti-cancer treatment. In addition, these molecules appear capable of increasing tumor immunogenicity through the increase of cancer antigens and the activation of cytotoxic activity of CD8 cells leading to an increased putative activity of ICIs when associated in concomitant or sequential therapeutic schedules.

9. Conclusions

This systematic review has summarized the current study of the main classes of drugs which improve the activity of the ICIs. The assessment of drugs able to modify the tumor immune microenvironment in addition to ICIs is a field of research, which is currently undergoing a significant escalation. Despite the encouraging results, only chemotherapy has currently adhered to clinical practice for this specific use. Curiously, most of these molecules are characterized by a high level of safety and already consolidated clinical use for indications other than those considered in this study. These features should allow for the possibility of undertaking more extensive and well-designed studies. At the same time, the possibility of new side effects due to the combinatorial strategies or the potential amplification of the well-known ICIs side effects [103,104] should be carefully monitored.

Funding: This research received no external funding.

Conflicts of Interest: The Authors declare no conflicts of interests.

References

1. Gandhi, L.; Rodríguez-Abreu, D.; Gadgeel, S.; Esteban, E.; Felip, E.; De Angelis, F.; Domine, M.; Clingan, P.; Hochmair, M.J.; Powell, S.F.; et al. Pembrolizumab plus Chemotherapy in Metastatic Non-Small-Cell Lung Cancer. *N. Engl. J. Med.* **2018**, *378*, 2078–2092. [CrossRef]
2. Socinski, M.A.; Jotte, R.M.; Cappuzzo, F.; Orlandi, F.; Stroyakovskiy, D.; Nogami, N.; Rodríguez-Abreu, D.; Moro-Sibilot, D.; Thomas, C.A.; Barlesi, F.; et al. Atezolizumab for First-Line Treatment of Metastatic Nonsquamous NSCLC. *N. Engl. J. Med.* **2018**, *378*, 2288–2301. [CrossRef]
3. Antonia, S.J.; Villegas, A.; Daniel, D.; Vicente, D.; Murakami, S.; Hui, R.; Yokoi, T.; Chiappori, A.; Lee, K.H.; de Wit, M.; et al. Durvalumab after Chemoradiotherapy in Stage III Non-Small-Cell Lung Cancer. *N. Engl. J. Med.* **2017**, *377*, 1919–1929. [CrossRef]
4. Wolchok, J.D.; Chiarion-Sileni, V.; Gonzalez, R.; Rutkowski, P.; Grob, J.J.; Cowey, C.L.; Lao, C.D.; Wagstaff, J.; Schadendorf, D.; Ferrucci, P.F.; et al. Overall Survival with Combined Nivolumab and Ipilimumab in Advanced Melanoma. *N. Engl. J. Med.* **2017**, *377*, 1345–1356. [CrossRef] [PubMed]
5. Cella, D.; Grünwald, V.; Escudier, B.; Hammers, H.J.; George, S.; Nathan, P.; Grimm, M.O.; Rini, B.I.; Doan, J.; Ivanescu, C.; et al. Patient-reported outcomes of patients with advancedrenalcell carcinoma treated withnivolumabplusipilimumabversussunitinib (CheckMate214): A randomised, phase 3 trial. *Lancet Oncol.* **2019**, *20*, 297–310. [CrossRef]
6. Balar, A.V.; Castellano, D.; O'Donnell, P.H.; Grivas, P.; Vuky, J.; Powles, T.; Plimack, E.R.; Hahn, N.M.; de Wit, R.; Pang, L.; et al. First-linepembrolizumabin cisplatin-ineligible patients with locally advanced and unresectable or metastaticurothelialcancer (KEYNOTE-052): A multicentre, single-arm, phase 2 study. *Lancet Oncol.* **2017**, *18*, 1483–1492. [CrossRef]
7. Borghaei, H.; Paz-Ares, L.; Horn, L.; Spigel, D.R.; Steins, M.; Ready, N.E.; Chow, L.Q.; Vokes, E.E.; Felip, E.; Holgado, E.; et al. Nivolumab versus Docetaxel in Advanced Nonsquamous Non-Small-Cell Lung Cancer. *N. Engl. J. Med.* **2015**, *373*, 1627–1639. [CrossRef]

8. Kanjanapan, Y.; Day, D.; Wang, L.; Al-Sawaihey, H.; Abbas, E.; Namini, A.; Siu, L.L.; Hansen, A.; Razak, A.A.; Spreafico, A.; et al. Hyperprogressive disease in early-phase immunotherapy trials: Clinical predictors and association with immune-related toxicities. *Cancer* **2019**, *125*, 1341–1349. [CrossRef] [PubMed]
9. Chuong, M.; Chang, E.T.; Choi, E.Y.; Mahmood, J.; Lapidus, R.G.; Davila, E.; Carrier, F. Exploring the Concept of Radiation "Booster Shot" in Combination with an Anti-PD-L1 mAb to Enhance Anti-Tumor Immune Effects in Mouse Pancreas Tumors. *J. Clin. Oncol. Res.* **2017**, *5*, 1058.
10. Meng, X.; Feng, R.; Yang, L.; Xing, L.; Yu, J. The Role of Radiation Oncology in Immuno-Oncology. *Oncologist* **2019**, *24*, S42–S52. [CrossRef]
11. Ivanov, I.I.; Honda, K. Intestinal commensal microbes as immune modulators. *Cell. Host Microbe.* **2012**, *12*, 496–508. [CrossRef] [PubMed]
12. Lynch, S.V.; Pedersen, O. The Human Intestinal Microbiome in Health and Disease. *N. Engl. J. Med.* **2016**, *375*, 2369–2379. [CrossRef]
13. Roy, S.; Trinchieri, G. Microbiota: A key orchestrator of cancer therapy. *Nat. Rev. Cancer* **2017**, *5*, 271–285. [CrossRef] [PubMed]
14. Routy, B.; Le Chatelier, E.; Derosa, L.; Duong, C.P.M.; Alou, M.T.; Daillère, R.; Fluckiger, A.; Messaoudene, M.; Rauber, C.; Roberti, M.P.; et al. Gut microbiome influences efficacy of PD-1-based immunotherapy against epithelial tumors. *Science* **2018**, *359*, 91–97. [CrossRef] [PubMed]
15. Vétizou, M.; Pitt, J.M.; Daillère, R.; Lepage, P.; Waldschmitt, N.; Flament, C.; Rusakiewicz, S.; Routy, B.; Roberti, M.P.; Duong, C.P.; et al. Anticancer immunotherapy by CTLA-4 blockade relies on the gut microbiota. *Science* **2015**, *350*, 1079–1084. [CrossRef] [PubMed]
16. Pitt, J.M.; Vétizou, M.; Gomperts, B.I.; Lepage, P.; Chamaillard, M.; Zitvogel, L. Enhancing the clinical coverage and anticancer efficacy of immune checkpoint blockade through manipulation of the gut microbiota. *Oncoimmunology* **2016**, *6*, e1132137. [CrossRef] [PubMed]
17. Dubin, K.; Callahan, M.K.; Ren, B.; Khanin, R.; Viale, A.; Ling, L.; No, D.; Gobourne, A.; Littmann, E.; Huttenhower, C.; et al. Intestinal microbiome analyses identify melanoma patients at risk for checkpoint-blockade-induced colitis. *Nat Commun.* **2016**, *7*, e10391. [CrossRef] [PubMed]
18. Sivan, A.; Corrales, L.; Hubert, N.; Williams, J.B.; Aquino-Michaels, K.; Earley, Z.M.; Benyamin, F.W.; Lei, Y.M.; Jabri, B.; Alegre, M.L.; et al. Commensal Bifidobacterium promotes antitumor immunity and facilitates anti-PD-L1 efficacy. *Science* **2015**, *350*, 1084–1089. [CrossRef]
19. Chaput, N.; Lepage, P.; Coutzac, C.; Soularue, E.; Le Roux, K.; Monot, C.; Boselli, L.; Routier, E.; Cassard, L.; Collins, M.; et al. Baseline gut micro biota predicts clinical response and colitis in metastatic melanoma patients treated with ipilimumab. *Ann. Oncol.* **2017**, *28*, 1368–1379. [CrossRef] [PubMed]
20. Frankel, A.E.; Coughlin, L.A.; Kim, J.; Froehlich, T.W.; Xie, Y.; Frenkel, E.P.; Koh, A.Y. Metagenomic Shotgun Sequencing and Unbiased Metabolomic Profiling Identify Specific Human Gut Microbiota and Metabolites Associated with Immune Checkpoint Therapy Efficacy in Melanoma Patients. *Neoplasia* **2017**, *19*, 848–855. [CrossRef] [PubMed]
21. Gopalakrishnan, V.; Spencer, C.N.; Nezi, L.; Reuben, A.; Andrews, M.C.; Karpinets, T.V.; Prieto, P.A.; Vicente, D.; Hoffman, K.; Wei, S.C.; et al. Gut microbiome modulates response to anti-PD-1 immunotherapy in melanoma patients. *Science* **2018**, *359*, 97–103. [CrossRef] [PubMed]
22. Matson, V.; Fessler, J.; Bao, R.; Chongsuwat, T.; Zha, Y.; Alegre, M.L.; Luke, J.J.; Gajewski, T.F. The commensal microbiome is associated with anti-PD-1 efficacy in metastatic melanoma patients. *Science* **2018**, *359*, 104–108. [CrossRef]
23. Emens, L.A.; Middleton, G. The interplay of immunotherapy and chemotherapy: Harnessing potential synergies. *Cancer Immunol. Res.* **2015**, *5*, 436–443. [CrossRef] [PubMed]
24. Pfirschke, C.; Engblom, C.; Rickelt, S.; Cortez-Retamozo, V.; Garris, C.; Pucci, F.; Yamazaki, T.; Poirier-Colame, V.; Newton, A.; Redouane, Y.; et al. Immunogenic Chemotherapy Sensitizes Tumors to Checkpoint Blockade Therapy. *Immunity* **2016**, *44*, 343–354. [CrossRef] [PubMed]
25. Song, W.; Shen, L.; Wang, Y.; Liu, Q.; Goodwin, T.J.; Li, J.; Dorosheva, O.; Liu, T.; Liu, R.; Huang, L. Synergistic and low adverse effect cancer immunotherapy by immunogenic chemotherapy and locally expressed PD-L1 trap. *Nat. Commun.* **2018**, *9*, 2237. [CrossRef]
26. Mkrtichyan, M.; Najjar, Y.G.; Raulfs, E.C.; Abdalla, M.Y.; Samara, R.; Rotem-Yehudar, R.; Cook, L.; Khleif, S.N. Anti-PD-1 synergizes with cyclophosphamide to induce potent anti-tumor vaccine effects through novel mechanisms. *Eur. J. Immunol.* **2011**, *41*, 2977–2986. [CrossRef]

27. Merlano, M.C.; Merlotti, A.M.; Licitra, L.; Denaro, N.; Fea, E.; Galizia, D.; Di Maio, M.; Fruttero, C.; Curcio, P.; Vecchio, S.; et al. Activation of immune responses in patients with relapsed-metastatic head and neck cancer (CONFRONT phase I-II trial): Multimodality immunotherapy with avelumab, short-course radiotherapy, and cyclophosphamide. *Clin. Transl. Radiat. Oncol.* **2018**, *12*, 47–52. [CrossRef]
28. Cui, S. Immunogenic Chemotherapy Sensitizes Renal Cancer to Immune Checkpoint Blockade Therapy in Preclinical Models. *Med. Sci. Monit.* **2017**, *23*, 3360–3366. [CrossRef]
29. VanDer Kraak, L.; Goel, G.; Ramanan, K.; Kaltenmeier, C.; Zhang, L.; Normolle, D.P.; Freeman, G.J.; Tang, D.; Nason, K.S.; Davison, J.M.; et al. 5-Fluorouracil upregulates cell surface B7-H1 (PD-L1) expression in gastrointestinal cancers. *J. Immunother. Cancer* **2016**, *4*, 65. [CrossRef]
30. Guo, Z.; Wang, H.; Meng, F.; Li, J.; Zhang, S. Combined Trabectedin and anti-PD1 antibody produces a synergistic antitumor effect in a murine modelofovarian cancer. *J. Transl. Med.* **2015**, *13*, 247. [CrossRef]
31. Peng, J.; Hamanishi, J.; Matsumura, N.; Abiko, K.; Murat, K.; Baba, T.; Yamaguchi, K.; Horikawa, N.; Hosoe, Y.; Murphy, S.K.; et al. Chemotherapy Induces Programmed Cell Death-Ligand 1 Overexpression via the Nuclear Factor-κB to Foster an Immunosuppressive Tumor Microenvironment in OvarianCancer. *Cancer Res.* **2015**, *75*, 5034–5045. [CrossRef]
32. Mesnage, S.J.L.; Auguste, A.; Genestie, C.; Dunant, A.; Pain, E.; Drusch, F.; Gouy, S.; Morice, P.; Bentivegna, E.; Lhomme, C.; et al. Neoadjuvant chemotherapy (NACT) increases immune infiltration and programmed death-ligand 1 (PD-L1) expression in epithelialovariancancer (EOC). *Ann. Oncol.* **2017**, *28*, 651–657. [CrossRef]
33. Kok, M.; Voorwerk, L.; Horlings, H.; Sikorska, K.; van der Vijver, K.; Slagter, M.; Warren, S.; Ong, S.; Wiersma, T.; Russell, N.; et al. Adaptive phase II randomized trial of nivolumab after induction treatment in triple negative breast cancer (TONIC trial): Final response data stage I and first translational data. *J. Clin. Oncol.* **2018**, *36*, 1012. [CrossRef]
34. Loibl, S.; Untch, M.; Burchardi, N.; Huober, J.B.; Blohmer, J.U.; Grischke, E.M.; Furlanetto, J.; Tesch, H.; Hanusch, C.; Rezai, M.; et al. Randomized phase II neoadjuvant study (GeparNuevo) to investigate the addition of durvalumab to a taxane-anthracycline containing chemotherapy in triple negative breast cancer (TNBC). *J. Clin. Oncol.* **2018**, *36*, 104. [CrossRef]
35. NCT03585465: Nivolumab in Combination with Metronomic Chemotherapy in Paediatrics Refractory/Relapsing Solid Tumors or Lymphoma. Available online: https://clinicaltrials.gov/ct2/show/NCT03585465 (accessed on 30 October 2018).
36. NCT03683407: Effect of Chemotherapy on TMB in NSCLC. Available online: https://clinicaltrials.gov/ct2/show/NCT03683407 (accessed on 30 October 2018).
37. Lanitis, E.; Irving, M.; Coukos, G. Targeting the tumor vasculature to enhance T cell activity. *Curr. Opin. Immunol.* **2015**, *33*, 55–63. [CrossRef] [PubMed]
38. Stockmann, C.; Schadendorf, D.; Klose, R.; Helfrich, I. The impact of the immune system on tumor: Angiogenesis and vascular remodeling. *Front. Oncol.* **2014**, *4*, e69. [CrossRef] [PubMed]
39. Nuti, M.; Zizzari, I.G.; Botticelli, A.; Rughetti, A.; Marchetti, P. The ambitious role of anti angiogenesis molecules: Turning a cold tumor into a hot one. *Cancer Treat. Rev.* **2018**, *70*, 41–46. [CrossRef] [PubMed]
40. Hodi, F.S.; Lawrence, D.; Lezcano, C.; Wu, X.; Zhou, J.; Sasada, T.; Zeng, W.; Giobbie-Hurder, A.; Atkins, M.B.; Ibrahim, N.; et al. Bevacizumab plus ipilimumab in patients with metastatic melanoma. *Cancer Immunol. Res.* **2014**, *2*, 632–642. [CrossRef] [PubMed]
41. Ozaki, Y.; Matsumoto, K.; Takahashi, M.; Mukohara, T.; Futamura, M.; Masuda, N.; Tsurutani, J.; Yoshimura, K.; Minami, H.; Takano, T. Phase II study of a combination therapy of nivolumab, bevacizumab and paclitaxel in patients with HER2-negative metastatic breast cancer as a first-line treatment (WJOG9917B, NEWBEAT trial). *J. Clin. Oncol.* **2018**, *36*, TPS1110. [CrossRef]
42. Liu, J.F.; Herold, C.; Luo, W.; Penson, R.; Horowitz, N.; Konstantinopoulos, P.; Castro, C.; Curtis, J.; Matulonis, U.A.; Cannistra, S.; et al. A phase 2 trial of combination nivolumab and bevacizumab in recurrent ovarian cancer. *Ann. Oncol.* **2018**, *29*, viii332–viii358. [CrossRef]
43. Rizvi, N.A.; Antonia, S.J.; Shepherd, F.A.; Chow, L.Q.; Goldman, J.; Shen, Y.; Chen, A.C.; Gettinger, S. Nivolumab (Anti-PD-1; BMS-936558, ONO-4538) Maintenance as Monotherapy or in Combination With Bevacizumab (BEV) for Non-Small Cell Lung Cancer (NSCLC) Previously Treated With Chemotherapy. *Int. J. Radiat. Oncol. Biol. Phys.* **2014**, *90*, S32. [CrossRef]

44. Motzer, R.J.; Powles, T.; Atkins, M.B.; Escudier, B.; McDermott, D.F.; Suarez, C.; Bracarda, S.; Stadler, W.M.; Donskov, F.; Lee, J.L.; et al. IMmotion151: A Randomized Phase III Study of Atezolizumab Plus Bevacizumab vs. Sunitinib in Untreated Metastatic Renal Cell Carcinoma (mRCC). *J. Clin. Oncol.* **2018**, *36*, 578. [CrossRef]
45. NCT024243324: A Study of Ramucirumab Plus Pembrolizumab in Participants with Gastric or GEJ Adenocarcinoma, NSCLC, Transitional Cell Carcinoma of the Urothelium, or Biliary Tract Cancer. Available online: https://clinicaltrials.gov/ct2/show/NCT02443324 (accessed on 30 October 2018).
46. Chau, I.; Penel, N.; Arkenau, H.T.; Santana-Davila, R.; Calvo, E.; Soriano, A.O.; Mi, G.; Jin, J.; Ferry, D.; Herbst, R.S.; et al. Safety and antitumor activity of ramucirumab plus pembrolizumab in treatment naïve advanced gastric or gastroesophageal junction (G/GEJ) adenocarcinoma: Preliminary results from a multi-disease phase I study (JVDF). *J. Clin. Oncol.* **2018**, *36*, 101. [CrossRef]
47. Amin, A.; Plimack, E.R.; Ernstoff, M.S.; Lewis, L.D.; Bauer, T.M.; McDermott, D.F.; Carducci, M.; Kollmannsberger, C.; Rini, B.I.; Heng, D.Y.C.; et al. Safety and efficacy of nivolumab in combination with sunitinib or pazopanib in advanced or metastatic renal cell carcinoma: The CheckMate 016 study. *J. Immunother. Cancer* **2018**, *6*, 109. [CrossRef] [PubMed]
48. Yu, X.; Harden, K.; Gonzalez, L.C.; Francesco, M.; Chiang, E.; Irving, B.; Tom, I.; Ivelja, S.; Refino, C.J.; Clark, H.; et al. The surface protein TIGIT suppresses T cell activation by promoting the generation of mature immunoregulatory dendritic cells. *Nat. Immunol.* **2009**, *10*, 48–57. [CrossRef]
49. Mahoney, K.M.; Rennert, P.D.; Freeman, G.J. Combination cancer immunotherapyand new immunomodulatory targets. *Nat. Rev. Drug Discov.* **2015**, *14*, 561–584. [CrossRef] [PubMed]
50. Hung, A.L.; Maxwell, R.; Theodros, D.; Belcaid, Z.; Mathios, D.; Luksik, A.S.; Kim, E.; Wu, A.; Xia, Y.; Garzon-Muvdi, T.; et al. TIGITand PD-1 dual checkpoint blockade enhances antitumor immunity and survival in GBM. *Oncoimmunology* **2018**, *7*, e1466769. [CrossRef] [PubMed]
51. NCT03563716: A Study of MTIG7192A in Combination withAtezolizumab in Chemotherapy-Naïve Patients with Locally Advanced or Metastatic Non-Small Cell Lung Cancer. Available online: https://clinicaltrials.gov/ct2/show/NCT03563716 (accessed on 30 October 2018).
52. Melero, I.; Berman, D.M.; Aznar, M.A.; Korman, A.J.; Perez Gracia, J.L.; Haanen, J. Evolving synergistic combinations of targeted immunotherapies to combat cancer. *Nat. Rev. Cancer* **2015**, *15*, 457–472. [CrossRef]
53. Woo, S.R.; Turnis, M.E.; Goldberg, M.V.; Bankoti, J.; Selby, M.; Nirschl, C.J.; Bettini, M.L.; Gravano, D.M.; Vogel, P.; Liu, C.L.; et al. Immune inhibitory molecules LAG-3 and PD-1 synergistically regulate T-cell function to promote tumoral immune escape. *Cancer Res.* **2012**, *72*, 917–927. [CrossRef]
54. Ascierto, P.A.; Bono, P.; Bhatia, S.; Melero, I.; Nyakas, M.S.; Svane, I.; Callahan, M.K.; Gajewski, T.; Gomez-Roca, C.A.; Hodi, F.S.; et al. Initial efficacy of anti-lymphocyte activation gene-3 (anti–LAG-3; BMS-986016) in combination with nivolumab (nivo) in pts with melanoma (MEL) previously treated with anti–PD-1/PD-L1 therapy. *J. Clin. Oncol.* **2017**, *35*, 9520. [CrossRef]
55. Hong, D.S.; Schoffski, P.; Calvo, A.; Sarantopoulos, J.; De Olza, M.O.; Carvajal, R.D.; Prawira, A.; Kyi, C.; Esaki, T.; Akerley, W.L.; et al. Phase I/II study of LAG525 ± spartalizumab (PDR001) in patients (pts) with advanced malignancies. *J. Clin. Oncol.* **2018**, *36*, 3012. [CrossRef]
56. Anderson, A.C.; Joller, N.; Kuchroo, V.K. Lag-3, Tim-3, and TIGIT: Co-inhibitory receptors with specialized functions in immune regulation. *Immunity* **2016**, *44*, 989–1004. [CrossRef] [PubMed]
57. NCT02817633: A Phase 1 Study of TSR-022, an Anti-TIM-3 Monoclonal Antibody, in Patients with Advanced Solid Tumors (AMBER). Available online: https://clinicaltrials.gov/ct2/show/NCT02817633 (accessed on 30 October 2018).
58. Ribas, A.; Dummer, R.; Puzanov, I.; VanderWalde, A.; Andtbacka, R.H.I.; Michielin, O.; Olszanski, A.J.; Malvehy, J.; Cebon, J.; Fernandez, E.; et al. Oncolytic Virotherapy Promotes Intratumoral T Cell Infiltration and Improves Anti-PD-1 Immunotherapy. *Cell* **2017**, *170*, 1109. [CrossRef] [PubMed]
59. La Rocca, C.J.; Warner, S.G. Oncolytic viruses and checkpoint inhibitors: Combination therapy in clinical trials. *Clin. Transl. Med.* **2018**, *7*, 35. [CrossRef]
60. Chesney, J.; Puzanov, I.; Collichio, F.; Singh, P.; Milhem, M.M.; Glaspy, J.; Hamid, O.; Ross, M.; Friedlander, P.; Garbe, C.; et al. Randomized, Open-Label Phase II Study Evaluating the Efficacy and Safety of TalimogeneLaherparepvec in Combination With Ipilimumab Versus Ipilimumab Alone in Patients With Advanced, Unresectable Melanoma. *J. Clin. Oncol.* **2018**, *36*, 1658–1667. [CrossRef]

61. NCT02263508: Pembrolizumab with or without TalimogeneLaherparepvec or TalimogeneLaherparepvec Placebo in Unresected Melanoma (KEYNOTE-034). Available online: https://clinicaltrials.gov/ct2/show/NCT02263508 (accessed on 30 October 2018).
62. Andtbacka, R.H.I.; Ross, M.I.; Agarwala, S.S.; Taylor, M.H.; Vetto, J.T.; Neves, R.I.; Daud, A.; Khong, H.T.; Ungerleider, R.S.; Tanaka, M.; et al. Final results of a phase II multicenter trial of HF10, a replication-competent HSV-1 oncolytic virus, and ipilimumab combination treatment in patients with stage IIIB-IV unresectable or metastatic melanoma. *J. Clin. Oncol.* **2017**, *35*, 9510. [CrossRef]
63. NCT02798406: Combination Adenovirus + Pembrolizumab to Trigger Immune Virus Effects (CAPTIVE). Available online: https://clinicaltrials.gov/ct2/show/NCT02798406 (accessed on 30 October 2018).
64. Haddad, D. Genetically Engineered Vaccinia Viruses As Agents for Cancer Treatment, Imaging, and Transgene Delivery. *Front. Oncol.* **2017**, *7*, 96. [CrossRef] [PubMed]
65. Anthoney, A.; Samson, A.; West, E.; Turnbull, S.J.; Scott, K.; Tidswell, E.; Kingston, J.; Johnpulle, M.; Noutch, S.; Bendjama, K.; et al. Single intravenous preoperative administration of the oncolytic virus Pexa-Vec to prime anti-tumor immunity. *J. Clin. Oncol.* **2018**, *36*, 3092. [CrossRef]
66. NCT03206073: A Phase I/II Study of Pexa-Vec Oncolytic Virus in Combination with Immune Checkpoint Inhibition in Refractory Colorectal Cancer. Available online: https://clinicaltrials.gov/ct2/show/NCT03206073 (accessed on 30 October 2018).
67. NCT02977156: Immunization Strategy with Intra-tumoral Injections of Pexa-Vec With Ipilimumab in Metastatic/Advanced Solid Tumors. (ISI-JX). Available online: https://clinicaltrials.gov/ct2/show/NCT02977156 (accessed on 30 October 2018).
68. NCT02307149: Intratumoral CAVATAK (CVA21) and Ipilimumab in Patients with Advanced Melanoma (VLA-013 MITCI) (MITCI). Available online: https://clinicaltrials.gov/ct2/show/NCT02307149 (accessed on 30 October 2018).
69. Silk, A.W.; Kaufman, H.; Gabrail, N.; Mehnert, J.; Bryan, J.; Norrell, J.; Medina, D.; Bommareddy, P.; Shafren, D.; Grose, M.; et al. Phase 1b study of intratumoralCoxsackievirus A21 (CVA 21) and systemic pembrolizumab in a dvanced melanoma patients: Interim results of the CAPRA clinical trial. *Cancer Res.* **2017**, *77*, CT026. [CrossRef]
70. Mahalingam, D.; Fountzilas, C.; Moseley, J.L.; Noronha, N.; Cheetham, K.; Dzugalo, A.; Nuovo, G.; Gutierrez, A.; Arora, S.P.; et al. A study of REOLYSIN in combination with pembrolizumab and chemotherapy in patients (pts) with relapsed metastatic adenocarcinoma of the pancreas (MAP). *J. Clin. Oncol.* **2017**, *35*, e15753. [CrossRef]
71. NCT02620423: Study of Pembrolizumab with REOLYSIN® and Chemotherapy in Patients with Advanced Pancreatic Adenocarcinoma. Available online: https://clinicaltrials.gov/ct2/show/NCT02620423 (accessed on 30 October 2018).
72. Frederick, D.T.; Piris, A.; Cogdill, A.P.; Cooper, Z.A.; Lezcano, C.; Ferrone, C.R.; Mitra, D.; Boni, A.; Newton, L.P.; Liu, C.; et al. BRAF inhibition is associated with enhanced melanoma antigen expression and a more favorable tumor microenvironment in patients with metastatic melanoma. *Clin. Cancer Res.* **2013**, *19*, 1225–1231. [CrossRef]
73. Comin-Anduix, B.; Chodon, T.; Sazegar, H.; Matsunaga, D.; Mock, S.; Jalil, J.; Escuin-Ordinas, H.; Chmielowski, B.; Koya, R.C.; Ribas, A.; et al. The oncogenic BRAF kinase inhibitor PLX4032/RG7204 does not affect the viability or function of human lymphocytes across a wide range of concentrations. *Clin. Cancer Res.* **2010**, *16*, 6040–6048. [CrossRef] [PubMed]
74. Wilmott, J.S.; Long, G.V.; Howle, J.R.; Haydu, L.E.; Sharma, R.N.; Thompson, J.F.; Kefford, R.F.; Hersey, P.; Scolyer, R.A. Selective BRAF inhibitors induce marked T-cell infiltration into human metastatic melanoma. *Clin. Cancer Res.* **2012**, *18*, 1386–1394. [CrossRef] [PubMed]
75. Bradley, S.D.; Chen, Z.; Melendez, B.; Talukder, A.; Khalili, J.S.; Rodriguez-Cruz, T.; Liu, S.; Whittington, M.; Deng, W.; Li, F.; et al. BRAFV600E co-opts a conserved MHC class I internalization pathway to diminish antigen presentation and CD8+ T-cell recognition of melanoma. *Cancer Immunol. Res.* **2015**, *3*, 602–609. [CrossRef]
76. Koya, R.C.; Mok, S.; Otte, N.; Blacketor, K.J.; Comin-Anduix, B.; Tumeh, P.C.; Minasyan, A.; Graham, N.A.; Graeber, T.G.; Chodon, T.; et al. BRAF inhibitor vemurafenib improves the antitumor activity of adoptive cell immunotherapy. *Cancer Res.* **2012**, *72*, 3928–3937. [CrossRef]

77. Knight, D.A.; Ngiow, S.F.; Li, M.; Parmenter, T.; Mok, S.; Cass, A.; Haynes, N.M.; Kinross, K.; Yagita, H.; Koya, R.C.; et al. Host immunity contributes to the anti-melanoma activity of BRAF inhibitors. *J. Clin. Investig.* **2016**, *126*, 402–403. [CrossRef]
78. Hooijkaas, A.; Gadiot, J.; Morrow, M.; Stewart, R.; Schumacher, T.; Blank, C.U. Selective BRAF inhibition decreases tumor-resident lymphocyte frequencies in a mouse model of human melanoma. *Oncoimmunology* **2012**, *1*, 609–617. [CrossRef]
79. Cooper, Z.A.; Juneja, V.R.; Sage, P.T.; Frederick, D.T.; Piris, A.; Mitra, D.; Lo, J.A.; Hodi, F.S.; Freeman, G.J.; Bosenberg, M.W.; et al. Response to BRAF inhibition in melanoma is enhanced when combined with immune checkpoint blockade. *Cancer Immunol. Res.* **2014**, *2*, 643–654. [CrossRef]
80. Hu-Lieskovan, S.; Mok, S.; Moreno, B.H.; Tsoi, J.; Faja, L.R.; Goedert, L.; Pinheiro, E.M.; Koya, R.C.; Graeber, T.G.; Comin-Anduix, B.; et al. Improved antitumor activity of immunotherapy with BRAF and MEK inhibitors in BRAFV600E melanoma. *Sci. Transl. Med.* **2015**, *7*, 279ra41. [CrossRef]
81. Ribas, A.; Hodi, F.S.; Callahan, M.; Konto, C.; Wolchok, J. Hepatotoxicity with combination of vemurafenib and ipilimumab. *N. Engl. J. Med.* **2013**, *368*, 1365–1366. [CrossRef]
82. Minor, D.R.; Puzanov, I.; Callahan, M.K.; Hug, B.A.; Hoos, A. Severe gastrointestinal toxicity with administration of trametinib in combination with dabrafenib and ipilimumab. *Pigment Cell Melanoma Res.* **2015**, *28*, 611–612. [CrossRef] [PubMed]
83. Puzanov, I.; Callahan, M.; Gerald, P.; Linette, G.; Luke, J.J.; Sosmanet, J.A.; Wolchok, J.D.; Hamid, O.; Minor, D.R.; Orford, K.W.; et al. Phase 1 study of the BRAF inhibitor dabrafenib (D) with or without the MEK inhibitor trametinib (T) in combination with ipilimumab (Ipi) for V600E/K mutation–positive unresectable or metastatic melanoma (MM). *J. Clin. Oncol.* **2014**, *32*, 2511. [CrossRef]
84. NCT01656642: A Phase 1b Study of Atezolizumab in Combination with BRAFV600-Mutation Positive Metastatic Melanoma. Available online: https://clinicaltrials.gov/ct2/show/NCT01656642 (accessed on 30 October 2018).
85. Ribas, A.; Hodi, F.; Lawrence, D.; Atkinson, V.; Starodub, A.; Carlino, M.S.; Fisher, R.A.; Long, G.V.; Miller, W.H.; Huang, Y.; et al. Pembrolizumab (pembro) in combination with dabrafenib (D) and trametinib (T) for BRAF-mutant advanced melanoma: Phase 1 KEYNOTE-022 study. *J. Clin. Oncol.* **2016**, *34*, 3014. [CrossRef]
86. Sullivan, R.J.; Gonzalez, R.; Lewis, K.D.; Hamid, O.; Infante, J.R.; Patel, M.R.; Hodi, F.S.; Wallin, J.; Pitcher, B.; Cha, E.; et al. Atezolizumab (A) + cobimetinib (C) + vemurafenib (V) in BRAFV600-mutant metastatic melanoma (mel): Updated safety and clinical activity. *J. Clin. Oncol.* **2017**, *35*, 3063. [CrossRef]
87. Larmonier, N.; Janikashvili, N.; La Casse, C.J.; Larmonier, C.B.; Cantrell, J.; Situ, E.; Lundeen, T.; Bonnotte, B.; Katsanis, E. Imatinib mesylate inhibits CD4+ CD25+ regulatory T cell activity and enhances active immunotherapy against BCR-ABL-tumors. *J. Immunol.* **2008**, *181*, 6955–6963. [CrossRef] [PubMed]
88. Ménard, C.; Blay, J.Y.; Borg, C.; Michiels, S.; Ghiringhelli, F.; Robert, C.; Nonn, C.; Chaput, N.; Taïeb, J.; Delahaye, N.F.; et al. Natural killer cell IFN-gamma levels predict long-term survival with imatinib mesylate therapy in gastrointestinal stromal tumor-bearing patients. *Cancer Res.* **2009**, *69*, 3563–3569. [CrossRef] [PubMed]
89. Balachandran, V.P.; Cavnar, M.J.; Zeng, S.; Bamboat, Z.M.; Ocuin, L.M.; Obaid, H.; Sorenson, E.C.; Popow, R.; Ariyan, C.; Rossi, F.; et al. Imatinib potentiates antitumor T cell responses in gastrointestinal stromal tumor through the inhibition of Ido. *Nat. Med.* **2011**, *17*, 1094–1100. [CrossRef] [PubMed]
90. Seifert, A.M.; Zeng, S.; Zhang, J.Q.; Kim, T.S.; Cohen, N.A.; Beckman, M.J.; Medina, B.D.; Maltbaek, J.H.; Loo, J.K.; Crawley, M.H.; et al. PD-1/PD-L1 Blockade Enhances T-cell Activity and Antitumor Efficacy of Imatinib in Gastrointestinal Stromal Tumors. *Clin. Cancer Res.* **2017**, *23*, 454–465. [CrossRef]
91. NCT01738139: Ipilimumab and Imatinib Mesylate in Treating Participants with Metastatic or Unresectable Solid Tumors. Available online: https://clinicaltrials.gov/ct2/show/NCT01738139 (accessed on 30 October 2018).
92. Reilley, M.J.; Bailey, A.; Subbiah, V.; Janku, F.; Naing, A.; Falchook, G.; Karp, D.; Piha-Paul, S.; Tsimberidou, A.; Fu, S.; et al. Phase I clinical trial of combination imatinib and ipilimumab in patients with advanced malignancies. *J. Immunother. Cancer* **2017**, *5*, 35. [CrossRef]
93. Cash, H.; Shay, S.; Moree, E.; Cariso, A.; Uppaluri, R.; Van Waes, C.; Allen, C. mTOR and MEK1/2 inhibition differentially modulate tumor growth and the immune microenvironment in syngeneic models of oral cavity cancer. *Onco. Target* **2015**, *6*, 36400–36417. [CrossRef]

94. Moore, E.C.; Cash, H.A.; Caruso, A.M.; Uppaluri, R.; Hodge, J.W.; Van Waes, C.; Allen, C.T. Enhanced tumor control with combination mTOR and PD-L1 inhibition in syngeneic oral cavity cancers. *Cancer Immunol. Res.* **2016**, *4*, 611–620. [CrossRef]
95. Goel, S.; De Cristo, M.J.; Watt, A.C.; Brin Jones, H.; Sceneay, J.; Li, B.B.; Khan, N.; Ubellacker, J.M.; Xie, S.; Metzger-Filho, O.; et al. CDK4/6 inhibition triggers anti-tumour immunity. *Nature* **2017**, *548*, 471–475. [CrossRef]
96. Zhang, J.; Bu, X.; Wang, H.; Zhu, Y.; Geng, Y.; Nihira, N.T.; Tan, Y.; Ci, Y.; Wu, F.; Dai, X.; et al. Cyclin D-CDK4 kinase destabilizes PD-L1 via cullin 3-SPOP to control cancer immune surveillance. *Nature* **2018**, *553*, 91–95. [CrossRef]
97. Teo, Z.L.; Versaci, S.; Dushyanthen, S.; Caramia, F.; Savas, P.; Mintoff, C.P.; Zethoven, M.; Virassamy, B.; Luen, S.J.; McArthur, G.A.; et al. Combined CDK4/6 and PI3Kα Inhibition Is Synergistic and Immunogenic in Triple-Negative Breast Cancer. *Cancer Res.* **2017**, *77*, 6340–6352. [CrossRef]
98. NCT02130466: A Study of the Safety and Efficacy of Pembrolizumab (MK-3475) in Combination with Trametinib and Dabrafenib in Participants with Advanced Melanoma (MK-3475-022/KEYNOTE-022). Available online: https://clinicaltrials.gov/ct2/show/NCT02130466 (accessed on 30 October 2018).
99. Nanda, V.G.Y.; Peng, W.; Hwu, P.; Davies, M.A.; Ciliberto, G.; Fattore, L.; Malpicci, D.; Aurisicchio, L.; Ascierto, P.A.; Croce, C.M.; et al. Melanoma and immunotherapy bridge 2015. Naples, Italy. 1–5 December 2015. *J. Transl. Med.* **2016**, *14* (Suppl. 1), 65. [CrossRef] [PubMed]
100. Borg, C.; Terme, M.; Taïeb, J.; Ménard, C.; Flament, C.; Robert, C.; Maruyama, K.; Wakasugi, H.; Angevin, E.; Thielemans, K.; et al. Novel mode of action of c-kit tyrosine kinase inhibitors leading to NK cell-dependent antitumor effects. *J. Clin.Investig.* **2004**, *114*, 379–388. [CrossRef] [PubMed]
101. Van Dongen, M.; Savage, N.D.; Jordanova, E.S.; Briaire-de Bruijn, I.H.; Walburg, K.V.; Ottenhoff, T.H.; Hogendoorn, P.C.; van der Burg, S.H.; Gelderblom, H.; van Hall, T. Anti-inflammatory M2 type macrophages characterize metastasized and tyrosine kinase inhibitor-treated gastrointestinal stromal tumors. *Int. J. Cancer* **2010**, *127*, 899–909. [CrossRef]
102. Loukinova, E.; Dong, G.; Enamorado-Ayalya, I.; Thomas, G.R.; Chen, Z.; Schreiber, H.; VanWaes, C. Growth regulated oncogene-alpha expression by murine squamous cell carcinoma promotes tumor growth, metastasis, leukocyte infiltration and angiogenesis by a host CXC receptor-2 dependent mechanism. *Oncogene* **2000**, *19*, 3477–3486. [CrossRef] [PubMed]
103. Moslehi, J.J.; Salem, J.E.; Sosman, J.A.; Lebrun-Vignes, B.; Johnson, D.B. Increased reporting of fatal immune checkpoint inhibitor-associated myocarditis. *Lancet* **2018**, *391*, 933. [CrossRef]
104. Tajiri, K.; Ieda, M. Cardiac Complications in Immune Checkpoint Inhibition Therapy. *Front. Cardiovasc. Med.* **2019**, *6*, 3. [CrossRef] [PubMed]

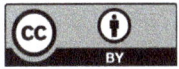

© 2019 by the authors. Licensee MDPI, Basel, Switzerland. This article is an open access article distributed under the terms and conditions of the Creative Commons Attribution (CC BY) license (http://creativecommons.org/licenses/by/4.0/).

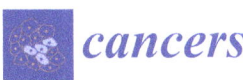

Review

Damage-Associated Molecular Patterns Modulation by microRNA: Relevance on Immunogenic Cell Death and Cancer Treatment Outcome

María Julia Lamberti [1,2,*], Annunziata Nigro [2], Vincenzo Casolaro [2], Natalia Belén Rumie Vittar [1] and Jessica Dal Col [2,*]

[1] INBIAS, CONICET-UNRC, Río Cuarto, Córdoba 5800, Argentina; nrumievittar@exa.unrc.edu.ar
[2] Department of Medicine, Surgery and Dentistry 'Scuola Medica Salernitana', University of Salerno, Baronissi, 84081 Salerno, Italy; annnigro@unisa.it (A.N.); vcasolaro@unisa.it (V.C.)
* Correspondence: mlamberti@exa.unrc.edu.ar (M.J.L.); jdalcol@unisa.it (J.D.C.)

Citation: Lamberti, M.J.; Nigro, A.; Casolaro, V.; Rumie Vittar, N.B.; Dal Col, J. Damage-Associated Molecular Patterns Modulation by microRNA: Relevance on Immunogenic Cell Death and Cancer Treatment Outcome. *Cancers* 2021, *13*, 2566. https://doi.org/10.3390/cancers13112566

Academic Editor: Vita Golubovskaya

Received: 1 April 2021
Accepted: 18 May 2021
Published: 24 May 2021

Publisher's Note: MDPI stays neutral with regard to jurisdictional claims in published maps and institutional affiliations.

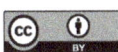

Copyright: © 2021 by the authors. Licensee MDPI, Basel, Switzerland. This article is an open access article distributed under the terms and conditions of the Creative Commons Attribution (CC BY) license (https://creativecommons.org/licenses/by/4.0/).

Simple Summary: Inside the cell, damage-associated molecular pattern molecules (DAMPs) play several physiological functions, but when they are released or translocated to the extracellular space, they gain additional immunogenic roles. Thus, DAMPs are considered key hallmarks of immunogenic cell death (ICD) in cancer, a functionally unique regulated form of stress-mediated cell death that activates the immune system response against tumor cells. Several epigenetic modulators of DAMPs have been reported. In this review, we aimed to provide an overview of the effects of microRNAs (miRNAs) on the expression of DAMPs and the putative link between miRNA, DAMPs, and cell death, focused on ICD. Overall, we propose that miRNAs, by targeting DAMPs, play critical roles in the regulation of both cell death and immune-associated mechanisms in cancer, while evidence of their potential involvement in ICD is limited. Finally, we discuss emerging data regarding the impact of miRNAs' modulation on cancer treatment outcome.

Abstract: Immunogenic cell death (ICD) in cancer is a functionally unique regulated form of stress-mediated cell death that activates both the innate and adaptive immune response against tumor cells. ICD makes dying cancer cells immunogenic by improving both antigenicity and adjuvanticity. The latter relies on the spatiotemporally coordinated release or exposure of danger signals (DAMPs) that drive robust antigen-presenting cell activation. The expression of DAMPs is often constitutive in tumor cells, but it is the initiating stressor, called ICD-inducer, which finally triggers the intracellular response that determines the kinetics and intensity of their release. However, the contribution of cell-autonomous features, such as the epigenetic background, to the development of ICD has not been addressed in sufficient depth. In this context, it has been revealed that several microRNAs (miRNAs), besides acting as tumor promoters or suppressors, can control the ICD-associated exposure of some DAMPs and their basal expression in cancer. Here, we provide a general overview of the dysregulation of cancer-associated miRNAs whose targets are DAMPs, through which new molecular mediators that underlie the immunogenicity of ICD were identified. The current status of miRNA-targeted therapeutics combined with ICD inducers is discussed. A solid comprehension of these processes will provide a framework to evaluate miRNA targets for cancer immunotherapy.

Keywords: miRNA; immunogenic cell death; cancer

1. Introduction

Under physiological homeostasis, cell death involved in the continuous cellular turnover is non-immunogenic or even tolerogenic. This silence mechanism is imperative given that the activation of an immune response against dead cell-associated antigens would have autoimmune-related catastrophic consequences [1]. On the other hand, the death of infected or tumor cells under specific treatment conditions can elicit a robust antigen-specific immune response. This type of death that enhances the immunogenic potential of dying cells has been termed since 2005 as Immunogenic Cell Death (ICD) [2,3]. In the context of cancer therapies, several chemotherapeutics (doxorubicin, cisplatin, oxaliplatin), radiotherapy, oncolytic virus therapy, and photodynamic therapy have been characterized as ICD-inducers [4]. Innate and adaptive immune responses elicited by such anti-cancer agents are now deemed essential for an optimal therapeutic outcome, highlighting the clinical relevance of ICD.

Formerly, ICD was exclusively described in terms of immunogenic extrinsic or intrinsic apoptosis, but recently, with the increasing knowledge of cell death mechanisms, many non-apoptotic cell death processes have been involved in immune activation, including necroptosis, pyroptosis, and ferroptosis [5]. However, ICD cannot be considered only as a cellular death event given its strong dependence on the complex cellular communication between dying and immune cells [6]. In fact, for ICD to be successfully promoted, an exact combination of damage-associated molecular patterns (DAMPs) must be released/exposed in a spatiotemporally coordinated sequence and recognized by immune cells [7]. DAMPs are molecules that exert intracellular physiological functions, but gain additional immunogenic properties when they are exposed to the extracellular environment. Thanks to this peculiarity, DAMPs have been defined as ICD hallmarks. In this context, the immunogenicity of dying tumor cells is dependent on two main factors: antigenicity (conferred by tumor-associated antigens, cancer-testis antigen, and/or neo-epitopes) and adjuvanticity (provided by DAMPs) [8,9]. Accordingly, the inhibition of various processes involved in DAMPs' expression, emission, and sensing could support the neoplastic cell full escape from immune recognition and elimination and potentiate malignant lethal progression.

Interestingly, several epigenetic modulators that suppress or activate genes encoding ICD-associated DAMPs have been discovered. They cause variations in gene expression through chromatin remodeling mechanisms, for example, DNA methylation and histone modification, and the generation of non-coding RNAs (ncRNAs), including long non-coding RNAs (lncRNAs), circular RNAs (circRNAs), and microRNAs (miRNAs) [10].

A recent review from Cruickshank et al. [8] recapitulated the evidence linking epigenetic modifications and ICD. In this review, our efforts are focused on extending that previous work by providing an overview of the current knowledge of miRNAs targeting ICD hallmarks and, thus, their potential involvement in ICD regulation and outcomes. We present a summary of the known miRNAs involved in DAMP modulation within tumors. Finally, we contextualize these findings in the design of novel therapeutic strategies.

Accumulating evidence indicates that several miRNAs can act as oncogenes (here termed oncomiRNAs) or tumor suppressor miRNAs by directly targeting different DAMPs, whose expression is frequently altered across human cancers. These observations lead us to forming the initial hypothesis that reestablishing the normal regulation of DAMP expression would constitute an important and clinically relevant goal to restore immunogenicity and to counteract immune evasion, which often results in the acquisition of chemoresistance and in tumor progression. However, as often happens in biological processes, the same molecules can perform completely different functions depending on the spatiotemporal context and/or the stimuli/insults to which the cell is subjected. Hence, DAMPs can both suppress cell death and promote the immunogenicity of cancer cells, according to tumor microenvironmental conditions. Therefore, we aimed here to provide a comprehensive and exhaustive overview of the effects of miRNAs on the expression of DAMPs, to help identify commonalities and differences that indicate possible interrelationships between miRNA, DAMPs, and cell death, with a special focus on ICD.

2. Immunogenic Cell Death

According to current models, cells undergoing ICD release or expose DAMPs on their surface can function as adjuvants for the innate immune system activation [9]. Most of these molecules have primarily non-immunological roles in the intracellular compartment before their mobilization by ICD. The adequate immunogenic response relies on the ability of specific stimuli to damage cells lethally while inducing the spatiotemporally coordinated emission of those DAMPs [11].

At the very beginning of the well-described ICD sequence, in a pre-apoptotic stage, the endoplasmic reticulum (ER) chaperone calreticulin (CRT) is translocated to the membrane before the cells exhibit phosphatidylserine residues [12]. Ecto-CRT mobilization works as an immunogenic "eat-me" signal for dendritic cells (DCs). This step is essential for an appropriate induction of ICD [12,13]. ICD also involves autophagy for optimal ATP active secretion. This autophagy-dependent release of ATP requires accumulation of ATP in autolysosomes [14]. In the extracellular space, ATP acts as a "find-me" signal for DCs and the consequent activation of the inflammasome to promote the release of the pro-inflammatory cytokine, interleukin (IL)-1β [15,16]. Doxorubicin [17] and PDT-treated cancer cells [18] also upregulate a type I interferon (IFN-1) signaling cascade resulting in C-X-C motif chemokine ligand 10 (CXCL10) secretion and finally in DC maturation. Although they are usually located inside the cells, heat shock proteins 70 and 90 (Hsp70 and Hsp90), under ICD, can be expressed at the surface of the cell membrane or released in the extracellular microenvironment and participate in immune stimulation [11,19]. In the late stages of apoptosis, high-mobility group box 1 (HMGB1) is passively released and binds Toll-Like Receptor 4 (TLR4) on DCs to increase antigen presentation [20].

The main objective of inducing ICD is to overcome the immunosuppressive phenotype of the tumor microenvironment through the restitution of the three signals between DC-T cell interaction, all of them mandatory for immunogenic T cell activation: (a) signal 1: antigen presentation; (b) signal 2: co-stimulation; and (c) signal 3: production of stimulatory cytokines [21]. Along this process, DCs engulf fragments of the stressed/dying cell and incorporate antigenic peptides into MHCs (antigenicity). During antigen presentation, the maturation signals triggered by DAMPs (adjuvanticity) lead to optimal activation of T cells, which finally detect and eliminate cancer cells in a highly precise, antigen-specific fashion [22] (Figure 1).

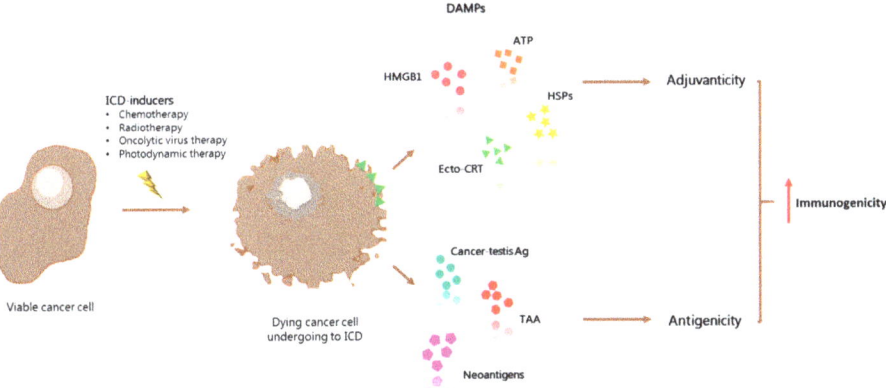

Figure 1. ICD-antitumor effect relies on the enhancement of adjuvanticity and antigenicity of tumor cells. In the tumor microenvironment, immunogenic cell death (ICD) triggered by several ICD-inducers plays a major role in stimulating antitumor immune response. Its lethal action leads to the release of tumor associated antigens (TAAs), cancer testis antigens, and neoantigens, which ultimately increases antigenicity. The concomitant exposure of damage-associated molecular patterns (DAMPs), such as ATP, calreticulin (CRT), HMGB1, and Hsps (Hsp70, Hsp90), confers a robust adjuvanticity to dying cancer cells. Both antigenicity and adjuvanticity enhancement leads to an exacerbated immunogenicity of ICD-undergoing tumor cells.

Linking the immunogenic potential of ICD with an immunotherapy regimen is a promising approach for antitumor treatment. In this sense, we have recently summarized the findings suggesting the use of ICD as a strategy to optimize the current vaccine design for cancer immunotherapy [4,23]. Unfortunately, immunosuppression exerted by the tumor microenvironment limits the potential success of this strategy. In line with these observations, we propose here to identify which immune-activating or immunosuppressive ICD hallmarks are epigenetically targeted by miRNAs.

3. Epigenetic Regulation by miRNA

Over the last years, many studies have been conducted that support the idea that genetic information can be tightly regulated by non-coding RNAs (ncRNAs). ncRNAs do not code for proteins, and can be classified into long non-coding RNAs (lncRNAs), circular RNAs (circRNAs), and microRNAs (miRNAs). Among these ncRNAs, here we focus on post-transcriptional regulation of the expression of ICD molecular mediators by miRNAs.

The main function of miRNAs is to repress protein production, working as post-transcriptional regulators of mRNA. The miRNA biogenesis initiates with the generation of a large primary transcript (pri-miRNA), mainly transcribed by RNA polymerase II, which is 5′ capped and 3′ polyadenylated. The pri-miRNAs are then cleaved into precursor miRNAs (pre-miRNAs) that consist of around 85 nucleotides exhibiting a stem-loop structure. This cleavage is made by a microprocessor complex, composed of the RNA-binding protein DGCR8 and the type III RNase Drosha. Pre-miRNAs are then transported from the nucleus to cytoplasm by the Ran/GTP/Exportin 5 complex, where they are processed by another RNase III enzyme, Dicer, to a 20–22-nucleotide miRNA:miRNA* duplex. The * denotes the passenger strand, which is degraded, while the other complementary strand is the mature or guide strand. The mature/guided miRNA is then incorporated into a protein complex termed RNA-induced silencing complex (RISC) and guides RISC to target mRNA. miRNAs exert their effects by complementary base-pair binding to a short 7–8 nucleotide "seed" region typically located in the 3′ untranslated region (UTR) of the mRNA that they inhibit [24]. Importantly, one miRNA may regulate many targeted genes, while one gene may be targeted by many miRNAs [25].

Nowadays, it is well known that transcriptional control changes, chromosomal abnormalities, epigenetic changes, and defects in the miRNA biogenesis machinery may lead to an aberrant miRNA expression in human cancers. It has been described that this dysregulation affects one or more of the hallmarks of cancer described by Hanahan and Weinberg [26]. Thus, in a cancer context, depending on their target genes and the environmental conditions, miRNAs could function as either oncogenes (termed here oncomiRNAs) or tumor suppressors [27].

Current evidence sheds more light on the functional properties of miRNAs and opens new paradigms that need to be further explored [25]. In this sense, it has been demonstrated that miRNAs can act in different cellular locations (cytoplasm, mitochondrion, nucleus, and exosomes) [28–30] and even bind their targets in different binding sites (5′UTR, coding region, and 3′UTR) [31,32]. Several additional non-canonical binding clusters independent of seed region have been discovered [33]. It has also been reported that, under certain circumstances, instead of repression, miRNAs activate their target expression [34]. Finally, possible interactions have been observed between other ncRNAs and miRNA:mRNA complexes [35].

4. Epigenetic Regulation of ICD-Hallmarks by miRNA

Given their well-known contributions to cell death control [36] and autophagy [37], miRNAs may easily be envisioned to play key roles in the processes regulating ICD.

In the following section, we recapitulate the current data supporting epigenetic regulation of DAMPs by miRNAs. In particular, we have only focused on studies in which direct miRNA:mRNA interactions have been experimentally validated, e.g., by gene reporter or target protector-mediated assays [38]. Given that both miRNAs and DAMPs roles are so much context-dependent, we propose a classification of miRNA function (as tumor suppressor or oncomiRNA) solely based on factual experimental evidence. Surprisingly, we notice that they mainly function as tumor suppressors. For miRNA nomenclature, we decided to adapt and unify miRNA names and accession numbers according to the miRBase database, the primary repository for published miRNA, freely available at http://www.mirbase.org/ (accessed on 25 January 2021). All data are summarized in Table 1 and schematized in Figure 2.

Table 1. miRNA directly targets DAMPs and their tumor suppressor or oncomiRNA associated roles. According to the miRBase nomenclature, miRNAs are named with the abbreviation "miR" followed by a dash and a number. These are preceded by a prefix representing the species (for example, "hsa" for *Homo sapiens*). Each miRNA is also identified by its miRBase accession number and, if available, the type of its dysregulation reported in the tumor model analyzed, according to which it may be classified as tumor suppressor or oncomiRNA. For each targeted DAMP, the effects of its regulation are also described (↓ decrease/inhibition; ↑ increase/activation).

miRNA	miRBase Accession Number	Dysregulation in Cancer vs. Normal Counterparts	Target DAMP	miRNA Binding Site in Target Gene	Cancer Type	Effects	Role	Reference
hsa-let-7e-5p	MIMAT0000066	Not evaluated	HMGB1	3′UTR	Thyroid cancer	↓ Migration ↓ Invasion	Tumor suppressor	Ding et al., 2019 [39]
hsa-miR-107	MIMAT0000104	Downregulation (tissues and cell lines)	HMGB1	3′UTR	Breast cancer	↓ Migration ↓ Proliferation ↓ Autophagy	Tumor suppressor	Ai et al., 2018 [40]
hsa-miR-1179	MIMAT0005824	Downregulation (tissues and cell lines)	HMGB1	3′UTR	Gastric cancer	↓ Proliferation ↓ Invasion	Tumor suppressor	Li et al., 2019 [41]
hsa-miR-1284	MIMAT0005941	Downregulation (tissues and cell lines)	HMGB1	Not reported	Cervical cancer	↓ Proliferation ↓ Invasion ↑ Cisplatin-induced apoptosis	Tumor suppressor	Chen & Li, 2018 [42]
hsa-miR-129-5p	MIMAT0000242	Not evaluated	HMGB1	3′UTR	Breast cancer	↓ Irradiation-induced autophagy ↑ Radiosensitivity	Tumor suppressor	Luo et al., 2015 [43]
		Not evaluated		Not evaluated	Breast cancer	↓ Autophagy ↑ Paclitaxel-induced apoptosis	Tumor suppressor	Shi et al., 2019 [44]
		Not evaluated		Not reported	Colon cancer	↓ Proliferation	Tumor suppressor	Wu et al., 2018 [45]
		Downregulation (tissues and cell lines)		3′UTR	Gastric cancer	↓ Proliferation ↑ Apoptosis	Tumor suppressor	Feng et al., 2020 [46]
		Downregulation (cell lines)		3′UTR	Gastric cancer	↓ Proliferation ↓ Epithelial-mesenchymal transition	Tumor suppressor	Wang et al., 2019 [47]
		Not evaluated		3′UTR	Hepatocellular carcinoma	↓ Migration ↓ Invasion	Tumor suppressor	Zhang et al., 2017 [48]
		Downregulation (tissues)		3′UTR	Osteosarcoma	↓ Proliferation ↑ Apoptosis	Tumor suppressor	Liu et al., 2017 [49]

Table 1. Cont.

miRNA	miRBase Accession Number	Dysregulation in Cancer vs. Normal Counterparts	Target DAMP	miRNA Binding Site in Target Gene	Cancer Type	Effects	Role	Reference
hsa-miR-142-3p	MIMAT0000434	Downregulation (tissues)	HMGB1	3′UTR	Glioma	↓ Proliferation ↓ Invasion	Tumor suppressor	Zhang et al., 2018 [50]
		Not evaluated		3′UTR	Non-small-cell lung cancer	↓ Starvation-induced autophagy ↑ Cisplatin and doxorubicin-chemosensitivity	Tumor suppressor	Chen et al., 2017 [51]
		Downregulation (tissues and cell lines)		3′UTR	Non-small-cell lung cancer	↓ Proliferation ↑ Apoptosis	Tumor suppressor	Xiao & Lu, 2015 [52]
		Downregulation (tissues)		3′UTR	Osteosarcoma	↓ Proliferation ↑ Apoptosis	Tumor suppressor	Liu et al., 2017 [49]
		Not evaluated	Hsp70	3′UTR	Pancreatic ductal adenocarcinoma	↓ Proliferation	Tumor suppressor	MacKenzie et al., 2013 [53]
hsa-miR-181b-5p	MIMAT0000257	Not evaluated	HMGB1	3′UTR	Acute myeloid leukemia	↑ Doxorubicin or cytarabine-induced apoptosis	Tumor suppressor	Lu et al., 2014 [54]
hsa-miR-193a-3p	MIMAT0000459	Not evaluated	HMGB1	3′UTR	Lung cancer	↓ Proliferation ↓ Migration	Tumor suppressor	Wu et al., 2018 [55]
hsa-miR-200a-5p	MIMAT0001620	Downregulation (tissues)	HMGB1	3′UTR	Hepatocellular carcinoma	Not determined	Tumor suppressor	Li et al., 2017 [56]
hsa-miR-200c-3p	MIMAT0000617	Not evaluated		3′UTR	Breast cancer	↓ Invasion ↓ Migration	Tumor suppressor	Chang et al., 2014 [57]
		Not evaluated	HMGB1	Not evaluated	Lung cancer	↓ Invasion ↓ Migration ↓ Epithelial-mesenchymal transition	Tumor suppressor	Liu et al., 2017 [58]
hsa-miR-205-5p	MIMAT0000266	Downregulation (tissues). Moreover, it is downregulated in metastatic compared to non-metastatic cancer	HMGB1	3′UTR	Triple-negative breast cancer	↓ Invasion ↓ Migration ↓ Proliferation	Tumor suppressor	Wang et al., 2019 [59]

Table 1. Cont.

miRNA	miRBase Accession Number	Dysregulation in Cancer vs. Normal Counterparts	Target DAMP	miRNA Binding Site in Target Gene	Cancer Type	Effects	Role	Reference
hsa-miR-218-5p	MIMAT0000275	Downregulation Paclitaxel-resistant compared to non-drug resistant cells (cell lines)	HMGB1	3'UTR	Endometrial carcinoma	↓ Autophagy ↑ Paclitaxel-chemosensitivity	Tumor suppressor	Ran et al., 2015 [60]
		Not evaluated		3'UTR	Lung cancer	↓ Invasion ↓ Migration	Tumor suppressor	Zhang et al., 2013 [61]
		Non evaluated		3'UTR	Prostate cancer	↓ Invasion ↓ Migration ↓ Proliferation ↑ Apoptosis	Tumor suppressor	Zhang et al., 2019 [62]
hsa-miR-223-3p	MIMAT0000280	Not evaluated	Hsp90	3'UTR	Osteosarcoma	↓ Proliferation ↑ Apoptosis ↑ Cell cycle G0/G1 arrest	Tumor suppressor	Li et al., 2012 [63]
hsa-miR-223-5p	MIMAT0004570	Downregulation (tissues and cell lines)	Hsp70	3'UTR	Osteosarcoma	↑ Cisplastin-induced apoptosis	Tumor suppressor	Tang et al., 2018 [64]
hsa-miR-320a-3p	MIMAT0000510	Downregulation (tissues)	HMGB1	3'UTR	Hepatocellular carcinoma	↓ Invasion ↓ Migration	Tumor suppressor	Lv et al., 2017 [65]
hsa-miR-325	MIMAT0000771	Downregulation (tissues)	HMGB1	3'UTR	Non-small cell lung cancer	↓ Invasion ↓ Proliferation	Tumor suppressor	Yao et al., 2015 [66]
hsa-miR-27a-3p	MIMAT0000084	Upregulation (tissues)	Calreticulin	3'UTR	Colorectal cancer	↓ Mitoxantrone and oxaliplain-induced apoptosis ↓ Autophagy ↓ MCH-1 expression ↓ Dendritic cell maturation ↓ In situ immune cells infiltration ↑ Tumor growth ↑ Liver metastasis	Onco-miRNA	Colangelo et al., 2016a and b [67,68]
hsa-miR-27b-3p	MIMAT0000419	Not evaluated	Hsp90	3'UTR	Non-small-cell lung carcinoma	↓ Migration ↓ Invasion	Tumor suppressor	Dong et al., 2019 [69]
hsa-miR-34a-3p	MIMAT0004557	Not evaluated	HMGB1	3'UTR	Retinoblastoma	↑ Etoposide and carboplatin-induced apoptosis ↓ Starvation-induced autophagy	Tumor suppressor	Liu et al., 2014 [70]

167

Table 1. Cont.

miRNA	miRBase Accession Number	Dysregulation in Cancer vs. Normal Counterparts	Target DAMP	miRNA Binding Site in Target Gene	Cancer Type	Effects	Role	Reference
hsa-miR-34a-5p	MIMAT0000255	Downregulation (cell lines)		3′UTR	Acute Myeloid Leukemia	↑ Apoptosis ↓ Autophagy	Tumor suppressor	Liu et al., 2017 [58]
		Downregulation (tissues)	HMGB1	3′UTR	Cervical (CaCx) and colorectal (CRC) cancers	↓ Invasion ↓ Migration ↓ Proliferation	Tumor suppressor	Chandrasekaran et al., 2016 [71]
		Downregulation (tissues and cell lines)		3′UTR	Cutaneous squamous cell carcinoma	↓ Invasion ↓ Migration ↓ Proliferation	Tumor suppressor	Li et al., 2017 [72]
hsa-miR-361-5p	MIMAT0000703	Downregulation (tissues and cell lines)	Hsp90	3′UTR	Cervical cancer	↓ Epithelial-mesenchymal transition ↓ Invasion	Tumor suppressor	Xu et al., 2020 [73]
hsa-miR-449a	MIMAT0001541	Downregulation (tissues and cell lines)	HMGB1	3′UTR	Non-small cell lung cancer	↓ Invasion ↓ Migration ↓ Proliferation	Tumor suppressor	Wu et al., 2019 [74]
		Downregulation (cell lines)		3′UTR	Gastric cancer	↓ Migration ↓ Proliferation ↑ Apoptosis	Tumor suppressor	Tian et al., 2018 [75]
hsa-miR-505-3p	MIMAT0002876	Downregulation (tissues and cell lines)	HMGB1	3′UTR	Hepatocellular carcinoma	↓ Proliferation ↓ Invasion ↓ Epithelial-mesenchymal transition	Tumor suppressor	Lu et al., 2016 [76]
		Not evaluated		Non evaluated	Hepatocellular carcinoma	↑ Doxorubicin-induced apoptosis	Tumor suppressor	Lu et al., 2018 [77]
		Downregulation (tissues)		3′UTR	Osteosarcoma	↓ Invasion ↓ Migration ↓ Proliferation	Tumor suppressor	Liu et al., 2017 [78]
hsa-miR-519d-3p	MIMAT0002853	Downregulation (tissues)	HMGB1	3′UTR	Lung cancer	↓ Invasion ↓ Migration ↓ Proliferation	Tumor suppressor	Ye et al., 2020 [79]
hsa-miR-548b-3p	MIMAT0003254	Downregulation (tissues and cell lines)	HMGB1	3′UTR	Hepatocellular carcinoma	↓ Invasion ↓ Migration ↓ Proliferation ↑ Apoptosis	Tumor suppressor	Yun et al., 2019 [80]

Table 1. Cont.

miRNA	miRBase Accession Number	Dysregulation in Cancer vs. Normal Counterparts	Target DAMP	miRNA Binding Site in Target Gene	Cancer Type	Effects	Role	Reference
hsa-miR-628-3p	MIMAT0003297	Not evaluated	Hsp90	3′UTR	Non-small-cell lung carcinoma	↓ Migration ↑ Apoptosis	Tumor suppressor	Pan et al., 2018 [81]
hsa-miR-665	MIMAT0004952	Downregulation (tissues and cell lines)	HMGB1	3′UTR	Retinoblastoma	↓ Invasion ↓ Migration ↓ Proliferation ↑ Apoptosis	Tumor suppressor	Wang et al., 2019 [82]

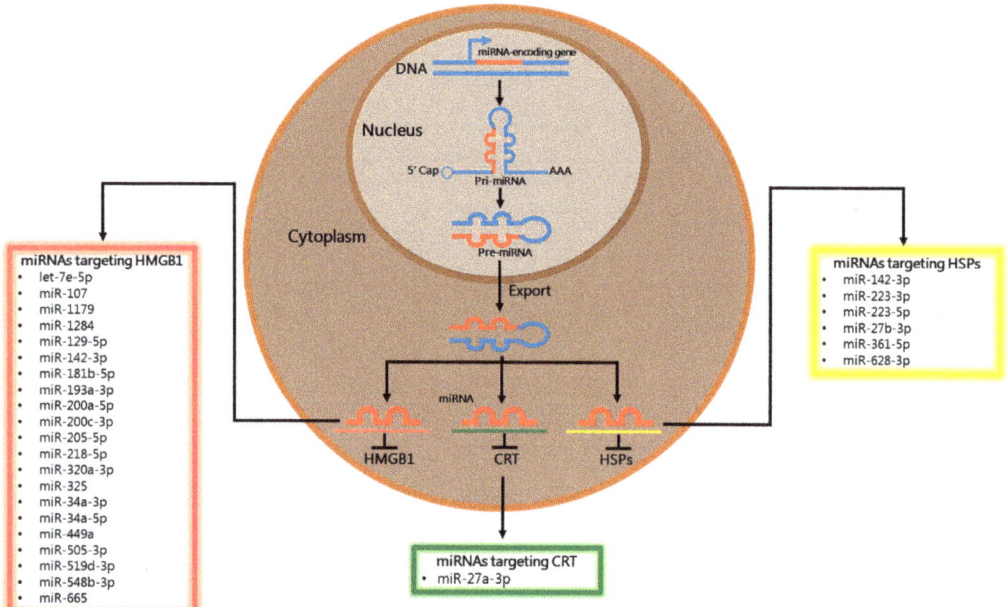

Figure 2. Immunogenic Cell Death-hallmarks targeted by miRNAs. The miRNA processing pathway initiates with the transcription of the primary miRNA (pri-miRNA) and its cleavage to generate the pre-miRNA. Then, pre-miRNA is exported from the nucleus to the cytoplasm, where it is cleaved to its mature miRNA. The functional strand of the mature miRNA has the major role to silence target mRNAs through different mechanisms. In this review, we summarize miRNAs that target well-known Immunogenic Cell Death-associated DAMPs, such as calreticulin (CRT), HMGB1, and Hsps (Hsp70, Hsp90).

4.1. Calreticulin

Calreticulin (CRT) is a chaperone protein mainly located in the lumen of the endoplasmic reticulum (ER). Given its high capacity of buffering calcium, it modulates calcium signaling and homeostasis [83]. Through these functions, CRT has important biological regulatory roles inside and outside the ER, and is involved in cancer, wound healing, cardiogenesis, autoimmune diseases, and neurological diseases [84].

In addition, CRT can be translocated to the surface of stressed and dying cells [12]. Exposure of CRT on the cell surface is a major factor in ICD, as it serves as an "eat me" engulfment signal for DCs, thus promoting the presentation of tumor-associated antigens to T cells [12]. In the context of cancer, CRT was identified as a direct target of miR-27a-3p. The role of this miRNA seems controversial, as it has been previously assigned with both anti-tumor [85–87] and pro-tumor properties [88,89]. miR-27a-3p downregulates CRT expression by inhibiting target mRNA translation [67]. It was also demonstrated that the miR-27a-3p throught targeting CRT modulates MHC class I surface exposure, and that, in particular, high miR-27a-3p concomitant with low CRT expression associates with enhanced tumor growth in vivo, colorectal cancer stage, development of metastasis, and impairment of CD8[+] T-cell infiltration [67]. When colorectal cancer cells were subjected to ICD inducers (mitoxantrone and oxaliplatin), miR-27a-3p blocked CRT exposure, as well as ATP and HMGB1 secretion. Upon chemotherapeutic treatment, miR-27a-3p levels were inversely correlated with induction of apoptosis (by ICD inducers) and autophagy (by chloroquine). In parallel, soluble factors released by miR-27a-3p overexpressing tumor cells subjected to ICD failed to induce DC functional and phenotypic maturation [68]. The investigations of Colangelo et al. [67,68] discussed in this section support the idea that the miR-27a-3p/CRT axis modulates the ICD program, especially by blocking the initial interaction between DCs and ICD-subjected tumor cells.

Collectively, data recapitulated here suggest that miR-27a can be postulated as an oncomiRNA in colorectal cancer, where its expression was shown to be upregulated, and that it may support tumor progression through downregulation of CRT-dependent immunostimulation.

4.2. Heat Shock Proteins

Heat-shock proteins (Hsps) are a group of molecular chaperones whose main cellular function is to ensure the precise (re)folding of proteins in stress conditions. They are usually located in the intracellular space wherein they exert prominent cytoprotective functions. Importantly, many tumors overexpress Hsps, presumably as an adaptive response to a "stressful" niche where they develop [90]. However, the ability of Hsps to contribute chaperoned peptides for antigen processing and MHC-restricted presentation has not yet been elucidated [91].

Under some circumstances, for example during ICD, at least two members of this family, Hsp70 and Hsp90, can be expressed at the cell surface, where they exhibit immunostimulatory properties [92,93]. Therefore, miRNAs that target Hsps expression are likely to have a significant impact on the tumor phenotype.

In pancreatic ductal adenocarcinoma, miR-142-3p inhibited cell proliferation by negatively regulating Hsp70 expression [53]. In addition to its proliferative role in cancer, Hsp70 was associated with chemoresistance. In this context, it was reported that miR-223-5p suppressed the chemoresistance of osteosarcoma cells to cisplatin through JNK/Jun signaling by downregulating Hsp70 expression; however, expression of miR-223-5p was reduced in osteosarcoma biopsies compared with paired non-tumor tissues [64]. Interestingly, also in an in vitro osteosarcoma model, ectopic expression of miR-223-3p, through Hsp90 downregulation, inhibited cell proliferation by inducing cell cycle arrest and apoptosis [63]. miR-27b-3p and miR-628-3p directly targeted Hsp90, resulting in suppression of non-small-cell lung carcinoma migration and invasion, and promoted apoptosis [69,81]. In addition, the lncRNA KCNQ1OT1 modulated Hsp90 expression by blocking miR-27b-3p [69]. The expression of miR-361-5p in cervical cancer was also downregulated by a lncRNA NEAT1, whereas its negative modulation of Hsp90 inhibited invasion and epithelial-mesenchymal transition (EMT) [73].

miRNAs described here act on the overall expression of Hsps, but the effects on postransductional modification and surface translocation are not revealed. However, the potential contribution of these miRNAs in modulating Hsps expression in the context of ICD remains an unmet question; thus, it is not yet elucidated whether they can play in favor of or against immunogenicity.

4.3. HMGB1

HMGB1 is a non-histone chromatin-binding protein that regulates different cellular functions according to its cellular localization. Within the nucleus, HMGB1 is involved in many DNA events (repair, transcription, stability, telomerase maintenance). In the cytoplasm, membrane, or extracellular space, several studies have demonstrated its ability to regulate cell proliferation, apoptosis, autophagy, inflammation, invasion, metastasis, and immunity, among others [94]. Paradoxically, HMGB1 has been attributed with both pro- and anti-tumoral properties. Relative to its immune functions, HMGB1 has been described as both a suppressor and an activator, which depends on receptors, targeted cells, and redox state [95].

A series of studies have demonstrated that miRNAs participate in the regulation of HMGB1 expression. By targeting HMGB1, miR-548b-3p [80] and miR-320-3p [65] suppressed hepatocellular carcinoma (HCC) cell proliferation, metastasis, and invasion while inducing apoptosis. In addition, HMGB1 expression was downregulated in HCC specimens and cell lines, which correlated with poor prognosis. Along this line, downregulation of miR-325 [66] and miR-449a [74] correlated with poor prognosis in lung cancer patients, as these miRNAs negatively targeted HMGB1, resulting in decreased cell migration, invasion, and/or proliferation. It was also discovered that miR-107 [40] and miR-1179 [41], whose expression was downregulated in breast cancer and gastric cancer, respectively, inhibited autophagy, proliferation, and/or migration of tumor cells by directly suppressing HMGB1. While miR-1284 downregulation in cervical cancer tissues and cell lines correlated with poor survival, the miR-1284/HMGB1 axis suppressed proliferation and invasion [42]. Restoration of miR-665, by directly targeting HMGB1, suppressed cell proliferation, colony formation, migration, and invasion, and induced cell apoptosis in retinoblastoma [82]. Similar effects of let-7e-5p were observed in thyroid cancer, whereas similar effects were observed in thyroid cancer but through let-7e-5p [39].

Both mature sequences of mir-34a were shown to target HMGB1 directly. Antitumor events were promoted by the miR-34a-5p/HMGB1 axis in acute myeloid leukemia [96], cutaneous squamous cell carcinoma [72], cervical cancer, and colorectal cancers [71], and similar effects were exerted by miR-34a-3p/HMGB1 in retinoblastoma [70]. In acute myeloid leukemia, miR-181b-5p was significantly decreased, especially in relapsed/refractory patients. Upregulation of miR-181b-5p increased the chemosensitivity of leukemia cells and promoted drug-induced apoptosis via negative modulation of HMGB1 expression [54]. When a miR-200c-3p mimic was transfected into lung [58] and breast cancer cells [57], there was a significant decrease in cell migration, invasion, and epithelial to mesenchymal transition (EMT). These changes were associated in part with the downregulation of HMGB1 by miR-200c-3p. In triple negative breast cancer, the downregulation of miR-205-5p was negatively associated with progression and metastasis, and cell growth and EMT were inhibited by the miR-205-5p/HMGB1 axis [59].

The antitumor role of the miR-129-5p/HMGB1 axis was studied in osteosarcoma [45], hepatocellular carcinoma [48], breast cancer [43,44], gastric cancer [46,47], and colon cancer [45]. Downregulation of this miRNA expression was also reported in cancer cells lines and primary cancers, compared to their normal counterparts [46]. In these reports, ectopic expression of miR-129-5p was found to suppress migration, invasion, proliferation, and EMT, while it enhanced apoptosis, radio-, and chemosensitivity through HMGB1 downregulation. In addition, the miR-505-3p/HMGB1 axis exerted a negative impact on tumor progression in osteosarcoma [78], hepatocellular carcinoma [76,77], and gastric cancer [75].

Interestingly, it was found that the miRNA/HMGB1 axis was modulated by long noncoding RNAs (lncRNAs) and circular RNAs (circRNAs), most of them upregulated in cancer tissues. The lncRNA prostate cancer-associated transcript 1 (PCAT-1) [48] and MALAT1 [45,49] inhibited reversed miRNA-dependent HMGB1 downregulation. Likewise, the lncRNA UCA1 exerted pro-tumoral activity in lung cancer, acting mechanistically by upregulating HMGB1 expression through miR-193a-3p inhibition [55]. The lncRNA PCA3 [62] downregulated the expression of miR-218-5p, whose negative targeting of HMGB1 was evaluated in endometrial carcinoma [60], lung cancer [61], and prostate cancer [62], leading to a decrease in tumor proliferation, migration, invasion, and chemoresistance. miR-142-3p has also been identified as a microRNA that suppressed HMGB1 expression in non-small-cell lung carcinoma [51,52] and glioma [50], therefore playing a major role in reducing tumor cell proliferation, invasion, apoptosis, and drug resistance (to cisplatin). Along this line, the lncRNA TP73-AS1 upregulated HMGB1 expression through sponging miR-142-3p [50] and also miR-200a-5p [56]. Finally, the circRNA circ_0007385 enhanced cell proliferation, migration, invasion, and chemoresistance in lung cancer through upregulating miR-519d-3p and thus downregulating HMGB1 [79].

Overall, the data recapitulated in the last two sections suggest that, at least in the described phenotypes, the cytoprotective roles of HMGB1, Hsp70, and Hsp90 were more relevant than their immunostimulatory properties. Indeed, their targeting miRNAs appeared to repress pro-tumoral phenotypes by directly inhibiting their expression, thereby functioning as potential tumor suppressors. Moreover, some of these miRNAs were shown to be downregulated in tumors compared to their normal counterparts (Table 1). These findings might enhance our knowledge of the molecular mechanisms underlying malignant progression, making miRNAs promising targets for therapeutic intervention.

5. Modulation of Therapeutic Outcome through Targeting DAMPs by miRNA

Nowadays, drug resistance represents a main obstacle in the clinical setting, leading to relapse and metastasis in several cancer types. Therefore, new and more innovative approaches are required to treat these malignancies efficiently. The new knowledge on miRNA molecular actions and their involvement in cancer-associated mechanisms has opened new perspectives in the development of more effective therapeutic strategies. As miRNAs modulate multiple signaling pathways associated with therapy response, modification in miRNA expression can lead to significant changes in disease evolution and cancer outcome. Over the last few decades, numerous studies have been published on miRNA regulation of the cancer treatment response [97]. Compelling evidence has shown that the fundamental mechanisms of resistance to different anticancer drugs might be attributed to aberrantly expressed miRNAs in a wide range of malignancies [98]. Some miRNAs that have been described above as tumor suppressors have also been shown to modulate the sensitivity to chemotherapeutic agents.

By directly targeting HMGB1, several miRNAs may synergistically promote chemosensitivity, increasing drug pro-apoptotic activity often impaired by HMGB1-promoted autophagy. Of those, Lu et al. reported that tumor cells exhibit greatly enhanced apoptosis-related sensitivity to doxorubicin or cytarabine after transfection with the miR-181b mimic [54], and, in line with this, Chen & Li showed that miR-1284 enhanced cisplatin-induced apoptosis [42]. Ectopic expression of miR-505-3p was shown to enhance doxorubicin-induced cell death and caspase-3 dependent apoptosis, via inactivation of the Akt pathway [77]. The PI3K/Akt/mTOR pathway has been implicated in HMGB1-mediated autophagy, which was shown to play an important pro-survival role and contribute to chemoresistance [99]. Moreover, Chen et al. reported that miR-142-3p overexpression inhibited autophagy by activating the PI3K/Akt/mTOR pathway through HMGB1, and thus resulting in the increase of cisplatin and doxorubicin-chemosensitivity [51]. In addition, HMGB1-mediated autophagic resistance to paclitaxel was identified by Ran et al., whereas upregulation of miR-218-5p could restore chemosensitivity [60]. Consistently, miR-129-5p was found to increase apoptosis during paclitaxel treatment, and the improvement in sensitivity was associated with inhibition of autophagy [44]. Liu et al. demonstrated that miR-34a-3p-mediated inhibition of autophagy could sensitize cells to etoposide and carboplatin-induced apoptosis [70]. Similarly, Tang et al. precisely described a feedback loop formed by miR-223-5p, Hsp70, and the JNK/Jun signaling pathway associated with the modulation of cisplatin-resistance [64].

Interestingly, most of the miRNAs with tumor suppressor functions are found downregulated in various cancer types compared to normal tissues: miR-505-3p in hepatocellular carcinoma [76] and osteosarcoma [78], miR-1284 in cervical cancer [42], miR-129-5p in osteosarcoma [49], miR-142-3p in non-small-cell lung cancer [52] and in osteosarcoma [49], and miR-223-5p in osteosarcoma [64], among others. This aberrant expression is closely implicated in cancer treatment resistance. However, even when the aberrant expression of those miRNA induced a substantial upregulation of ICD-associated DAMPs, none of the above-mentioned reports have explored its association with the induction of ICD. Elucidation of those features would require more targeted assays, which would allow us to obtain a more comprehensive view about the epigenetic modulation occurring in cancer cells undergoing ICD.

6. Therapeutic Combination of ICD and miRNAs: A New Opportunity

Innovative therapeutic approaches including miRNA-based agents together with current standard treatment modalities could importantly benefit cancer patients. Targeting miRNAs by restoring their expression seems to be an attractive tool for emerging, more effective individualized therapies. However, there are still significant challenges to overcome to ensure the efficient delivery of miRNA to the tumor in vivo, for example, off-target effects, poor serum stability, and ineffective, poorly selective cellular entry. Hence, the development of novel drug delivery systems with the capacity to target-directed transport and protection of such cargos is mandatory [100].

In the face of these challenges, two different delivery systems have been designed in order to combine miRNA and ICD-inducer administration.

Phung et al. successfully fabricated nanoparticles (NPs) for target-specific co-delivery of low-dose doxorubicin and miR-200c to cancer cells [101]. These mixed NPs were composed of two co-polymers: poly(D,L-lactide-co-glycolide)-polyethyleneimine (PLGA-PEI) and folic acid (FA)-conjugated PLGA-block-poly(ethylene glycol) (PLGA-PEG-FA). Doxorubicin was encapsulated by the hydrophobic core formed by PLGA, whereas the negative charges of miR-200c were electrostatically absorbed by the cationic backbone of PEI. PEI cytotoxicity was reduced by PEG, which also conferred stability and the way to introduce folic acid (FA) [102]. Despite conferring pH and temperature stability, permeability, non-immunogenicity, capacity to be tagged, among other advantages, FA is extremely important in this system because it may increase the proper and selective uptake by tumor cells in both in vitro and especially in vivo settings. This is because folate receptors are overexpressed in numerous cancer types compared to corresponding normal tissues [103]. This configuration was in fact successful because it protected miR-200c from degradation in serum. In addition, the complete NPs were well tolerated by hosts, probably due, at least in part, to the substantially low dose of doxorubicin used [101].

Surprisingly, although miR-200c has been shown to downregulate HMGB1 expression directly [57,58], this new NP-based platform that combined miR-200c and doxorubicin promoted ICD via the translocation of CRT to the cell surface and the release of HMGB1 in vitro and in vivo. Accordingly, DAMPs' modulation was accomplished by DCs' phenotypic maturation. In addition, T cell antitumor activity was enhanced, partially due to downregulation of PD-L1 by miR-200c [101].

Recently, Wang et al. designed another type of nanocarrier to deliver both miR-1284 and cisplatin [104]. They generated liposomes composed of distearoylphosphatidylcholine (DSPC) succinylphosphatidylethanolamine (DSPE-mPEG), distearoyl-N-(3-carboxy-propionoylpoly (ethyleneglycol) succinyl) phosphatidylethanolamine (DSPE-PEG-COOH), and 1,2-dioleoyl-3-trimethylammoniumpropane (DOTAP) to be loaded with 10% of cisplatin and surface-conjugated with the CD59 antibody. The presence of anti-CD59 on the NP surface conferred tumor selective accumulation properties, as CD59 has been shown to be overexpressed in cancer and associated with immune escape events [105]. This cationic liposome was able to bind the negatively charged miR-1284 electrostatically.

The pharmacokinetic analysis of the formulation indicated that the nanocarrier-based system prolonged the blood circulation of the drugs. The anticancer effects were only assessed in vitro and demonstrated a full internalization of the complex by tumor cells. As expected and according to previous results [42], co-delivery of miR-1284 and cisplatin synergistically inhibited cell viability and promoted apoptosis by HMGB1 downregulation [104]. Given these promising results, future in vivo analysis should be done to evaluate the pre-clinical efficacy of this formulation. The impact of this combination should also be studied in the context of ICD, given that cisplatin was shown to be an ICD inducer [4].

Together, these results provide guidance for a promising combination strategy to improve the clinical use and the immunostimulatory efficiency of ICD-inducing drugs and develop an effective and safe cancer therapeutic option.

7. Future Challenges

Understanding the regulation of ICD hallmarks is pivotal for a better exploitation of the different effects characterizing ICD inducers. In this review, we summarized studies that have reported that numerous miRNAs contributed to DAMP modulation, acting as either oncogenic miRNAs or tumor suppressor miRNAs. However, it is important to note that there is not much evidence regarding miRNA modulation by ICD, although it was reported that different miRNAs could contribute to ICD inducers therapeutic activities. Outstanding questions exist: Does a miRNA signature associated with ICD actually exist? Do specific miRNAs play a role in ICD in cancer cells?

As mentioned above, ICD-associated pathways are not tumor-exclusive. For that reason, when evaluating the role of an immunity modulator, it is necessary to integrate fully the different cellular actors and the molecular crosstalk established between them. In this scenario, it was demonstrated that miRNAs could be involved in the paracrine dialogue governing inter-cellular signaling within the tumor microenvironment. In this sense, dysregulation of endogenous miRNAs can be induced in immune cells by cancer cell-released DAMPs or miRNAs derived from cancer cells that can directly affect immune cell functions. Unlu et al. demonstrated that miR-34c and miR-214 were specifically upregulated in human PBMCs following incubation with conditioned media or tumor cell lysate from stressed cells, as part of the inflammatory response. In particular, the presence of HMGB1 within the paracrine stimulus was strongly associated with miRNA modulation [106]. Frank et al. provided evidence that miR-375 transfer from tumor cells to macrophages is crucial to alter the tumor-associated macrophage phenotype and the subsequent development of a tumor-promoting microenvironment [107]. Moreover, tumor-secreted miR-21 and miR-29a also can function by another mechanism, by binding as ligands to the Toll-like receptor (TLR) 8, in immune cells, triggering a TLR-mediated prometastatic inflammatory response that ultimately may lead to tumor growth and metastasis. Thus, by acting as paracrine agonists of TLRs, secreted miRNAs are key regulators of the tumor microenvironment and are implicated in tumor–immune system communication [108]. Intriguingly, recently, Lee J et al. generated in the laboratory two distinct modified single-stranded RNAs (ssRNAs) and showed their ability to induce immunogenic cell death in different types of cancer cell lines. In particular, those ssRNA promoted DAMP release and consequent impact on cytokine secretion by immature DCs [109]. We have recently discovered that the employment of immunogenic tumor cell lysates as a tumor antigen source in the development of DC-based vaccines influenced the miRNA profile in DCs. Therefore, we wonder: Could cancer cells undergoing ICD exploit specific miRNAs to communicate with the tumor immune microenvironment? Could cancer cell-derived miRNAs become messengers for DCs during ICD?

These questions compelled us to match several multifaceted interactions to understand the effects of environmental factors on miRNA expression more comprehensively. In this sense, a novel discipline termed "molecular pathological epidemiology" (MPE) has been proposed as a comprehensive approach to precision medicine. MPE protocols include a multilevel research platform to integrate molecular pathologies, immune response, and clinical outcomes in cancer. The application of in vivo pathology together with new multi-omics techniques might contribute to a more profound understanding of miRNA heterogeneous regulation, their role in tumor biology and therapeutic response, and the putative link with the endogenous/exogenous environment (diet, drugs, including ICD-inducing agents, microbiota, and germline genetics), further supporting the design of targeted, personalized therapies [110,111].

8. Conclusions

The discovery of miRNAs has deepened our knowledge of human diseases, especially cancer and its supporting epigenetic mechanisms. In this article, we have reviewed the evidence regarding the effects of miRNAs on the expression of DAMP mRNAs in different cancer types. Initially, we expected to identify several oncomiRNAs targeting DAMPs whose ectopic inhibition could promote and/or restore the immunogenic potential of therapeutic agents. Surprisingly, our hypothesis was only valid for CRT targeting, whereas miRNA-based downregulation of other DAMPs was in fact associated with suppressed cancer properties. We propose several reasons to explain, at least in part, these unexpected data. First of all, most DAMPs which were shown to be regulated by miRNAs are classified as constitutive (cDAMPs); hence, they are present inside healthy cells, and are released following immunogenic stimulus, exerting their proinflammatory functions in the extracellular space. Their ICD-associated modulation is mainly post-translational, whereas miRNA regulation is exerted at a pre-translational level. However, it seems possible that downregulation by miRNAs in cancer cells could temporarily limit their release and so their immunogenic roles. Further studies should be done in order to clarify this hypothesis. In contrast to cDAMPs, inducible DAMPs (iDAMPs) are not present in healthy cells but are induced and/or altered upon cell death (e.g., type 1 IFN). As far as we know, the regulation of iDAMPs by miRNAs has not yet been determined.

Secondly, when studying miRNAs, it is important to consider the relative promiscuity of their targets. As stated above, a given miRNA may have thousands of targets with significant differences in function. Even in the presence of restoration-of-function assays, this would lead to paradoxical conclusions about the role of miRNAs, in that a single miRNA may theoretically impact in opposite ways within the cell by targeting effectors with opposite functions. Moreover, interpretation of this paradox is even more complex when considering that miRNAs probably show different functions depending on the environment in which they are expressed.

However, given miRNAs' role in regulating cellular processes as cell death and autophagy, but also different immune escape mechanisms modulating antigen processing/presentation and immune inhibitory molecules in different types of cancer cells, it remains reasonable to speculate their involvement in ICD. This is especially true if we consider that miRNAs are implicated in tumor–immune system communication, a key feature of ICD.

Author Contributions: Investigation, M.J.L., J.D.C., V.C.; writing—original draft preparation, M.J.L., A.N.; writing—review and editing, M.J.L., J.D.C., N.B.R.V., V.C.; review and editing, V.C., J.D.C., N.B.R.V.; supervision, M.J.L., J.D.C. All authors have read and agreed to the published version of the manuscript.

Funding: This research was funded by: Italian Ministry of Health (Young Researcher Grant GR-2011-02350476 to J.D.C.), "Fondazione con il Sud" (Brains2South 2015 PDR-0224 to J.D.C.), Agencia Nacional de Promoción Científica y Tecnológica (PICT-2017-1755 to M.J.L.), and Regione Campania, POR FESR 2014/20 RarePlatNet Project (Az. 1.2, CUP B63D18000380007 to V.C.).

Acknowledgments: M.J.L. holds a Fondazione Umberto Veronesi fellowship, A.N. holds a triennial fellowship from Regional Operational Program FSE 2014-2020-Axis III-Specific Objective 14 "Increasing the skills of the workforce and facilitating mobility, work teaching/reintegration (RA 10.4)".

Conflicts of Interest: The authors declare no conflict of interest.

References

1. Van Kempen, T.S.; Wenink, M.H.; Leijten, E.F.A.; Radstake, T.R.D.J.; Boes, M. Perception of Self: Distinguishing Autoimmunity from Autoinflammation. *Nat. Rev. Rheumatol.* **2015**, *11*, 483–492. [CrossRef] [PubMed]
2. Galluzzi, L.; Buqué, A.; Kepp, O.; Zitvogel, L.; Kroemer, G. Immunogenic Cell Death in Cancer and Infectious Disease. *Nat. Rev. Immunol.* **2017**, *17*, 97–111. [CrossRef]
3. Casares, N.; Pequignot, M.O.; Tesniere, A.; Ghiringhelli, F.; Roux, S.; Chaput, N.; Schmitt, E.; Hamai, A.; Hervas-Stubbs, S.; Obeid, M.; et al. Caspase-Dependent Immunogenicity of Doxorubicin-Induced Tumor Cell Death. *J. Exp. Med.* **2005**, *202*, 1691–1701. [CrossRef]
4. Lamberti, M.J.; Nigro, A.; Mentucci, F.M.; Rumie Vittar, N.B.; Casolaro, V.; Dal Col, J. Dendritic Cells and Immunogenic Cancer Cell Death: A Combination for Improving Antitumor Immunity. *Pharmaceutics* **2020**, *12*, 256. [CrossRef]
5. Tang, R.; Xu, J.; Zhang, B.; Liu, J.; Liang, C.; Hua, J.; Meng, Q.; Yu, X.; Shi, S. Ferroptosis, Necroptosis, and Pyroptosis in Anticancer Immunity. *J. Hematol. Oncol.* **2020**, *13*, 110. [CrossRef] [PubMed]
6. Legrand, A.J.; Konstantinou, M.; Goode, E.F.; Meier, P. The Diversification of Cell Death and Immunity: Memento Mori. *Mol. Cell* **2019**, *76*, 232–242. [CrossRef] [PubMed]
7. Krysko, D.V.; Garg, A.D.; Kaczmarek, A.; Krysko, O.; Agostinis, P.; Vandenabeele, P. Immunogenic Cell Death and DAMPs in Cancer Therapy. *Nat. Rev. Cancer* **2012**, *12*, 860–875. [CrossRef] [PubMed]
8. Cruickshank, B.; Giacomantonio, M.; Marcato, P.; McFarland, S.; Pol, J.; Gujar, S. Dying to Be Noticed: Epigenetic Regulation of Immunogenic Cell Death for Cancer Immunotherapy. *Front. Immunol.* **2018**, *9*, 654. [CrossRef] [PubMed]

9. Bloy, N.; Garcia, P.; Laumont, C.M.; Pitt, J.M.; Sistigu, A.; Stoll, G.; Yamazaki, T.; Bonneil, E.; Buqué, A.; Humeau, J.; et al. Immunogenic Stress and Death of Cancer Cells: Contribution of Antigenicity vs Adjuvanticity to Immunosurveillance. *Immunol. Rev.* **2017**, *280*, 165–174. [CrossRef]
10. Portela, A.; Esteller, M. Epigenetic Modifications and Human Disease. *Nat. Biotechnol.* **2010**, *28*, 1057–1068. [CrossRef] [PubMed]
11. Fucikova, J.; Kepp, O.; Kasikova, L.; Petroni, G.; Yamazaki, T.; Liu, P.; Zhao, L.; Spisek, R.; Kroemer, G.; Galluzzi, L. Detection of Immunogenic Cell Death and Its Relevance for Cancer Therapy. *Cell Death Dis.* **2020**, *11*, 1013. [CrossRef] [PubMed]
12. Obeid, M.; Tesniere, A.; Ghiringhelli, F.; Fimia, G.M.; Apetoh, L.; Perfettini, J.-L.; Castedo, M.; Mignot, G.; Panaretakis, T.; Casares, N.; et al. Calreticulin Exposure Dictates the Immunogenicity of Cancer Cell Death. *Nat. Med.* **2007**, *13*, 54–61. [CrossRef]
13. Panaretakis, T.; Kepp, O.; Brockmeier, U.; Tesniere, A.; Bjorklund, A.-C.; Chapman, D.C.; Durchschlag, M.; Joza, N.; Pierron, G.; van Endert, P.; et al. Mechanisms of Pre-Apoptotic Calreticulin Exposure in Immunogenic Cell Death. *EMBO J.* **2009**, *28*, 578–590. [CrossRef]
14. Martins, I.; Wang, Y.; Michaud, M.; Ma, Y.; Sukkurwala, A.Q.; Shen, S.; Kepp, O.; Métivier, D.; Galluzzi, L.; Perfettini, J.-L.; et al. Molecular Mechanisms of ATP Secretion during Immunogenic Cell Death. *Cell Death Differ.* **2014**, *21*, 79–91. [CrossRef]
15. Aymeric, L.; Apetoh, L.; Ghiringhelli, F.; Tesniere, A.; Martins, I.; Kroemer, G.; Smyth, M.J.; Zitvogel, L. Tumor Cell Death and ATP Release Prime Dendritic Cells and Efficient Anticancer Immunity. *Cancer Res.* **2010**, *70*, 855–858. [CrossRef]
16. Ghiringhelli, F.; Apetoh, L.; Tesniere, A.; Aymeric, L.; Ma, Y.; Ortiz, C.; Vermaelen, K.; Panaretakis, T.; Mignot, G.; Ullrich, E.; et al. Activation of the NLRP3 Inflammasome in Dendritic Cells Induces IL-1beta-Dependent Adaptive Immunity against Tumors. *Nat. Med.* **2009**, *15*, 1170–1178. [CrossRef]
17. Sistigu, A.; Yamazaki, T.; Vacchelli, E.; Chaba, K.; Enot, D.P.; Adam, J.; Vitale, I.; Goubar, A.; Baracco, E.E.; Remédios, C.; et al. Cancer Cell-Autonomous Contribution of Type I Interferon Signaling to the Efficacy of Chemotherapy. *Nat. Med.* **2014**, *20*, 1301–1309. [CrossRef]
18. Lamberti, M.J.; Mentucci, F.M.; Roselli, E.; Araya, P.; Rivarola, V.A.; Rumie Vittar, N.B.; Maccioni, M. Photodynamic Modulation of Type 1 Interferon Pathway on Melanoma Cells Promotes Dendritic Cell Activation. *Front. Immunol.* **2019**, *10*, 2614. [CrossRef] [PubMed]
19. Spisek, R.; Charalambous, A.; Mazumder, A.; Vesole, D.H.; Jagannath, S.; Dhodapkar, M.V. Bortezomib Enhances Dendritic Cell (DC)-Mediated Induction of Immunity to Human Myeloma via Exposure of Cell Surface Heat Shock Protein 90 on Dying Tumor Cells: Therapeutic Implications. *Blood* **2007**, *109*, 4839–4845. [CrossRef]
20. Yamazaki, T.; Hannani, D.; Poirier-Colame, V.; Ladoire, S.; Locher, C.; Sistigu, A.; Prada, N.; Adjemian, S.; Catani, J.P.; Freudenberg, M.; et al. Defective Immunogenic Cell Death of HMGB1-Deficient Tumors: Compensatory Therapy with TLR4 Agonists. *Cell Death Differ.* **2014**, *21*, 69–78. [CrossRef]
21. Yatim, N.; Cullen, S.; Albert, M.L. Dying Cells Actively Regulate Adaptive Immune Responses. *Nat. Rev. Immunol.* **2017**, *17*, 262–275. [CrossRef] [PubMed]
22. Zelenay, S.; Reis e Sousa, C. Adaptive Immunity after Cell Death. *Trends Immunol.* **2013**, *34*, 329–335. [CrossRef] [PubMed]
23. Montico, B.; Nigro, A.; Casolaro, V.; Dal Col, J. Immunogenic Apoptosis as a Novel Tool for Anticancer Vaccine Development. *Int. J. Mol. Sci.* **2018**, *19*, 594. [CrossRef] [PubMed]
24. Denzler, R.; McGeary, S.E.; Title, A.C.; Agarwal, V.; Bartel, D.P.; Stoffel, M. Impact of MicroRNA Levels, Target-Site Complementarity, and Cooperativity on Competing Endogenous RNA-Regulated Gene Expression. *Mol. Cell* **2016**, *64*, 565–579. [CrossRef] [PubMed]
25. Ni, W.-J.; Leng, X.-M. Dynamic MiRNA-MRNA Paradigms: New Faces of MiRNAs. *Biochem. Biophys. Rep.* **2015**, *4*, 337–341. [CrossRef] [PubMed]
26. Hanahan, D.; Weinberg, R.A. Hallmarks of Cancer: The Next Generation. *Cell* **2011**, *144*, 646–674. [CrossRef] [PubMed]
27. Peng, Y.; Croce, C.M. The Role of MicroRNAs in Human Cancer. *Signal Transduct. Target. Ther.* **2016**, *1*, 15004. [CrossRef]
28. Barrey, E.; Saint-Auret, G.; Bonnamy, B.; Damas, D.; Boyer, O.; Gidrol, X. Pre-MicroRNA and Mature MicroRNA in Human Mitochondria. *PLoS ONE* **2011**, *6*, e20220. [CrossRef]
29. Valadi, H.; Ekström, K.; Bossios, A.; Sjöstrand, M.; Lee, J.J.; Lötvall, J.O. Exosome-Mediated Transfer of MRNAs and MicroRNAs Is a Novel Mechanism of Genetic Exchange between Cells. *Nat. Cell Biol.* **2007**, *9*, 654–659. [CrossRef]
30. Liang, H.; Zhang, J.; Zen, K.; Zhang, C.-Y.; Chen, X. Nuclear MicroRNAs and Their Unconventional Role in Regulating Non-Coding RNAs. *Protein Cell* **2013**, *4*, 325–330. [CrossRef]
31. Brümmer, A.; Hausser, J. MicroRNA Binding Sites in the Coding Region of MRNAs: Extending the Repertoire of Post-Transcriptional Gene Regulation. *Bioessays News Rev. Mol. Cell. Dev. Biol.* **2014**, *36*, 617–626. [CrossRef]
32. Lytle, J.R.; Yario, T.A.; Steitz, J.A. Target MRNAs Are Repressed as Efficiently by MicroRNA-Binding Sites in the 5′ UTR as in the 3′ UTR. *Proc. Natl. Acad. Sci. USA* **2007**, *104*, 9667–9672. [CrossRef] [PubMed]
33. Helwak, A.; Kudla, G.; Dudnakova, T.; Tollervey, D. Mapping the Human MiRNA Interactome by CLASH Reveals Frequent Noncanonical Binding. *Cell* **2013**, *153*, 654–665. [CrossRef]
34. Vasudevan, S.; Tong, Y.; Steitz, J.A. Switching from Repression to Activation: MicroRNAs Can up-Regulate Translation. *Science* **2007**, *318*, 1931–1934. [CrossRef] [PubMed]
35. Yoon, J.-H.; Abdelmohsen, K.; Gorospe, M. Functional Interactions among MicroRNAs and Long Noncoding RNAs. *Semin. Cell Dev. Biol.* **2014**, *34*, 9–14. [CrossRef]

36. Shirjang, S.; Mansoori, B.; Asghari, S.; Duijf, P.H.G.; Mohammadi, A.; Gjerstorff, M.; Baradaran, B. MicroRNAs in Cancer Cell Death Pathways: Apoptosis and Necroptosis. *Free Radic. Biol. Med.* **2019**, *139*, 1–15. [CrossRef]
37. Shan, C.; Chen, X.; Cai, H.; Hao, X.; Li, J.; Zhang, Y.; Gao, J.; Zhou, Z.; Li, X.; Liu, C.; et al. The Emerging Roles of Autophagy-Related MicroRNAs in Cancer. *Int. J. Biol. Sci.* **2021**, *17*, 134–150. [CrossRef] [PubMed]
38. Thomson, D.W.; Bracken, C.P.; Goodall, G.J. Experimental Strategies for MicroRNA Target Identification. *Nucleic Acids Res.* **2011**, *39*, 6845–6853. [CrossRef]
39. Ding, C.; Yu, H.; Shi, C.; Shi, T.; Qin, H.; Cui, Y. MiR-Let-7e Inhibits Invasion and Magration and Regulates HMGB1 Expression in Papillary Thyroid Carcinoma. *Biomed. Pharmacother.* **2019**, *110*, 528–536. [CrossRef]
40. Ai, H.; Zhou, W.; Wang, Z.; Qiong, G.; Chen, Z.; Deng, S. MicroRNAs-107 Inhibited Autophagy, Proliferation, and Migration of Breast Cancer Cells by Targeting HMGB1. *J. Cell. Biochem.* **2019**, *120*, 8696–8705. [CrossRef]
41. Li, Y.; Qin, C. MiR-1179 Inhibits the Proliferation of Gastric Cancer Cells by Targeting HMGB1. *Hum. Cell* **2019**, *32*, 352–359. [CrossRef]
42. Chen, J.; Li, G. MiR-1284 Enhances Sensitivity of Cervical Cancer Cells to Cisplatin via Downregulating HMGB1. *Biomed. Pharmacother.* **2018**, *107*, 997–1003. [CrossRef]
43. Luo, J.; Chen, J.; He, L. Mir-129-5p Attenuates Irradiation-Induced Autophagy and Decreases Radioresistance of Breast Cancer Cells by Targeting HMGB1. *Med. Sci. Monit.* **2015**, *21*, 4122–4129. [CrossRef] [PubMed]
44. Shi, Y.; Gong, W.; Lu, L.; Wang, Y.; Ren, J. Upregulation of MiR-129-5p Increases the Sensitivity to Taxol through Inhibiting HMGB1-Mediated Cell Autophagy in Breast Cancer MCF-7 Cells. *Braz. J. Med. Biol. Res.* **2019**, *52*, e8657. [CrossRef]
45. Wu, Q.; Meng, W.-Y.; Jie, Y.; Zhao, H. LncRNA MALAT1 Induces Colon Cancer Development by Regulating MiR-129-5p/HMGB1 Axis. *J. Cell. Physiol.* **2018**, *233*, 6750–6757. [CrossRef] [PubMed]
46. Feng, J.; Guo, J. MiR-129-5p Inhibits Proliferation of Gastric Cancer Cells through Targeted Inhibition on HMGB1 Expression. *Eur. Rev. Med. Pharmacol. Sci.* **2020**, *24*, 3665–3673. [PubMed]
47. Wang, S.; Chen, Y.; Yu, X.; Lu, Y.; Wang, H.; Wu, F.; Teng, L. MiR-129-5p Attenuates Cell Proliferation and Epithelial Mesenchymal Transition via HMGB1 in Gastric Cancer. *Pathol. Res. Pract.* **2019**, *215*, 676–682. [CrossRef]
48. Zhang, D.; Cao, J.; Zhong, Q.; Zeng, L.; Cai, C.; Lei, L.; Zhang, W.; Liu, F. Long Noncoding RNA PCAT-1 Promotes Invasion and Metastasis via the MiR-129-5p-HMGB1 Signaling Pathway in Hepatocellular Carcinoma. *Biomed. Pharmacother.* **2017**, *95*, 1187–1193. [CrossRef] [PubMed]
49. Liu, K.; Huang, J.; Ni, J.; Song, D.; Ding, M.; Wang, J.; Huang, X.; Li, W. MALAT1 Promotes Osteosarcoma Development by Regulation of HMGB1 via MiR-142-3p and MiR-129-5p. *Cell Cycle* **2017**, *16*, 578–587. [CrossRef]
50. Zhang, R.; Jin, H.; Lou, F. The Long Non-Coding RNA TP73-AS1 Interacted With MiR-142 to Modulate Brain Glioma Growth Through HMGB1/RAGE Pathway. *J. Cell. Biochem.* **2018**, *119*, 3007–3016. [CrossRef]
51. Chen, Y.; Zhou, X.; Qiao, J.; Bao, A. MiR-142-3p Overexpression Increases Chemo-Sensitivity of NSCLC by Inhibiting HMGB1-Mediated Autophagy. *Cell. Physiol. Biochem.* **2017**, *41*, 1370–1382. [CrossRef]
52. Xiao, P.; Liu, W.-L. MiR-142-3p Functions as a Potential Tumor Suppressor Directly Targeting HMGB1 in Non-Small-Cell Lung Carcinoma. *Int. J. Clin. Exp. Pathol.* **2015**, *8*, 10800–10807.
53. MacKenzie, T.N.; Mujumdar, N.; Banerjee, S.; Sangwan, V.; Sarver, A.; Vickers, S.; Subramanian, S.; Saluja, A.K. Triptolide Induces the Expression of MiR-142-3p: A Negative Regulator of Heat Shock Protein 70 and Pancreatic Cancer Cell Proliferation. *Mol. Cancer Ther.* **2013**, *12*, 1266–1275. [CrossRef] [PubMed]
54. Lu, F.; Zhang, J.; Ji, M.; Li, P.; Du, Y.; Wang, H.; Zang, S.; Ma, D.; Sun, X.; Ji, C. MiR-181b Increases Drug Sensitivity in Acute Myeloid Leukemia via Targeting HMGB1 and Mcl-1. *Int. J. Oncol.* **2014**, *45*, 383–392. [CrossRef] [PubMed]
55. Wu, H.; Zhou, C. Long Non-Coding RNA UCA1 Promotes Lung Cancer Cell Proliferation and Migration via MicroRNA-193a/HMGB1 Axis. *Biochem. Biophys. Res. Commun.* **2018**, *496*, 738–745. [CrossRef] [PubMed]
56. Li, S.; Huang, Y.; Huang, Y.; Fu, Y.; Tang, D.; Kang, R.; Zhou, R.; Fan, X. The Long Non-Coding RNA TP73-AS1 Modulates HCC Cell Proliferation through MiR-200a-Dependent HMGB1/RAGE Regulation. *J. Exp. Clin. Cancer Res.* **2017**, *36*, 51. [CrossRef]
57. Chang, B.; Wang, D.; Xing, J.; Yang, S.; Chu, Q.; Yu, S. MiR-200c Inhibits Metastasis of Breast Cancer Cells by Targeting HMGB1. *J. Huazhong Univ. Sci. Technol. Med. Sci.* **2014**, *34*, 201–206. [CrossRef] [PubMed]
58. Liu, P.-L.; Liu, W.-L.; Chang, J.-M.; Chen, Y.-H.; Liu, Y.-P.; Kuo, H.-F.; Hsieh, C.-C.; Ding, Y.-S.; Chen, W.-W.; Chong, I.-W. MicroRNA-200c Inhibits Epithelial-Mesenchymal Transition, Invasion, and Migration of Lung Cancer by Targeting HMGB1. *PLoS ONE* **2017**, *12*, e0180844. [CrossRef]
59. Wang, L.; Kang, F.; Wang, J.; Yang, C.; He, D. Downregulation of MiR-205 Contributes to Epithelial–Mesenchymal Transition and Invasion in Triple-Negative Breast Cancer by Targeting HMGB1–RAGE Signaling Pathway. *Anticancer Drugs* **2019**, *30*, 225–232. [CrossRef]
60. Ran, X.; Yang, J.; Liu, C.; Zhou, P.; Xiao, L.; Zhang, K. MiR-218 Inhibits HMGB1-Mediated Autophagy in Endometrial Carcinoma Cells during Chemotherapy. *Int. J. Clin. Exp. Pathol.* **2015**, *8*, 6617–6626. [PubMed]
61. Zhang, C.; Ge, S.; Hu, C.; Yang, N.; Zhang, J. MiRNA-218, a New Regulator of HMGB1, Suppresses Cell Migration and Invasion in Non-Small Cell Lung Cancer. *Acta Biochim. Biophys. Sin.* **2013**, *45*, 1055–1061. [CrossRef]
62. Zhang, G.; He, X.; Ren, C.; Lin, J.; Wang, Q. Long Noncoding RNA PCA3 Regulates Prostate Cancer through Sponging MiR-218-5p and Modulating High Mobility Group Box 1. *J. Cell. Physiol.* **2019**, *234*, 13097–13109. [CrossRef] [PubMed]

63. Li, G.; Cai, M.; Fu, D.; Chen, K.; Sun, M.; Cai, Z.; Cheng, B. Heat Shock Protein 90B1 Plays an Oncogenic Role and Is a Target of MicroRNA-223 in Human Osteosarcoma. *Cell. Physiol. Biochem.* **2012**, *30*, 1481–1490. [CrossRef]
64. Tang, Q.; Yuan, Q.; Li, H.; Wang, W.; Xie, G.; Zhu, K.; Li, D. MiR-223/Hsp70/JNK/JUN/MiR-223 Feedback Loop Modulates the Chemoresistance of Osteosarcoma to Cisplatin. *Biochem. Biophys. Res. Commun.* **2018**, *497*, 827–834. [CrossRef]
65. Lv, G.; Wu, M.; Wang, M.; Jiang, X.; Du, J.; Zhang, K.; Li, D.; Ma, N.; Peng, Y.; Wang, L.; et al. MiR-320a Regulates High Mobility Group Box 1 Expression and Inhibits Invasion and Metastasis in Hepatocellular Carcinoma. *Liver Int.* **2017**, *37*, 1354–1364. [CrossRef] [PubMed]
66. Yao, S.; Zhao, T.; Jin, H. Expression of MicroRNA-325-3p and Its Potential Functions by Targeting HMGB1 in Non-Small Cell Lung Cancer. *Biomed. Pharmacother.* **2015**, *70*, 72–79. [CrossRef]
67. Colangelo, T.; Polcaro, G.; Ziccardi, P.; Pucci, B.; Muccillo, L.; Galgani, M.; Fucci, A.; Milone, M.R.; Budillon, A.; Santopaolo, M.; et al. Proteomic Screening Identifies Calreticulin as a MiR-27a Direct Target Repressing MHC Class I Cell Surface Exposure in Colorectal Cancer. *Cell Death Dis.* **2016**, *7*, e2120. [CrossRef]
68. Colangelo, T.; Polcaro, G.; Ziccardi, P.; Muccillo, L.; Galgani, M.; Pucci, B.; Rita Milone, M.; Budillon, A.; Santopaolo, M.; Mazzoccoli, G.; et al. The MiR-27a-Calreticulin Axis Affects Drug-Induced Immunogenic Cell Death in Human Colorectal Cancer Cells. *Cell Death Dis.* **2016**, *7*, e2108. [CrossRef]
69. Dong, Z.; Yang, P.; Qiu, X.; Liang, S.; Guan, B.; Yang, H.; Li, F.; Sun, L.; Liu, H.; Zou, G.; et al. KCNQ1OT1 Facilitates Progression of Non-small-cell Lung Carcinoma via Modulating MiRNA-27b-3p/HSP90AA1 Axis. *J. Cell. Physiol.* **2019**, *234*, 11304–11314. [CrossRef]
70. Liu, K.; Huang, J.; Xie, M.; Yu, Y.; Zhu, S.; Kang, R.; Cao, L.; Tang, D.; Duan, X. MIR34A Regulates Autophagy and Apoptosis by Targeting HMGB1 in the Retinoblastoma Cell. *Autophagy* **2014**, *10*, 442–452. [CrossRef]
71. Chandrasekaran, K.S.; Sathyanarayanan, A.; Karunagaran, D. Downregulation of HMGB1 by MiR-34a Is Sufficient to Suppress Proliferation, Migration and Invasion of Human Cervical and Colorectal Cancer Cells. *Tumor Biol.* **2016**, *37*, 13155–13166. [CrossRef]
72. Li, S.; Luo, C.; Zhou, J.; Zhang, Y. MicroRNA-34a Directly Targets High-mobility Group Box 1 and Inhibits the Cancer Cell Proliferation, Migration and Invasion in Cutaneous Squamous Cell Carcinoma. *Exp. Ther. Med.* **2017**, *14*, 5611–5618. [CrossRef] [PubMed]
73. Xu, D.; Dong, P.; Xiong, Y.; Yue, J.; Konno, Y.; Ihira, K.; Kobayashi, N.; Todo, Y.; Watari, H. MicroRNA-361-Mediated Inhibition of HSP90 Expression and EMT in Cervical Cancer Is Counteracted by Oncogenic LncRNA NEAT1. *Cells* **2020**, *9*, 632. [CrossRef] [PubMed]
74. Wu, D.; Liu, J.; Chen, J.; He, H.; Ma, H.; Lv, X. MiR-449a Suppresses Tumor Growth, Migration, and Invasion in Non-Small Cell Lung Cancer by Targeting a HMGB1-Mediated NF-KB Signaling Pathway. *Oncol. Res. Featur. Preclin. Clin. Cancer Ther.* **2019**, *27*, 227–235. [CrossRef]
75. Tian, L.; Wang, Z.; Hao, J.; Zhang, X. MiR-505 Acts as a Tumor Suppressor in Gastric Cancer Progression through Targeting HMGB1. *J. Cell. Biochem.* **2019**, *120*, 8044–8052. [CrossRef] [PubMed]
76. Lu, L.; Qiu, C.; Li, D.; Bai, G.; Liang, J.; Yang, Q. MicroRNA-505 Suppresses Proliferation and Invasion in Hepatoma Cells by Directly Targeting High-Mobility Group Box 1. *Life Sci.* **2016**, *157*, 12–18. [CrossRef] [PubMed]
77. Lu, L.; Zhang, D.; Xu, Y.; Bai, G.; Lv, Y.; Liang, J. MiR-505 Enhances Doxorubicin-Induced Cytotoxicity in Hepatocellular Carcinoma through Repressing the Akt Pathway by Directly Targeting HMGB1. *Biomed. Pharmacother.* **2018**, *104*, 613–621. [CrossRef]
78. Liu, Y.-J.; Li, W.; Chang, F.; Liu, J.-N.; Lin, J.-X.; Chen, D.-X. MicroRNA-505 Is Downregulated in Human Osteosarcoma and Regulates Cell Proliferation, Migration and Invasion. *Oncol. Rep.* **2017**, *39*, 491–500. [CrossRef]
79. Ye, Y.; Zhao, L.; Li, Q.; Xi, C.; Li, Y.; Li, Z. Circ_0007385 Served as Competing Endogenous for MiR-519d-3p to Suppress Malignant Behaviors and Cisplatin Resistance of Non-small Cell Lung Cancer Cells. *Thorac. Cancer* **2020**, *11*, 2196–2208. [CrossRef]
80. Yun, Z.; Meng, F.; Jiang, P.; Yue, M.; Li, S. MicroRNA-548b Suppresses Aggressive Phenotypes of Hepatocellular Carcinoma by Directly Targeting High-Mobility Group Box 1 MRNA. *Cancer Manag. Res.* **2019**, *11*, 5821–5834. [CrossRef]
81. Pan, J.; Jiang, F.; Zhou, J.; Wu, D.; Sheng, Z.; Li, M. HSP90: A Novel Target Gene of MiRNA-628-3p in A549 Cells. *BioMed Res. Int.* **2018**, *2018*, 1–10. [CrossRef]
82. Wang, S.; Du, S.; Lv, Y.; Zhang, F.; Wang, W. MicroRNA-665 Inhibits the Oncogenicity of Retinoblastoma by Directly Targeting High-Mobility Group Box 1 and Inactivating the Wnt/β-Catenin Pathway. *Cancer Manag. Res.* **2019**, *11*, 3111–3123. [CrossRef]
83. Kwon, M.S.; Park, C.S.; Choi, K.; Ahnn, J.; Kim, J.I.; Eom, S.H.; Kaufman, S.J.; Song, W.K. Calreticulin Couples Calcium Release and Calcium Influx in Integrin-Mediated Calcium Signaling. *Mol. Biol. Cell* **2000**, *11*, 1433–1443. [CrossRef]
84. Wang, W.-A.; Groenendyk, J.; Michalak, M. Calreticulin Signaling in Health and Disease. *Int. J. Biochem. Cell Biol.* **2012**, *44*, 842–846. [CrossRef]
85. Yan, X.; Yu, H.; Liu, Y.; Hou, J.; Yang, Q.; Zhao, Y. MiR-27a-3p Functions as a Tumor Suppressor and Regulates Non-Small Cell Lung Cancer Cell Proliferation via Targeting HOXB8. *Technol. Cancer Res. Treat.* **2019**, *18*, 1533033819861971. [CrossRef]
86. Tang, H.; Xu, X.; Xiao, W.; Liao, Y.; Xiao, X.; Li, L.; Li, K.; Jia, X.; Feng, H. Silencing of MicroRNA-27a Facilitates Autophagy and Apoptosis of Melanoma Cells through the Activation of the SYK-Dependent MTOR Signaling Pathway. *J. Cell. Biochem.* **2019**, *120*, 13262–13274. [CrossRef]

87. Li, J.-M.; Zhou, J.; Xu, Z.; Huang, H.-J.; Chen, M.-J.; Ji, J.-S. MicroRNA-27a-3p Inhibits Cell Viability and Migration through down-Regulating DUSP16 in Hepatocellular Carcinoma. *J. Cell. Biochem.* **2018**, *119*, 5143–5152. [CrossRef]
88. Xu, C.; Cheng, H.; Li, N.; Zhou, N.; Tang, X. Relationship between MicroRNA-27a and Efficacy of Neoadjuvant Chemotherapy in Gastric Cancer and Its Mechanism in Gastric Cancer Cell Growth and Metastasis. *Biosci. Rep.* **2019**, *39*. [CrossRef]
89. Mu, Y.; Zhang, L.; Chen, X.; Chen, S.; Shi, Y.; Li, J. Silencing MicroRNA-27a Inhibits Proliferation and Invasion of Human Osteosarcoma Cells through the SFRP1-Dependent Wnt/β-Catenin Signaling Pathway. *Biosci. Rep.* **2019**, *39*. [CrossRef] [PubMed]
90. Ciocca, D.R.; Calderwood, S.K. Heat Shock Proteins in Cancer: Diagnostic, Prognostic, Predictive, and Treatment Implications. *Cell Stress Chaperones* **2005**, *10*, 86–103. [CrossRef]
91. Binder, R.J. Functions of Heat Shock Proteins in Pathways of the Innate and Adaptive Immune System. *J. Immunol.* **2014**, *193*, 5765–5771. [CrossRef] [PubMed]
92. Garrido, C.; Gurbuxani, S.; Ravagnan, L.; Kroemer, G. Heat Shock Proteins: Endogenous Modulators of Apoptotic Cell Death. *Biochem. Biophys. Res. Commun.* **2001**, *286*, 433–442. [CrossRef]
93. Rodríguez, M.E.; Cogno, I.S.; Milla Sanabria, L.S.; Morán, Y.S.; Rivarola, V.A. Heat Shock Proteins in the Context of Photodynamic Therapy: Autophagy, Apoptosis and Immunogenic Cell Death. *Photochem. Photobiol. Sci. Off. J. Eur. Photochem. Assoc. Eur. Soc. Photobiol.* **2016**, *15*, 1090–1102. [CrossRef]
94. He, S.-J.; Cheng, J.; Feng, X.; Yu, Y.; Tian, L.; Huang, Q. The Dual Role and Therapeutic Potential of High-Mobility Group Box 1 in Cancer. *Oncotarget* **2017**, *8*, 64534–64550. [CrossRef] [PubMed]
95. Kang, R.; Zhang, Q.; Zeh, H.J.; Lotze, M.T.; Tang, D. HMGB1 in Cancer: Good, Bad, or Both? *Clin. Cancer Res. Off. J. Am. Assoc. Cancer Res.* **2013**, *19*, 4046–4057. [CrossRef]
96. Liu, L.; Ren, W.; Chen, K. MiR-34a Promotes Apoptosis and Inhibits Autophagy by Targeting HMGB1 in Acute Myeloid Leukemia Cells. *Cell. Physiol. Biochem.* **2017**, *41*, 1981–1992. [CrossRef]
97. Ratti, M.; Lampis, A.; Ghidini, M.; Salati, M.; Mirchev, M.B.; Valeri, N.; Hahne, J.C. MicroRNAs (MiRNAs) and Long Non-Coding RNAs (LncRNAs) as New Tools for Cancer Therapy: First Steps from Bench to Bedside. *Target. Oncol.* **2020**, *15*, 261–278. [CrossRef]
98. Acunzo, M.; Romano, G.; Wernicke, D.; Croce, C.M. MicroRNA and Cancer–a Brief Overview. *Adv. Biol. Regul.* **2015**, *57*, 1–9. [CrossRef]
99. Yang, L.; Yu, Y.; Kang, R.; Yang, M.; Xie, M.; Wang, Z.; Tang, D.; Zhao, M.; Liu, L.; Zhang, H.; et al. Up-Regulated Autophagy by Endogenous High Mobility Group Box-1 Promotes Chemoresistance in Leukemia Cells. *Leuk. Lymphoma* **2012**, *53*, 315–322. [CrossRef] [PubMed]
100. Costa, D.F.; Torchilin, V.P. Micelle-like Nanoparticles as SiRNA and MiRNA Carriers for Cancer Therapy. *Biomed. Microdevices* **2018**, *20*, 59. [CrossRef] [PubMed]
101. Phung, C.D.; Nguyen, H.T.; Choi, J.Y.; Pham, T.T.; Acharya, S.; Timilshina, M.; Chang, J.-H.; Kim, J.-H.; Jeong, J.-H.; Ku, S.K.; et al. Reprogramming the T Cell Response to Cancer by Simultaneous, Nanoparticle-Mediated PD-L1 Inhibition and Immunogenic Cell Death. *J. Control. Release* **2019**, *315*, 126–138. [CrossRef] [PubMed]
102. Harris, J.M.; Chess, R.B. Effect of Pegylation on Pharmaceuticals. *Nat. Rev. Drug Discov.* **2003**, *2*, 214–221. [CrossRef]
103. Zwicke, G.L.; Mansoori, G.A.; Jeffery, C.J. Utilizing the Folate Receptor for Active Targeting of Cancer Nanotherapeutics. *Nano Rev.* **2012**, *3*, 18496. [CrossRef] [PubMed]
104. Wang, L.; Liang, T.-T. CD59 Receptor Targeted Delivery of MiRNA-1284 and Cisplatin-Loaded Liposomes for Effective Therapeutic Efficacy against Cervical Cancer Cells. *AMB Express* **2020**, *10*, 54. [CrossRef]
105. Afshar-Kharghan, V. The Role of the Complement System in Cancer. *J. Clin. Investig.* **2017**, *127*, 780–789. [CrossRef] [PubMed]
106. Unlu, S.; Tang, S.; Na Wang, E.; Martinez, I.; Tang, D.; Bianchi, M.E.; Iii, H.J.Z.; Lotze, M.T. Damage Associated Molecular Pattern Molecule-Induced MicroRNAs (DAMPmiRs) in Human Peripheral Blood Mononuclear Cells. *PLoS ONE* **2012**, *7*, e38899. [CrossRef]
107. Frank, A.C.; Ebersberger, S.; Fink, A.F.; Lampe, S.; Weigert, A.; Schmid, T.; Ebersberger, I.; Syed, S.N.; Brüne, B. Apoptotic Tumor Cell-Derived MicroRNA-375 Uses CD36 to Alter the Tumor-Associated Macrophage Phenotype. *Nat. Commun.* **2019**, *10*, 1135. [CrossRef]
108. Fabbri, M.; Paone, A.; Calore, F.; Galli, R.; Gaudio, E.; Santhanam, R.; Lovat, F.; Fadda, P.; Mao, C.; Nuovo, G.J.; et al. MicroRNAs Bind to Toll-like Receptors to Induce Prometastatic Inflammatory Response. *Proc. Natl. Acad. Sci. USA* **2012**, *109*, E2110–E2116. [CrossRef]
109. Lee, J.; Lee, Y.; Xu, L.; White, R.; Sullenger, B.A. Differential Induction of Immunogenic Cell Death and Interferon Expression in Cancer Cells by Structured SsRNAs. *Mol. Ther. J. Am. Soc. Gene Ther.* **2017**, *25*, 1295–1305. [CrossRef]
110. Ogino, S.; Nowak, J.A.; Hamada, T.; Phipps, A.I.; Peters, U.; Milner, D.A.; Giovannucci, E.L.; Nishihara, R.; Giannakis, M.; Garrett, W.S.; et al. Integrative Analysis of Exogenous, Endogenous, Tumour and Immune Factors for Precision Medicine. *Gut* **2018**, *67*, 1168–1180. [CrossRef] [PubMed]
111. Ogino, S.; Nowak, J.A.; Hamada, T.; Milner, D.A.; Nishihara, R. Insights into Pathogenic Interactions Among Environment, Host, and Tumor at the Crossroads of Molecular Pathology and Epidemiology. *Annu. Rev. Pathol.* **2019**, *14*, 83–103. [CrossRef]

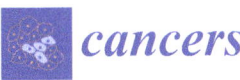

Review

The Functional Crosstalk between Myeloid-Derived Suppressor Cells and Regulatory T Cells within the Immunosuppressive Tumor Microenvironment

Maximilian Haist *, Henner Stege, Stephan Grabbe and Matthias Bros

Department of Dermatology, University Medical Center of the Johannes Gutenberg University, 55131 Mainz, Germany; Henner.Stege@unimedizin-mainz.de (H.S.); stephan.grabbe@unimedizin-mainz.de (S.G.); mbros@uni-mainz.de (M.B.)
* Correspondence: Maximilian.Haist@unimedizin-mainz.de; Tel.: +49-6131-17-8793

Simple Summary: Immunotherapy improved the therapeutic landscape for patients with advanced cancer diseases. However, many patients do not benefit from immunotherapy. The bidirectional crosstalk between myeloid-derived suppressor cells (MDSC) and regulatory T cells (Treg) contributes to immune evasion, limiting the success of immunotherapy by checkpoint inhibitors. This review aims to outline the current knowledge of the role and the immunosuppressive properties of MDSC and Treg within the tumor microenvironment (TME). Furthermore, we will discuss the importance of the functional crosstalk between MDSC and Treg for immunosuppression, issuing particularly the role of cell adhesion molecules. Lastly, we will depict the impact of this interaction for cancer research and discuss several strategies aimed to target these pathways for tumor therapy.

Abstract: Immune checkpoint inhibitors (ICI) have led to profound and durable tumor regression in some patients with metastatic cancer diseases. However, many patients still do not derive benefit from immunotherapy. Here, the accumulation of immunosuppressive cell populations within the tumor microenvironment (TME), such as myeloid-derived suppressor cells (MDSC), tumor-associated macrophages (TAM), and regulatory T cells (Treg), contributes to the development of immune resistance. MDSC and Treg expand systematically in tumor patients and inhibit T cell activation and T effector cell function. Numerous studies have shown that the immunosuppressive mechanisms exerted by those inhibitory cell populations comprise soluble immunomodulatory mediators and receptor interactions. The latter are also required for the crosstalk of MDSC and Treg, raising questions about the relevance of cell–cell contacts for the establishment of their inhibitory properties. This review aims to outline the current knowledge on the crosstalk between these two cell populations, issuing particularly the potential role of cell adhesion molecules. In this regard, we further discuss the relevance of β2 integrins, which are essential for the differentiation and function of leukocytes as well as for MDSC–Treg interaction. Lastly, we aim to describe the impact of such bidirectional crosstalk for basic and applied cancer research and discuss how the targeting of these pathways might pave the way for future approaches in immunotherapy.

Keywords: myeloid-derived suppressor cells; regulatory T cells; crosstalk; tumor microenvironment; tumor immune evasion; immunotherapy; cell–cell contact; β2 integrins; CD18; CD11

1. Introduction

Immunotherapy with immune checkpoint inhibitors (ICI) has emerged as a promising treatment for many different types of cancer [1], since it has demonstrated stable and impressive tumor regressions even at an advanced stage of disease [1]. However, a large number of cancer patients do not derive benefit from ICI therapy, which is presumably due to an intrinsic or acquired resistance [2]. Increasing evidence suggests that an immunologically active TME is an important predictor for the therapeutic responsiveness toward ICI. Here, it has been demonstrated that both tumor-related factors, e.g., a high mutational load of the tumor cells [3,4], the presence of neoantigens [5,6], microsatellite instability [7,8], and host factors, i.e., the frequency, composition, and activation status [9,10] of tumor-infiltrating lymphocytes (TIL), are predictive for the responsiveness toward ICI treatment. Particularly referring to the activation status of TIL, it has been documented that the extent of programmed cell death 1 ligand 1 (PD-L1) expression on tumor cells correlates with objective response rates in melanoma and non-small cell lung cancer [11–13]. Hence, PD-L1 expression levels are also applied in the clinical setting to optimize patient stratification prior to the introduction of ICI therapy. However, both the extent of cytotoxic T-lymphocyte (CTL) infiltration into the tumor and PD-L1 expression on tumor cells do not always correlate with clinical benefit [14]. So far, the various immunosuppressive mechanisms, being present both locally within the tumor microenvironment (TME) and in lymphoid organs, have been identified as major factors mediating immune resistance [15]. Next to the immunosuppressive effects conferred by soluble mediators and leukocyte receptor interactions, the extensive infiltration of the tumor by immunosuppressive cell populations, such as tumor-associated macrophages (TAM) [16,17], myeloid-derived suppressor cells (MDSC) [18], and regulatory T cells (Treg) [19,20], has been identified as a major driver of the pro-tumorigenic transformation in the TME. The presence of these immunosuppressive cells hampers effector T cell induction and recruitment as well as the capability of both natural killer (NK) cells and antigen-presenting cells (APC) to exert effective tumor surveillance, consequently leading to a profound inhibition of the anti-tumor immune response [21]. Thus, the understanding of this immunosuppressive network mediating tumor immune evasion, via cell–cell interactions and by the secretion of soluble immunomodulatory mediators, is essential for the development of novel strategies overcoming immune resistance in cancer treatment.

Recent observations in different cancer models suggest a crosstalk between MDSC and Treg, but its character remains incompletely defined [21–23]. As the crosstalk between MDSC and Treg has recently been proposed to be a powerful barrier counter-acting antitumoral immune responses, this review is dedicated to give insights into the potential role of cell–cell contacts as a prerequisite for the immunosuppressive mechanisms in the TME, leading to tumor immune evasion. This in consequence facilitates cancer progression and the development of metastases [24].

Furthermore, we aim to delineate the relevance of metabolic pathways and soluble mediators for the functional interaction of MDSC and Treg, according to the current state of scientific research. Since β2 integrins are known to be key regulators of cell adhesion and cell signaling, they are essential for immune cell functions [25]. Accordingly, β2 integrins may constitute potential mediators of the crosstalk between MDSC and Treg [26]. Hence, this review additionally aims to outline the potential role of β2 integrins in this critical cell–cell interaction within an immunosuppressive TME.

2. The Immunosuppressive TME

The TME is a complex milieu being composed of a heterogeneous assemblage of distinct tumor—and host cell types such as cancer-associated fibroblasts (CAF), endothelial cells, pericytes, and immune cells that constitute the tumor parenchyma and tumor stroma [14,27]. These various cell types exhibit an extensive crosstalk that dynamically regulates the phenotype and function of the individual cells within the TME. This allows the establishment of a chronic pro-inflammatory state that favors the establishment of a tumor-supportive microenvironment [14,28–30]. Thus, it is increasingly evident that the crosstalk between cancer cells and cells of the neoplastic stroma in the TME enables tumor cells to evade host immunosurveillance and thereby supports tumor growth, progression, and metastasis [14,31]. Moreover, the regulatory signaling conveyed by soluble mediators and cell–cell interactions is considered essential in controlling the individual cell function and orchestrating the collective activity within the tumor network [14].

2.1. Immunomodulatory Mediators Shape the TME

In the context of immunotherapy, the mutual interactions of tumor-infiltrating immune cells have become an increasingly important area of research, as these cells shape the unique properties of the TME [2]. The tumor-infiltrating immune cells include both tumor-promoting as well as tumor-killing subclasses [14]. Here, it has been shown that tumor infiltration by T cells (mainly CTL) and NK cells correlates with overall prognosis and with the response to ICI treatment [32]. However, in the course of tumor development, a chronic inflammatory state is frequently being induced, which includes the elevation of pro-inflammatory mediators, the infiltration of regulatory immune cells, and the recruitment of endothelial cells and fibroblasts [30,33]. The accumulation of both pro-inflammatory mediators, including cytokines (e.g., interleukin (IL-1, IL-6); tumor-necrosis-factor-alpha, (TNF-α)), chemokines (CC-chemokine ligand 2 (CCL2), and C-X-C motif ligand 2; (CXCL-2)), prostaglandines (prostaglandine E2 (PGE2)) and growth factors (e.g., transforming growth factor-β (TGF-β), granulocyte-macrophage colony-stimulating factor (GM-CSF)), orchestrate the crosstalk between the various cells within the TME. In concert with these soluble mediators, cell–cell-based interactions such as the programmed death protein (PD)-1/PD-ligand (L)-1 axis contribute to the intense crosstalk between the immunosuppressive cell populations, subsequently enhancing the tumor-supporting capacity of the TME, which tips the scale toward immunosuppression and tumor angiogenesis [30]. Altogether, these mechanisms antagonize the cancer-directed immune responses and effectively impair the lytic machinery of TIL in the TME [24,34].

2.2. Cellular Composition of the TME

Notably, MDSC, TAM, and Treg are the major cellular components of the immunosuppressive TME. It has been demonstrated that the release of pro-inflammatory cytokines within the TME promotes the immunosuppressive potential of regulatory myeloid cells, such as tumor-associated neutrophils (TAN) [35–37], TAM [27,33,38–40], MDSC [28,41,42] and regulatory dendritic cells (DC) [43–45]. Consequently, a strong tumor infiltration by myeloid cells—being the most abundant cell types within the TME [46]—correlates with rapid tumor growth and a poor prognosis [32]. Here, TAM primarily serves to promote tumor growth and progression via the generation of angiogenetic factors such as vascular endothelial growth factor (VEGF), and the secretion of immunomodulatory cytokines (e.g., IL-6, IL8 and IL-10) [38]. These cytokines generated by TAM and tumor cells promote an aberrant activation of myelopoiesis, resulting in a defective differentiation of myeloid progenitor cells toward MDSC, which exert a strong pro-tumor activity [46,47]. In particular, it has been shown that MDSC suppress both CTL and NK cell activity via immunomodulatory mediators, including IL-1, IL-6, reactive oxygen species (ROS), and nitric oxide (NO) [14,48–50]. Hence, the proliferation, activation, and retention of highly immunosuppressive MDSC are not only induced by the chronic inflammatory state within the TME, but it further enhances these conditions, thus creating a positive feedback loop [34,51]. In this context, recent studies revealed that MDSC can modulate the de novo induction, development, and activation of Treg, thus further amplifying the immunosuppressive character in the TME [24]. CD4$^+$CD25^{hi} Forkhead-Box-Protein P3 (FoxP3)$^+$ Treg cells are frequently found in the course of tumor progression and counteract APC activity, T cell activation, and anti-tumor functions of effector T cells (Teff) [24,52]. Therefore, similar to MDSC, clinical reports confirmed a negative correlation between the frequency of Treg, the patient's individual prognosis, and the response to ICI treatment [24].

Next to their direct immunosuppressive effects, MDSC and Treg implicitly contribute to the establishment of a TME being characterized by hypoxia, the accumulation of lactic acid, and adenosine (ADO). These factors prevent APC maturation, impair Teff functions, and thus counteract the tumoricidal functions of activated immune effector cells [14,24,46,53]. Since MDSC and Treg systemically expand in the course of tumor development and strongly impair T cell driven anti-tumor immune responses, a detailed characterization of the phenotype and immunosuppressive functions of these cells will be provided in the following section.

3. Myeloid-Derived Suppressor Cells

Immature myeloid cells, which are generated in the bone marrow (BM) of healthy individuals in response to acute infection, stress, or trauma, regularly differentiate into mature myeloid cells, such as polymorphonuclear neutrophils (PMN) and monocytes, without exerting immunosuppression [49]. In contrast, neoplastic cells, tumor-associated stroma cells, and a frequently observed inflammation within the TME favor the aberrant activation of myelopoiesis that results in the expansion and recruitment of immature myeloid cells to the tumor site [50]. Indeed, a prominent effect of this "tumor-driven macroenvironment" is the accumulation of highly suppressive, immature myeloid cells in the tumor. Owing to their common myeloid origin and suppressive properties, these cells were termed MDSC.

3.1. MDSC Subsets and Their Immunophenotypes

MDSC have first been identified in tumor-bearing mice as immature myeloid cells characterized by the co-expression of CD11b and Gr-1, comprising the lineage markers Ly6G and Ly6C [49,54]. Unlike other myeloid cells, MDSC exhibit a larger diversity of phenotypes, which complicates their identification and characterization [24]. This heterogeneity is in part due to the unique inflammatory milieu present within different tumor entities [41]. Further contributing to the high plasticity of MDSC phenotypes are the temporal variations in the context of tumor-immune editing, as the TME is subject to permanent modulations in the course of the malignant transformation [39,55].

There are currently two main subsets of MDSC to be distinguished: granulocytic (G)-MDSC and monocytic (M)-MDSC [56]. G-MDSC represents the predominant subset of MDSC in the majority of tumor patients and tumor animal models (approximately 75%) compared with M-MDSC (approximately 25%) [57,58]. However, G-MDSC are considered to be less suppressive than M-MDSC when evaluated on a per-cell basis [49,58,59]. This observation was confirmed in human studies, demonstrating a tight correlation between M-MDSC numbers and the inhibition of T cell activation [60].

Murine G-MDSC are generally characterized as $CD11b^+$, $Ly-6G^+$, $Ly-6C^{low}$ (collectively termed as $Gr-1^{high}$), and $CD49^-$, whereas murine M-MDSC are defined as $CD11b^+$, $Ly6G^-$, $Ly-6C^{high}$ ($Gr-1^{high}$), and $CD49^+$, while expressing F4/80, CD115, or CCR2 at varying extents [49]. Due to the polymorphonuclear morphology of G-MDSC and the expression of CD11b and Ly6G, their relationship to PMN is an ongoing issue [24,61]. However, as compared to PMN, G-MDSC show a diminished phagocytic activity, produce higher levels of ROS, and suppress T cell activation upon activation (Table 1) [61]. Therefore, the assessment of these distinctive immunosuppressive properties is important for a definite characterization of G-MDSC, since no distinctive G-MDSC marker set has been established yet [24,62].

Leaving alone the vast heterogeneity in murine MDSC phenotypes, the definition of specific markers for MDSC in humans remains another important issue. Human MDSC are commonly found to be $CD11b^+$, $CD33^+$, and $HLA-DR^-$ [63,64], and the majority of G-MDSC is $CD15^+$, whereas CD14 expression is predominantly confined to M-MDSC (Table 1) [24,65]. However, MDSC subsets in humans have yet not been defined consistently with respect to surface marker expression [60].

Despite conflicting reports about MDSC surface marker expression, the clinical value of MDSC has readily been demonstrated: Recent reports highlighted that the frequency of MDSC per se may reflect the tumor burden of cancer patients, thus showing a strong correlation between a high MDSC frequency and a poor prognosis [64,66,67]. On the other hand, the tumor itself may influence the composition of the MDSC compartment. In general, G-MDSC have been found to be the main MDSC subset in patients with renal cell carcinoma [68], whereas M-MDSC constitute the dominant immunosuppressive MDSC subpopulation in melanomas or head–neck cancer [60,65]. However, since none of the aforementioned individual markers are unique to a distinct MDSC subset, the definitive identification of human MDSC subsets requires the assessment of their employed suppressive mechanisms [41,55].

Table 1. Phenotypic definitions and functional characteristics of different myeloid cell types present within solid tumors.

Characteristics	PMN	TAN	G-MDSC	M-MDSC	TAM
Murine marker subsets	$CD11b^+$ $CD11c^-$ $Ly6C^{low}$ $Ly6G^+$ $CD101^+$ $F4/80^-$ $CD115^-$	$CD11b^+$ $Ly6C^{low}$ $Ly6G^+$ $PD-L1^+$ $CD170^{high}$	$CD11b^+$ $Gr-1^+$ $Ly6G^+$ $Ly6C^{low}$ $CD115^{low}$ $CD49^-$	$CD11b^+$ $Gr-1^+$ $Ly6C^{high}$ $Ly6G^-$ $CD49d^+$ $CD115^{high}$	$CD11b^+$ $F4/80^+$ $CD206^+$ $CD163^+$ $CD36^+$ $MHC-II^{low}$ $IL-10R^+$ $CD124^+$
Human marker subsets	$CD11b^+$ $CD66b^+$ $CD15^+$ $CD14^-$ $CD16^+$ $CD62L^+$ $CXCR1^+$	$CD45^+$ $CD33^+$ $CD11b^+$ $HLA-DR^-$ $CD66b^+$ $PD-L1^+$ $CD170^{high}$ $LOX-1^+$	$CD33^+$ $CD11b^+$ $HLA-DR^-$ $CD15^+$ $STAT-3^{high}$ $CD66b^+$ $CD244^+$ $S100A9^+$ $LOX-1^+$	$CD33^+$ $CD11b^+$ HLA-DR- $CD14^+$ $STAT-3^{high}$ $CD124^+$ $S100A9^+$	$CD14^+$ $CD68^+$ $CD205^+$ $CD163^+$ $CD36^+$ $HLA-DR^{low}$ $IL-10R^+$ $PD-L1^+$ $STAT-3^{low}$
Maturation stage	predominantly mature	predominantly mature	Immature	Immature	Mature
Potent inductors	GM-CSF	TGF-β	G-CSF IL-6	M-CSF IL-6	IL-4 IL-10 TGF-β Hypoxia
Inhibition of T cell proliferation	Ø	↑	↑	↑↑	↑
ROS	↑	↑	↑↑	↓	Ø
MPO	↑	↑	↑↑	Ø	Ø
Arginase-1	Ø	↑	↑↑	↑	↑
NO	Ø	↓	↓	↑↑	↑
NETosis	↑	↑	Ø	Ø	Ø
IL-8	↑	↑	Ø	Ø	↑↑
Immune cell polarization in response to stimulation	TAN, G-MDSC, APC-like-PMN	PMN	TAN, PMN (?)	TAM, DC	Functional polarization (M1 and M2 phenotype)

Ø: no significant effect; ↓: lower expression/activity compared to the other listed cell types; ↑: higher expression/activity compared to the other cell types; ↑↑: strongest expression/activity among the listed cell types; MPO = myeloperoxidase; NET = neutrophil extracellular traps.

3.2. Myeloid Cell Plasticity within Tumors

Of note, MDSC entering the TME may have the plasticity to interconvert between different phenotypes. In particular, it has been shown that MDSC might convert into TAM, DC, or TAN depending on the conditions present in the TME (Figure 1) [36,49,50]. For example, the culture of tumor-derived MDSC in the absence of tumor-derived factors was repetitively shown to result in the generation of mature macrophages, PMN, and DC [50,69–71], whereas the presence of tumor-derived factors or the adoptive transfer of MDSC into tumor-bearing hosts promoted their differentiation into immunosuppressive macrophages [49,69]. Hence, TAN and TAM may constitute differentiated MDSC or represent a pro-tumorigenic subset of mature PMN and macrophages polarized by soluble mediators [24,49,53].

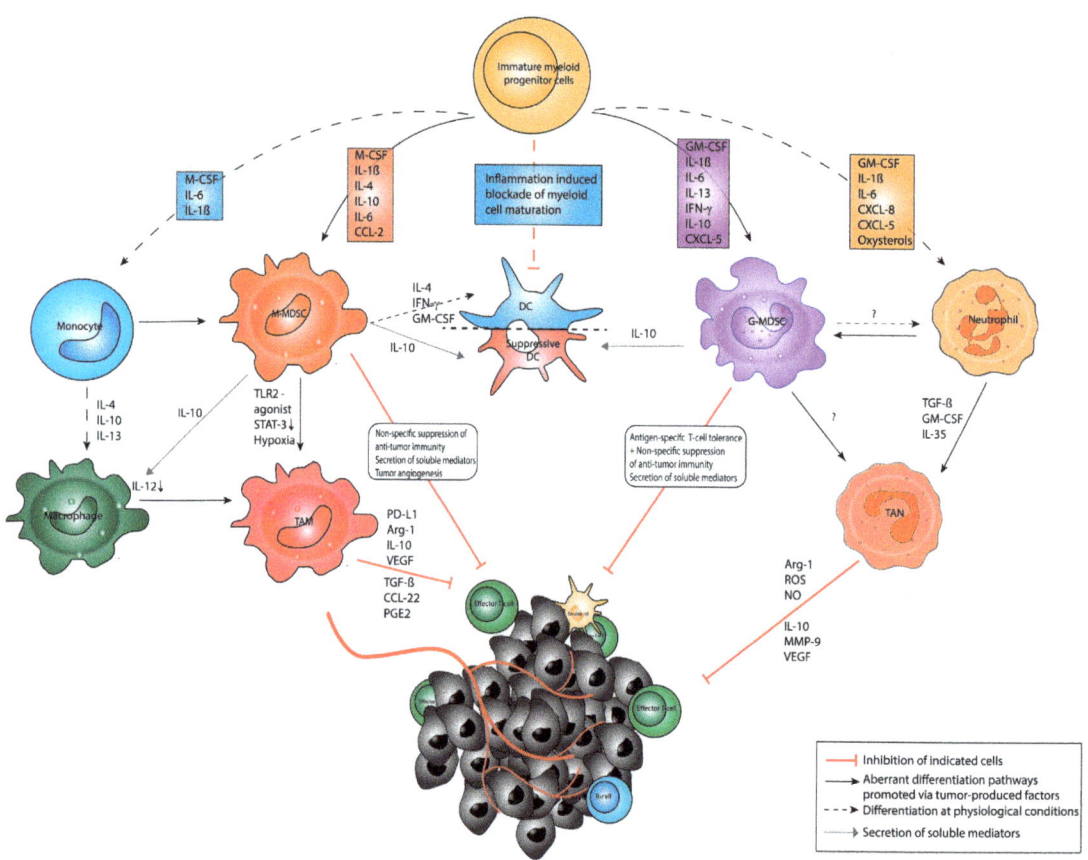

Figure 1. Myeloid cell plasticity in cancer. Myeloid cell types originate from hematopoietic stem cells and multipotent immature myeloid progenitor cells in the bone marrow (BM). The differentiation toward the matured cell line (i.e., polymorphonuclear neutrophils (PMN)) is promoted by soluble mediators and chemokines. In cancer patients, the differentiation pathways are strongly affected by factors produced in the tumor microenvironment (TME) by stromal cells, immune cells, and tumor cells (e.g., granulocyte-macrophage colony-stimulating factor (GM-CSF), interleukin (IL)-1β, IL-6, IL-10, IL-23, interferon-gamma (IFN-γ)). In particular, the TME promotes the polarization of macrophages toward immunosuppressive tumor-associated macrophages (TAM), which confer the inhibition of effector T cells (Teff) within the TME via various mechanisms [72]. PMN within the TME frequently show a polarization toward immunosuppressive TAN, which is driven by soluble factors such as transforming growth factor-β (TGF-β). Tumor-associated neutrophils (TAN) confer immunosuppression via multiple mechanisms. The most prominent effect of the aberrant differentiation includes the accumulation of granulocytic (G-MDSC) and monocytic (M-MDSC) myeloid-derived suppressor cells. Myeloid cells may act as an integrated system in the context of tumor immunity [49]. Depending on the structural composition of the TME, myeloid cells polarize from MDSC toward TAM or TAN or promote the tolerization of DC in the context of a nutrient-depleted, hypoxic, inflamed TME. Under normoxic conditions, IFN-γ and TNF-α have been found to reverse this polarization and promote MDSC differentiation toward immunogenic DC and inflammatory M1 macrophages. It remains questioned if MDSC and TAN undergo an irreversible polarization or can polarize to anti-tumor PMN [24].

Despite the phenotypical similarities of the various (immunosuppressive) myeloid cell types, recent reports highlighted, that these can be discriminated by transcriptomic and multi-omics approaches: Referring to the granulocytic cell line in particular, Fridlender et al. revealed cell-specific transcriptome signatures of PMN, G-MDSC, and TAN, confirming the existence of three distinct phenotypes [62]. Moreover, G-MDSC have shown a higher immunosuppressive activity, expressed higher levels of CD115 and CD244, and lower levels of CXCR1 than PMN [61,73]. G-MDSC exerted less phagocytic activity, show a smaller chemotactic response, expressed higher levels of Arginase (Arg)-1 and myeloperoxidase (MPO), and showed a higher production of ROS [49,73].

Likewise, M-MDSC, despite their similarity in morphology and phenotype with other monocytic cell populations, are a functionally distinct population. Particularly, they showed a strong expression of inducible NO-synthase (iNOS) and Arg-1, which explains their highly immunosuppressive character [49,74]. In parallel, it has been reported that hypoxia and hypoxia inducible factor 1α (HIF-1α) within the TME might be key drivers for the upregulation of immunosuppressive Arg-1 and iNOS in M-MDSC and may promote the differentiation of CD11b$^+$ Ly6C$^+$ M-MDSC into immunosuppressive TAM [53,75]. Since the polarization toward a macrophage M2 phenotype is more likely in MDSC at the tumor site compared to spleen-derived MDSC, it remains an issue to clarify whether the origin of MDSC within the TME might determine the modulation of their phenotype [24,53].

Collectively, these findings provide a mechanistic link between different myeloid cells and indicate that MDSC have the plasticity to interconvert between different phenotypes depending on the specific conditions present within the TME (see Figure 1) [24,53]. However, knowledge of the factors that govern the interconversion of the various granulocytic and monocytic (immunosuppressive) cell types is still far from being complete. Therefore, in vivo strategies and multi-omics approaches are vital to elucidate (combinations of) TME-derived factors that may induce the differentiation, expansion, activation, and interconversion of MDSC populations [24,76].

3.3. Mechanisms of Tumor-Induced MDSC Accumulation

Evidence suggests that the release of tumor-derived soluble mediators, such as GM-CSF, VEGF, or IL-6 impairs the myeloid compartment and thus contributes to defective myeloid cell maturation. Moreover, it has been proposed that the relative amounts of G-CSF and M-CSF present within the bone marrow may account for the different shares of the aforementioned MDSC subsets [59]. Here, Waight et al. reported that G-CSF facilitates the accumulation of G-MDSC in the TME, subsequently promoting tumor growth. Moreover, tumor-derived CCL2, CCL12, CXCL5, S100A8, and S100A9 promote the recruitment of immature myeloid cells to the tumor stroma, facilitating the enrichment of both MDSC subpopulations within the TME [49,77–79]. Tumor-derived TGF-β has also been found to regulate MDSC accumulation and the polarization of other myeloid cell populations, such as tumor-infiltrating PMN toward an immunosuppressive phenotype [80]. Furthermore, soluble factors such as IL-1β, IL-6, and S100A9 [81,82], and T cell-derived cytokines such as IFN-γ, IL-4, IL10, and IL-13 have been reported to promote immunosuppressive MDSC [83].

The regulation of the integrated myeloid cell network via tumor-derived soluble mediators is controlled on multiple levels via the activation of various transcription factors. Here, the Toll-like receptor (TLR) family, namely TLR-4, which is triggered by S100A8 and S100A9 proteins, contributes to myeloid cell development via the downstream induction of nuclear factor-kB (NFκB), thus supporting the mobilization of myeloid cells to sites of inflammation and their inflammation-driven suppressive potency [49,84]. Other suppressive properties of MDSC are controlled by signal transducer and activator of transcription (STAT)-1 and STAT-6, which regulate myeloid cells by inducing iNOS and Arg-1 expression [69,83].

Further, STAT-3 has been identified as a crucial regulator of MDSC expansion that conveys the recruitment of MDSC to the tumor site by upregulating the pro-inflammatory S100A8 and S100A9 proteins [85]. Hence, S100A9 protein has been proposed as a potential marker characterizing human CD14$^+$ HLA-DR$^-$ M-MDSC. STAT-3 has also been reported to induce the upregulation of NADPH oxidase (Nox) components, thereby adding up to the immunosuppressive features of MDSC, such as ROS production [49,86]. However, an unsolved question remains: How do these molecular markers relate to the suppressive function of MDSC? Hence, the most definitive characterization of MDSC remains their immunosuppressive function, which will be addressed in the following section.

4. Immunosuppressive Properties of MDSC

MDSC are considered key regulators of immune responses in many pathophysiological conditions, including anti-tumor immune responses. G-MDSC and M-MDSC apply antigen-specific and antigen-non-specific mechanisms to regulate immune responses and thus inhibit Teff via a plethora of mechanisms [24]: In peripheral lymphoid organs, the MDSC-mediated suppression of CTL usually requires antigen presentation by MDSC and direct MDSC/T cell contact [87,88]. Otherwise, at the tumor site [53,89] and in the periphery [90], MDSC can suppress nearby T cells in an antigen-independent manner. Although none of these mechanisms are exclusively used by either MDSC subpopulation, it has been demonstrated that ROS generation is characteristic for G-MDSC, whereas Arg-1 expression and the generation of NO has primarily been found in M-MDSC [50,58,75].

4.1. Depletion of Nutrients

MDSC confer immunosuppression by various mechanisms (Figure 2), such as the depletion of nutrients. This involves the Arg-1-dependent consumption of L-arginine and deprivation of L-cysteine via its consumption and sequestration in MDSC [91], which causes the proliferative arrest of antigen-activated T cells due to the downregulation of the TCR (T cell receptor) complex and a cell cycle arrest in the G0-G1 phase [49,68]. This phenomenon could be reversed by the replenishment of L-arginine in vitro, but more importantly, in vivo studies reported that the depletion of G-MDSC re-established T cell growth, emphasizing their role in cancer immunosuppression [92]. The inhibition of T cell activation is further enhanced via the consumption of L-tryptophan by MDSC-derived indoleamine-2,3-dioxygenase (IDO) and the subsequent accumulation of kynurenines [93]. Additionally, it was shown that the ADO-generating ectoenzymes CD39 and CD73 are upregulated by MDSC upon HIF-1α induction [94]. ADO impedes Teff function via A2A-receptor (A2AR) and promotes TAM and MDSC suppressive functions via A2BR [95,96]. Whereas the depletion of nutrients and oxygen within the TME comprises T cell function [97,98], tumor hypoxia and lactate accumulation drive HIF-1α stabilization in MDSC, thus upregulating PD-L1 expression and promoting a metabolic switch to fatty acid oxidation (FAO). FAO further induces Arg-1 expression, NO, and peroxynitrite generation, resulting in Teff impairment [99].

4.2. Oxidative Stress

Another suppressive mechanisms is the generation of oxidative stress via ROS and reactive nitrogen species [49]. The production of ROS is mediated by Nox-2. Here, studies conducted by Corzo et al. found an upregulation of ROS in G-MDSC isolated from seven different murine tumor models and in tumor-derived G-MDSC obtained from patients with head neck cancer [86]. Interestingly, in the absence of ROS production, G-MDSC did not only lose their ability to confer T cell hyporesponsiveness in vivo, they also differentiated into mature DC [86]. On the other hand, MDSC themselves are protected from the cytotoxic ROS effects by induction of the antioxidant nuclear factor erythroid related factor 2 (Nrf2) and the accumulation of the ROS scavenger phosphoenolpyruvate (PEP) [100]. Peroxynitrite is produced by the cooperative activities of Nox-2, Arg-1, and iNOS [24,101]. Peroxynitrites can cause the nitration of several proteins in tumor and immune cells including the TCR, leading to subsequent TCR desensitization and T cell apoptosis [49]. Moreover, nitration mediates several molecular blocks in T cells, including conformational changes in the TCR–CD8 complex, which renders CTL unresponsive to antigen-specific stimulation [87]. Furthermore, it was found that peroxynitrite interferes with IL-2 receptor signaling [102] and leads to the nitration of CCL-2 chemokines. Consequently, antigen-specific CTLs do not infiltrate into the tumor but instead remain in the tumor-surrounding stroma [79]. Notably, iNOS-driven NO generation may further induce cyclooxygenase-2 (COX-2) activity, resulting in an enhanced PGE2 production, which serves as a potent inductor of IDO, Arg-1, IL-10, and VEGF secretion by MDSC [98]. Lastly, it has been documented that MDSC counteract the upregulation of CD44 and CD162 by T cells in an NO-dependent manner, thus impairing T cell extravasation and tissue infiltration [103,104].

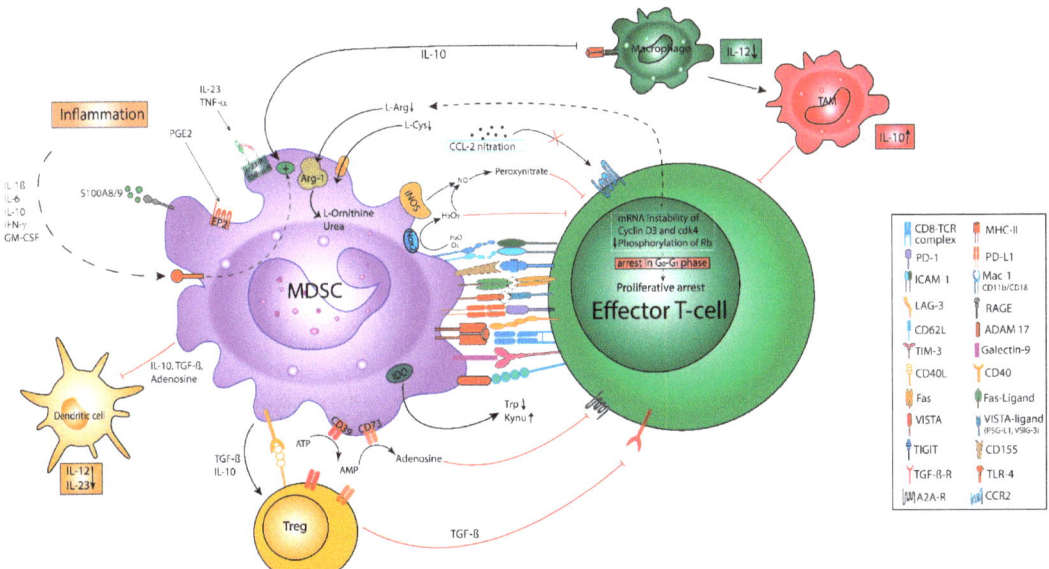

Figure 2. MDSC-mediated inhibition of T cell activation and proliferation. Direct inhibition of Teff involves cell–cell contacts (e.g., via checkpoint molecules), which induce proliferative arrest apoptosis, a reduced migratory activity, and attenuated T cell recirculation. T cell activation is further inhibited via soluble mediators and metabolic pathways: MDSC contribute to L-arginine and L-cysteine depletion in the TME, which causes proliferative arrest via mRNA instability of cyclin-dependent kinase 4 (cdk4), reduced phosphorylation of retinoblastoma protein (Rb), and the loss of the T cell receptor (TCR) ζ-chain on Teff. G-MDSC express high levels of NADPH oxidase (Nox)-2, mediating ROS-dependent inhibition of Teff. The cooperative activities of Nox-2, Arginase (Arg)-1, and inducible nitric oxide synthase (iNOS) generate peroxynitrite, which drives protein nitration resulting in desensitization of the TCR and the interference with IL-2 receptor signaling. The consumption of L-tryptophan and the accumulation of kynurenines in the TME add up to the inhibition of Teff and regulatory T cells (Treg) induction. CD39 and CD73 degrade extracellular ATP to adenosine, which enhances T cell inhibition and Treg induction. Indirect mechanisms of MDSC-mediated immunosuppression include the induction and expansion of Treg both via cell–cell contact-dependent mechanisms and soluble mediators (e.g., TGF-β, IL-10, prostaglandine-E2; PGE2; and A2A-receptor mediated signaling). Likewise, MDSC imprint a tolerogenic function in DC via IL-10, TGF-β, and adenosine. Both the accumulation of Treg and TAM add up to Teff inhibition within the TME. Macrophages are skewed toward an M2 phenotype via IL-10, thus impairing IL-12 production. Tumor-derived soluble factors contribute to STAT3-mediated upregulation of proteins including Nox-2, cell survival proteins (Cyclin D1), or S100A8/9, promoting MDSC accumulation (via S100A8/9 ligation to RAGE), survival, and immunosuppression.

4.3. Receptor-Mediated Inhibition

The interference with lymphocyte trafficking and viability is another immunosuppressive mechanism exerted by MDSC: Here, the expression of membrane-bound ADAM-metallopeptidase domain 17 (ADAM17) on MDSC decreased CD62 ligand (CD62L) expression on CD4+ and CD8+ T cells, thereby limiting the recirculation into lymph nodes [105]. Furthermore, several checkpoint molecules were shown to be critically involved in MDSC-mediated immunosuppression: Among these, PD-L1 and CTLA-4 are prominent negative regulators of T cell functions [106]. PD-L1 exerts its effects via ligation of PD-1 on T cells, resulting in T cell anergy and apoptosis [104], promoting the induction and function of Treg [107] and thus contributing to tumor immune evasion. Treg express CTLA-4, which mainly interacts with CD80/CD86 as expressed by APC-like DC. This interaction causes an impairment of APC-dependent T cell activation [108], enhances the immunosuppressive properties of Treg, and augments peripheral tolerance [109]. Blocking checkpoint molecules via monoclonal antibodies has in fact proven to restore effective anti-tumor immune responses in many patients with advanced malignancies. This effect has been attributed in part to the blockade of MDSC-mediated immunosuppression of Teff [104].

Youn and coworkers additionally suggested that PD-L2 might add up to MDSC-induced T cell inhibition, since PD-L2-/PD-1 interaction skewed T cells toward T-helper cells type 2 (Th2) [61,110,111].

Notably, more recent observations revealed the pivotal role of additional checkpoint molecules, such as the V domain-containing immunoglobulin suppressor of T-cell activation (VISTA), Galectin-9 (Gal-9), and CD155 for MDSC-mediated immunosuppression [112]. In particular, VISTA has been reported to enhance the inhibition of T cell [113,114] and B cell responses [115] by MDSC, whereas a blockade of VISTA allowed for the restoration of a protective anti-tumor response [116,117]. Next, it has been documented that Gal-9-expression on MDSC induced T cell apoptosis via ligation to the checkpoint protein T cell immunoglobulin and mucin domain-containing protein (TIM)-3 [118]. Gal-9 has been also been reported to promote a suppressive TME by enhancing the degradation of stimulator of interferon genes (STING) [119]. As suggested by Dardalhon et al., the interaction of TIM-3+, IFN-γ-secreting T cells with Gal-9+ MDSC might add up to both MDSC expansion and immunosuppressive functions [120]. Last, recent observations indicated that CD155 might also be involved in MDSC-mediated T cell inhibition, since it may serve as a ligand for T-cell Ig and ITIM domain (TIGIT), which is found on T and NK cells promoting the immunosuppressive functions of Treg [121,122]. Despite conflicting reports about the role of Fas-(L)igand-Fas signaling for MDSC homeostasis and function [90,123], it is well documented that MDSC are able to induce T cell apoptosis via FasL [124]. Next to the T cell-specific inhibition, MDSC also interfere with NK cell cytotoxicity via receptor-mediated mechanisms, e.g., the interaction of membrane-bound TGF-β with the NK cell receptor NKp30 [49,125,126].

4.4. Induction of Protolerogenic APC

Additionally, MDSC promote immunosuppression indirectly by the interaction with other cells of the myeloid cell lineage, such as the inhibition of conventional DC and macrophages. This observation further complicates the understanding of the myeloid cell network within tumors, since myeloid cells engage with each other but also have the plasticity to transdifferentiate between different phenotypes. The interdependency of cells in the myeloid linage can be exemplified by the IL-10 and cell–cell contact-mediated mechanisms by which MDSC decrease macrophage IL-12 production, tipping them toward an M2-like phenotype [127]. This initiates a positive feedback loop, as macrophages themselves promote IL-10 synthesis in MDSC, further enhancing the shift toward an M2-like phenotype [49]. An inflamed TME enhances the infiltration of MDSC into the tumor, promotes TLR-4 signaling, the expression of CD14 on MDSC, and their activation. Thus, inflammation is considered a key driver of MDSC and macrophage crosstalk within the TME [128]. Next to the interaction between MDSC and macrophages, MDSC impair DC function via the production of IL-10, which inhibits IL-12 production in DC and the subsequent DC-mediated activation of T cells [49,129]. Adding up more recently to the wide array of immunosuppressive features, it has been observed that MDSC significantly enhance their immunosuppressive potential via the activation and expansion of Treg populations [49]. The character of this interaction is discussed in the following after a brief presentation of Treg characteristics.

5. Regulatory T Cells

It has been shown that regulatory T cells play a crucial role in regulating the homeostasis of the immune system and maintaining tolerance [130]. Moreover, Treg have been found to limit the anti-tumor immune response. In accordance, the number of Treg circulating in the blood of cancer patients and the infiltration of Treg into the tumor have been documented to be closely related to the progression and prognosis of multiple cancer entities [20]. More interestingly, the extent of Treg infiltration into human tumors has been proposed to show an inverse correlation with the response to ICI therapy [131,132]. Not least, this observation emphasizes the importance of Treg in the understanding of the anti-tumor immunity and thus the development of novel therapeutic approaches.

5.1. Characteristics and Classification of Treg

Treg are defined as a T helper cell subpopulation characterized by the co-expression of CD4, CD25, and in large parts of FoxP3, which inhibit the activation and differentiation of CD4$^+$ and CD8$^+$ T cells, subsequently impairing reactivity against autologous and tumor-expressed antigens [130,133,134]. According to their biological properties, Treg are generally divided into two groups: natural (n) regulatory T cells and induced (i) regulatory T cells, which commonly express FoxP3 [135]. Whereas nTreg develop in the thymus and exert their inhibitory activity for maintaining immune tolerance largely through intercellular contact, iTreg are derived from peripheral naïve tumor antigen-specific T cells, which are induced by TME-derived cytokines and other soluble mediators [130]. However, both types of Treg act in a tumor-antigen specific manner [136]. In contrast to Th cells and CTL, which rely largely on glycolysis, glucose transporter (GLUT)-1 expression, and on mammalian target of rapamycin (mTOR) signaling, to sustain their metabolic activity, Treg express low levels of GLUT-1, are negatively regulated by mTOR, and depend largely on oxidative phosphorylation and FAO to sustain their metabolic and suppressive activity [98,137,138].

5.2. Immunosuppressive Properties of Treg

Treg use several mechanisms to inhibit the anti-tumor immune activity of Teff, NK cells, and DC, thus driving tumor progression. First, it has been shown that Treg-derived soluble mediators, such as IL-10, TGF-β, and IL-35, suppress antigen presentation by DC, promote T cell exhaustion and CTL dysfunction [139,140]. Next, it has been reported that Treg largely interfere with the cell metabolism both within the TME and in secondary lymphatic organs, inhibiting the proliferation of Teff by the competitive consumption of IL-2 [136]. Additionally, the expression of the ectonucleotidases CD39 and CD73 enables Treg to hydrolyze extracellular adenosine triphosphate (ATP) into adenosine monophosphate (AMP) and subsequently to immunosuppressive ADO, which inhibits Teff via engagement with the A2AR [141]. Moreover, the intercellular transfer of cyclic AMP (cAMP) to Teff via gap junctions is considered another metabolic mechanism of Treg to inhibit an effective anti-tumor immune response [130]. Similar to TAM and MDSC, Treg contribute to Arg-1 mediated arginine depletion within the TME [142]. In contrast to Teff, Treg are largely unaffected by limitations of either glutamine or leucine within the TME [143]. Treg counterbalance the high ROS levels within the TME via antioxidants such as glutathione. In agreement, the removal of this ROS-inactivating mechanism in Treg significantly impaired their inhibitory activity [144]. Lastly, Treg hampered Teff and NK cell function and activity via immunosuppressive receptor interactions and the application of cytotoxic enzymes [145]. In particular, Treg are capable of killing effector cells using granzymes or perforins and orchestrate the quiescence of memory T cells by inhibiting effector programs via checkpoint molecules such as cytotoxic T-lymphocyte-associated protein 4 (CTLA-4) [130,146]. Furthermore, Treg hamper anti-tumor immunity via the interaction of CTLA-4 with the co-stimulatory receptors CD80 and CD86, which are expressed by APC-like DC, resulting in the inhibition of their T cell stimulatory capacity [130,147]. In the course of this interaction, it has been found that Treg might enhance immunosuppression via the upregulation of IDO and Arg-1 on APC, which impaired the induction of Teff and in turn also inhibited mTOR signaling in Treg [148,149].

Recent reports indicate that the interaction of Treg with MDSC might further contribute to the immunosuppressive activity and potential of Treg, forming a positive feedback loop that facilitates the enforcement of their suppressive activity [130], as described in the following.

6. Functional Crosstalk between MDSC and Treg

The interactions of MDSC and Treg in different cancer models have been proposed to play a critical role in shaping the TME (Table 2) [21]. Although a strong influx of MDSC and Treg has been described for many different tumor entities, there is only little evidence yet for a direct mechanistic link between these major immunoregulatory cell populations. Here, different modes of interactions have been proposed, namely those conferred by soluble mediators, metabolic cooperations, or cell–cell contacts (Figure 3) [21]. Furthermore, it has been suggested that MDSC promote both the conversion of naïve CD4$^+$ T cells toward iTreg and the expansion of nTreg [150–152].

Table 2. A selection of important mediators in the functional crosstalk between MDSC and Treg.

Receptors/Soluble Mediators	Cell Type	Species	Disease Model, Immune State	Observations	Reference
TGF-β	Treg and MDSC	mouse	Murine colitis	■ Treg-derived TGF-β enhanced Arg-1, PD-L1, and iNOS expression on MDSC, thus promoting their immunosuppressive properties ■ MDSC themselves showed a stronger induction of Treg after TGF-β stimulation	[153]
PD-1/PD-L1, IL-10	Treg, MDSC and CD4$^+$ T cells	mouse	Ret-melanoma	■ Depletion of Treg downregulated PD-L1 expression on MDSC and inhibited IL-10 production ■ Diminished PD-L1 expression on MDSC led to a reduced inhibition of CD4$^+$ T cells ■ iNOS expression was not affected by Treg depletion	[154]
IL-10, TGF-β	MDSC and Treg	mouse	Metastatic colon cancer	■ MDSC mediated Treg induction via IL-10 and TGF-β ■ Treg induction was independent of NO-mediated immunosuppression by MDSC	[151]
Cell-cell contacts (receptors not specified)	MDSC and Treg	mouse	Pancreatic ductal Adeno-Carcinoma	■ Physical interactions between MDSC and Treg (video-microscopic analysis) ■ $^+$MDSC mediated Treg induction and immunosuppression via cell–cell contacts (transwell system)	[21]
CD40/CD40L	MDSC and Treg	mouse	B16-OVA Melanoma	■ CD40-deficient MDSC failed to induce Treg (after adoptive transfer) ■ anti-CD40 antibody treatment promoted the differentiation of MDSC toward DC and macrophages	[155]
CD80/CTLA-4	MDSC and Treg	mouse	Ovarian carcinoma	■ MDSC enhanced the immunosuppressive properties of Treg via the engagement of CTLA-4 with CD80 ■ CD80 depletion led to a significant reduction in tumor growth	[156]
Mac-1	MDSC and T cells	human	Acute systemic inflammation	■ Mac-1 and ROS production were required for the inhibition of T cell function by a suppressive subset of human PMN	[157]

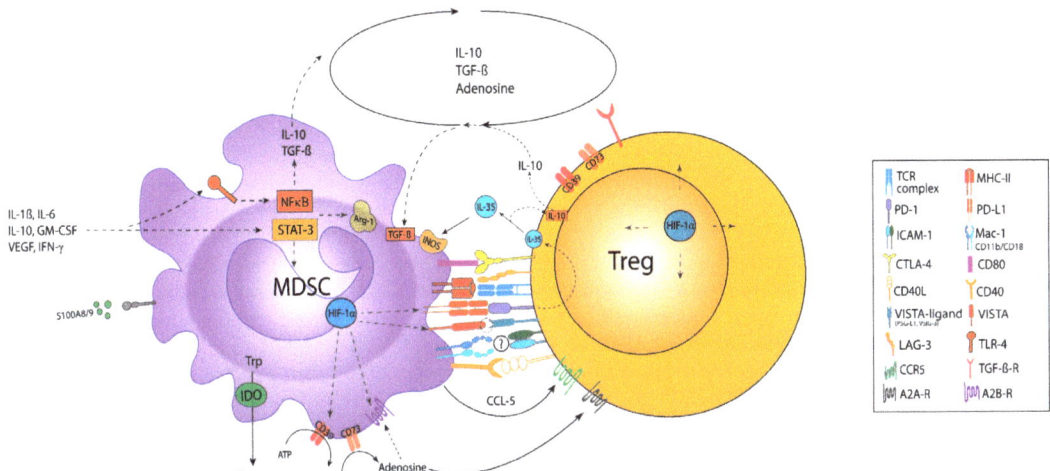

Figure 3. Crosstalk of MDSC and Treg. MDSC and Treg interactions are enhanced by soluble mediators, a close metabolic cooperation, and cell–cell interactions. Particularly, MDSC-derived IL-10 and TGF-β promote Treg induction, proliferation, and activation. The secretion of TGF-β and IL-10 by Treg enhances the generation of these cytokines in MDSC, establishing a positive feedback loop. IL-10 and TGF-β promote the expression of immunosuppressive receptors (e.g., PD-L1) and enzymes (e.g., Arg-1, iNOS, and CD73) on MDSC. Autocrine IL-35 secretion by Treg, which is promoted via the PD-L1-PD-1 pathway, contributes to enhanced IL-10 secretion. The cooperative generation of adenosine (ADO) via the CD39/73 axis and the IDO-mediated accumulation of kynurenines (Kynu) further serve as important mechanisms of the bidirectional crosstalk. First, ADO prevents the maturation of MDSC via A2B-receptor (A2BR) stimulation. A2A-receptor (A2AR) stimulation augments the proliferation and immunosuppressive potential of Treg. Indoleamine-2,3-dioxygenase (IDO)-mediated depletion of tryptophan (Trp) and the Kynu accumulation in the TME add up to the induction of Treg and the recruitment of MDSC to the tumor site. Checkpoint molecules contribute to the crosstalk between MDSC and Treg via PD-L1/PD-1, CD80/CTLA-4, MHC-II/LAG-3, V domain-containing immunoglobulin suppressor of T-cell activation (VISTA)-Ligand/VISTA, Gal-9/TIM-3 (not shown), or CD155/TIGIT (not shown) interaction, promoting the suppressive activities of MDSC and Treg. Notably, CD80 expression is upregulated after direct MDSC–Treg interaction. In addition, CD40–CD40L interaction is involved in MDSC-mediated immunosuppression and Treg expansion at the tumor site. Lastly, the interaction of CD11b/CD18 on MDSC with intercellular adhesion molecule (ICAM)-1 expressed by Treg might enhance MDSC-derived ROS generation. Here, it seems plausible that the engagement of other β2 integrins might also be involved in the crosstalk between MDSC and Treg, e.g., lymphocyte function-associated antigen-1 (LFA-1) on Treg with ICAM-1 on MDSC. The inflammatory and hypoxic TME further enhances MDSC/Treg interaction via mediators, such as IL-1β, IL-6, IL-10, IFN-γ, GM-CSF, or VEGF, which enhance the secretion of IL-10 and TGF-β or promote STAT-3 signaling, contributing to the upregulation of cell surface molecules (e.g., PD-L1, CD80, Mac-1) and enzymes (CD39, Nox-2 or Arg-1) involved in the bidirectional positive feedback loops.

6.1. Functional Interactions Based on Soluble Mediators

Soluble mediators in the TME are considered vital for orchestrating the regulatory tumor immune network. It has been shown as early as 2005 that MDSC promote Treg proliferation in vivo in a TGF-β-dependent manner [158]. Subsequent reports further revealed that IFN-γ and IL-10 are required for the production of both TGF-β and IL-10 by MDSC in tumor-bearing mice [125,151,159]. Additionally, it has been found that IFN-γ and IL-10 upregulated ligands for several co-stimulatory molecules on MDSC (e.g., CD86 and PD-L1). In concert with the aforementioned molecules, the production of soluble mediators (IL-10 and TGF-β) may provide signals for the induction of Treg [151]. Therefore, the authors concluded that MDSC mediate Treg development and subsequent immunosuppression within the TME through a combination of pathways dependent on TGF-β and/or IL-10, which may also involve cell–cell contacts. In the same study, the authors observed that Treg induction and other immunosuppressive mechanisms exerted by MDSC (e.g., NO production) are independent pathways, since iNOS-deficient MDSC lost their suppressive activity but not the ability to induce Treg.

Conversely, Lee and coworkers observed in a murine model of colitis that Treg mediated MDSC proliferation and potentiated their immunosuppressive function via the secretion of TGF-β. This interaction established a positive feedback loop, which mutually enhanced the immunosuppressive capacities of both immune cell populations [153]. More specifically, the authors found that an impaired TGF-β secretion by Treg led to a reduced expression of Arg-1, PD-L1, and iNOS in M-MDSC, resulting in a diminished suppressive activity and a reduced ability of MDSC to induce Treg. Additionally, they documented a significantly stronger G-MDSC accumulation in mice with functionally impaired Treg, suggesting that Treg are important for maintaining normal proportions of MDSC subsets [153].

In another report, IL-35, a heterodimer of EBV-induced gene 3 (EBI3) and of IL-12p35, has been identified as an inhibitory cytokine generated by nTreg, which promoted IL-10 secretion and CD39 expression by iTreg, and NO production in MDSC [160,161]. In turn, IL-10 augmented PD-L1 expression by MDSC, thereby enhancing their immunosuppressive capacity. Notably, the combination signals transduced by PD-L1 and CD169 on MDSC were found to be essential for an induction of IL-35-producing nTreg [162]. Thus, it was suggested that IL-35 generation might establish another positive feedback loop between MDSC and Treg, contributing to the suppressive capacities of Treg [160].

Umansky et al. further found that CCL-5-secretion by M-MDSC resulted in a direct CCR5-dependent recruitment of Treg, indicating that chemokines also add up to MDSC–Treg interaction in the TME [163].

6.2. Metabolic Crosstalk between MDSC and Treg

The TME is predominantly characterized by hypoxia, ADO accumulation, a decreased pH, and low tryptophan levels [49]. ADO is derived from ATP being released by apoptotic cancer cells and subsequently degraded in the TME by the CD39/CD73 ectonucleotidase axis [164]. MDSC and Treg have been found to express high levels of CD39 and CD73, thereby contributing to the accumulation of ADO [141,164,165]. ADO serves as a potent immunosuppressive molecule, inhibiting effector immune cell populations via different adenosine receptors (A1, A2A, A2B, and A3). Next to its immunosuppressive role for effector immune cells, it has been observed that ADO might also augment the proliferation and immunosuppressive properties of Treg via A2AR. Of note, it has been reported that TGF-β can even further induce the expression of CD39 and CD73 on MDSC, promoting ADO accumulation in the TME [95]. In accordance with these observations, ADO production serves as an additional mechanism promoting MDSC-mediated immunosuppression, since ADO augmented the accumulation of MDSC within tumor lesions and their immunosuppressive activity [165,166]. Here, in vitro experiments have shown that A2B receptor stimulation of bone marrow hematopoietic cells prevents the differentiation of these progenitor cells into mature myeloid cells [165]. In agreement, the blockade of A2B receptor with a selective antagonist reduced the number of tumor-infiltrating MDSC and improved T cell-mediated immune surveillance in a melanoma model [95]. Hence, these reports suggest that the cooperative ATP degradation by MDSC and Treg might promote the positive feedback loop between these two immunosuppressive cell populations.

Next to the pivotal role of ADO, tumor hypoxia might further augment ADO-driven effects on MDSC accumulation and Treg-suppressive activity [49]. In particular, it has been found that an upregulation of CD73 on both tumor-infiltrating MDSC and Treg could be induced by hypoxia-inducible factor (HIF)-1α [49]. Moreover, the upregulation of HIF-1α by myeloid cells within the TME has been shown to induce the expression of the A2B receptor, causing a differentiation arrest of myeloid cells, subsequently promoting the accumulation of MDSC [167]. HIF-1α also enhanced the expression of PD-L1, thereby promoting the suppressive capacities of MDSC and their interaction with Treg [168]. Taken together, hypoxic conditions, which are characteristic for the TME, induced the accumulation of MDSC and Treg at the tumor site, stimulated Treg induction, and produced the capacities of both cell types to effectively inhibit the anti-tumor responses by reinforcing their functional crosstalk [169].

COX-2 mediated PGE2 generation has been suggested as another enhancer of Treg and MDSC immunosuppressive properties. On the one hand, autocrine PGE2 secretion by MDSC resulted in an enhanced IL-10 secretion and IDO expression in MDSC [98]. On the other hand, PGE2 is known to enhance FoxP3 expression in Treg and thus promotes their inhibitory activity [170].

Lastly, it has been found that M-MDSC express high levels of IDO in chronic lymphocytic leukemia (CLL). IDO is known to catabolize the rate-limiting step of the kynurenine pathway, which resulted in lower tryptophan levels and the accumulation of kynurenines within the TME [171]. Both the depletion of L-tryptophan and the accumulation of kynurenines suppressed T cell activation and induced Treg in vitro [93,172]. IDO-overexpressing tumors were further shown to exhibit a more aggressive growth as well as enhanced Treg and MDSC accumulation [173]. These findings are indicative of a link between IDO, Treg, and MDSC. Indeed, the depletion of Treg in mice bearing IDO-producing tumors significantly reduced the number of tumor-infiltrating MDSC and prevented their migration as assessed in vitro. Hence, IDO-induced Treg may play an important role in the recruitment and activation of MDSC [173].

6.3. Cell–Cell-Dependent Crosstalk between MDSC and Treg

In addition to soluble mediators mediating MDSC–Treg crosstalk, the interactions of MDSC and Treg have also been proposed to be regulated by direct cell–cell contacts. More recently, Siret and coworkers found that the accumulation of both immunosuppressive cell populations in a pancreatic ductal adenocarcinoma model (PDAC) was associated with a strong expression of CD40, PD-L1, and CD124 by MDSC, whereas Treg expressed CTLA-4, CD103, CCR5, and TGF-β-receptor at high levels [21]. Here, the depletion of MDSC led to a significant reduction of intratumoral Treg, thus confirming, that MDSC have the ability to promote the de novo generation and recruitment of Treg [21,152]. Notably, in the same study, videomicroscopic analyses demonstrated a physical interaction of both cell populations. When using a transwell system to separate CD4$^+$ T-cells and MDSC, no induction of Treg was observed, suggesting that the MDSC-mediated induction of Treg indeed required cell–cell interactions [21]. However, the authors could not identify cell surface receptors mediating this interaction [173].

By contrast, Fujimura and coworkers observed an upregulation of PD-L1 on tumor-infiltrating MDSC in a ret-melanoma model and thus proposed that PD-L1/PD-1 interaction might contribute to the immunosuppressive activities of Treg and the inhibition of T cell proliferation [22]. In particular, the authors could show that the depletion of Treg led to the downregulation of the inhibitory receptors PD-L1, CD276, and B7-H4 on MDSC. These findings suggest that the presence of Treg promoted the acquisition of a more immunosuppressive MDSC phenotype characterized by elevated PD-L1 levels, augmented IL-10, and reduced IFN-γ secretion, contributing to tumor growth [154]. However, iNOS expression by MDSC has not been found to be modified by the presence of Treg.

Vice versa, it has been observed that MDSC enhanced the immunosuppressive properties of Treg in a mouse ovarian cancer model through the interaction of CTLA-4 with CD80 on MDSC [156]. Here, the authors observed an upregulation of CD80-expression by MDSC after direct interaction with Treg. Notably, tumor growth has been retarded upon CD80 knockout or antibody-mediated blockade of either CD80 or CTLA-4 [156]. The importance of checkpoint receptors for MDSC–Treg interaction has been further documented in numerous studies analyzing the role of VISTA, TIM-3, TIGIT, and the lymphocyte-activation gene 3 (LAG-3) as negative regulators of T cell function (Figure 3).

For example, Xu and coworkers suggested that VISTA, which is known to either engage in homotypic interactions or with Selectin P ligand (PSGL-1) as expressed by

MDSC [114], might mediate the crosstalk between MDSC and Treg, thus enhancing their immunosuppressive capacity [174]. More interestingly, the antibody-mediated blockade of VISTA impaired the induction and suppressive function of Treg and reduced the overall number of MDSC [116,175]. LAG-3 (CD223) is known as a co-inhibitory regulator of T cells, Treg, and DC, which is induced upon activation and allows for high-affinity binding to MHCII on myeloid APC [176]. The interaction of LAG-3 with MHCII subsequently prohibits the binding of the same MHC molecule to the TCR and thus suppresses T cell activation and cytokine secretion, thereby ensuring homeostasis [177]. In this regard, Pinton and coworkers found that MDSC confer immunosuppression upon MHCII/LAG-3 interaction [178], whereas the blockade of LAG-3 increased the number of Teff [179]. Interestingly, both MHCII expression on MDSC and LAG-3 expression on T cells have been found to be upregulated upon MDSC-T cell interaction [180]. As LAG-3 is essential for maximal Treg suppressive function, including the secretion of the immunosuppressive cytokines IL-10 and TGF-ß [181], the induction of Treg [182], and their differentiation toward a regulatory phenotype [183], it is conceivable that LAG-3/MHCII interaction between Treg and MDSC could mutually enhance their immunosuppressive activity. Notably, a strong cooperative effect between LAG-3, PD-1, and CTLA-4 has been elucidated in recent reports, highlighting the relevance of the interplay between these checkpoint molecules in the regulation of tumor immunity [184,185].

TIM-3, another important checkpoint molecule regulating T cell homeostasis, has also been found to be critically involved in MDSC–Treg interaction. In particular, it has been documented that TIM-3$^+$ Treg conferred stronger immunosuppressive capacities via increased IL-10 production and the inhibition of CTL as compared to their TIM-3$^-$-counterparts [186,187]. Moreover, Dardalhon et al. suggested that the interaction of MDSC-expressed Gal-9 and TIM-3 on Treg might drive MDSC expansion and suppressive activity [120], whereas a blockade of TIM-3 restored anti-tumor immunity by decreasing Treg numbers, their inhibitory capacity, and MDSC-mediated T cell inhibition [188]. More recently, Wu and coworkers reported that the interaction of TIGIT and CD155 on MDSC might equally be involved in Treg–MDSC crosstalk [121,189], as it added up to the immunoregulatory functions of Treg [190] and MDSC [122].

Next to Treg/MDSC interaction based on the checkpoint molecules and their ligands, it has been reported that the interaction of CD40 on MDSC with CD40L expressed by T cells is required to induce T cell tolerance and Treg accumulation [155]. Namely, the authors observed that CD40-deficient MDSC adoptively transferred to melanoma-burdened mice failed to induce Treg in vivo, suggesting that the CD40/CD40L axis might be crucial for MDSC-mediated inhibition of Teff as well as the expansion of Treg [155]. In accordance with previous reports, the authors specifically identified M-MDSC to activate Treg via the CD40/CD40L axis, whereas G-MDSC failed to do so [155]. Interestingly, the antibody-mediated blockade of CD40 could reverse MDSC-mediated immunosuppression and promote the differentiation of MDSC into DC and macrophages [155]. Although the results may be contradictory at first glance, because CD40 is commonly known to induce adaptive immunity [191], the observations could reveal a crucial mechanism mediating MDSC immunosuppression. Moreover, it has been reported that a combination treatment of IL-2 and agonistic CD40 antibodies elicited synergistic anti-tumor immune responses coincident with the depletion of both Treg and MDSC in primary renal cell carcinomas [192]. This effect has been attributed in part to Fas–FasL mediated apoptosis [104], which is implicated in the regulation of both MDSC and Treg turnover. As for the strong interconnection of MDSC and Treg in the mutual regulation of apoptosis, it is conceivable that FasL–Fas interaction might further be involved in MDSC–Treg interaction, although the exact character of this interaction yet remains undefined.

Altogether, these findings confirm a tight crosstalk between tumor-infiltrating MDSC and Treg, especially within the TME, which is mediated by soluble mediators, metabolic pathways (such as ADO, IDO, and hypoxia) and cell–cell interactions. The aforementioned studies could demonstrate that the blockade of either cell surface receptor may not only reverse the immunosuppressive activity of the targeted cell population but more importantly might even weaken immunosuppression conferred by the interacting cell population. Thus, the targeting of key molecules involved in the establishment of the positive feedback loop might similarly reveal this potentiating character.

7. The Role of β2 Integrins for the Immune Regulatory Tumor Network and Tumor Progression

Due to their crucial functions in leukocyte biology, it has been reasoned that β2 integrins might be involved in the immune–cell crosstalk within the immunosuppressive regulatory network. β2 integrins are heterodimeric surface receptors composed of a variable α-(CD11a-CD11d), which determines ligand specificity, and a common abundantly expressed β-subunit (CD18) [193–195]. So far, β2 integrins are classified into four different heterodimeric receptors, namely lymphocyte function-associated antigen-1 (LFA-1; CD11a/CD18 engagement), macrophage-1-antigen (Mac-1, also termed complement receptor type 3 (CR-3); CD11b/CD18), CR-4 (CD11c/CD18), and the heterodimer of CD11d/CD18.

7.1. β2 Integrins Are Critical for Leukocyte Functions

Being specifically expressed by leukocytes, β2 integrins confer essential functions in mediating adhesion to other cells (LFA-1) and components of the extracellular matrix (ECM), orchestrate the uptake of extracellular material (Mac-1/CR-3) such as complement-opsonized pathogens, and modulate cell signaling (CR-4) [193]. Moreover, β2 integrins are critically involved in the differentiation of immune cells [196], the migration into inflammatory tissues [197], as well as the extent and character of immune responses. β2 integrins interact with various surface receptors, e.g., intercellular adhesion molecules (ICAM1-5), vascular cell adhesion protein (VCAM)-1, platelet endothelial cell adhesion molecule (PECAM-1), receptor for advanced glycation end products (RAGE), and CD40L [198,199]. In particular, β2 integrins are considered critical components for the formation of the immunological synapse between APC and T cells and the intercellular communication of immune cells in general [193,200]. Here, observations indicated that the interaction between LFA-1 on DC and T cell expressed ICAM-1 lowered the threshold required for T cell stimulation [201]. Thus, β2 integrin deficiency resulted in elevated thresholds for TCR activation and subsequently promoted tolerance in vitro and in vivo [202].

7.2. β2 Integrins and Treg

However, β2 integrins also regulate the polarization of CD4$^+$ T cells: Singh and coworkers found that CD11a$^{-/-}$ and thereby LFA-1-deficient mice presented with decreased frequencies of CD4$^+$CD25$^+$ Treg, even when stimulated under Treg-promoting conditions, but T cells rather differentiated toward Th17-cells. Further, T cells resembling nTreg according to their phenotype, derived from CD11a$^{-/-}$ mice, conferred a diminished suppressive activity on stimulated naïve T cells [203,204]. Next to CD11a, CD11b might be involved in the regulation of the Treg/Th 17 balance as well [205]. These observations suggest an important role of β2 integrins in Treg differentiation and function [204]. Here, Wang and coworkers demonstrated that the TGF-ß secretion of Treg required the expression of CD18 [206] and that LFA-1 is essential for an effective inhibition of T cell proliferation [207]. In accordance with these findings, the importance of LFA-1, expressed on T cells, for the induction of tolerance and the suppression of inflammation has been documented in various autoimmune diseases, such as experimental autoimmune encephalitis (EAE) [208,209], systemic sclerosis [210,211], rheumatoid arthritis, psoriasis [193,212], or systemic lupus erythematosus [213,214]. Notably, in most of these diseases, expression levels of CD11a on T cells inversely correlated with the severity of the disease [213,215,216]. In order to exert immunosuppressive functions, Treg express high levels of ICAM-1, P-Selectin, and the integrin a4b1 (very late antigen-4; VLA-4) allowing the quick migration to the site of inflammation [217]. Here, β2 integrins may control the homing and migration of Treg during inflammatory conditions, whereas the absence of β2 integrins impairs Treg infiltration into inflamed tissues [218,219]. Given the essential role of β2 integrins in conferring the suppression of effector cell functions in these pathophysiological models, it is plausible that integrins might also contribute to the inhibition of anti-tumor immune responses [220]. Indeed, in the context of tumor immunity, it has been shown that tumor-infiltrating Treg expressed significantly higher levels of Integrin αE (CD103) than peripheral Tregs and that CD103$^+$ Treg displayed a more suppressive phenotype [221]. In accordance with these findings, it has been noted that patients suffering from leukocyte adhesion deficiency-1 (LAD1), a hereditary disease characterized by a mutation-dependent loss of CD18 expression—suffered from reoccurring severe infections (attributed to a loss of PMN functions) and renal or intestinal autoimmune disease [222].

7.3. β2 Integrins in (Immunomodulatory) Myeloid Cells

The inability of the immune system of LAD1 patients to control infectious diseases mainly results from the functional defects of PMN, monocytes, and macrophages, which constitute the first line of cellular innate immunity [223]. Here, previous studies revealed that CD11b$^{-/-}$ mice were characterized by a strong lung infiltration of PMN in a model of polymicrobial sepsis [224]. However, these mice showed higher bacterial counts and a stronger systemic inflammation, which is indicative of the attenuated killing activity of CD11b-deficient leukocytes [224]. In particular, it has been found that PMN showed a strong functional impairment to kill pathogens in various infection models, such as pulmonary infections with *S. pneumoniae* [225] and *Aspergillus fumigatus* [226], whereas the recruitment and migration into infected lungs was not affected. Moreover, observations from LAD-1 patients suggested that PMN functionality might equally require an integrin-dependent cell–cell contact with other immune cells. Here, it has been found that PMN from LAD-1 patients have indeed not been able to suppress the proliferation of T cells, whereas CD18-expressing PMN could effectively suppress T cell proliferation, while ROS production and degranulation were intact in both PMN populations. Accordingly, the blockade of ICAM-1 reduced T cell suppression by approximately 50%, suggesting that additional molecules might be involved in Mac-1/ICAM interaction [227].

In contrast to the well-established role of β2 integrins on myeloid cell types for T cell interaction and infection control, the role of β2 integrins for MDSC is still rather elusive and has mostly been investigated in the context of tumor development. Observations in various cancer entities have found that the infiltration of CD11b$^+$ myeloid cells supports tumor progression and is thus correlated with tumor size, lymph node metastasis, and poor prognosis, which has largely been attributed to the immunosuppressive function of TAM and MDSC [228]. Accordingly, Zhang and coworkers reported that CD11b$^{-/-}$ mice showed a reduced infiltration of myeloid cells in intestinal adenoma and an attenuated tumor growth [229]. Other observations revealed that a systemic application of CD11b blocking antibodies after radiation increased anti-tumor immune responses, which has been explained by a reduced myeloid cell migration to the tumor site and an attenuated support of tumor neovascularization [230]. With regard to the role of β2-integrins for tumor neovascularization, Soloviev and coworkers found that CD11b$^{-/-}$ mice displayed an impaired infiltration of myeloid cells in the tumor tissue, subsequently resulting in an attenuated VEGF secretion and thus attenuated neovascularization [231,232]. This observation is in line with the finding that MDSC produce pro-angiogenic factors and proteases that endorse angiogenesis and metastases of tumors [164] and that β2 integrins are particularly upregulated on MDSC in hypoxic tissues [233].

However, the role of (β2) integrins in regulating the migration of MDSC and the release of their progenitors from the BM is less clear: It has been found that CD11b deficiency impaired MDSC recruitment to intestinal tumors [229]. Moreover, myeloid progenitor cells in the BM express β2 integrins and the integrin VLA-4 [234]. b2 integrins have been found to be involved in the mobilization of myeloid progenitor cells from the BM to the blood and might confer synergistic effects with VLA-4 [235], enabling the release and trafficking of those myeloid progenitors into the vascular microenvironment [236–238].

In particular, it has been reported that VLA-4 promotes the homing of CD34+ progenitor cells to sites of active tumor neovascularization. Conversely, blocking of VLA-4 impaired the adhesion of myeloid progenitor cells to the tumor endothelia, the infiltration into the tumor, and resulted in a reduced blood vessel density [238,239]. Notably, β2 integrins have been suggested to mediate the IL-8-induced mobilization of myeloid progenitor cells [237], which is indicative for the involvement of MDSC. On the other hand, VLA-4 deficient mice show a strong increase in circulating progenitor cells, suggesting an early release from the BM and the inability of progenitors to infiltrate into tissues [240]. Moreover, Schmid et al. reported that CD11b does not affect myeloid cell recruitment to tumors but rather regulates macrophage polarization [241].

Despite conflicting reports about the exact role of β2 integrins for myeloid cell release from the BM and their ability to migrate or infiltrate into tumor tissue, CD11b has been demonstrated to determine a wide range of MDSC-suppressive functions other than affecting cell recruitment. Hence, it is possible that a cell-specific blockade of β2 integrins might yet show unrecognized effects on tumor immunity [220].

Similar to MDSC, there are divergent reports on the role of β2 integrins for TAM. First, it has been shown that the ligation of β2 integrins in macrophages might impair type I interferon receptor activation, TLR signaling, and induced IL-10 expression, thus enhancing their immunosuppressive capacities [242]. Additionally, the VLA-4 has been reported to be essentially involved in the polarization of macrophages toward an immunesuppressive phenotype via the induction of IL-10, TGF-ß, and Arg-1 [243]. Thus, tumor growth was significantly impaired in mice lacking VLA-4 [243]. In contrast, Schmid et al. demonstrated that a pharmacological activation of CD11b promoted the pro-inflammatory macrophage polarization, which in turn impaired tumor growth in murine and human cancer models [241].

7.4. Role of β2 Integrins for MDSC/T Cell Interaction

Yet, the role of β2 integrins and their ligands for the interaction of MDSC with other immune cells within the tumor micro- and macroenvironment is not well defined to date [193]. In this respect, it has been found that MDSC interact with CTL via the β2 integrin Mac-1 and the integrin β1 (CD29) [24]. The antibody-mediated blockade of either integrin abrogated ROS production by MDSC and diminished MDSC-mediated suppression of CTL [101], suggesting that (β2) integrins might be involved in MDSC/T cell interaction. In accordance with this study, a previous report noted that MDSC were unable to suppress T cell-proliferation in the absence of physical contact [227]. Furthermore, it has been observed that the antibody-mediated blockade of CD11b prevented MDSC suppressive activity [227]. Similarly, it has been noted that CD18 expression is involved in Treg suppressive function. Here, Wang and coworkers showed that a reduced expression of β2 integrins disrupts the interaction between Treg and DC, which impaired Treg proliferation and TGF-ß production [206].

The trafficking of MDSC and Treg to the tumor site is mediated via VLA-4 and β2 integrins [217,238]. Thus, Foubert and coworkers found that tumors derived from VLA-4-deficient mice had reduced frequencies of MDSC but increased numbers of CD8+ T cells and DC [243]. The induction of β2 integrins and their ligands (e.g., ICAM-1) can be enhanced via the ligation of PSGL-1 [193], which is expressed on both MDSC and Treg [244]. Consequently, PSGL-1 might enhance the migration of either cell type into inflamed tissues [245] and also promote immunosuppressive properties via the ligation of VISTA (see Section 4). Notably, both LFA-1 and Mac-1 have been implicated in Treg [207] and MDSC induction [246] and survival.

Moreover, β2 integrins play a pivotal role in the communication of tumor cells and myeloid cells (e.g., MDSC, TAM, and PMN) within the TME [247], which induce tolerance and thus support tumor growth and progression. Although recent reports have focused on other immune cell interactions mediated by β2 integrins, such as the establishment of the immunological synapse between APC and T cells [248], it seems plausible that β2 integrins might also be involved in the crosstalk between MDSC and Treg. However, a more profound understanding of the role of β2 integrins in the TME, especially with regard to their potential function in regulatory immune cells, is still required. As b2 integrins might mediate multiple possible interactions between different immune cells, a cell-type-specific assessment of the role of the different β2 integrins in orchestrating the tumor immune network is required. This might reveal a more specific insight into their pathophysiological role and enable the development of new therapeutic strategies aiming at a cell-type-specific inhibition of the involved molecules.

8. Inhibition of the Immune Regulatory Network for Tumor Therapy

The emergence of ICI in cancer immunotherapy has been a remarkable breakthrough in cancer treatment. In particular, immune checkpoint inhibitors targeting PD-1, PD-L1, or CTLA-4 have been found to restore anti-tumor immune responses in some cancer entities, thus leading to profound therapeutic improvements in patients with advanced cancer diseases. This has been attributed in large parts to the blockade of immune checkpoints either on tumor cells (PD-L1) and Teff (PD-1, CTLA-4).

To date, ICI has been approved for the treatment of several advanced malignancies, including malignant melanoma, Merkel cell carcinoma, non-small cell lung cancer, and head–neck cancer [249]. However, a number of patients do not derive benefit from ICI treatment. This discrepancy in the patients' responses toward ICI is partly explained by immune-suppressive effects, which are elicited by the diverse character of the immune milieu that exists within the TME, since patients with immunologically anergic tumors are likely to be non-responsive to ICI therapy [250]. Most notably, recent reports suggest that MDSC-mediated immunosuppression substantially contributes to tumor immune evasion [28,251].

Although the identity of MDSC is still a subject of controversial discussion, it is well recognized that these immature myeloid cells play a pivotal role in the inhibition of an efficient anti-tumor immune response, the polarization and recruitment of other immunosuppressive cell populations, and thus the regulation of the immunosuppressive tumor network. Despite the common expression of checkpoint molecules such as PD-L1 on MDSC or CTLA-4 on Treg, it has been observed that anti-PD-L1 and anti-CTLA-4 treatments could only restore an efficient anti-tumor immune response in about 10% of metastatic tumor cases entirely, thus leading to a clinical complete response [252–256]. Hence, it has been speculated that the various immunosuppressive mechanisms exerted by MDSC might rather be addressed in a combinational approach and in a more specific way in order to contribute to a realignment of the immune regulatory network.

Therefore, recent strategies aimed to specifically target MDSC, hence improving the therapeutic efficiency of ICI and restoring anti-tumor immunity in cancer patients. So far, four different approaches have been proposed to directly target MDSC in a combination therapy with ICI, namely (i) a reduction of MDSC frequency by low-dose chemotherapy (paclitaxel, cisplatin, or 5-fluorouracil) or the tyrosine kinase and STAT-3 inhibitor Sunitinib, (ii) the blockade of MDSC recruitment via CCR5 and CXCR2 antagonists, and CSF-1R inhibition, (iii) the inhibition of immunosuppression conferred by MDSC via COX-2 inhibitors, phosphodiesterase-5 inhibitors, or A2AR inhibitors and (iv) the promotion of MDSC differentiation to mature antigen-presenting (non-suppressive) macrophages and DC using all-trans retinoic acid (ATRA) [249,250].

It has been reported in various preclinical tumor models that the targeting of MDSC potentiated the effect of ICI and led to a significantly increased survival [249,250]. Notably, monotherapy with ICI or an adjuvant MDSC-targeting drug was not as efficient as a combination of both approaches, emphasizing the synergistic effects of a combination therapy. In particular, the co-application of the histone deacetylase inhibitor entinostat with anti-PD-1 and anti-CLTA-4 checkpoint inhibitors resulted in an inhibition of MDSC activity, an improved infiltration and effector function of CTL, and a strong regression of the tumor in various cancer models [257–259]. Similarly, in a murine pancreatic cancer model, targeting CXCR2 in combination with anti-PD1 treatment revealed that the inhibition of MDSC trafficking into the tumor could equally restore intra-tumoral T cell infiltration and improve ICI efficacy in terms of overall survival [260]. Additional immunotherapeutic agents, including drugs that target either checkpoint molecules, such as TIM-3 [261], LAG-3 [176], or VISTA [262] or immune-metabolic checkpoints such as adenosine (A2A-receptor antagonist, CD73 or CD39 inhibitors) and IDO, yielded promising results in preclinical tumor models [263–265] and are currently evaluated in conjunction with anti-PD-1/L1 treatments [254].

9. Conclusions and Outlook

In this review, we have outlined that the level of MDSC-mediated immunosuppression might not only be determined by the quantitative amount of MDSC infiltration into the tumor and the extent of their immunosuppressive activity, but it might equally involve the quality of their functional crosstalk with other immunosuppressive cells within the TME. This assumption is in accordance with previous reports suggesting that MDSC-mediated immunosuppression needs to be re-evaluated in the context of the functionally closely interconnected network of immune cells within the TME. In particular, a growing body of evidence describes a tight crosstalk between tumor-infiltrating MDSC and Treg within the TME, which is mediated by cell–cell interactions, soluble mediators, and metabolic pathways. This bidirectional crosstalk enhances synergies among both cell types and thereby amplifies the immuno-suppressive effects of the individual cell population. As a result, MDSC and Treg in the TME are inextricably interconnected such that functions of either population are impacted by the other one [24]. This co-dependency benefits the tumor, but it also implies that therapies that target one population may also reduce the immunosuppressive activity of the other cell population (i.e., the application of anti-PD-L1 or anti-CTLA-4 inhibitors in the clinical setting). Therefore, we propose that targeting of the bidirectional crosstalk between MDSC and Treg might tip the scale toward the restoration of an efficient anti-tumor immune response. Most notably, the targeting of cell surface molecules involved in the direct physical interaction of both MDSC and Treg, such as the checkpoint receptors PD-1/PD-L1, LAG-3/MHCII, VISTA/VISTA-L, TIM-3/Gal-9, and CD80/CTLA-4, and receptor pairs, such as CD40/CD40L or Mac-1/ICAM-1, might be promising approaches to enhance the efficacy of immunotherapy.

Moreover, it is conclusive that targeting those cell surface receptors might further be promising, because it seems plausible that the formation of cell–cell interactions might additionally contribute to the efficacy of receptor-independent mechanisms (e.g., paracrine signaling), as they enable a close proximity of immune cells for a limited period of time, thereby improving the directionality of secreted mediators, such as TGF-β, IL-10, or ADO toward the relevant target cell. As for the strong interdependency of cells within the myeloid cell line, it might further be suggested that targeting of the aforementioned receptors on MDSC (e.g., PD-L1) might as well promote the polarization of TAM toward the inflammatory M1 phenotype [49], consequently adding up to the restoration of an effective anti-tumor immunity.

Despite the lack of specific markers that reflect either the phenotype or the functional polarization of MDSC, the application of new multi-omics techniques might prospectively contribute to a more profound understanding of MDSC heterogeneity, their role in tumor progression, and enable the application of selective MDSC-targeting therapies [250]. Therefore, strategies targeting MDSC populations in general and more particularly their crosstalk with Treg, as part of a combination therapy to enhance ICI potency, should be considered as another promising step in the development toward a generation of immunotherapies with improved therapeutic response and outcome.

Author Contributions: Writing review and editing by M.H., H.S., S.G. and M.B.; figures designed by M.H.; supervision by S.G. and M.B. All authors have read and agreed to the published version of the manuscript.

Funding: M.H. is supported by the TransMed Jumpstart Program funded by the Else-Kröner Fresenius Foundation (EKFF). S.G. and M.B. are funded by the German Research Council (SFB 1066, B4, B5). S.G. is funded by the German Research Council (TR156, B11).

Institutional Review Board Statement: Not applicable.

Informed Consent Statement: Not applicable.

Data Availability Statement: Not applicable.

Conflicts of Interest: The authors declare no conflict of interest.

Abbreviations

A2AR	Adenosine A2 Receptor
ADAM17	ADAM Metallopeptidase Domain 17
ADO	Extracellular adenosine
AMP	Adenosine monophosphate
APC	Antigen-presenting cells
Arg-1	Arginase-1
ATP	Adenosine triphosphate
ATRA	All-trans retinoic acid
BM	Bone marrow
CAF	Cancer-associated fibroblasts
cAMP	Cyclical adenosine monophosphate
CCL	CC-chemokine ligand
CD	Cluster of differentiation
CD62L	CD62 Ligand
Cdk4	Cyclin-dependent kinase 4
CLL	Chronic lymphocytic leukemia
COX-2	Cyclooxygenase 2
CR	Complement receptor
CTL	Cytotoxic T-lymphocyte
CTLA-4	Cytotoxic T-lymphocyte-associated protein 4
CXCL	C-X-C motif chemokine ligand
EBI3	EBV-induced gene 3
ECM	Extracellular matrix
EP2	Receptor for prostaglandine E2
FAO	Fatty acid oxidation
FoxP3	Forkhead-Box-Protein P3
Gal-9	Galectin-9
G-CSF	Granulocyte-colony stimulating factor
GM-CSF	Granulocyte-macrophage-colony-stimulating factor
GLUT	Glucose transporter
G-MDSC	Granulocytic (polymorphonuclear) MDSC
HIF-1a	Hypoxia-inducible factor 1 alpha
ICAM	Intercellular adhesion molecule
ICI	Immune Checkpoint Inhibitors
IDO	Indoleamine-2,3-dioxygenase
IFN-γ	Interferon-gamma
Ig	Immunoglobulin
IL	Interleukin
iNOS	Inducible NO-synthase
Kynu	Kynurenines
LAD1	Lymphocyte adhesion deficiency type 1
LAG-3	Lymphocyte-activation gene 3
LFA-1	Leucocyte function associated molecule-1
M-CSF	Macrophage colony-stimulating factor
MDSC	Myeloid-derived suppressor cells

MHC	Major histocompatibility complex
M-MDSC	Monocytic MDSC
MPO	Myeloperoxidase
mTOR	Mammalian target of rapamycin
NET	Neutrophil extracellular traps
NFkB	Nuclear factor kappa-light-chain-enhancer of activated B-cells
NK-cells	Natural killer cells
NO	Nitric oxide
Nox	NADPH-oxidase
Nrf2	Nuclear factor erythroid 2-related factor 2
PD-1	Programmed death protein
PDAC	Pancreatic ductal adenocarcinoma
Pdk-1	Protein-3-phophoinositid-dependant proteinkinase 1
PD-L1	Programmed death ligand protein 1
PECAM	Platelet endothelial cell adhesion molecule
PEP	Phosphoenolpyruvate
PGE2	Prostaglandin E2
PMN	Polymorphonuclear neutrophils
PSGL-1	P-selectin glycoprotein ligand-1
RAGE	Receptor for advanced glycation end products
Rb	Retinoblastoma protein
ROS	Reactive oxygen species
STAT	Signal transducer and activator of transcription
STING	Stimulator of interferon genes
TAM	Tumor-associated macrophages
TAN	Tumor-associated neutrophils
TCR	T cell receptor complex
Teff	Effector-T cells
TGF-β	Transforming-growth factor beta
TIGIT	T-cell Ig and ITIM domain
TIL	Tumor-infiltrating lymphocytes
TIM-3	T cell immunoglobulin and mucin domain-containing protein 3
TLR	Toll-like receptor
TME	Tumor microenvironment
TNF-α	Tumor-necrosis factor alpha
Treg	Regulatory T cells
Trp	L-Tryptophan
VCAM	Vascular cell adhesion molecule
VEGF	Vascular endothelial growth factor
VISTA	V-domain Ig suppressor of T cell activation
VLA-4	Very late antigen-4 (Integrin α4β1)

References

1. Dougan, M.; Dranoff, G. Immune therapy for cancer. *Annu. Rev. Immunol.* **2009**, *27*, 83–117. [CrossRef] [PubMed]
2. Harder, N.; Schonmeyer, R.; Nekolla, K.; Meier, A.; Brieu, N.; Vanegas, C.; Madonna, G.; Capone, M.; Botti, G.; Ascierto, P.A.; et al. Automatic discovery of image-based signatures for ipilimumab response prediction in malignant melanoma. *Sci. Rep.* **2019**, *9*, 7449. [CrossRef] [PubMed]
3. Snyder, A.; Makarov, V.; Merghoub, T.; Yuan, J.; Zaretsky, J.M.; Desrichard, A.; Walsh, L.A.; Postow, M.A.; Wong, P.; Ho, T.S.; et al. Genetic basis for clinical response to CTLA-4 blockade in melanoma. *N. Engl. J. Med.* **2014**, *371*, 2189–2199. [CrossRef] [PubMed]
4. Wu, Y.; Xu, J.; Du, C.; Wu, Y.; Xia, D.; Lv, W.; Hu, J. The Predictive Value of Tumor Mutation Burden on Efficacy of Immune Checkpoint Inhibitors in Cancers: A Systematic Review and Meta-Analysis. *Front. Oncol.* **2019**, *9*, 1161. [CrossRef]
5. Zappasodi, R.; Wolchok, J.D.; Merghoub, T. Strategies for Predicting Response to Checkpoint Inhibitors. *Curr. Hematol. Malig. Rep.* **2018**, *13*, 383–395. [CrossRef]
6. Rizvi, N.A.; Hellmann, M.D.; Snyder, A.; Kvistborg, P.; Makarov, V.; Havel, J.J.; Lee, W.; Yuan, J.; Wong, P.; Ho, T.S.; et al. Cancer immunology. Mutational landscape determines sensitivity to PD-1 blockade in non-small cell lung cancer. *Science* **2015**, *348*, 124–128. [CrossRef] [PubMed]

7. Schrock, A.B.; Ouyang, C.; Sandhu, J.; Sokol, E.; Jin, D.; Ross, J.S.; Miller, V.A.; Lim, D.; Amanam, I.; Chao, J.; et al. Tumor mutational burden is predictive of response to immune checkpoint inhibitors in MSI-high metastatic colorectal cancer. *Ann. Oncol.* **2019**, *30*, 1096–1103. [CrossRef]
8. Kim, J.Y.; Kronbichler, A.; Eisenhut, M.; Hong, S.H.; van der Vliet, H.J.; Kang, J.; Shin, J.I.; Gamerith, G. Tumor Mutational Burden and Efficacy of Immune Checkpoint Inhibitors: A Systematic Review and Meta-Analysis. *Cancers* **2019**, *11*, 1798. [CrossRef]
9. Daud, A.I.; Loo, K.; Pauli, M.L.; Sanchez-Rodriguez, R.; Sandoval, P.M.; Taravati, K.; Tsai, K.; Nosrati, A.; Nardo, L.; Alvarado, M.D.; et al. Tumor immune profiling predicts response to anti-PD-1 therapy in human melanoma. *J. Clin. Investig.* **2016**, *126*, 3447–3452. [CrossRef]
10. Maccalli, C.; Giannarelli, D.; Capocefalo, F.; Pilla, L.; Fonsatti, E.; Di Giacomo, A.M.; Parmiani, G.; Maio, M. Immunological markers and clinical outcome of advanced melanoma patients receiving ipilimumab plus fotemustine in the NIBIT-M1 study. *Oncoimmunology* **2016**, *5*, e1071007. [CrossRef]
11. Topalian, S.L.; Hodi, F.S.; Brahmer, J.R.; Gettinger, S.N.; Smith, D.C.; McDermott, D.F.; Powderly, J.D.; Carvajal, R.D.; Sosman, J.A.; Atkins, M.B.; et al. Safety, activity, and immune correlates of anti-PD-1 antibody in cancer. *N. Engl. J. Med.* **2012**, *366*, 2443–2454. [CrossRef]
12. Larkin, J.; Chiarion-Sileni, V.; Gonzalez, R.; Grob, J.J.; Cowey, C.L.; Lao, C.D.; Schadendorf, D.; Dummer, R.; Smylie, M.; Rutkowski, P.; et al. Combined Nivolumab and Ipilimumab or Monotherapy in Untreated Melanoma. *N. Engl. J. Med.* **2015**, *373*, 23–34. [CrossRef] [PubMed]
13. Gibney, G.T.; Weiner, L.M.; Atkins, M.B. Predictive biomarkers for checkpoint inhibitor-based immunotherapy. *Lancet Oncol.* **2016**, *17*, e542–e551. [CrossRef]
14. Hanahan, D.; Weinberg, R.A. Hallmarks of cancer: The next generation. *Cell* **2011**, *144*, 646–674. [CrossRef] [PubMed]
15. Ji, R.R.; Chasalow, S.D.; Wang, L.; Hamid, O.; Schmidt, H.; Cogswell, J.; Alaparthy, S.; Berman, D.; Jure-Kunkel, M.; Siemers, N.O.; et al. An immune-active tumor microenvironment favors clinical response to ipilimumab. *Cancer Immunol. Immunother.* **2012**, *61*, 1019–1031. [CrossRef]
16. Salmi, S.; Siiskonen, H.; Sironen, R.; Tyynela-Korhonen, K.; Hirschovits-Gerz, B.; Valkonen, M.; Auvinen, P.; Pasonen-Seppanen, S. The number and localization of CD68+ and CD163+ macrophages in different stages of cutaneous melanoma. *Melanoma Res.* **2019**, *29*, 237–247. [CrossRef]
17. Fujimura, T.; Kambayashi, Y.; Fujisawa, Y.; Hidaka, T.; Aiba, S. Tumor-Associated Macrophages: Therapeutic Targets for Skin Cancer. *Front. Oncol.* **2018**, *8*, 3. [CrossRef]
18. Ai, L.; Mu, S.; Wang, Y.; Wang, H.; Cai, L.; Li, W.; Hu, Y. Prognostic role of myeloid-derived suppressor cells in cancers: A systematic review and meta-analysis. *BMC Cancer* **2018**, *18*, 1220. [CrossRef]
19. Shang, B.; Liu, Y.; Jiang, S.J.; Liu, Y. Prognostic value of tumor-infiltrating FoxP3+ regulatory T cells in cancers: A systematic review and meta-analysis. *Sci. Rep.* **2015**, *5*, 15179. [CrossRef]
20. Colombo, M.P.; Piconese, S. Regulatory-T-cell inhibition versus depletion: The right choice in cancer immunotherapy. *Nat. Rev. Cancer* **2007**, *7*, 880–887. [CrossRef]
21. Siret, C.; Collignon, A.; Silvy, F.; Robert, S.; Cheyrol, T.; Andre, P.; Rigot, V.; Iovanna, J.; van de Pavert, S.; Lombardo, D.; et al. Deciphering the Crosstalk Between Myeloid-Derived Suppressor Cells and Regulatory T Cells in Pancreatic Ductal Adenocarcinoma. *Front. Immunol.* **2019**, *10*, 3070. [CrossRef] [PubMed]
22. Fujimura, T.; Kambayashi, Y.; Aiba, S. Crosstalk between regulatory T cells (Tregs) and myeloid derived suppressor cells (MDSCs) during melanoma growth. *Oncoimmunology* **2012**, *1*, 1433–1434. [CrossRef]
23. Centuori, S.M.; Trad, M.; LaCasse, C.J.; Alizadeh, D.; Larmonier, C.B.; Hanke, N.T.; Kartchner, J.; Janikashvili, N.; Bonnotte, B.; Larmonier, N.; et al. Myeloid-derived suppressor cells from tumor-bearing mice impair TGF-beta-induced differentiation of CD4+CD25+FoxP3+ Tregs from CD4+CD25-FoxP3- T cells. *J. Leukoc. Biol.* **2012**, *92*, 987–997. [CrossRef] [PubMed]
24. Lindau, D.; Gielen, P.; Kroesen, M.; Wesseling, P.; Adema, G.J. The immunosuppressive tumour network: Myeloid-derived suppressor cells, regulatory T cells and natural killer T cells. *Immunology* **2013**, *138*, 105–115. [CrossRef] [PubMed]
25. Grabbe, S.; Varga, G.; Beissert, S.; Steinert, M.; Pendl, G.; Seeliger, S.; Bloch, W.; Peters, T.; Schwarz, T.; Sunderkotter, C.; et al. Beta2 integrins are required for skin homing of primed T cells but not for priming naive T cells. *J. Clin. Investig.* **2002**, *109*, 183–192. [CrossRef] [PubMed]
26. Lin, A.; Lore, K. Granulocytes: New Members of the Antigen-Presenting Cell Family. *Front. Immunol.* **2017**, *8*, 1781. [CrossRef]
27. Beury, D.W.; Parker, K.H.; Nyandjo, M.; Sinha, P.; Carter, K.A.; Ostrand-Rosenberg, S. Cross-talk among myeloid-derived suppressor cells, macrophages, and tumor cells impacts the inflammatory milieu of solid tumors. *J. Leukoc. Biol.* **2014**, *96*, 1109–1118. [CrossRef] [PubMed]
28. Ostrand-Rosenberg, S.; Fenselau, C. Myeloid-Derived Suppressor Cells: Immune-Suppressive Cells That Impair Antitumor Immunity and Are Sculpted by Their Environment. *J. Immunol.* **2018**, *200*, 422–431. [CrossRef]
29. Wang, M.; Zhao, J.; Zhang, L.; Wei, F.; Lian, Y.; Wu, Y.; Gong, Z.; Zhang, S.; Zhou, J.; Cao, K.; et al. Role of tumor microenvironment in tumorigenesis. *J. Cancer* **2017**, *8*, 761–773. [CrossRef]
30. Wang, D.; DuBois, R.N. Immunosuppression associated with chronic inflammation in the tumor microenvironment. *Carcinogenesis* **2015**, *36*, 1085–1093. [CrossRef]
31. Joyce, J.A.; Pollard, J.W. Microenvironmental regulation of metastasis. *Nat. Rev. Cancer* **2009**, *9*, 239–252. [CrossRef]

32. Lanitis, E.; Dangaj, D.; Irving, M.; Coukos, G. Mechanisms regulating T-cell infiltration and activity in solid tumors. *Ann. Oncol.* **2017**, *28*, xii18–xii32. [CrossRef] [PubMed]
33. Noy, R.; Pollard, J.W. Tumor-associated macrophages: From mechanisms to therapy. *Immunity* **2014**, *41*, 49–61. [CrossRef] [PubMed]
34. Umansky, V.; Shevchenko, I.; Bazhin, A.V.; Utikal, J. Extracellular adenosine metabolism in immune cells in melanoma. *Cancer Immunol. Immunother.* **2014**, *63*, 1073–1080. [CrossRef] [PubMed]
35. Mishalian, I.; Granot, Z.; Fridlender, Z.G. The diversity of circulating neutrophils in cancer. *Immunobiology* **2017**, *222*, 82–88. [CrossRef] [PubMed]
36. Rosales, C. Neutrophil: A Cell with Many Roles in Inflammation or Several Cell Types? *Front. Physiol.* **2018**, *9*, 113. [CrossRef] [PubMed]
37. Galdiero, M.R.; Bonavita, E.; Barajon, I.; Garlanda, C.; Mantovani, A.; Jaillon, S. Tumor associated macrophages and neutrophils in cancer. *Immunobiology* **2013**, *218*, 1402–1410. [CrossRef]
38. Lin, Y.; Xu, J.; Lan, H. Tumor-associated macrophages in tumor metastasis: Biological roles and clinical therapeutic applications. *J. Hematol. Oncol.* **2019**, *12*, 76. [CrossRef]
39. Biswas, S.K.; Mantovani, A. Macrophage plasticity and interaction with lymphocyte subsets: Cancer as a paradigm. *Nat. Immunol.* **2010**, *11*, 889–896. [CrossRef]
40. Biswas, S.K.; Allavena, P.; Mantovani, A. Tumor-associated macrophages: Functional diversity, clinical significance, and open questions. *Semin. Immunopathol.* **2013**, *35*, 585–600. [CrossRef]
41. Parker, K.H.; Beury, D.W.; Ostrand-Rosenberg, S. Myeloid-Derived Suppressor Cells: Critical Cells Driving Immune Suppression in the Tumor Microenvironment. *Adv. Cancer Res.* **2015**, *128*, 95–139. [CrossRef] [PubMed]
42. Kumar, V.; Patel, S.; Tcyganov, E.; Gabrilovich, D.I. The Nature of Myeloid-Derived Suppressor Cells in the Tumor Microenvironment. *Trends Immunol.* **2016**, *37*, 208–220. [CrossRef] [PubMed]
43. DeVito, N.C.; Plebanek, M.P.; Theivanthiran, B.; Hanks, B.A. Role of Tumor-Mediated Dendritic Cell Tolerization in Immune Evasion. *Front. Immunol.* **2019**, *10*, 2876. [CrossRef] [PubMed]
44. Liu, Q.; Zhang, C.; Sun, A.; Zheng, Y.; Wang, L.; Cao, X. Tumor-educated CD11bhighIalow regulatory dendritic cells suppress T cell response through arginase I. *J. Immunol.* **2009**, *182*, 6207–6216. [CrossRef]
45. Enk, A.H.; Jonuleit, H.; Saloga, J.; Knop, J. Dendritic cells as mediators of tumor-induced tolerance in metastatic melanoma. *Int. J. Cancer* **1997**, *73*, 309–316. [CrossRef]
46. Schupp, J.; Krebs, F.K.; Zimmer, N.; Trzeciak, E.; Schuppan, D.; Tuettenberg, A. Targeting myeloid cells in the tumor sustaining microenvironment. *Cell. Immunol.* **2019**, *343*, 103713. [CrossRef]
47. Murdoch, C.; Muthana, M.; Coffelt, S.B.; Lewis, C.E. The role of myeloid cells in the promotion of tumour angiogenesis. *Nat. Rev. Cancer* **2008**, *8*, 618–631. [CrossRef]
48. Qian, B.Z.; Pollard, J.W. Macrophage diversity enhances tumor progression and metastasis. *Cell* **2010**, *141*, 39–51. [CrossRef] [PubMed]
49. Gabrilovich, D.I.; Ostrand-Rosenberg, S.; Bronte, V. Coordinated regulation of myeloid cells by tumours. *Nat. Rev. Immunol.* **2012**, *12*, 253–268. [CrossRef]
50. Gabrilovich, D.I.; Nagaraj, S. Myeloid-derived suppressor cells as regulators of the immune system. *Nat. Rev. Immunol.* **2009**, *9*, 162–174. [CrossRef]
51. Meyer, C.; Sevko, A.; Ramacher, M.; Bazhin, A.V.; Falk, C.S.; Osen, W.; Borrello, I.; Kato, M.; Schadendorf, D.; Baniyash, M.; et al. Chronic inflammation promotes myeloid-derived suppressor cell activation blocking antitumor immunity in transgenic mouse melanoma model. *Proc. Natl. Acad. Sci. USA* **2011**, *108*, 17111–17116. [CrossRef]
52. Najafi, M.; Farhood, B.; Mortezaee, K. Contribution of regulatory T cells to cancer: A review. *J. Cell. Physiol.* **2019**, *234*, 7983–7993. [CrossRef]
53. Corzo, C.A.; Condamine, T.; Lu, L.; Cotter, M.J.; Youn, J.I.; Cheng, P.; Cho, H.I.; Celis, E.; Quiceno, D.G.; Padhya, T.; et al. HIF-1alpha regulates function and differentiation of myeloid-derived suppressor cells in the tumor microenvironment. *J. Exp. Med.* **2010**, *207*, 2439–2453. [CrossRef]
54. Peranzoni, E.; Zilio, S.; Marigo, I.; Dolcetti, L.; Zanovello, P.; Mandruzzato, S.; Bronte, V. Myeloid-derived suppressor cell heterogeneity and subset definition. *Curr. Opin. Immunol.* **2010**, *22*, 238–244. [CrossRef]
55. Dunn, G.P.; Bruce, A.T.; Ikeda, H.; Old, L.J.; Schreiber, R.D. Cancer immunoediting: From immunosurveillance to tumor escape. *Nat. Immunol.* **2002**, *3*, 991–998. [CrossRef]
56. Bronte, V.; Brandau, S.; Chen, S.H.; Colombo, M.P.; Frey, A.B.; Greten, T.F.; Mandruzzato, S.; Murray, P.J.; Ochoa, A.; Ostrand-Rosenberg, S.; et al. Recommendations for myeloid-derived suppressor cell nomenclature and characterization standards. *Nat. Commun* **2016**, *7*, 12150. [CrossRef]
57. Schmielau, J.; Finn, O.J. Activated granulocytes and granulocyte-derived hydrogen peroxide are the underlying mechanism of suppression of t-cell function in advanced cancer patients. *Cancer Res.* **2001**, *61*, 4756–4760.
58. Youn, J.I.; Nagaraj, S.; Collazo, M.; Gabrilovich, D.I. Subsets of myeloid-derived suppressor cells in tumor-bearing mice. *J. Immunol.* **2008**, *181*, 5791–5802. [CrossRef]

59. Dolcetti, L.; Peranzoni, E.; Ugel, S.; Marigo, I.; Fernandez Gomez, A.; Mesa, C.; Geilich, M.; Winkels, G.; Traggiai, E.; Casati, A.; et al. Hierarchy of immunosuppressive strength among myeloid-derived suppressor cell subsets is determined by GM-CSF. *Eur. J. Immunol.* **2010**, *40*, 22–35. [CrossRef]
60. Mandruzzato, S.; Solito, S.; Falisi, E.; Francescato, S.; Chiarion-Sileni, V.; Mocellin, S.; Zanon, A.; Rossi, C.R.; Nitti, D.; Bronte, V.; et al. IL4Ralpha+ myeloid-derived suppressor cell expansion in cancer patients. *J. Immunol.* **2009**, *182*, 6562–6568. [CrossRef]
61. Youn, J.I.; Collazo, M.; Shalova, I.N.; Biswas, S.K.; Gabrilovich, D.I. Characterization of the nature of granulocytic myeloid-derived suppressor cells in tumor-bearing mice. *J. Leukoc. Biol.* **2012**, *91*, 167–181. [CrossRef]
62. Fridlender, Z.G.; Sun, J.; Mishalian, I.; Singhal, S.; Cheng, G.; Kapoor, V.; Horng, W.; Fridlender, G.; Bayuh, R.; Worthen, G.S.; et al. Transcriptomic analysis comparing tumor-associated neutrophils with granulocytic myeloid-derived suppressor cells and normal neutrophils. *PLoS ONE* **2012**, *7*, e31524. [CrossRef]
63. Poschke, I.; Mougiakakos, D.; Hansson, J.; Masucci, G.V.; Kiessling, R. Immature immunosuppressive CD14+HLA-DR-/low cells in melanoma patients are Stat3hi and overexpress CD80, CD83, and DC-sign. *Cancer Res.* **2010**, *70*, 4335–4345. [CrossRef]
64. Solito, S.; Falisi, E.; Diaz-Montero, C.M.; Doni, A.; Pinton, L.; Rosato, A.; Francescato, S.; Basso, G.; Zanovello, P.; Onicescu, G.; et al. A human promyelocytic-like population is responsible for the immune suppression mediated by myeloid-derived suppressor cells. *Blood* **2011**, *118*, 2254–2265. [CrossRef]
65. Filipazzi, P.; Valenti, R.; Huber, V.; Pilla, L.; Canese, P.; Iero, M.; Castelli, C.; Mariani, L.; Parmiani, G.; Rivoltini, L. Identification of a new subset of myeloid suppressor cells in peripheral blood of melanoma patients with modulation by a granulocyte-macrophage colony-stimulation factor-based antitumor vaccine. *J. Clin. Oncol.* **2007**, *25*, 2546–2553. [CrossRef]
66. Diaz-Montero, C.M.; Salem, M.L.; Nishimura, M.I.; Garrett-Mayer, E.; Cole, D.J.; Montero, A.J. Increased circulating myeloid-derived suppressor cells correlate with clinical cancer stage, metastatic tumor burden, and doxorubicin-cyclophosphamide chemotherapy. *Cancer Immunol. Immunother.* **2009**, *58*, 49–59. [CrossRef]
67. Raychaudhuri, B.; Rayman, P.; Ireland, J.; Ko, J.; Rini, B.; Borden, E.C.; Garcia, J.; Vogelbaum, M.A.; Finke, J. Myeloid-derived suppressor cell accumulation and function in patients with newly diagnosed glioblastoma. *Neuro Oncol.* **2011**, *13*, 591–599. [CrossRef]
68. Rodriguez, P.C.; Ernstoff, M.S.; Hernandez, C.; Atkins, M.; Zabaleta, J.; Sierra, R.; Ochoa, A.C. Arginase I-producing myeloid-derived suppressor cells in renal cell carcinoma are a subpopulation of activated granulocytes. *Cancer Res.* **2009**, *69*, 1553–1560. [CrossRef]
69. Kusmartsev, S.; Gabrilovich, D.I. STAT1 signaling regulates tumor-associated macrophage-mediated T cell deletion. *J. Immunol.* **2005**, *174*, 4880–4891. [CrossRef]
70. Narita, Y.; Wakita, D.; Ohkur, T.; Chamoto, K.; Nishimura, T. Potential differentiation of tumor bearing mouse CD11b+Gr-1+ immature myeloid cells into both suppressor macrophages and immunostimulatory dendritic cells. *Biomed. Res.* **2009**, *30*, 7–15. [CrossRef]
71. Li, Q.; Pan, P.Y.; Gu, P.; Xu, D.; Chen, S.H. Role of immature myeloid Gr-1+ cells in the development of antitumor immunity. *Cancer Res.* **2004**, *64*, 1130–1139. [CrossRef] [PubMed]
72. Jaillon, S.; Ponzetta, A.; Di Mitri, D.; Santoni, A.; Bonecchi, R.; Mantovani, A. Neutrophil diversity and plasticity in tumour progression and therapy. *Nat. Rev. Cancer* **2020**, *20*, 485–503. [CrossRef] [PubMed]
73. Brandau, S.; Trellakis, S.; Bruderek, K.; Schmaltz, D.; Steller, G.; Elian, M.; Suttmann, H.; Schenck, M.; Welling, J.; Zabel, P.; et al. Myeloid-derived suppressor cells in the peripheral blood of cancer patients contain a subset of immature neutrophils with impaired migratory properties. *J. Leukoc. Biol.* **2011**, *89*, 311–317. [CrossRef]
74. Mantovani, A.; Sozzani, S.; Locati, M.; Allavena, P.; Sica, A. Macrophage polarization: Tumor-associated macrophages as a paradigm for polarized M2 mononuclear phagocytes. *Trends Immunol.* **2002**, *23*, 549–555. [CrossRef]
75. Movahedi, K.; Guilliams, M.; Van den Bossche, J.; Van den Bergh, R.; Gysemans, C.; Beschin, A.; De Baetselier, P.; Van Ginderachter, J.A. Identification of discrete tumor-induced myeloid-derived suppressor cell subpopulations with distinct T cell-suppressive activity. *Blood* **2008**, *111*, 4233–4244. [CrossRef]
76. Kotsakis, A.; Harasymczuk, M.; Schilling, B.; Georgoulias, V.; Argiris, A.; Whiteside, T.L. Myeloid-derived suppressor cell measurements in fresh and cryopreserved blood samples. *J. Immunol. Methods* **2012**, *381*, 14–22. [CrossRef]
77. Shojaei, F.; Wu, X.; Zhong, C.; Yu, L.; Liang, X.H.; Yao, J.; Blanchard, D.; Bais, C.; Peale, F.V.; van Bruggen, N.; et al. Bv8 regulates myeloid-cell-dependent tumour angiogenesis. *Nature* **2007**, *450*, 825–831. [CrossRef]
78. Huang, B.; Lei, Z.; Zhao, J.; Gong, W.; Liu, J.; Chen, Z.; Liu, Y.; Li, D.; Yuan, Y.; Zhang, G.M.; et al. CCL2/CCR2 pathway mediates recruitment of myeloid suppressor cells to cancers. *Cancer Lett.* **2007**, *252*, 86–92. [CrossRef]
79. Molon, B.; Ugel, S.; Del Pozzo, F.; Soldani, C.; Zilio, S.; Avella, D.; De Palma, A.; Mauri, P.; Monegal, A.; Rescigno, M.; et al. Chemokine nitration prevents intratumoral infiltration of antigen-specific T cells. *J. Exp. Med.* **2011**, *208*, 1949–1962. [CrossRef]
80. Sinha, P.; Clements, V.K.; Fulton, A.M.; Ostrand-Rosenberg, S. Prostaglandin E2 promotes tumor progression by inducing myeloid-derived suppressor cells. *Cancer Res.* **2007**, *67*, 4507–4513. [CrossRef]
81. Bunt, S.K.; Sinha, P.; Clements, V.K.; Leips, J.; Ostrand-Rosenberg, S. Inflammation induces myeloid-derived suppressor cells that facilitate tumor progression. *J. Immunol.* **2006**, *176*, 284–290. [CrossRef]
82. Sinha, P.; Okoro, C.; Foell, D.; Freeze, H.H.; Ostrand-Rosenberg, S.; Srikrishna, G. Proinflammatory S100 proteins regulate the accumulation of myeloid-derived suppressor cells. *J. Immunol.* **2008**, *181*, 4666–4675. [CrossRef]

83. Gallina, G.; Dolcetti, L.; Serafini, P.; De Santo, C.; Marigo, I.; Colombo, M.P.; Basso, G.; Brombacher, F.; Borrello, I.; Zanovello, P.; et al. Tumors induce a subset of inflammatory monocytes with immunosuppressive activity on CD8+ T cells. *J. Clin. Investig.* **2006**, *116*, 2777–2790. [CrossRef]
84. Liu, Y.; Xiang, X.; Zhuang, X.; Zhang, S.; Liu, C.; Cheng, Z.; Michalek, S.; Grizzle, W.; Zhang, H.G. Contribution of MyD88 to the tumor exosome-mediated induction of myeloid derived suppressor cells. *Am. J. Pathol.* **2010**, *176*, 2490–2499. [CrossRef]
85. Cheng, P.; Corzo, C.A.; Luetteke, N.; Yu, B.; Nagaraj, S.; Bui, M.M.; Ortiz, M.; Nacken, W.; Sorg, C.; Vogl, T.; et al. Inhibition of dendritic cell differentiation and accumulation of myeloid-derived suppressor cells in cancer is regulated by S100A9 protein. *J. Exp. Med.* **2008**, *205*, 2235–2249. [CrossRef]
86. Corzo, C.A.; Cotter, M.J.; Cheng, P.; Cheng, F.; Kusmartsev, S.; Sotomayor, E.; Padhya, T.; McCaffrey, T.V.; McCaffrey, J.C.; Gabrilovich, D.I. Mechanism regulating reactive oxygen species in tumor-induced myeloid-derived suppressor cells. *J. Immunol.* **2009**, *182*, 5693–5701. [CrossRef]
87. Nagaraj, S.; Gupta, K.; Pisarev, V.; Kinarsky, L.; Sherman, S.; Kang, L.; Herber, D.L.; Schneck, J.; Gabrilovich, D.I. Altered recognition of antigen is a mechanism of CD8+ T cell tolerance in cancer. *Nat. Med.* **2007**, *13*, 828–835. [CrossRef]
88. Watanabe, S.; Deguchi, K.; Zheng, R.; Tamai, H.; Wang, L.X.; Cohen, P.A.; Shu, S. Tumor-induced CD11b+Gr-1+ myeloid cells suppress T cell sensitization in tumor-draining lymph nodes. *J. Immunol.* **2008**, *181*, 3291–3300. [CrossRef]
89. Doedens, A.L.; Stockmann, C.; Rubinstein, M.P.; Liao, D.; Zhang, N.; DeNardo, D.G.; Coussens, L.M.; Karin, M.; Goldrath, A.W.; Johnson, R.S. Macrophage expression of hypoxia-inducible factor-1 alpha suppresses T-cell function and promotes tumor progression. *Cancer Res.* **2010**, *70*, 7465–7475. [CrossRef]
90. Sinha, P.; Chornoguz, O.; Clements, V.K.; Artemenko, K.A.; Zubarev, R.A.; Ostrand-Rosenberg, S. Myeloid-derived suppressor cells express the death receptor Fas and apoptose in response to T cell-expressed FasL. *Blood* **2011**, *117*, 5381–5390. [CrossRef]
91. Srivastava, M.K.; Sinha, P.; Clements, V.K.; Rodriguez, P.; Ostrand-Rosenberg, S. Myeloid-derived suppressor cells inhibit T-cell activation by depleting cystine and cysteine. *Cancer Res.* **2010**, *70*, 68–77. [CrossRef] [PubMed]
92. Zea, A.H.; Rodriguez, P.C.; Atkins, M.B.; Hernandez, C.; Signoretti, S.; Zabaleta, J.; McDermott, D.; Quiceno, D.; Youmans, A.; O'Neill, A.; et al. Arginase-producing myeloid suppressor cells in renal cell carcinoma patients: A mechanism of tumor evasion. *Cancer Res.* **2005**, *65*, 3044–3048. [CrossRef] [PubMed]
93. Platten, M.; Nollen, E.A.A.; Rohrig, U.F.; Fallarino, F.; Opitz, C.A. Tryptophan metabolism as a common therapeutic target in cancer, neurodegeneration and beyond. *Nat. Rev. Drug Discov.* **2019**, *18*, 379–401. [CrossRef] [PubMed]
94. Li, L.; Wang, L.; Li, J.; Fan, Z.; Yang, L.; Zhang, Z.; Zhang, C.; Yue, D.; Qin, G.; Zhang, T.; et al. Metformin-Induced Reduction of CD39 and CD73 Blocks Myeloid-Derived Suppressor Cell Activity in Patients with Ovarian Cancer. *Cancer Res.* **2018**, *78*, 1779–1791. [CrossRef] [PubMed]
95. Iannone, R.; Miele, L.; Maiolino, P.; Pinto, A.; Morello, S. Blockade of A2b adenosine receptor reduces tumor growth and immune suppression mediated by myeloid-derived suppressor cells in a mouse model of melanoma. *Neoplasia* **2013**, *15*, 1400–1409. [CrossRef] [PubMed]
96. Morello, S.; Miele, L. Targeting the adenosine A2b receptor in the tumor microenvironment overcomes local immunosuppression by myeloid-derived suppressor cells. *Oncoimmunology* **2014**, *3*, e27989. [CrossRef]
97. Macintyre, A.N.; Gerriets, V.A.; Nichols, A.G.; Michalek, R.D.; Rudolph, M.C.; Deoliveira, D.; Anderson, S.M.; Abel, E.D.; Chen, B.J.; Hale, L.P.; et al. The glucose transporter Glut1 is selectively essential for CD4 T cell activation and effector function. *Cell Metab.* **2014**, *20*, 61–72. [CrossRef]
98. Guerra, L.; Bonetti, L.; Brenner, D. Metabolic Modulation of Immunity: A New Concept in Cancer Immunotherapy. *Cell Rep.* **2020**, *32*, 107848. [CrossRef]
99. Hossain, F.; Al-Khami, A.A.; Wyczechowska, D.; Hernandez, C.; Zheng, L.; Reiss, K.; Valle, L.D.; Trillo-Tinoco, J.; Maj, T.; Zou, W.; et al. Inhibition of Fatty Acid Oxidation Modulates Immunosuppressive Functions of Myeloid-Derived Suppressor Cells and Enhances Cancer Therapies. *Cancer Immunol. Res.* **2015**, *3*, 1236–1247. [CrossRef]
100. Ohl, K.; Fragoulis, A.; Klemm, P.; Baumeister, J.; Klock, W.; Verjans, E.; Boll, S.; Mollmann, J.; Lehrke, M.; Costa, I.; et al. Nrf2 Is a Central Regulator of Metabolic Reprogramming of Myeloid-Derived Suppressor Cells in Steady State and Sepsis. *Front. Immunol.* **2018**, *9*, 1552. [CrossRef]
101. Kusmartsev, S.; Nefedova, Y.; Yoder, D.; Gabrilovich, D.I. Antigen-specific inhibition of CD8+ T cell response by immature myeloid cells in cancer is mediated by reactive oxygen species. *J. Immunol.* **2004**, *172*, 989–999. [CrossRef] [PubMed]
102. Mazzoni, A.; Bronte, V.; Visintin, A.; Spitzer, J.H.; Apolloni, E.; Serafini, P.; Zanovello, P.; Segal, D.M. Myeloid suppressor lines inhibit T cell responses by an NO-dependent mechanism. *J. Immunol.* **2002**, *168*, 689–695. [CrossRef] [PubMed]
103. Schouppe, E.; Mommer, C.; Movahedi, K.; Laoui, D.; Morias, Y.; Gysemans, C.; Luyckx, A.; De Baetselier, P.; Van Ginderachter, J.A. Tumor-induced myeloid-derived suppressor cell subsets exert either inhibitory or stimulatory effects on distinct CD8+ T-cell activation events. *Eur. J. Immunol.* **2013**, *43*, 2930–2942. [CrossRef] [PubMed]
104. Groth, C.; Hu, X.; Weber, R.; Fleming, V.; Altevogt, P.; Utikal, J.; Umansky, V. Immunosuppression mediated by myeloid-derived suppressor cells (MDSCs) during tumour progression. *Br. J. Cancer* **2019**, *120*, 16–25. [CrossRef]
105. Hanson, E.M.; Clements, V.K.; Sinha, P.; Ilkovitch, D.; Ostrand-Rosenberg, S. Myeloid-derived suppressor cells down-regulate L-selectin expression on CD4+ and CD8+ T cells. *J. Immunol.* **2009**, *183*, 937–944. [CrossRef]

106. Juneja, V.R.; McGuire, K.A.; Manguso, R.T.; LaFleur, M.W.; Collins, N.; Haining, W.N.; Freeman, G.J.; Sharpe, A.H. PD-L1 on tumor cells is sufficient for immune evasion in immunogenic tumors and inhibits CD8 T cell cytotoxicity. *J. Exp. Med.* **2017**, *214*, 895–904. [CrossRef]
107. Neumann, K.; Ostmann, A.; Breda, P.C.; Ochel, A.; Tacke, F.; Paust, H.J.; Panzer, U.; Tiegs, G. The co-inhibitory molecule PD-L1 contributes to regulatory T cell-mediated protection in murine crescentic glomerulonephritis. *Sci. Rep.* **2019**, *9*, 2038. [CrossRef]
108. Chambers, C.A.; Kuhns, M.S.; Egen, J.G.; Allison, J.P. CTLA-4-mediated inhibition in regulation of T cell responses: Mechanisms and manipulation in tumor immunotherapy. *Annu. Rev. Immunol.* **2001**, *19*, 565–594. [CrossRef]
109. Tai, X.; Van Laethem, F.; Pobezinsky, L.; Guinter, T.; Sharrow, S.O.; Adams, A.; Granger, L.; Kruhlak, M.; Lindsten, T.; Thompson, C.B.; et al. Basis of CTLA-4 function in regulatory and conventional CD4(+) T cells. *Blood* **2012**, *119*, 5155–5163. [CrossRef]
110. Vanderstraeten, A.; Luyten, C.; Verbist, G.; Tuyaerts, S.; Amant, F. Mapping the immunosuppressive environment in uterine tumors: Implications for immunotherapy. *Cancer Immunol. Immunother.* **2014**, *63*, 545–557. [CrossRef]
111. Rozali, E.N.; Hato, S.V.; Robinson, B.W.; Lake, R.A.; Lesterhuis, W.J. Programmed death ligand 2 in cancer-induced immune suppression. *Clin. Dev. Immunol.* **2012**, *2012*, 656340. [CrossRef] [PubMed]
112. Petrova, V.; Arkhypov, I.; Weber, R.; Groth, C.; Altevogt, P.; Utikal, J.; Umansky, V. Modern Aspects of Immunotherapy with Checkpoint Inhibitors in Melanoma. *Int. J. Mol. Sci.* **2020**, *21*, 2367. [CrossRef]
113. Wang, L.; Jia, B.; Claxton, D.F.; Ehmann, W.C.; Rybka, W.B.; Mineishi, S.; Naik, S.; Khawaja, M.R.; Sivik, J.; Han, J.; et al. VISTA is highly expressed on MDSCs and mediates an inhibition of T cell response in patients with AML. *Oncoimmunology* **2018**, *7*, e1469594. [CrossRef] [PubMed]
114. Deng, J.; Li, J.; Sarde, A.; Lines, J.L.; Lee, Y.C.; Qian, D.C.; Pechenick, D.A.; Manivanh, R.; Le Mercier, I.; Lowrey, C.H.; et al. Hypoxia-Induced VISTA Promotes the Suppressive Function of Myeloid-Derived Suppressor Cells in the Tumor Microenvironment. *Cancer Immunol. Res.* **2019**, *7*, 1079–1090. [CrossRef]
115. Green, K.A.; Wang, L.; Noelle, R.J.; Green, W.R. Selective Involvement of the Checkpoint Regulator VISTA in Suppression of B-Cell, but Not T-Cell, Responsiveness by Monocytic Myeloid-Derived Suppressor Cells from Mice Infected with an Immunodeficiency-Causing Retrovirus. *J. Virol.* **2015**, *89*, 9693–9698. [CrossRef]
116. Le Mercier, I.; Chen, W.; Lines, J.L.; Day, M.; Li, J.; Sergent, P.; Noelle, R.J.; Wang, L. VISTA Regulates the Development of Protective Antitumor Immunity. *Cancer Res.* **2014**, *74*, 1933–1944. [CrossRef]
117. Kondo, Y.; Ohno, T.; Nishii, N.; Harada, K.; Yagita, H.; Azuma, M. Differential contribution of three immune checkpoint (VISTA, CTLA-4, PD-1) pathways to antitumor responses against squamous cell carcinoma. *Oral Oncol.* **2016**, *57*, 54–60. [CrossRef]
118. Sakuishi, K.; Jayaraman, P.; Behar, S.M.; Anderson, A.C.; Kuchroo, V.K. Emerging Tim-3 functions in antimicrobial and tumor immunity. *Trends Immunol.* **2011**, *32*, 345–349. [CrossRef]
119. Zhang, C.X.; Huang, D.J.; Baloche, V.; Zhang, L.; Xu, J.X.; Li, B.W.; Zhao, X.R.; He, J.; Mai, H.Q.; Chen, Q.Y.; et al. Galectin-9 promotes a suppressive microenvironment in human cancer by enhancing STING degradation. *Oncogenesis* **2020**, *9*, 65. [CrossRef]
120. Dardalhon, V.; Anderson, A.C.; Karman, J.; Apetoh, L.; Chandwaskar, R.; Lee, D.H.; Cornejo, M.; Nishi, N.; Yamauchi, A.; Quintana, F.J.; et al. Tim-3/galectin-9 pathway: Regulation of Th1 immunity through promotion of CD11b+Ly-6G+ myeloid cells. *J. Immunol.* **2010**, *185*, 1383–1392. [CrossRef]
121. Harjunpaa, H.; Guillerey, C. TIGIT as an emerging immune checkpoint. *Clin. Exp. Immunol.* **2020**, *200*, 108–119. [CrossRef] [PubMed]
122. Sarhan, D.; Cichocki, F.; Zhang, B.; Yingst, A.; Spellman, S.R.; Cooley, S.; Verneris, M.R.; Blazar, B.R.; Miller, J.S. Adaptive NK Cells with Low TIGIT Expression Are Inherently Resistant to Myeloid-Derived Suppressor Cells. *Cancer Res.* **2016**, *76*, 5696–5706. [CrossRef]
123. Peyvandi, S.; Buart, S.; Samah, B.; Vetizou, M.; Zhang, Y.; Durrieu, L.; Polrot, M.; Chouaib, S.; Benihoud, K.; Louache, F.; et al. Fas Ligand Deficiency Impairs Tumor Immunity by Promoting an Accumulation of Monocytic Myeloid-Derived Suppressor Cells. *Cancer Res.* **2015**, *75*, 4292–4301. [CrossRef] [PubMed]
124. Zhu, J.; Powis de Tenbossche, C.G.; Cane, S.; Colau, D.; van Baren, N.; Lurquin, C.; Schmitt-Verhulst, A.M.; Liljestrom, P.; Uyttenhove, C.; Van den Eynde, B.J. Resistance to cancer immunotherapy mediated by apoptosis of tumor-infiltrating lymphocytes. *Nat. Commun* **2017**, *8*, 1404. [CrossRef] [PubMed]
125. Hoechst, B.; Voigtlaender, T.; Ormandy, L.; Gamrekelashvili, J.; Zhao, F.; Wedemeyer, H.; Lehner, F.; Manns, M.P.; Greten, T.F.; Korangy, F. Myeloid derived suppressor cells inhibit natural killer cells in patients with hepatocellular carcinoma via the NKp30 receptor. *Hepatology* **2009**, *50*, 799–807. [CrossRef] [PubMed]
126. Elkabets, M.; Ribeiro, V.S.; Dinarello, C.A.; Ostrand-Rosenberg, S.; Di Santo, J.P.; Apte, R.N.; Vosshenrich, C.A. IL-1beta regulates a novel myeloid-derived suppressor cell subset that impairs NK cell development and function. *Eur. J. Immunol.* **2010**, *40*, 3347–3357. [CrossRef] [PubMed]
127. Sinha, P.; Clements, V.K.; Bunt, S.K.; Albelda, S.M.; Ostrand-Rosenberg, S. Cross-talk between myeloid-derived suppressor cells and macrophages subverts tumor immunity toward a type 2 response. *J. Immunol.* **2007**, *179*, 977–983. [CrossRef]
128. Ostrand-Rosenberg, S.; Sinha, P. Myeloid-derived suppressor cells: Linking inflammation and cancer. *J. Immunol.* **2009**, *182*, 4499–4506. [CrossRef]
129. Hu, C.E.; Gan, J.; Zhang, R.D.; Cheng, Y.R.; Huang, G.J. Up-regulated myeloid-derived suppressor cell contributes to hepatocellular carcinoma development by impairing dendritic cell function. *Scand. J. Gastroenterol.* **2011**, *46*, 156–164. [CrossRef]

130. Li, C.; Jiang, P.; Wei, S.; Xu, X.; Wang, J. Regulatory T cells in tumor microenvironment: New mechanisms, potential therapeutic strategies and future prospects. *Mol. Cancer* **2020**, *19*, 116. [CrossRef]
131. Olbryt, M.; Rajczykowski, M.; Widlak, W. Biological Factors behind Melanoma Response to Immune Checkpoint Inhibitors. *Int. J. Mol. Sci.* **2020**, *21*, 4071. [CrossRef] [PubMed]
132. Imbert, C.; Montfort, A.; Fraisse, M.; Marcheteau, E.; Gilhodes, J.; Martin, E.; Bertrand, F.; Marcellin, M.; Burlet-Schiltz, O.; Peredo, A.G.; et al. Resistance of melanoma to immune checkpoint inhibitors is overcome by targeting the sphingosine kinase-1. *Nat. Commun* **2020**, *11*, 437. [CrossRef] [PubMed]
133. van der Veeken, J.; Gonzalez, A.J.; Cho, H.; Arvey, A.; Hemmers, S.; Leslie, C.S.; Rudensky, A.Y. Memory of Inflammation in Regulatory T Cells. *Cell* **2016**, *166*, 977–990. [CrossRef]
134. Li, M.O.; Rudensky, A.Y. T cell receptor signalling in the control of regulatory T cell differentiation and function. *Nat. Rev. Immunol.* **2016**, *16*, 220–233. [CrossRef] [PubMed]
135. Wing, J.B.; Tanaka, A.; Sakaguchi, S. Human FOXP3(+) Regulatory T Cell Heterogeneity and Function in Autoimmunity and Cancer. *Immunity* **2019**, *50*, 302–316. [CrossRef]
136. Ahmadzadeh, M.; Pasetto, A.; Jia, L.; Deniger, D.C.; Stevanovic, S.; Robbins, P.F.; Rosenberg, S.A. Tumor-infiltrating human CD4(+) regulatory T cells display a distinct TCR repertoire and exhibit tumor and neoantigen reactivity. *Sci. Immunol.* **2019**, *4*. [CrossRef]
137. Delgoffe, G.M.; Kole, T.P.; Zheng, Y.; Zarek, P.E.; Matthews, K.L.; Xiao, B.; Worley, P.F.; Kozma, S.C.; Powell, J.D. The mTOR kinase differentially regulates effector and regulatory T cell lineage commitment. *Immunity* **2009**, *30*, 832–844. [CrossRef]
138. Michalek, R.D.; Gerriets, V.A.; Jacobs, S.R.; Macintyre, A.N.; MacIver, N.J.; Mason, E.F.; Sullivan, S.A.; Nichols, A.G.; Rathmell, J.C. Cutting edge: Distinct glycolytic and lipid oxidative metabolic programs are essential for effector and regulatory CD4+ T cell subsets. *J. Immunol.* **2011**, *186*, 3299–3303. [CrossRef]
139. Sawant, D.V.; Yano, H.; Chikina, M.; Zhang, Q.; Liao, M.; Liu, C.; Callahan, D.J.; Sun, Z.; Sun, T.; Tabib, T.; et al. Adaptive plasticity of IL-10(+) and IL-35(+) Treg cells cooperatively promotes tumor T cell exhaustion. *Nat. Immunol.* **2019**, *20*, 724–735. [CrossRef]
140. Sullivan, J.A.; Tomita, Y.; Jankowska-Gan, E.; Lema, D.A.; Arvedson, M.P.; Nair, A.; Bracamonte-Baran, W.; Zhou, Y.; Meyer, K.K.; Zhong, W.; et al. Treg-Cell-Derived IL-35-Coated Extracellular Vesicles Promote Infectious Tolerance. *Cell Rep.* **2020**, *30*, 1039–1051.e5. [CrossRef]
141. Ohta, A.; Kini, R.; Ohta, A.; Subramanian, M.; Madasu, M.; Sitkovsky, M. The development and immunosuppressive functions of CD4(+) CD25(+) FoxP3(+) regulatory T cells are under influence of the adenosine-A2A adenosine receptor pathway. *Front. Immunol.* **2012**, *3*, 190. [CrossRef]
142. Rodriguez, P.C.; Quiceno, D.G.; Ochoa, A.C. L-arginine availability regulates T-lymphocyte cell-cycle progression. *Blood* **2007**, *109*, 1568–1573. [CrossRef]
143. Nakaya, M.; Xiao, Y.; Zhou, X.; Chang, J.H.; Chang, M.; Cheng, X.; Blonska, M.; Lin, X.; Sun, S.C. Inflammatory T cell responses rely on amino acid transporter ASCT2 facilitation of glutamine uptake and mTORC1 kinase activation. *Immunity* **2014**, *40*, 692–705. [CrossRef] [PubMed]
144. Kurniawan, H.; Franchina, D.G.; Guerra, L.; Bonetti, L.; Baguet, L.S.; Grusdat, M.; Schlicker, L.; Hunewald, O.; Dostert, C.; Merz, M.P.; et al. Glutathione Restricts Serine Metabolism to Preserve Regulatory T Cell Function. *Cell Metab.* **2020**, *31*, 920–936.e7. [CrossRef] [PubMed]
145. Sarhan, D.; Hippen, K.L.; Lemire, A.; Hying, S.; Luo, X.; Lenvik, T.; Curtsinger, J.; Davis, Z.; Zhang, B.; Cooley, S.; et al. Adaptive NK Cells Resist Regulatory T-cell Suppression Driven by IL37. *Cancer Immunol. Res.* **2018**, *6*, 766–775. [CrossRef] [PubMed]
146. Kalia, V.; Penny, L.A.; Yuzefpolskiy, Y.; Baumann, F.M.; Sarkar, S. Quiescence of Memory CD8(+) T Cells Is Mediated by Regulatory T Cells through Inhibitory Receptor CTLA-4. *Immunity* **2015**, *42*, 1116–1129. [CrossRef]
147. Ihara, F.; Sakurai, D.; Takami, M.; Kamata, T.; Kunii, N.; Yamasaki, K.; Iinuma, T.; Nakayama, T.; Motohashi, S.; Okamoto, Y. Regulatory T cells induce CD4(-) NKT cell anergy and suppress NKT cell cytotoxic function. *Cancer Immunol. Immunother.* **2019**, *68*, 1935–1947. [CrossRef]
148. Newton, R.; Priyadharshini, B.; Turka, L.A. Immunometabolism of regulatory T cells. *Nat. Immunol.* **2016**, *17*, 618–625. [CrossRef] [PubMed]
149. Cobbold, S.P.; Adams, E.; Farquhar, C.A.; Nolan, K.F.; Howie, D.; Lui, K.O.; Fairchild, P.J.; Mellor, A.L.; Ron, D.; Waldmann, H. Infectious tolerance via the consumption of essential amino acids and mTOR signaling. *Proc. Natl. Acad. Sci. USA* **2009**, *106*, 12055–12060. [CrossRef]
150. Serafini, P.; Mgebroff, S.; Noonan, K.; Borrello, I. Myeloid-derived suppressor cells promote cross-tolerance in B-cell lymphoma by expanding regulatory T cells. *Cancer Res.* **2008**, *68*, 5439–5449. [CrossRef]
151. Huang, B.; Pan, P.Y.; Li, Q.; Sato, A.I.; Levy, D.E.; Bromberg, J.; Divino, C.M.; Chen, S.H. Gr-1+CD115+ immature myeloid suppressor cells mediate the development of tumor-induced T regulatory cells and T-cell anergy in tumor-bearing host. *Cancer Res.* **2006**, *66*, 1123–1131. [CrossRef]
152. Fujimura, T.; Mahnke, K.; Enk, A.H. Myeloid derived suppressor cells and their role in tolerance induction in cancer. *J. Dermatol. Sci.* **2010**, *59*, 1–6. [CrossRef]
153. Lee, C.R.; Kwak, Y.; Yang, T.; Han, J.H.; Park, S.H.; Ye, M.B.; Lee, W.; Sim, K.Y.; Kang, J.A.; Kim, Y.C.; et al. Myeloid-Derived Suppressor Cells Are Controlled by Regulatory T Cells via TGF-beta during Murine Colitis. *Cell Rep.* **2016**, *17*, 3219–3232. [CrossRef] [PubMed]

154. Fujimura, T.; Ring, S.; Umansky, V.; Mahnke, K.; Enk, A.H. Regulatory T cells stimulate B7-H1 expression in myeloid-derived suppressor cells in ret melanomas. *J. Investig. Dermatol.* **2012**, *132*, 1239–1246. [CrossRef]
155. Pan, P.Y.; Ma, G.; Weber, K.J.; Ozao-Choy, J.; Wang, G.; Yin, B.; Divino, C.M.; Chen, S.H. Immune stimulatory receptor CD40 is required for T-cell suppression and T regulatory cell activation mediated by myeloid-derived suppressor cells in cancer. *Cancer Res.* **2010**, *70*, 99–108. [CrossRef] [PubMed]
156. Yang, R.; Cai, Z.; Zhang, Y.; Yutzy, W.H.T.; Roby, K.F.; Roden, R.B. CD80 in immune suppression by mouse ovarian carcinoma-associated Gr-1+CD11b+ myeloid cells. *Cancer Res.* **2006**, *66*, 6807–6815. [CrossRef]
157. Pillay, J.; Kamp, V.M.; van Hoffen, E.; Visser, T.; Tak, T.; Lammers, J.W.; Ulfman, L.H.; Leenen, L.P.; Pickkers, P.; Koenderman, L. A subset of neutrophils in human systemic inflammation inhibits T cell responses through Mac-1. *J. Clin. Investig.* **2012**, *122*, 327–336. [CrossRef] [PubMed]
158. Ghiringhelli, F.; Puig, P.E.; Roux, S.; Parcellier, A.; Schmitt, E.; Solary, E.; Kroemer, G.; Martin, F.; Chauffert, B.; Zitvogel, L. Tumor cells convert immature myeloid dendritic cells into TGF-beta-secreting cells inducing CD4+CD25+ regulatory T cell proliferation. *J. Exp. Med.* **2005**, *202*, 919–929. [CrossRef] [PubMed]
159. Hoechst, B.; Ormandy, L.A.; Ballmaier, M.; Lehner, F.; Kruger, C.; Manns, M.P.; Greten, T.F.; Korangy, F. A new population of myeloid-derived suppressor cells in hepatocellular carcinoma patients induces CD4(+)CD25(+)Foxp3(+) T cells. *Gastroenterology* **2008**, *135*, 234–243. [CrossRef] [PubMed]
160. Kochetkova, I.; Golden, S.; Holderness, K.; Callis, G.; Pascual, D.W. IL-35 stimulation of CD39+ regulatory T cells confers protection against collagen II-induced arthritis via the production of IL-10. *J. Immunol.* **2010**, *184*, 7144–7153. [CrossRef]
161. Lian, M.; Zhang, J.; Zhao, L.; Chen, X.; Peng, Y.; Wang, Q.; Chen, S.; Ma, X. Interleukin-35 Regulates Immune Microenvironment of Autoimmune Hepatitis Through Inducing the Expansion of Myeloid-Derived Suppressor Cells. *Front. Immunol.* **2019**, *10*, 2577. [CrossRef] [PubMed]
162. Seyerl, M.; Kirchberger, S.; Majdic, O.; Seipelt, J.; Jindra, C.; Schrauf, C.; Stockl, J. Human rhinoviruses induce IL-35-producing Treg via induction of B7-H1 (CD274) and sialoadhesin (CD169) on DC. *Eur. J. Immunol.* **2010**, *40*, 321–329. [CrossRef] [PubMed]
163. Schlecker, E.; Stojanovic, A.; Eisen, C.; Quack, C.; Falk, C.S.; Umansky, V.; Cerwenka, A. Tumor-infiltrating monocytic myeloid-derived suppressor cells mediate CCR5-dependent recruitment of regulatory T cells favoring tumor growth. *J. Immunol.* **2012**, *189*, 5602–5611. [CrossRef] [PubMed]
164. Morello, S.; Pinto, A.; Blandizzi, C.; Antonioli, L. Myeloid cells in the tumor microenvironment: Role of adenosine. *Oncoimmunology* **2016**, *5*, e1108515. [CrossRef] [PubMed]
165. Ryzhov, S.; Novitskiy, S.V.; Goldstein, A.E.; Biktasova, A.; Blackburn, M.R.; Biaggioni, I.; Dikov, M.M.; Feoktistov, I. Adenosinergic regulation of the expansion and immunosuppressive activity of CD11b+Gr1+ cells. *J. Immunol.* **2011**, *187*, 6120–6129. [CrossRef] [PubMed]
166. Ryzhov, S.V.; Pickup, M.W.; Chytil, A.; Gorska, A.E.; Zhang, Q.; Owens, P.; Feoktistov, I.; Moses, H.L.; Novitskiy, S.V. Role of TGF-beta signaling in generation of CD39+CD73+ myeloid cells in tumors. *J. Immunol.* **2014**, *193*, 3155–3164. [CrossRef] [PubMed]
167. Yang, M.; Ma, C.; Liu, S.; Shao, Q.; Gao, W.; Song, B.; Sun, J.; Xie, Q.; Zhang, Y.; Feng, A.; et al. HIF-dependent induction of adenosine receptor A2b skews human dendritic cells to a Th2-stimulating phenotype under hypoxia. *Immunol. Cell Biol.* **2010**, *88*, 165–171. [CrossRef]
168. Noman, M.Z.; Desantis, G.; Janji, B.; Hasmim, M.; Karray, S.; Dessen, P.; Bronte, V.; Chouaib, S. PD-L1 is a novel direct target of HIF-1alpha, and its blockade under hypoxia enhanced MDSC-mediated T cell activation. *J. Exp. Med.* **2014**, *211*, 781–790. [CrossRef]
169. Chouaib, S.; Umansky, V.; Kieda, C. The role of hypoxia in shaping the recruitment of proangiogenic and immunosuppressive cells in the tumor microenvironment. *Contemp. Oncol.* **2018**, *22*, 7–13. [CrossRef]
170. Baratelli, F.; Lin, Y.; Zhu, L.; Yang, S.C.; Heuze-Vourc'h, N.; Zeng, G.; Reckamp, K.; Dohadwala, M.; Sharma, S.; Dubinett, S.M. Prostaglandin E2 induces FOXP3 gene expression and T regulatory cell function in human CD4+ T cells. *J. Immunol.* **2005**, *175*, 1483–1490. [CrossRef]
171. Moon, Y.W.; Hajjar, J.; Hwu, P.; Naing, A. Targeting the indoleamine 2,3-dioxygenase pathway in cancer. *J. Immunother. Cancer* **2015**, *3*, 51. [CrossRef] [PubMed]
172. Jitschin, R.; Braun, M.; Buttner, M.; Dettmer-Wilde, K.; Bricks, J.; Berger, J.; Eckart, M.J.; Krause, S.W.; Oefner, P.J.; Le Blanc, K.; et al. CLL-cells induce IDOhi CD14+HLA-DRlo myeloid-derived suppressor cells that inhibit T-cell responses and promote TRegs. *Blood* **2014**, *124*, 750–760. [CrossRef] [PubMed]
173. Holmgaard, R.B.; Zamarin, D.; Li, Y.; Gasmi, B.; Munn, D.H.; Allison, J.P.; Merghoub, T.; Wolchok, J.D. Tumor-Expressed IDO Recruits and Activates MDSCs in a Treg-Dependent Manner. *Cell Rep.* **2015**, *13*, 412–424. [CrossRef] [PubMed]
174. Xu, W.; Hieu, T.; Malarkannan, S.; Wang, L. The structure, expression, and multifaceted role of immune-checkpoint protein VISTA as a critical regulator of anti-tumor immunity, autoimmunity, and inflammation. *Cell. Mol. Immunol.* **2018**, *15*, 438–446. [CrossRef] [PubMed]
175. Liu, J.; Yuan, Y.; Chen, W.; Putra, J.; Suriawinata, A.A.; Schenk, A.D.; Miller, H.E.; Guleria, I.; Barth, R.J.; Huang, Y.H.; et al. Immune-checkpoint proteins VISTA and PD-1 nonredundantly regulate murine T-cell responses. *Proc. Natl. Acad. Sci. USA* **2015**, *112*, 6682–6687. [CrossRef] [PubMed]
176. Long, L.; Zhang, X.; Chen, F.; Pan, Q.; Phiphatwatchara, P.; Zeng, Y.; Chen, H. The promising immune checkpoint LAG-3: From tumor microenvironment to cancer immunotherapy. *Genes Cancer* **2018**, *9*, 176–189. [CrossRef]

177. Andrews, L.P.; Marciscano, A.E.; Drake, C.G.; Vignali, D.A. LAG3 (CD223) as a cancer immunotherapy target. *Immunol. Rev.* **2017**, *276*, 80–96. [CrossRef]
178. Pinton, L.; Solito, S.; Damuzzo, V.; Francescato, S.; Pozzuoli, A.; Berizzi, A.; Mocellin, S.; Rossi, C.R.; Bronte, V.; Mandruzzato, S. Activated T cells sustain myeloid-derived suppressor cell-mediated immune suppression. *Oncotarget* **2016**, *7*, 1168–1184. [CrossRef]
179. Macon-Lemaitre, L.; Triebel, F. The negative regulatory function of the lymphocyte-activation gene-3 co-receptor (CD223) on human T cells. *Immunology* **2005**, *115*, 170–178. [CrossRef]
180. Nagaraj, S.; Nelson, A.; Youn, J.I.; Cheng, P.; Quiceno, D.; Gabrilovich, D.I. Antigen-specific CD4(+) T cells regulate function of myeloid-derived suppressor cells in cancer via retrograde MHC class II signaling. *Cancer Res.* **2012**, *72*, 928–938. [CrossRef]
181. Wei, T.; Zhang, J.; Qin, Y.; Wu, Y.; Zhu, L.; Lu, L.; Tang, G.; Shen, Q. Increased expression of immunosuppressive molecules on intratumoral and circulating regulatory T cells in non-small-cell lung cancer patients. *Am. J. Cancer Res.* **2015**, *5*, 2190–2201. [PubMed]
182. Durham, N.M.; Nirschl, C.J.; Jackson, C.M.; Elias, J.; Kochel, C.M.; Anders, R.A.; Drake, C.G. Lymphocyte Activation Gene 3 (LAG-3) modulates the ability of CD4 T-cells to be suppressed in vivo. *PLoS ONE* **2014**, *9*, e109080. [CrossRef] [PubMed]
183. Huang, C.T.; Workman, C.J.; Flies, D.; Pan, X.; Marson, A.L.; Zhou, G.; Hipkiss, E.L.; Ravi, S.; Kowalski, J.; Levitsky, H.I.; et al. Role of LAG-3 in regulatory T cells. *Immunity* **2004**, *21*, 503–513. [CrossRef] [PubMed]
184. Woo, S.R.; Turnis, M.E.; Goldberg, M.V.; Bankoti, J.; Selby, M.; Nirschl, C.J.; Bettini, M.L.; Gravano, D.M.; Vogel, P.; Liu, C.L.; et al. Immune inhibitory molecules LAG-3 and PD-1 synergistically regulate T-cell function to promote tumoral immune escape. *Cancer Res.* **2012**, *72*, 917–927. [CrossRef] [PubMed]
185. He, Y.; Yu, H.; Rozeboom, L.; Rivard, C.J.; Ellison, K.; Dziadziuszko, R.; Suda, K.; Ren, S.; Wu, C.; Hou, L.; et al. LAG-3 Protein Expression in Non-Small Cell Lung Cancer and Its Relationship with PD-1/PD-L1 and Tumor-Infiltrating Lymphocytes. *J. Thorac. Oncol.* **2017**, *12*, 814–823. [CrossRef]
186. Sakuishi, K.; Ngiow, S.F.; Sullivan, J.M.; Teng, M.W.; Kuchroo, V.K.; Smyth, M.J.; Anderson, A.C. TIM3(+)FOXP3(+) regulatory T cells are tissue-specific promoters of T-cell dysfunction in cancer. *Oncoimmunology* **2013**, *2*, e23849. [CrossRef]
187. Anderson, A.C. Tim-3: An emerging target in the cancer immunotherapy landscape. *Cancer Immunol. Res.* **2014**, *2*, 393–398. [CrossRef]
188. Liu, J.F.; Wu, L.; Yang, L.L.; Deng, W.W.; Mao, L.; Wu, H.; Zhang, W.F.; Sun, Z.J. Blockade of TIM3 relieves immunosuppression through reducing regulatory T cells in head and neck cancer. *J. Exp. Clin. Cancer Res.* **2018**, *37*, 44. [CrossRef]
189. Wu, L.; Mao, L.; Liu, J.F.; Chen, L.; Yu, G.T.; Yang, L.L.; Wu, H.; Bu, L.L.; Kulkarni, A.B.; Zhang, W.F.; et al. Blockade of TIGIT/CD155 Signaling Reverses T-cell Exhaustion and Enhances Antitumor Capability in Head and Neck Squamous Cell Carcinoma. *Cancer Immunol. Res.* **2019**, *7*, 1700–1713. [CrossRef]
190. Joller, N.; Lozano, E.; Burkett, P.R.; Patel, B.; Xiao, S.; Zhu, C.; Xia, J.; Tan, T.G.; Sefik, E.; Yajnik, V.; et al. Treg cells expressing the coinhibitory molecule TIGIT selectively inhibit proinflammatory Th1 and Th17 cell responses. *Immunity* **2014**, *40*, 569–581. [CrossRef]
191. Byrne, K.T.; Vonderheide, R.H. CD40 Stimulation Obviates Innate Sensors and Drives T Cell Immunity in Cancer. *Cell Rep.* **2016**, *15*, 2719–2732. [CrossRef]
192. Weiss, J.M.; Subleski, J.J.; Back, T.; Chen, X.; Watkins, S.K.; Yagita, H.; Sayers, T.J.; Murphy, W.J.; Wiltrout, R.H. Regulatory T cells and myeloid-derived suppressor cells in the tumor microenvironment undergo Fas-dependent cell death during IL-2/αCD40 therapy. *J. Immunol.* **2014**, *192*, 5821–5829. [CrossRef] [PubMed]
193. Bednarczyk, M.; Stege, H.; Grabbe, S.; Bros, M. beta2 Integrins-Multi-Functional Leukocyte Receptors in Health and Disease. *Int. J. Mol. Sci.* **2020**, *21*, 1402. [CrossRef] [PubMed]
194. Takada, Y.; Ye, X.; Simon, S. The integrins. *Genome Biol.* **2007**, *8*, 215. [CrossRef] [PubMed]
195. Mitroulis, I.; Alexaki, V.I.; Kourtzelis, I.; Ziogas, A.; Hajishengallis, G.; Chavakis, T. Leukocyte integrins: Role in leukocyte recruitment and as therapeutic targets in inflammatory disease. *Pharmacol. Ther.* **2015**, *147*, 123–135. [CrossRef]
196. Urlaub, D.; Hofer, K.; Muller, M.L.; Watzl, C. LFA-1 Activation in NK Cells and Their Subsets: Influence of Receptors, Maturation, and Cytokine Stimulation. *J. Immunol.* **2017**, *198*, 1944–1951. [CrossRef]
197. Walling, B.L.; Kim, M. LFA-1 in T Cell Migration and Differentiation. *Front. Immunol.* **2018**, *9*, 952. [CrossRef]
198. Fan, Z.; Ley, K. Leukocyte arrest: Biomechanics and molecular mechanisms of beta2 integrin activation. *Biorheology* **2015**, *52*, 353–377. [CrossRef]
199. Rognoni, E.; Ruppert, R.; Fassler, R. The kindlin family: Functions, signaling properties and implications for human disease. *J. Cell Sci.* **2016**, *129*, 17–27. [CrossRef]
200. Zhou, M.; Todd, R.F., 3rd; van de Winkel, J.G.; Petty, H.R. Cocapping of the leukoadhesin molecules complement receptor type 3 and lymphocyte function-associated antigen-1 with Fc gamma receptor III on human neutrophils. Possible role of lectin-like interactions. *J. Immunol.* **1993**, *150*, 3030–3041.
201. Varga, G.; Nippe, N.; Balkow, S.; Peters, T.; Wild, M.K.; Seeliger, S.; Beissert, S.; Krummen, M.; Roth, J.; Sunderkotter, C.; et al. LFA-1 contributes to signal I of T-cell activation and to the production of T(h)1 cytokines. *J. Investig. Dermatol.* **2010**, *130*, 1005–1012. [CrossRef] [PubMed]
202. Wang, Y.; Shibuya, K.; Yamashita, Y.; Shirakawa, J.; Shibata, K.; Kai, H.; Yokosuka, T.; Saito, T.; Honda, S.; Tahara-Hanaoka, S.; et al. LFA-1 decreases the antigen dose for T cell activation in vivo. *Int. Immunol.* **2008**, *20*, 1119–1127. [CrossRef] [PubMed]

203. Marski, M.; Kandula, S.; Turner, J.R.; Abraham, C. CD18 is required for optimal development and function of CD4+CD25+ T regulatory cells. *J. Immunol.* **2005**, *175*, 7889–7897. [CrossRef] [PubMed]
204. Singh, K.; Gatzka, M.; Peters, T.; Borkner, L.; Hainzl, A.; Wang, H.; Sindrilaru, A.; Scharffetter-Kochanek, K. Reduced CD18 levels drive regulatory T cell conversion into Th17 cells in the CD18hypo PL/J mouse model of psoriasis. *J. Immunol.* **2013**, *190*, 2544–2553. [CrossRef]
205. Stevanin, M.; Busso, N.; Chobaz, V.; Pigni, M.; Ghassem-Zadeh, S.; Zhang, L.; Acha-Orbea, H.; Ehirchiou, D. CD11b regulates the Treg/Th17 balance in murine arthritis via IL-6. *Eur. J. Immunol.* **2017**, *47*, 637–645. [CrossRef] [PubMed]
206. Wang, H.; Peters, T.; Sindrilaru, A.; Kess, D.; Oreshkova, T.; Yu, X.Z.; Seier, A.M.; Schreiber, H.; Wlaschek, M.; Blakytny, R.; et al. TGF-beta-dependent suppressive function of Tregs requires wild-type levels of CD18 in a mouse model of psoriasis. *J. Clin. Investig.* **2008**, *118*, 2629–2639. [CrossRef]
207. Wohler, J.; Bullard, D.; Schoeb, T.; Barnum, S. LFA-1 is critical for regulatory T cell homeostasis and function. *Mol. Immunol.* **2009**, *46*, 2424–2428. [CrossRef]
208. Koboziev, I.; Karlsson, F.; Ostanin, D.V.; Gray, L.; Davidson, M.; Zhang, S.; Grisham, M.B. Role of LFA-1 in the activation and trafficking of T cells: Implications in the induction of chronic colitis. *Inflamm. Bowel Dis.* **2012**, *18*, 2360–2370. [CrossRef]
209. Gultner, S.; Kuhlmann, T.; Hesse, A.; Weber, J.P.; Riemer, C.; Baier, M.; Hutloff, A. Reduced Treg frequency in LFA-1-deficient mice allows enhanced T effector differentiation and pathology in EAE. *Eur. J. Immunol.* **2010**, *40*, 3403–3412. [CrossRef]
210. Wang, Y.; Shu, Y.; Xiao, Y.; Wang, Q.; Kanekura, T.; Li, Y.; Wang, J.; Zhao, M.; Lu, Q.; Xiao, R. Hypomethylation and overexpression of ITGAL (CD11a) in CD4(+) T cells in systemic sclerosis. *Clin. Epigenetics* **2014**, *6*, 25. [CrossRef]
211. Luo, Y.; Wang, Y.; Shu, Y.; Lu, Q.; Xiao, R. Epigenetic mechanisms: An emerging role in pathogenesis and its therapeutic potential in systemic sclerosis. *Int. J. Biochem. Cell Biol.* **2015**, *67*, 92–100. [CrossRef] [PubMed]
212. Guttman-Yassky, E.; Vugmeyster, Y.; Lowes, M.A.; Chamian, F.; Kikuchi, T.; Kagen, M.; Gilleaudeau, P.; Lee, E.; Hunte, B.; Howell, K.; et al. Blockade of CD11a by efalizumab in psoriasis patients induces a unique state of T-cell hyporesponsiveness. *J. Investig. Dermatol.* **2008**, *128*, 1182–1191. [CrossRef] [PubMed]
213. Faridi, M.H.; Khan, S.Q.; Zhao, W.; Lee, H.W.; Altintas, M.M.; Zhang, K.; Kumar, V.; Armstrong, A.R.; Carmona-Rivera, C.; Dorschner, J.M.; et al. CD11b activation suppresses TLR-dependent inflammation and autoimmunity in systemic lupus erythematosus. *J. Clin. Investig.* **2017**, *127*, 1271–1283. [CrossRef] [PubMed]
214. Gensterblum, E.; Renauer, P.; Coit, P.; Strickland, F.M.; Kilian, N.C.; Miller, S.; Ognenovski, M.; Wren, J.D.; Tsou, P.S.; Lewis, E.E.; et al. CD4+CD28+KIR+CD11a(hi) T cells correlate with disease activity and are characterized by a pro-inflammatory epigenetic and transcriptional profile in lupus patients. *J. Autoimmun.* **2018**, *86*, 19–28. [CrossRef]
215. Cao, L.Y.; Soler, D.C.; Debanne, S.M.; Grozdev, I.; Rodriguez, M.E.; Feig, R.L.; Carman, T.L.; Gilkeson, R.C.; Orringer, C.E.; Kern, E.F.; et al. Psoriasis and cardiovascular risk factors: Increased serum myeloperoxidase and corresponding immunocellular overexpression by Cd11b(+) CD68(+) macrophages in skin lesions. *Am. J. Transl. Res.* **2013**, *6*, 16–27.
216. Sanchez-Blanco, C.; Clarke, F.; Cornish, G.H.; Depoil, D.; Thompson, S.J.; Dai, X.; Rawlings, D.J.; Dustin, M.L.; Zamoyska, R.; Cope, A.P.; et al. Protein tyrosine phosphatase PTPN22 regulates LFA-1 dependent Th1 responses. *J. Autoimmun.* **2018**, *94*, 45–55. [CrossRef]
217. Kohm, A.P.; Carpentier, P.A.; Anger, H.A.; Miller, S.D. Cutting edge: CD4+CD25+ regulatory T cells suppress antigen-specific autoreactive immune responses and central nervous system inflammation during active experimental autoimmune encephalomyelitis. *J. Immunol.* **2002**, *169*, 4712–4716. [CrossRef]
218. Glatigny, S.; Duhen, R.; Arbelaez, C.; Kumari, S.; Bettelli, E. Integrin alpha L controls the homing of regulatory T cells during CNS autoimmunity in the absence of integrin alpha 4. *Sci. Rep.* **2015**, *5*, 7834. [CrossRef]
219. Haasken, S.; Auger, J.L.; Binstadt, B.A. Absence of beta2 integrins impairs regulatory T cells and exacerbates CD4+ T cell-dependent autoimmune carditis. *J. Immunol.* **2011**, *187*, 2702–2710. [CrossRef]
220. Harjunpää, H.; Llort Asens, M.; Guenther, C.; Fagerholm, S.C. Cell Adhesion Molecules and Their Roles and Regulation in the Immune and Tumor Microenvironment. *Front. Immunol.* **2019**, *10*, 1078. [CrossRef]
221. Anz, D.; Mueller, W.; Golic, M.; Kunz, W.G.; Rapp, M.; Koelzer, V.H.; Ellermeier, J.; Ellwart, J.W.; Schnurr, M.; Bourquin, C.; et al. CD103 is a hallmark of tumor-infiltrating regulatory T cells. *Int. J. Cancer* **2011**, *129*, 2417–2426. [CrossRef] [PubMed]
222. Moutsopoulos, N.M.; Konkel, J.; Sarmadi, M.; Eskan, M.A.; Wild, T.; Dutzan, N.; Abusleme, L.; Zenobia, C.; Hosur, K.B.; Abe, T.; et al. Defective neutrophil recruitment in leukocyte adhesion deficiency type I disease causes local IL-17-driven inflammatory bone loss. *Sci. Transl. Med.* **2014**, *6*, 229ra240. [CrossRef] [PubMed]
223. Anderson, D.C.; Schmalstieg, F.C.; Finegold, M.J.; Hughes, B.J.; Rothlein, R.; Miller, L.J.; Kohl, S.; Tosi, M.F.; Jacobs, R.L.; Waldrop, T.C.; et al. The severe and moderate phenotypes of heritable Mac-1, LFA-1 deficiency: Their quantitative definition and relation to leukocyte dysfunction and clinical features. *J. Infect. Dis.* **1985**, *152*, 668–689. [CrossRef] [PubMed]
224. Liu, J.R.; Han, X.; Soriano, S.G.; Yuki, K. The role of macrophage 1 antigen in polymicrobial sepsis. *Shock* **2014**, *42*, 532–539. [CrossRef] [PubMed]
225. Mizgerd, J.P.; Horwitz, B.H.; Quillen, H.C.; Scott, M.L.; Doerschuk, C.M. Effects of CD18 deficiency on the emigration of murine neutrophils during pneumonia. *J. Immunol.* **1999**, *163*, 995–999. [PubMed]
226. Teschner, D.; Cholaszczynska, A.; Ries, F.; Beckert, H.; Theobald, M.; Grabbe, S.; Radsak, M.; Bros, M. CD11b Regulates Fungal Outgrowth but Not Neutrophil Recruitment in a Mouse Model of Invasive Pulmonary Aspergillosis. *Front. Immunol.* **2019**, *10*, 123. [CrossRef]

227. Aarts, C.E.M.; Hiemstra, I.H.; Beguin, E.P.; Hoogendijk, A.J.; Bouchmal, S.; van Houdt, M.; Tool, A.T.J.; Mul, E.; Jansen, M.H.; Janssen, H.; et al. Activated neutrophils exert myeloid-derived suppressor cell activity damaging T cells beyond repair. *Blood Adv.* **2019**, *3*, 3562–3574. [CrossRef] [PubMed]
228. Kim, K.J.; Lee, K.S.; Cho, H.J.; Kim, Y.H.; Yang, H.K.; Kim, W.H.; Kang, G.H. Prognostic implications of tumor-infiltrating FoxP3+ regulatory T cells and CD8+ cytotoxic T cells in microsatellite-unstable gastric cancers. *Hum. Pathol.* **2014**, *45*, 285–293. [CrossRef]
229. Zhang, Q.Q.; Hu, X.W.; Liu, Y.L.; Ye, Z.J.; Gui, Y.H.; Zhou, D.L.; Qi, C.L.; He, X.D.; Wang, H.; Wang, L.J. CD11b deficiency suppresses intestinal tumor growth by reducing myeloid cell recruitment. *Sci. Rep.* **2015**, *5*, 15948. [CrossRef]
230. Ahn, G.O.; Tseng, D.; Liao, C.H.; Dorie, M.J.; Czechowicz, A.; Brown, J.M. Inhibition of Mac-1 (CD11b/CD18) enhances tumor response to radiation by reducing myeloid cell recruitment. *Proc. Natl. Acad. Sci. USA* **2010**, *107*, 8363–8368. [CrossRef]
231. Soloviev, D.A.; Hazen, S.L.; Szpak, D.; Bledzka, K.M.; Ballantyne, C.M.; Plow, E.F.; Pluskota, E. Dual role of the leukocyte integrin alphaMbeta2 in angiogenesis. *J. Immunol.* **2014**, *193*, 4712–4721. [CrossRef] [PubMed]
232. Sorrentino, C.; Miele, L.; Porta, A.; Pinto, A.; Morello, S. Myeloid-derived suppressor cells contribute to A2B adenosine receptor-induced VEGF production and angiogenesis in a mouse melanoma model. *Oncotarget* **2015**, *6*, 27478–27489. [CrossRef] [PubMed]
233. Kostlin-Gille, N.; Dietz, S.; Schwarz, J.; Spring, B.; Pauluschke-Frohlich, J.; Poets, C.F.; Gille, C. HIF-1alpha-Deficiency in Myeloid Cells Leads to a Disturbed Accumulation of Myeloid Derived Suppressor Cells (MDSC) During Pregnancy and to an Increased Abortion Rate in Mice. *Front. Immunol.* **2019**, *10*, 161. [CrossRef] [PubMed]
234. Teixido, J.; Hemler, M.E.; Greenberger, J.S.; Anklesaria, P. Role of beta 1 and beta 2 integrins in the adhesion of human CD34hi stem cells to bone marrow stroma. *J. Clin. Investig.* **1992**, *90*, 358–367. [CrossRef]
235. Papayannopoulou, T.; Priestley, G.V.; Nakamoto, B.; Zafiropoulos, V.; Scott, L.M.; Harlan, J.M. Synergistic mobilization of hemopoietic progenitor cells using concurrent beta1 and beta2 integrin blockade or beta2-deficient mice. *Blood* **2001**, *97*, 1282–1288. [CrossRef]
236. Watanabe, T.; Dave, B.; Heimann, D.G.; Lethaby, E.; Kessinger, A.; Talmadge, J.E. GM-CSF-mobilized peripheral blood CD34+ cells differ from steady-state bone marrow CD34+ cells in adhesion molecule expression. *Bone Marrow Transplant.* **1997**, *19*, 1175–1181. [CrossRef]
237. Pruijt, J.F.; van Kooyk, Y.; Figdor, C.G.; Lindley, I.J.; Willemze, R.; Fibbe, W.E. Anti-LFA-1 blocking antibodies prevent mobilization of hematopoietic progenitor cells induced by interleukin-8. *Blood* **1998**, *91*, 4099–4105. [CrossRef]
238. Talmadge, J.E.; Gabrilovich, D.I. History of myeloid-derived suppressor cells. *Nat. Rev. Cancer* **2013**, *13*, 739–752. [CrossRef]
239. Jin, H.; Su, J.; Garmy-Susini, B.; Kleeman, J.; Varner, J. Integrin alpha4beta1 promotes monocyte trafficking and angiogenesis in tumors. *Cancer Res.* **2006**, *66*, 2146–2152. [CrossRef]
240. Hidalgo, A.; Peired, A.J.; Weiss, L.A.; Katayama, Y.; Frenette, P.S. The integrin alphaMbeta2 anchors hematopoietic progenitors in the bone marrow during enforced mobilization. *Blood* **2004**, *104*, 993–1001. [CrossRef]
241. Schmid, M.C.; Khan, S.Q.; Kaneda, M.M.; Pathria, P.; Shepard, R.; Louis, T.L.; Anand, S.; Woo, G.; Leem, C.; Faridi, M.H.; et al. Integrin CD11b activation drives anti-tumor innate immunity. *Nat. Commun* **2018**, *9*, 5379. [CrossRef] [PubMed]
242. Wang, L.; Gordon, R.A.; Huynh, L.; Su, X.; Min, K.-H.P.; Han, J.; Arthur, J.S.; Kalliolias, G.D.; Ivashkiv, L.B. Indirect Inhibition of Toll-like Receptor and Type I Interferon Responses by ITAM-Coupled Receptors and Integrins. *Immunity* **2010**, *32*, 518–530. [CrossRef] [PubMed]
243. Foubert, P.; Kaneda, M.M.; Varner, J.A. PI3Kgamma Activates Integrin alpha4 and Promotes Immune Suppressive Myeloid Cell Polarization during Tumor Progression. *Cancer Immunol. Res.* **2017**, *5*, 957–968. [CrossRef] [PubMed]
244. Abadier, M.; Ley, K. P-selectin glycoprotein ligand-1 in T cells. *Curr. Opin. Hematol.* **2017**, *24*, 265–273. [CrossRef]
245. Angiari, S.; Rossi, B.; Piccio, L.; Zinselmeyer, B.H.; Budui, S.; Zenaro, E.; Della Bianca, V.; Bach, S.D.; Scarpini, E.; Bolomini-Vittori, M.; et al. Regulatory T cells suppress the late phase of the immune response in lymph nodes through P-selectin glycoprotein ligand-1. *J. Immunol.* **2013**, *191*, 5489–5500. [CrossRef]
246. Coxon, A.; Rieu, P.; Barkalow, F.J.; Askari, S.; Sharpe, A.H.; von Andrian, U.H.; Arnaout, M.A.; Mayadas, T.N. A Novel Role for the β2 Integrin CD11b/CD18 in Neutrophil Apoptosis: A Homeostatic Mechanism in Inflammation. *Immunity* **1996**, *5*, 653–666. [CrossRef]
247. Fagerholm, S.C.; Guenther, C.; Llort Asens, M.; Savinko, T.; Uotila, L.M. Beta2-Integrins and Interacting Proteins in Leukocyte Trafficking, Immune Suppression, and Immunodeficiency Disease. *Front. Immunol.* **2019**, *10*, 254. [CrossRef]
248. Benvenuti, F. The Dendritic Cell Synapse: A Life Dedicated to T Cell Activation. *Front. Immunol.* **2016**, *7*, 70. [CrossRef]
249. Weber, R.; Fleming, V.; Hu, X.; Nagibin, V.; Groth, C.; Altevogt, P.; Utikal, J.; Umansky, V. Myeloid-Derived Suppressor Cells Hinder the Anti-Cancer Activity of Immune Checkpoint Inhibitors. *Front. Immunol.* **2018**, *9*, 1310. [CrossRef]
250. Law, A.M.K.; Valdes-Mora, F.; Gallego-Ortega, D. Myeloid-Derived Suppressor Cells as a Therapeutic Target for Cancer. *Cells* **2020**, *9*, 561. [CrossRef]
251. De Cicco, P.; Ercolano, G.; Ianaro, A. The New Era of Cancer Immunotherapy: Targeting Myeloid-Derived Suppressor Cells to Overcome Immune Evasion. *Front. Immunol.* **2020**, *11*, 1680. [CrossRef] [PubMed]
252. Carlino, M.S.; Long, G.V.; Schadendorf, D.; Robert, C.; Ribas, A.; Richtig, E.; Nyakas, M.; Caglevic, C.; Tarhini, A.; Blank, C.; et al. Outcomes by line of therapy and programmed death ligand 1 expression in patients with advanced melanoma treated with pembrolizumab or ipilimumab in KEYNOTE-006: A randomised clinical trial. *Eur. J. Cancer* **2018**, *101*, 236–243. [CrossRef] [PubMed]

253. Keilholz, U.; Mehnert, J.M.; Bauer, S.; Bourgeois, H.; Patel, M.R.; Gravenor, D.; Nemunaitis, J.J.; Taylor, M.H.; Wyrwicz, L.; Lee, K.W.; et al. Avelumab in patients with previously treated metastatic melanoma: Phase 1b results from the JAVELIN Solid Tumor trial. *J. Immunother. Cancer* **2019**, *7*, 12. [CrossRef] [PubMed]
254. Page, D.B.; Bear, H.; Prabhakaran, S.; Gatti-Mays, M.E.; Thomas, A.; Cobain, E.; McArthur, H.; Balko, J.M.; Gameiro, S.R.; Nanda, R.; et al. Two may be better than one: PD-1/PD-L1 blockade combination approaches in metastatic breast cancer. *NPJ Breast Cancer* **2019**, *5*, 34. [CrossRef]
255. Ghatalia, P.; Zibelman, M.; Geynisman, D.M.; Plimack, E. Approved checkpoint inhibitors in bladder cancer: Which drug should be used when? *Ther. Adv. Med. Oncol.* **2018**, *10*, 1758835918788310. [CrossRef]
256. Motzer, R.J.; Tannir, N.M.; McDermott, D.F.; Aren Frontera, O.; Melichar, B.; Choueiri, T.K.; Plimack, E.R.; Barthelemy, P.; Porta, C.; George, S.; et al. Nivolumab plus Ipilimumab versus Sunitinib in Advanced Renal-Cell Carcinoma. *N. Engl. J. Med.* **2018**, *378*, 1277–1290. [CrossRef]
257. Orillion, A.; Hashimoto, A.; Damayanti, N.; Shen, L.; Adelaiye-Ogala, R.; Arisa, S.; Chintala, S.; Ordentlich, P.; Kao, C.; Elzey, B.; et al. Entinostat Neutralizes Myeloid-Derived Suppressor Cells and Enhances the Antitumor Effect of PD-1 Inhibition in Murine Models of Lung and Renal Cell Carcinoma. *Clin. Cancer Res.* **2017**, *23*, 5187–5201. [CrossRef]
258. Kim, K.; Skora, A.D.; Li, Z.; Liu, Q.; Tam, A.J.; Blosser, R.L.; Diaz, L.A., Jr.; Papadopoulos, N.; Kinzler, K.W.; Vogelstein, B.; et al. Eradication of metastatic mouse cancers resistant to immune checkpoint blockade by suppression of myeloid-derived cells. *Proc. Natl. Acad. Sci. USA* **2014**, *111*, 11774–11779. [CrossRef]
259. Christmas, B.J.; Rafie, C.I.; Hopkins, A.C.; Scott, B.A.; Ma, H.S.; Cruz, K.A.; Woolman, S.; Armstrong, T.D.; Connolly, R.M.; Azad, N.A.; et al. Entinostat Converts Immune-Resistant Breast and Pancreatic Cancers into Checkpoint-Responsive Tumors by Reprogramming Tumor-Infiltrating MDSCs. *Cancer Immunol. Res.* **2018**, *6*, 1561–1577. [CrossRef]
260. Steele, C.W.; Karim, S.A.; Leach, J.D.G.; Bailey, P.; Upstill-Goddard, R.; Rishi, L.; Foth, M.; Bryson, S.; McDaid, K.; Wilson, Z.; et al. CXCR2 Inhibition Profoundly Suppresses Metastases and Augments Immunotherapy in Pancreatic Ductal Adenocarcinoma. *Cancer Cell* **2016**, *29*, 832–845. [CrossRef]
261. Ngiow, S.F.; von Scheidt, B.; Akiba, H.; Yagita, H.; Teng, M.W.; Smyth, M.J. Anti-TIM3 antibody promotes T cell IFN-gamma-mediated antitumor immunity and suppresses established tumors. *Cancer Res.* **2011**, *71*, 3540–3551. [CrossRef] [PubMed]
262. Nowak, E.C.; Lines, J.L.; Varn, F.S.; Deng, J.; Sarde, A.; Mabaera, R.; Kuta, A.; Le Mercier, I.; Cheng, C.; Noelle, R.J. Immunoregulatory functions of VISTA. *Immunol. Rev.* **2017**, *276*, 66–79. [CrossRef] [PubMed]
263. Mittal, D.; Young, A.; Stannard, K.; Yong, M.; Teng, M.W.; Allard, B.; Stagg, J.; Smyth, M.J. Antimetastatic effects of blocking PD-1 and the adenosine A2A receptor. *Cancer Res.* **2014**, *74*, 3652–3658. [CrossRef] [PubMed]
264. Spira, A.I.; Hamid, O.; Bauer, T.M.; Borges, V.F.; Wasser, J.S.; Smith, D.C.; Clark, A.S.; Schmidt, E.V.; Zhao, Y.; Maleski, J.E.; et al. Efficacy/safety of epacadostat plus pembrolizumab in triple-negative breast cancer and ovarian cancer: Phase I/II ECHO-202 study. *J. Clin. Oncol.* **2017**, *35*, 1103. [CrossRef]
265. Smith, C.; Chang, M.Y.; Parker, K.H.; Beury, D.W.; DuHadaway, J.B.; Flick, H.E.; Boulden, J.; Sutanto-Ward, E.; Soler, A.P.; Laury-Kleintop, L.D.; et al. IDO is a nodal pathogenic driver of lung cancer and metastasis development. *Cancer Discov.* **2012**, *2*, 722–735. [CrossRef] [PubMed]

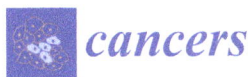

Review

Cancer Immunotherapy and Application of Nanoparticles in Cancers Immunotherapy as the Delivery of Immunotherapeutic Agents and as the Immunomodulators

Tilahun Ayane Debele [1], Cheng-Fa Yeh [1,2] and Wen-Pin Su [1,3,*]

1. Institute of Clinical Medicine, College of Medicine, National Cheng Kung University, No.138, Sheng Li Road, Tainan 704, Taiwan; z10803012@ncku.edu.tw (T.A.D.); u802091@gmail.com (C.-F.Y.)
2. Department of Internal Medicine, Chi Mei Medical Center, Tainan 710, Taiwan
3. Departments of Oncology and Internal Medicine, National Cheng Kung University Hospital, College of Medicine, National Cheng Kung University, Tainan 704, Taiwan
* Correspondence: wpsu@mail.ncku.edu.tw

Received: 30 November 2020; Accepted: 10 December 2020; Published: 15 December 2020

Simple Summary: Cancer becomes one of the major public health problems globally and the burden is expected to be increasing. Currently, both the medical and research communities have attempted an approach to nonconventional cancer therapies that can limit damage or loss of healthy tissues and be able to fully eradicate the cancer cells. In the last few decades, cancer immunotherapy becomes an important tactic for cancer treatment. Immunotherapy of cancer must activate the host's anti-tumor response by enhancing the innate immune system and the effector cell number, while, minimizing the host's suppressor mechanisms. However, many immunotherapies are still limited by poor therapeutic targeting and unwanted side effects. Hence, a deeper understanding of tumor immunology and antitumor immune responses is essential for further improvement of cancer immunotherapy. In addition, effective delivery systems are required to deliver immunotherapeutic agents to the site of interest (such as: to Tumor microenvironments, to Antigen-Presenting Cells, and to the other immune systems) to enhance their efficacy by minimizing off-targeted and unwanted cytotoxicity.

Abstract: In the last few decades, cancer immunotherapy becomes an important tactic for cancer treatment. However, some immunotherapy shows certain limitations including poor therapeutic targeting and unwanted side effects that hinder its use in clinics. Recently, several researchers are exploring an alternative methodology to overcome the above limitations. One of the emerging tracks in this field area is nano-immunotherapy which has gone through rapid progress and revealed considerable potentials to solve limitations related to immunotherapy. Targeted and stimuli-sensitive biocompatible nanoparticles (NPs) can be synthesized to deliver immunotherapeutic agents in their native conformations to the site of interest to enhance their antitumor activity and to enhance the survival rate of cancer patients. In this review, we have discussed cancer immunotherapy and the application of NPs in cancer immunotherapy, as a carrier of immunotherapeutic agents and as a direct immunomodulator.

Keywords: cancer; cancer immunotherapy; nanoparticles; immunotherapeutic agent; immunomodulators

1. Introduction

Cancer becomes one of a killer disease and its burden is anticipated to increase worldwide due to population growth, and lifestyles changes (such as smoking, poor diet, physical inactivity) [1,2]. According to global cancer observatory data (GLOBOCAN), 9.6 million deaths from cancer were estimated in 2018 [3]. The widely known conventional treatment methods for cancer include surgery, chemotherapy, and radiotherapy [4]. Due to the increasing knowledge of molecular and cancer biology, a notable change was observed in cancer treatment for the last few decades. However, conventional cancer treatment has certain limitations, which urges further research investigation. Recently, different research has been underway to improve the survival rate of cancer patients which includes immunotherapy, stem cell transplantation, and targeted cancer therapies [5–10].

Herein, we briefly discuss the application of nanoparticles (NPs) in the cancer immunotherapy as the carrier of immunotherapeutic agents and as the adjuvants to stimulate immune systems to eradicate cancer.

2. Nanoparticles and Nanoparticles-Based Drug Delivery Systems

The majority of drugs delivered through a different route of injection, encounter the physiological, biochemical, and chemical barriers [11]. Hence, it is important to know the physicochemical and biochemical nature of the pharmaceutical agents such as solubility, permeability, and metabolic stability which are crucial factors in the design of NPs for drug delivery systems [12]. In comparison to conventional drug formulation, NPs-based drug delivery systems are under extensive development for several applications including cancer treatment due to their unique physical, chemical, and structural properties. In the last few decades, the term nanomedicine is popularized to describe the application of nanotechnology, by exploiting the unique properties of nano-scale materials, in medicine for the diagnosis and treatment of disease.

Tumor blood vessels possess special characteristics in comparison to the normal blood vessels such as uncontrolled angiogenesis, aberrant vascular architecture, hypervascular permeability, and impaired lymphatic clearance from the interstitial space of tumor tissues (i.e., enhanced permeability and retention (EPR) effect) [13,14]. EPR effect is a crucial point in the drug delivery systems [15,16]. Several kinds of the literature showed that NPs with the diameter 10–100 nm in the bloodstream are too large to escape the vasculature and enter normal tissues or to be cleared by the kidneys, while NPs can easily escape and accumulate in the tumor tissues due to dysfunctional vasculature and defective lymphatics clearance [17].

The efficacy of nanoformulated pharmaceutical agents also determined based on NPs characteristics such as sizes, shapes, and surface charge [18,19]. As mentioned above, NPs with a diameter range of 10 to 100 nm are the best candidates for cancer therapy, as they can effectively deliver their cargo and achieve EPR effect, while NPs with smaller (<10 nm) and larger particle size (>200 nm) can be easily filtered by kidneys and phagocytosed by reticuloendothelial systems, respectively [20]. However, failures of NPs-based chemotherapy in clinical trials have raised some questions about the clinical relevance of the EPR effect and much more research investigation is required to understand the tumor microenvironment (TME). In addition, ligand-modified NPs are widely explored for the active tumor targeting that can enhance bioavailability and selective tumor accumulation which in turn enhance the therapeutic efficacy while reducing normal cytotoxicity.

Moreover, shape and surface charge are crucial in cellular uptake and bio-distribution of NPs. For example, unlike spherical NPs which vulnerable to protein adsorption, non-spherical NPs show less protein adsorption and prevent non-specific cellular phagocytosis which extends their stability and half-life in circulation [21]. Another important parameter is the surface charge of NPs which has a great effect on cellular uptake and in the induction of immune response. For example, cationic NPs show good transfection effects, and have a lysosomal escape tendency which helps to release cargo in the cytoplasm or other subcellular organelles [22]. However, due to their cationic nature, they adsorb more negatively charged serum proteins which hinders their bioavailability [23,24]. As the result, NPs are coated with hydrophilic materials such as polyethylene glycol (PEG), or polysaccharides such as dextran to minimize protein corona, which in turn enhance circulation half-life and its bioavailability [25–27].

NPs-based drug delivery shows a promising result in preclinical and clinical studies. Currently, approximately 50 nanopharmaceuticals agents are approved for cancer and other disease treatments by US FDA [28–30]. However, some nanomedicine products that have undergone extensive clinical trials were later withdrawn due to efficacy or safety concerns e.g., superparamagnetic iron oxide formulations Resovist and SINEREM [31,32].

2.1. The Application of Nanoparticles in Cancer Immunotherapy

The idea of cancer immunotherapy is boosting the antitumor activity of immune systems via tumor-specific immune activation or non-specific immune activation [4,33–36]. The cancer immunotherapy can be boosted via: (a) Increasing antigens presentation and induce specific cytotoxicity T-lymphocytes (CTLs) activity [37]. Naive $CD8^+$ T cells activated and induced antitumor immune response when their receptors recognize antigens presented by Antigen Presenting Cells (APCs) (such as DC) in the context of MHC-I molecules [38,39]. Activated CTLs secrete several cytokines such as interferon-gamma (IFN-γ), tumor necrosis factor-alpha (TNF-α) and the crucial cytolytic mediators (perforin, granzyme, etc.), which improve antigen presentation and mediate anti-tumor effects [40]. (b) Guiding T-cells to the tumor using a bispecific Antibody (bAbs). bAbs offers a unique opportunity to redirect specific immune effector cells to kill cancer cells [41,42]. bAbs can bind simultaneously two different antigens or epitopes to guide T cells to tumor cells, to inhibit two different signaling pathways, and to deliver cargos to the targeted sites [43]. (c) The downregulation of Treg cell, or MDSCs. The TME is enriched with cellular and acellular components that negatively influence cancer immunotherapy [44,45]. MDSC and Treg cells are major components of the immune-suppressive TME and promote T-cell dysfunction that in turn favors tumor progression [46,47]. Hence, downregulation of Treg cell or MDSCs via administration of specific antibodies for each cell is crucial in cancer immunotherapy [48–51].

Immunotherapy offers numerous advantages in comparison to the conventional standard cancer treatment available nowadays [52,53]. Of those, when appropriately stimulated, tumor-specific immune cells can target a microscopic disease, disseminate metastasis, and long-term control might completely remove cancer due to the memory cells [54–56].

Although immunotherapy is efficient to treat different types of cancer, still there is a certain challenge in delivery of immunotherapeutic agents which is expected to be resolved using NPs [57]. A major goal of the utilization of NPs in cancer immunotherapy is to improve therapeutic index by enhancing deliver of immunotherapeutic agents directly to the site of interests only, enhancing accumulation and potency at a region of interest, while simultaneously minimize the dose-dependent systemic toxicity [58]. Unlike delivering chemotherapeutic agents to tumor cells, which necessitates a high dose of nanoformulated drugs to kill all the target cells to be effective, lower concentrations of immune-stimulating drugs can be used to initiate an immune cell or organs (such leukocytes or lymphoid organs) response [59]. For example, Schmid et al. developed antibody-targeted NPs that bind to $CD8^+$ T cells in the blood, lymphoid tissues, and tumors of mice [60]. Synthesized NPs encapsulated with a SD-208, TGFβR1 inhibitor, or a TLR7/TLR8 agonist. Both in vitro and in vivo mice studies showed, successful targeting of $PD-1^+$ T cells in the circulation and in the tumor. Compared to the free drugs, NPs-encapsulated SD-208 enhances survival of mouse bearing colorectal cancer. In addition, synthesized NPs enabled PD-1-targeted delivery of a TLR7/8 agonist to the TME and tumor-infiltrating $CD8^+$ T cells were increased. Overall, this result shows that targeting tumor-infiltrating immune cells in the blood, rather than direct tumor cell targeting, is a better way to improve immunotherapeutic localization in tumors and to stimulate an antitumor response.

In summary, NPs based cancer treatment has a numerous advantage compared to conventional cancer therapy due to: (1) Nanoscale size with several surface characteristics to enhance drug accumulation at the site of interest via EPR effects, (2) Target tumor cells via active targeting which will minimize off-target normal cell toxicity, (3) Protect a therapeutic payload (such as protein, gene, small peptide) from biological degradation, (4) Enhance solubility of hydrophobic drugs and improves there bioavailability, (5) enhance in vivo stability and bioavailability, (6) prevents premature drug release, (7) used as theranostic, combined imaging and therapeutic applications and (8) stimuli, internal or external, programmed to release its cargo at the site of interest.

Furthermore, due to their effectiveness at eliciting cellular and humoral immune responses, NPs can be designed to activate the immune system that could form a gorgeous basis for cancer vaccine development [61,62]. As the result, several NPs are synthesized to deliver different types of immunotherapeutic agents to enhance their therapeutic efficacy, and some of them already shown satisfactory results in clinical trials [63].

2.1.1. Nanoparticles as the Carrier of Immunotherapeutic Agents

Over the last few decades, numerous studies and a large number of papers (Figure 1) have been published on nano-based therapies for cancer treatments. In the last two decades, the total number of papers related to 'nanoparticle + immunotherapy' on PubMed approximately doubled every two years which will be expected a rise similarly in the future.

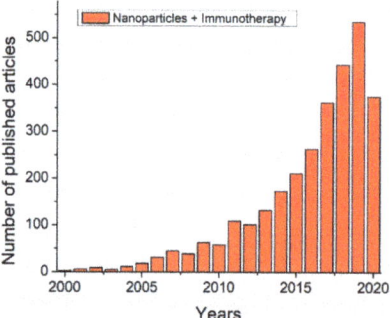

Figure 1. A number of published papers for the last two decades (i.e., 2000–2020) by searching on PubMed using key words "nanoparticles + immunotherapy".

NPs should be precisely designed to target region of interest preferentially from site of administration (common vaccine administration routes are mucosal or parenteral) in order to enhance the efficacy of immunotherapeutic agents [64,65]. NPs targeting lymphoid tissues, where the majority of immune cells are concentrated, would enhance the efficacy of immunotherapeutic agents due to direct access to immune cells [66–69].

Depending on their physicochemical characteristics, including particle size, hydrophobicity, shape, and surface charge, NPs can directly drain to the nearest lymph node, or stay in the injection site and attract migratory DC or macrophages [70]. Several kinds of the literature show that NPs with particle sizes > 100 nm tend to form depot and taken up by APCs and then draining to lymph nodes [71,72]. However, NPs with moderate particle size < 100 nm drained to lymph nodes via lymphatics and retained relatively for a long time, while NPs with small particle size (<10 nm) drain to blood capillaries [73,74]. Regarding the surface charge, negatively charged NPs drain to the lymph node was reported due to charge repulsion with negatively charged ECM, while, cationic NPs tend to form a depot, taken up by peripheral and migratory APCs or gradually draining to lymph node [75]. NPs with nearly neutral charge exhibited potential vector for tumor antigen because they targeted the draining lymph nodes after subcutaneous injection. However, they were weakly immune-stimulatory. In addition, the presence of PEG (PEGylation) on Surface of NPs significantly enhanced large particle size (~200 nm) drain to lymph node and uptake by DCs [76].

Moreover, targeted and stimuli sensitive biocompatible NP can be synthesized to deliver immunotherapeutic agents' in their native conformations to increase antigen uptake, processing, and presentation. For example, NPs can be synthesized for facilitating the cytosolic delivery of antigens, increasing cross-presentation via the MHC-I pathway, and thus inducing cytotoxic T-cell responses.

In addition, in the drug delivery system, it is possible to load or conjugate two or more than two drugs in the single nanocarriers as the co-delivery which will minimize dose related toxicity and enhance the activation of the immune response. For example, Song et al. developed the combined delivery of immunogenic chemotherapy and PD-L1 trap fusion protein using liposomal NPs [77]. They reported that PD-L1 trap is produced transiently and locally in the TME and oxaliplatin (OxP) boosts anti-PD-L1 therapy against murine colorectal cancer and exhibited reduced toxicity compared with non-nanoformulated ones (i.e., free PD-L1 antibodies and oxaliplatin).

In general, NP based drug delivery systems encompass a wide variety of nano-scale size materials including inorganic and Organic NPs in different forms [16].

2.1.2. Antigens and Adjuvants Delivery to Antigen Presenting Cells (APCs)

APCs used as the link between innate and adaptive immune responses by interacting with T cells [78]. APCs are primarily used to recognize and present tumorigenic antigens on their surface via MHC complexes to T cells to initiate an effective adaptive response [79]. However, due to enzymes susceptible of antigens in the body, they are not easily transferred to APCs which decreases its immunogenicity. Hence by using NPs it is possible to overcome this limitation. NPs can encapsulate and deliver cancer antigens to APCs without tumor antigen degradation by the intracellular enzyme. In addition, nanoformulated antigens are more efficiently taken up and processed by APCs than soluble vaccines to amplify T-cell responses due to intradermally or subcutaneously injected NPs drain to lymph nodes, in which APCs are in closeness to T cells [80].

Shen et al. encapsulated ovalbumin (OVA) antigen in the PLGA and deliver successfully to primary mouse bone marrow-derived dendritic cells (BMDCs) [81]. Their result showed that the MHC class I presentation of PLGA-encapsulated OVA stimulated T cell IL-2 secretion at a 1000-fold lower concentration than soluble antigen and 10-fold lower than antigen-coated latex beads.

Kranz et al. precisely designed RNA-lipoplexes (RNA-LPX) NPs with the particle size of ~200–320 nm, by optimally adjusting lipid: RNA ratio to precisely target DC using intravenous injection (Figure 2) [82]. The lipoplexes protect antigen-encoding RNA degradation by ribonucleases. In addition, RNA-LPX enhances cellular uptake and expression of the encoded antigens. Moreover, two transient waves of IFN-α were observed after the NP vaccine injection that led to better T-cell responses and produced vigorous and long-term antitumor effects.

Several kinds of literature showed that the targeted delivery of NPs formulated antigen into DC would enhance antigen presentation to T cells [83–86]. For example, Cruz et al. designed Pegylated PLGA NPs functionalized with TLR3/7 ligand to encapsulate OVA to target surface receptors of DC (i.e., CD40, DEC-205, and CD11c) to accomplish an effective cytotoxic T cell response [87]. In vitro cellular uptake study showed that TLR3/7 ligand targeted NP was more taken up by DC compared to non-targeted NP. Furthermore, high expression of IL-12, IFN-γ, and co-stimulatory molecules were observed in the ligand targeted NP in comparison to non-targeted NPs. Moreover, in vivo vaccination studies showed that ligand targeted NP consistently showed higher efficacy than non-targeted NP in stimulating $CD8^+$ T cell responses.

Some research finding shows that immune response will be enhanced by co-delivering of adjuvants along with tumor antigens due to efficient antigen cross-presentation and vigorous T-cell response for tumor immunotherapy [88–91]. For example, Kuai et al. synthesized high-density lipoprotein-mimicking nanodiscs for co-delivery of CpG adjuvant and neoantigens [92]. They reported that, synthesized nanodiscs elicited up to 47-fold greater frequencies of neoantigen-specific CTLs than soluble vaccines and 31-fold greater antigen-specific T-cell response compared to Montanide. Moreover, nanodiscs in combination with anti-PD-1 and anti-CTLA-4 therapy revealed better eradication of established cancer cells.

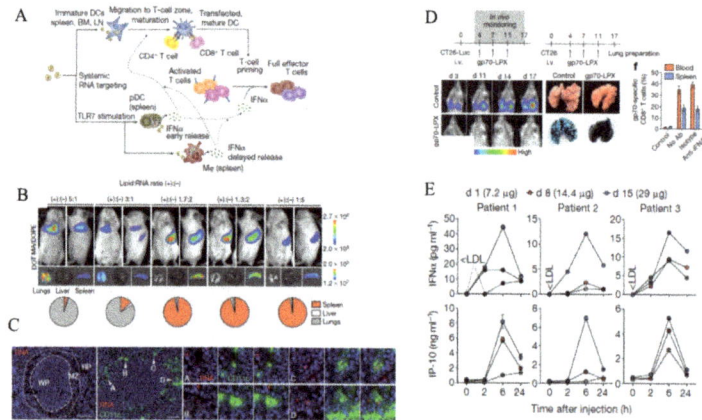

Figure 2. RNA-lipoplexes (RNA-LPX) delivery to DCs. (**A**) Mechanism action of RNA-LPX to induce anti-tumor immune responses, (**B**) Bioluminescence imaging of BALB/c mice, (**C**) Splenic localization of CD11c and Cy3 double-positive cells in BALB/c mice after 1 h of Cy3-labelled RNA-LPX i.v. injection, (**D**) in vivo studies in CT26 tumor bearing BALB/c mice immunized with gp70-LPX, and (**E**) Clinically administered RNA-LPX vaccines induce systemic INFα in dose-dependently manner. Reproduced with permission from [82]. Copyright 2016, Springer Nature.

Similarly, Liu et al. have been synthesized cell-penetrating peptide (CPP) decorated uniform-sized pristine NPs to deliver GM-CSF and IL-2 into tumor cells [93]. In vitro and in vivo (Figure 3) results revealed the programed promotions of multi-adjuvants on DC recruitment, antigen presentation, and T-cell activation. Furthermore, in vivo assessments revealed the satisfactory effects on tumor growth suppression, metastasis inhibition, and recurrence prevention.

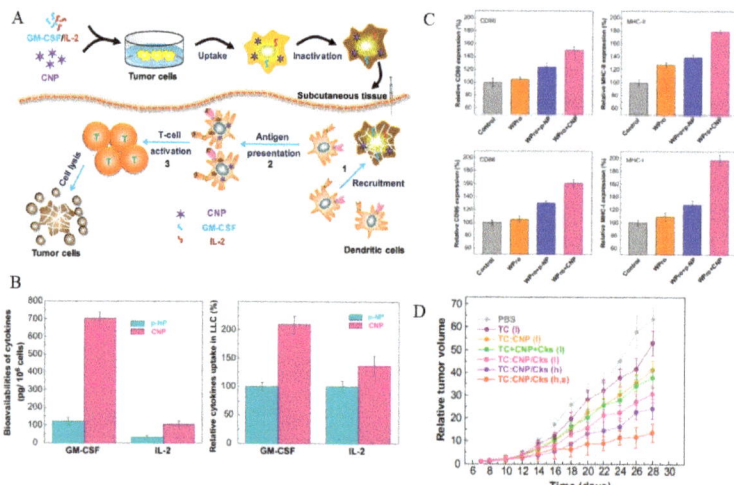

Figure 3. (**A**) Scheme of multi-adjuvant WCTV to initiate anti-tumor immunity, (**B**) bioavailability and cellular up take of GM-CSF and IL-2 in LLC cells after incubating with nanoparticles (NPs) for 24 h, (**C**) relative expressions of CD80, CD86, MHC II, and MHC-I molecules after treatment with whole tumor cell lysate protein (WPro), p-NP, and CNP for 24 h and (**D**) Relative tumor volume of LLC tumor bearing mice after immunization with multi-adjuvant WCTVs compared with other vaccine groups. Reproduced with permission from [93]. Copyright 2013, Elsevier Ltd.

2.1.3. Antigens and Adjuvants Delivery to Tumor Microenvironment (TME)

The TME comprised proliferating tumor cells, the tumor stroma, infiltrating inflammatory cells, apoptotic cancer cells, cancer-associated fibroblasts, myeloid-derived suppressor cells, tumor-associated macrophages, and a variety of associated tissue cells which are participating in the suppression of antitumor immunity [94]. These immunosuppressive cells secrete numerous soluble mediators including, Transforming growth factor-beta (TGF-β), Indoleamine 2,3-dioxygenase (IDO), arginase, prostaglandin E2 and nitric oxide synthase 2 (NOS2) [95–97]. By reducing the supply of indispensable amino acids (such as arginine (R) and Tryptophan (W)), IDO and arginase directly suppress T cell proliferation and differentiation [98]. The activity of arginase and IDO translates not only into amino acid deprivation but also in the production of metabolites (such as L-kynurenine and spermidine) capable of numerous physiologic effects [99,100]. For example, L-kynurenine derived from W, favors the differentiation of Treg cells and induces IDO expression in DCs. Similarly, TGF-β also alters activation, maturation, and differentiation of DCs, CD4$^+$, and CD8$^+$ T cells. In addition, PD-L1/PD-L2 expressed on tumor cells can engage PD-1 receptor on the surface of activated T cell and sends inhibitory signals via activating phosphatases, resulting in dephosphorylation of key elements in the T cell, leading to down-regulating proliferation, survival, and cytokine production [101]. Furthermore, the CTLA-4 receptor on tumor cells binds to co-stimulatory molecules on DCs and decreases antigen presentation. Moreover, there are an abundant accumulation of acellular components such as fibrosis, collagen, secreted protein acidic and rich in Cysteine (SPARC), and hyaluronan which alters the physicochemical properties of TME (including physical barriers, physical pressure (i.e., increase interstitial fluid pressure, change in metabolism, etc.) [102].

As mentioned above, although several immune effector cells are recruited to the TME, their anti-tumor activity is suppressed principally in response to tumor-derived signals [103]. Compared with normal tissue, TME has some unique characteristics, such as vascular abnormalities, hypoxia, increases in proteolytic activity, and an acidic microenvironment, which leads to treatment resistance [104]. Therefore, new approaches are demanded to overcome TME related immunosuppressive situations. Hence, targeting immunosuppressive cells (such as Treg) or Tumor-associated macrophage (TAM) in the TME using NPs could be the best tactics to prevent immunosuppression.

Sacchetti et al. designed ligand guided PEG-modified single-walled carbon nanotubes (PEG-SWCNTs) to target Treg-specific receptors in the TME [105]. They found that ligand targeted PEG-SWCNTs were preferentially up taken by Treg cell residing in the TME via glucocorticoid-induced TNFR-related receptor (GITR).

Similarly, Zhu et al. synthesized mannose targeted PEG-sheddable NPs to target TAM [106]. They reported that mannose-modified PEG-sheddable NPs was effectively targeted TAMs via the mannose-mannose receptor. As a result, more PEG-sheddable NPs accumulation was observed in TAM in comparison to non-sheddable PEG. This is maybe due to PEGylation which minimizes NPs opsonization and enhances its bioavailability.

In addition, NPs can be used to deliver anti-immunosuppressive factors, such as anti-TGF-β or TGF-β receptor inhibitor to the TME to increases the activation of the immune system. Park et al. synthesized liposomal polymeric gels (nLGs) to deliver IL-2 and TGF-β inhibitors (Figure 4) [107]. The author reported that IL-2 and TGF-β inhibitors were successfully delivered to the TME. In vivo results showed that nLGs treatment suppresses a tumor growth, improved survival rates, and enhanced the activity of NK cells and intratumoral-activated CD8$^+$ CTLs.

In summary, NPs can enhance anticancer immunity by regulating the TME either by inhibiting immunosuppression or by endorsing immune activation which could synergize with clinically established immunotherapeutic agents such as Immune Checkpoint Inhibitors (ICIs). Hence, targeting immune cells in the TME using nanoformulated therapeutic agents is the best tactic to activate antitumor immunity.

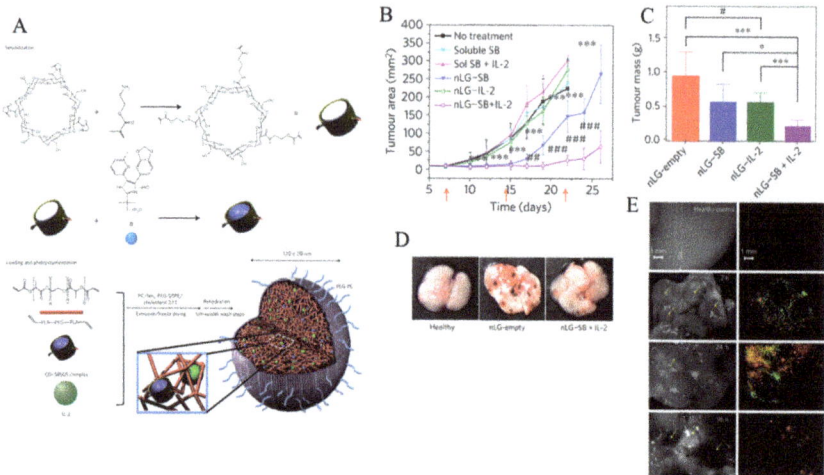

Figure 4. (**A**) The synthesis approach of the liposomal polymeric gel (nLG) particle system. (**B**) Plot of tumor area versus time. Red arrows indicate treatments (via intratumoral injection). ($p < 0.05$, *, $p < 0.001$, ***, By ANOVA with Turkey's multiple comparison test. $p < 0.05$, #, by two-tailed t-test. (**C**) Tumor masses vs nLG-treated groups, $p < 0.001$, ***, $p < 0.01$, **, $p < 0.05$, *, By ANOVA using Turkey's post-test. (**D**) Images of lung immediately before collection of lung-infiltrating lymphocytes from mice, (**E**) Uptake of lipid carrier (green) and rhodamine payload (red) around individual lung tumors at 2 h post injection. Reproduced with permission from [107]. Copyright 2012, Nature Publishing Group.

2.1.4. Immune Checkpoint Inhibitors (ICIs) Delivery

Immune checkpoints are surface proteins on immune cells that act as negative regulators of immune activation by various antigens, including tumor antigens [108]. Immune checkpoint molecules include PD-1, PD-L1/2, CTLA-4, T-cell immunoglobulin and mucin domain-containing-3 (TIM-3), and lymphocyte-activation gene 3 (LAG-3) [109,110]. Immune checkpoint molecules are widely expressed on both tumor cells and immune cells, which might be negatively regulated by tumor-specific T cells via receptor–ligand interactions, causing T-cell anergy or exhaustion [111,112]. Tumor cells evade destruction from the immune system by triggering immune checkpoint receptors, such as CTLA-4, PD-1, or PD-L1, that are expressed on T-cells and whose engagement inhibits T-lymphocyte function [113].

ICIs are monoclonal antibody that inhibits the receptors-ligands interaction and enhance immune-mediated cancer eradication. The development of ICIs lays a key foundation in cancer immunotherapy [114]. In 2018, James P. Allison and Tasuku Honjo were awarded a Nobel prize in physiology or medicine for the discovery of cytotoxic T-lymphocyte-associated antigen (CTLA-4), and programmed cell death protein 1/programmed cell death protein ligand 1 (PD-1/PD-L1), respectively [115]. According to literature report, anti-CTLA-4 antibody overcomes a block in essential costimulatory signals (i.e., CTLA-4 and CD28 competes for the same ligands CD80 and CD86; CTLA-4 has a higher affinity than CD28) that are required for activation of both naive T cells and resting clones, whereas PD-1/PD-L1 blockade seems to remove a barrier and enable T cell effector function at the tumor site [116,117]. As the result, ICIs including anti-CTLA-4 and anti-PD-1/PD-L1 Abs were developed to block these inhibitory pathways [118–120]. Currently, some of the ICIs including the anti-CTLA-4 agent, ipilimumab, Tremelimumab; anti-PD-1 agents, nivolumab and pembrolizumab; and anti-PDL-1 agent, Atezolizumab, Avelumab, Cemiplimab, Durvalumab, ipilimumab, and atezolizumab [121–123] have been approved for the treatment of certain types of cancer [124]. Mechanism action of ICIs are briefly summarized in Figure 5, [124]. Furthermore, in their current review paper, Vaddepally et al. have been briefly reviewed the majority of FDA-approved ICIs per national comprehensive cancer network guidelines [125].

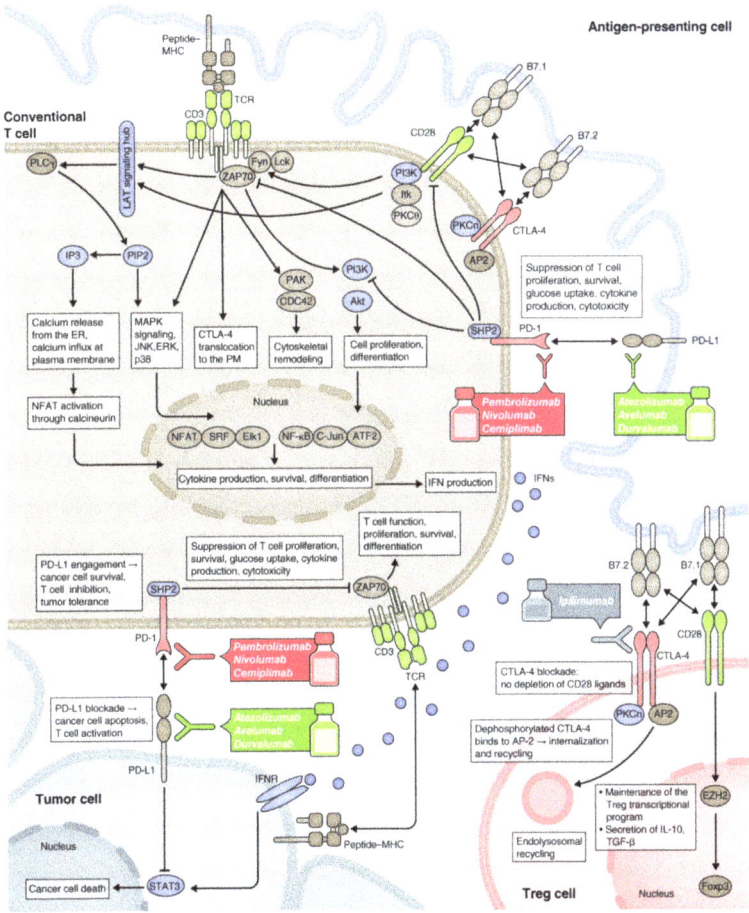

Figure 5. Mechanism action of Immune Checkpoint Inhibitors (ICIs). Reproduced with permission from the Journal of Cell Biology [124].

Even though a promising clinical data was obtained using ICIs, still, it shows certain limitations including an occurrence of immune-related adverse events, low response rate, and acquired resistance which is expected to be improved using NPs.

Wang et al. designed pH-sensitive microneedle (MN) patch for the sustained delivery of anti-PD1 (aPD1) (Figure 6) [126]. Glucose oxidase was used to generate acidic environments by converting glucose to glucuronic acid, leading to NPs self-dissociation, which in turn facilitates sustained aPD1 releases. The authors found that, at the same dose, pH-sensitive MN patch induces more immune responses compared to non-sensitive MN or free aPD1 using B16F10 mouse melanoma model. Furthermore, the author demonstrated that the aCTLA-4 and aPD1 co-loaded in MN patch shows synergistic effects.

Similarly, Wang et al. have been designed inflammation-triggered CpG DNA-based "nano-cocoons" for co-delivery of anti-PD-1 Ab and CpG oligodeoxynucleotides (CpG ODNs) (Figure 7) [127].The author reported that in comparison to free CpG nucleotides and aPD1, bioresponsive controlled release of CpG and aPD1 showed a considerable immune response and better therapeutic efficacy.

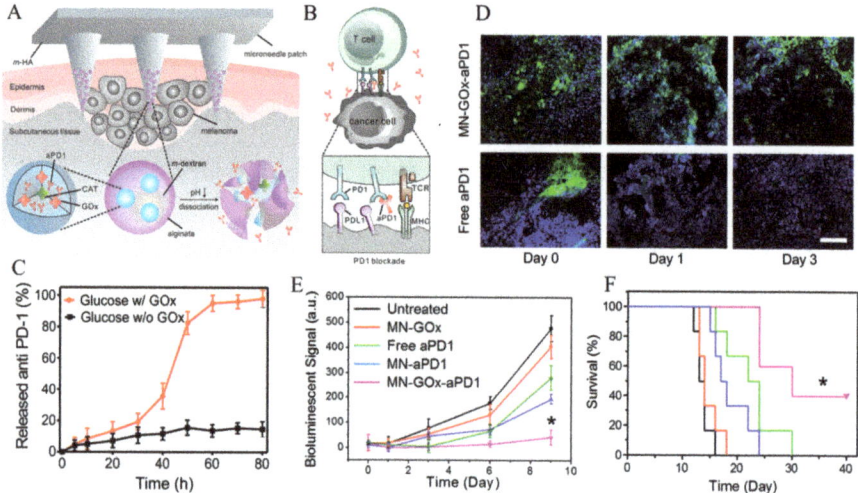

Figure 6. (**A**) Scheme of aPD1 delivery via microneedle (MN) patch, (**B**) Mechanism action of aPD1 to activate T-cell, (**C**) aPD1 release (%) from the MN patches in the presence of 100 mg/dL glucose solution at 37 °C, (**D**) Immunofluorescence staining of tumors treated with MN-GOx-aPD1 or free aPD1 at different time points (green: aPD1, blue: nucleus), (**E**) Bioluminescence signals vs. time after treatment with different groups, and (**F**) % Survival plot of mice after MN patch-assisted delivery of aPD1 therapy. P value: *, $p < 0.05$. Reproduced with permission from [126]. Copyright 2016, American Chemical Society.

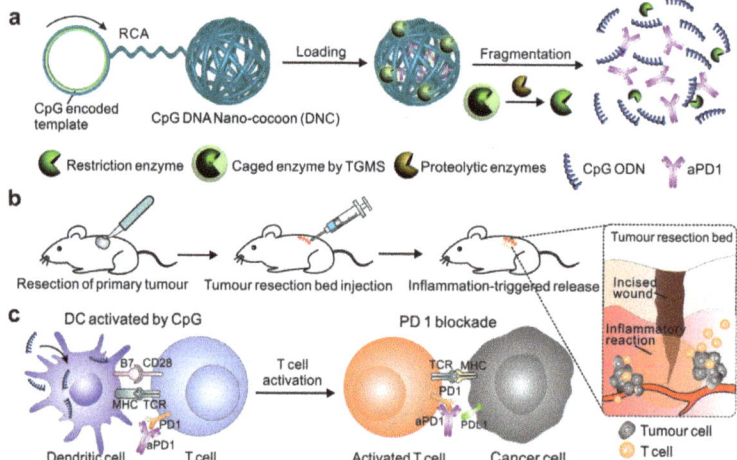

Figure 7. Schematic illustration of (**a**) aPD1 and caged restriction enzyme loaded DNA nanococoon (DNC), (**b**) In vivo tumor immunotherapy after primary tumor resection, local injection, and treatment of DNC-based delivery system and (**c**) Activation of DCs by CpG which in turn activates T cell response with aPD1 for PD 1 blockade. Reproduced with permission from [127]. Copyright 2016, WILEY-VCH Verlag GmbH & Co. KGaA, Weinheim.

Several researchers reported that patients with advanced cancer poorly respond to PD1/PD-L1 inhibitory therapy due to low TAA expression [128,129]. Epigenetic alteration like DNA hypermethylation, which is commonly seen at TAA promoter regions, plays an essential role in immune evasion of cancer cells during tumorigenesis [130]. Hence, epigenetic modulators, such as hypomethylation agents (HMAs), play a key role in the induction of TAA expression, which in turn increase antitumor immune response [131]. Ruan et al. synthesized a pH and reactive oxygen species (ROS) sensitive bioresponsive gel depot for co-delivery of aPD1 and Zebularine (Zeb), HMA [132]. The author reported that combination therapy enhances the immunogenicity of cancer cells and plays a crucial role in converting immunosuppressive TME.

Preclinical animal studies using cancer nanovaccines, nanoformulated TAA, or tumor-specific neoantigens, revealed promising therapeutic efficacy [133]. However, the clinical use of these nanovaccines has been limited due to immune evasion and suppression in the TME [134,135]. Some literature showed that high expression of immune checkpoints such as PD-L1 is responsible for the occurrence of tumor resistance to vaccine-mediated immune responses. Hence, it possible to overwhelm this limitation by combining with ICIs such as anti-PD-1, anti-PD-L1 or anti-CTLA4 Ab.

Kim et al. developed a small lipid nanoparticle (SLNP)-based nanovaccines embedded with antigen/adjuvant (OVA$_{PEP}$-SLNP@CpG), Figure 8 [136]. Synthesized nanovaccine showed high potent antitumor efficacy in both prophylactic and therapeutic E.G7 tumor models but induced T cell exhaustion by increasing PD-L1 expression, leading to tumor recurrence. However, by using mice that showed a good therapeutic response after the first cycle of immunization with the nanovaccine the author underwent a second cycle together with anti-PD-1 therapy. Their result revealed tumor relapse of suppressed, treatment sequence, and the timing of each modality is crucial in order to enhance antitumor efficacy using combinations of nanovaccines with ICIs.

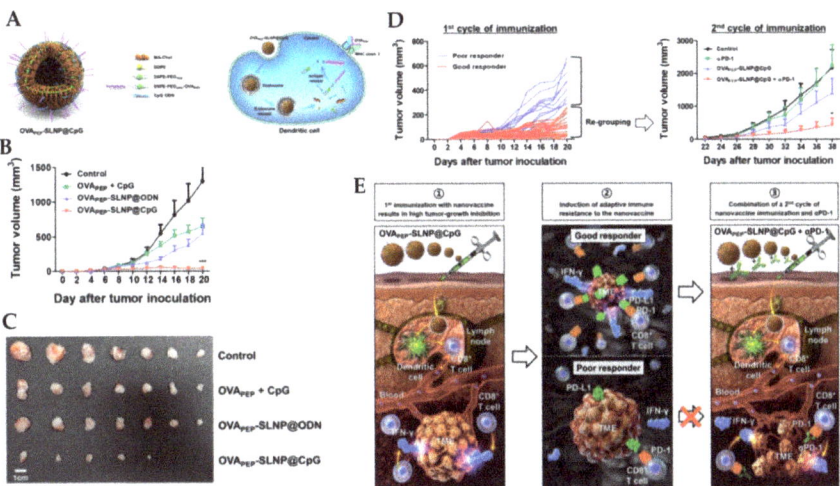

Figure 8. (**A**) Scheme and mechanism action of OVA$_{PEP}$-SLNP@CpG nanovaccine, (**B**) Therapeutic efficacy of OVA$_{PEP}$-SLNP@CpG nanovaccine in an established tumor model, (**C**) representative image of tumors. Scale bar = 1 cm, (**D**) First cycle and second cycle of immunization, (**E**) Overall process of sequential and timely combination strategy between cancer nanovaccine. $p < 0.001$, ***, $p < 0.05$, *, Reproduced with permission from [136]. Copyright 2020, Wiley-VCH Verlag GmbH & Co. KGaA, Weinheim.

Similarly, Fontana et al. have designed and assessed biohybrid nanovaccines in combination with anti-CTLA4 antibody [137]. The author observed, an increased activation of APCs and increased priming of CD8$^+$ T cells after nanovaccine injection. Most interestingly, treatment efficacy was increased

(87.5% of the animals responding, with 2 remissions) in the co-administration (nanovaccine with anti-CTLA4 antibody) compared to the checkpoint inhibitor alone in the B16.OVA model.

2.1.5. Nanoparticles as the Direct Immunomodulators

Immunomodulatory compounds such as cytokines, monoclonal antibodies and adjuvants have been used to reshape the TME and to initiate anti-tumor immunity; although there are certain limitations such as therapeutic efficacy and unwanted side effects during systemic administration, to use in clinics [138].

Immunomodulatory NPs can readily improve the therapeutic effects by enhancing immune stimulation and minimizing off-target side effects. As the result, more research works are undergoing to understand the mechanisms of NPs-Immuno-interactions which is highly important to know the immunomodulating potential of NPs, as the immunostimulating or as immunosuppression [139]. The function of NP in the immunomodulation depends on several factors that are intrinsic to NPs, such as surface chemistry, charge, size, and shape, besides extrinsic factors such as route of administration [140].

Several researchers have widely explored the immunomodulating effects of both polymeric and inorganic NPs [28,141,142]. Different evidence suggests that the immune system cells interact with NPs through Toll-like receptors (TLRs) [143,144]. TLRs are transmembrane proteins, expressed on APCs such as DCs and macrophages, which recognize specific molecular patterns that act as danger signals to the immune system [145]. Depending on the type of receptor and the type of stimuli, TLR engagement plays a great role both in the innate and adaptive immune response by altering several gene expressions.

Inorganic NPs such as Gold nanoparticles (AuNP), Titanium nanoparticles (TiNPs), iron nanoparticles (FeNPs), Zinc nanoparticles (ZnNPs), and silver nanoparticles (AgNPs) are the most stable and promising particles to modulate immune systems [146–148].

Vasilichin et al. investigated the influence of metal oxide NPs on innate immunity by testing TLR-4/6 mRNAs in the human monocyte cell line [149]. They found that all studied NPs activated TLR-6 expression, while AlOOH enhanced both TLR-4 and -6 expression.

Moreover, in human peripheral blood mononuclear cells, the administration of AuNPs activates immune-related genes depends on its physicochemical properties [150]. Lee et al. reported that gold nanorods (GNRs) and SiO_2-coated GNRs has a tendency to penetrate into macrophages to induce the release of inflammatory mediators (calcium (Ca), hydrogen peroxide, nitric oxide (NO), cytokines, prostaglandins, etc.) and the activation of immune response genes [151]. Both GNRs and SiO_2-coated GNRs have an immunostimulatory property to reinforce immune reactions via calcium—transcription factors pathway.

Fallarini et al. synthesized mono- and disaccharides coated AuNPs with a particle size of ~2 and 5 nm [152]. Their in vitro results showed that synthesized NPs initiate the immune response by activating the macrophages. However, unlike monosaccharide coated AuNPs, disaccharide coated tends to induce T cell proliferation and an increase in IL-2 levels. According to this report, the immunoactivity is strongly dependent on size, 5 nm AuNPs perform far better than 2 nm ones.

Lin et al. also reported that CpG modified AuNP induced macrophage and DC tumor infiltration and suppresses tumor growth compared with free CpG [153]. Similarly, Ahn et al. also reported that AuNP facilitates tumor-associated self-antigen delivery to DC and then activates the cells to facilitate cross-presentation and induce antigen-specific cytotoxic T cell responses [154].

AgNPs also trigger inflammatory reactions cascade involving the activation of macrophages, neutrophils, and helper T cells [155]. Subsequently, AgNPs enhance the expression of numerous types of cytokines [156,157]. Furthermore, different researchers have been investigated the effect of AgNPs as the immunological adjuvant using both in vitro and in vivo studies [158,159].

Xu et al. have investigated an adjuvant effect of AgNPs [160]. The in vivo result showed that serum antigen-specific IgG and IgE levels were increased, showing that AgNPs elicited $CD4^+$-mediated immune response. After 48h treatment with AgNPs, both the number of leukocytes and levels of cytokines TNF-α and IFN-γ was increased in abdominal lavage fluid of mice. Furthermore, the expression of the MHC complex class II molecule on the surface of peritoneal macrophages was significantly increased.

In addition, NPs can be designed as artificial APCs (aAPCs), that express surface features, that can activate immune cells or modulate the expression of pro- or anti-inflammatory genes [161,162]. This immunomodulatory behavior of NPs can enhance the therapeutic response of injected NPs by directly generating cytotoxic T cells. For example, Mandal et al. designed biocompatible and less-toxic anti-CD3 antibodies-modified artificial APCs based on poly (isocyano peptide) [163]. They found that synthesized aAPCs induce a more robust T cell response in comparison to free antibodies or PLGA particles. Similarly, Kosmides et al. designed and investigated the synergy between a PLGA-based aAPC and an aPD1 mAb [164]. Their in vitro results revealed that the combination of antigen-specific aAPC and aPD1 mAb induced IFN-γ secretion by $CD8^+$ T cells. In addition, in vivo results showed that combination treatment synergistically inhibits tumor growth, while either treatment alone had no effect.

3. Clinical Translation of Nano-Immunotherapy

In the last few decades, several researchers have deeply explored a regulatory mechanism of antitumor immunity, particularly the immune checkpoint pathways, which lays a basic foundation for the invention of ICIs, that have revolutionized cancer treatment [165,166]. However, different literature showed that the activity of ICIs as monotherapy is not satisfactory for all cancer patients [167]. To address this clinical challenge, the different researchers tried to combine NPs with immunotherapeutic agents or conventional cancer treatment with ICIs [168,169]. Several kind of the literature showed that, conventional cancer treatments such as chemotherapy, photodynamic therapy, and radiotherapy can initiate the immune system to elicit a specific antitumor immunity, due to its ability to induce immunogenic cell death, in addition, to directly killing cancer cells, which can induce a release of certain damage-associated molecular patterns (DAMPs) that can activate APCs [170]. Activated APCs in turn phagocytose dying tumor cells and present tumor antigens to initiate T cell responses [171]. By taking this into consideration, NPs-based chemotherapeutic agents or photosensitizer delivery can be used to exploit the ICD inducing properties to achieve potent antitumor efficacy in combination with immunotherapeutic agents such as ICIs [172]. Most importantly, NPs based drug delivery can enhance selective target delivery and reduce off-target cytotoxicity of chemotherapeutic or immunotherapeutic agents which in turn extends the therapeutic index, especially for combination therapy.

As briefly discussed above, targeting APCs, cancer cells or TME clearly indicates that NPs significantly improved the therapeutic efficacy of immunotherapeutic agents. Based on the progress made so far, nano-immunotherapy has been achieving remarkable results, some of them were approved by the FDA, and the majority of them are in the preclinical stage, for the treatment of cancer. The first nano-immunotherapy approved for the treatment of advanced triple-negative breast cancer (TNBC) was Atezolizumab (Tecentriq®), an ICI against PD-L1, in combination with albumin-bound paclitaxel NP (nab-paclitaxel) [173,174]. The result showed that atezolizumab plus nab-paclitaxel significantly prolonged progression-free survival (PFS) compared to nab-paclitaxel in the intent-to-treat population and the PD-L1 positive subgroup.

Furthermore, Hensify®/NBTXR3, 50 nm crystalline hafnium oxide (HfO_2) NP, received European market approval (CE Mark) in April 2019 for the treatment of locally advanced soft tissue sarcoma in combination with radiation therapy [175]. Hensify® is designed by Nanobiotix to physically destroy tumors and stimulate the immune system locally [176]. Nanobiotix is also running several clinical trials and has received US FDA approval to launch a combination trial with NBTXR3 and PD-1 antibodies to treat lung cancer (NCT03589339).

Similarly, the multicentre, randomized, open-label, phase 3 trial study was conducted as a first-line treatment for metastatic non-squamous non-small-cell lung cancer (IMpower130, NCT02367781) using

Atezolizumab in combination with carboplatin plus nab-paclitaxel chemotherapy compared with chemotherapy alone [177]. The result revealed that there were significant improvements in median overall survival (OS), 18.6 months in the atezolizumab plus chemotherapy group, 13.9 months in the chemotherapy group, median PFS 7.0 months in the atezolizumab plus chemotherapy group, and 5.5 months in the chemotherapy group.

Furthermore, there is the first randomized phase 3 JAVELIN Ovarian 200 trial (NCT02580058) study which is designed to demonstrate that Avelumab (human immunoglobulin G1 anti-PD-L1 monoclonal antibody) alone or in combination with Pegylated liposomal doxorubicin (PLD) is superior to PLD alone in prolonging OS in patients with platinum-resistant/platinum refractory ovarian cancer [178]. The results revealed that PLD combined with avelumab slightly improved OS (15.7), PFS (3.7), and objective response rate (ORR) (13.3) compared to either PLD (13.1, 3.5, and 4.2 for OS, PFS, and ORR, respectively) or avelumab (11.8, 1.9, and 3.7 for OS, PFS, and ORR, respectively) alone (Reference: ClinicalTrials.gov; NCT0258005). In addition, RNA formulated NPs alone or in combination with immunotherapeutic agents, such as ICIs, were also explored and the majority of them are under clinical trials as listed in Table 1. Moreover, in his recent review, Yang Shi was briefly reviewed several studies that are FDA approved or under clinical trials using nano-immunotherapy, such as NPs albumin-bound paclitaxel, Pegylated liposomal doxorubicin, mRNA nanovaccines, and WDVAX [179].

Table 1. FDA approved nano-Immunotherapy and studies under clinical trials to treat cancer [180–182].

Compound Name	Formulation Description	Mechanism of Action	Clinical Trials	Approved by the FDA	Ref
RNA-LPX (Lipoplex®)	RNA-lipoplexes	DC maturation, T cell response	Phase I (2016)		[82]
MRX34	miRNA-34a-loaded liposome	Downregulation of immune evasion tumor genes	Phase I (2016)		[183]
mRNA-4157	mRNA-4157 encapsulated in Lipids	induce neoantigen specific T cells and associated anti-tumor responses.	Phase I (2019)		[184]
Ferumoxytol (Ferahem®)	Iron oxide nanoparticles (IONP)	M2 Macrophage polarization to M1-like		Yes, for anemia and kidney diseases	[185]
PTX-LDE	Paclitaxel-loaded lipid core NPs	DC maturation	Phase II (2017)		[186,187]
Anti-EGFR-IL-dox	Doxorubicin-loaded anti-EGFR immunoliposomes	Block EGFR-mediated growth signaling and induce immunogenic cell death	Phase II (2016)		NCT02833766
JVRS-100	Cationic liposome incorporating plasmid DNA complex	Immune system stimulation	Phase I (2016)		NCT00860522
NBTXR3	Hafnium oxide nanoparticles in combination with anti-PD1	Enhance tumor cell death via electron production, induce immunogenic cell death leading to activation of the immune system	Phase I (2019)		[188], NCT03589339

In summary, several clinical and preclinical study results demonstrate that NPs are highly important in immunotherapy as the delivery of immunotherapeutic agents or as the direct immunomodulators. However, due to the multifactorial nature of cancer-immune interactions, identifying unique biomarkers are crucial to designing multifunctional NPs (i.e., which have a diagnostic and theranostic application). Hence, in order to design a novel biomarker-guided multifunctional and biocompatible NPs to enhance the efficacy and to promote clinical translation of nano-immunotherapy, a unique biomarker must be identified to distinguish which immune-activating or immunosuppressive cells or pathways are targeted.

4. Conclusions

Cancer immunotherapy is emerging as a beneficial tool for cancer treatment by activating the immune system to produce antitumor effects. However, there are some limitations to immunotherapy including poor therapeutic targeting and unwanted side effects. Currently, one of the emerging tracks in this field area is NPs-based immunotherapy which has a considerable potential to solve limitations related to immunotherapy. NPs plays a great role in cancer immunotherapy as the carrier of immunotherapeutic agents and as the direct immunomodulator. NPs based delivery of immunotherapeutic agents offers a great opportunity to minimize unwanted cytotoxicity through controlled release, dose-sparing, or enhanced tumor targeting capabilities. Hence, in the near future, as our knowledge enhanced to understand the detailed molecular mechanism of NPs-immune interaction, NP-based therapies will revolutionize and place NP-based immunotherapy at the forefront of immune-modulating therapeutics.

Author Contributions: T.A.D., conceived, designed, wrote and edited the review paper; C.-F.Y., funding and edited revised manuscript, W.-P.S., supervise, funding and edited the review paper. All authors have read and agreed to the published version of the manuscript.

Funding: This research was funded by the Ministry of Science and Technology, Taiwan; grants number: MOST- 110-2811-B-006-501, 108-2811-B-006-501, 108-2811-B-006-525, 109-2314-B-006-078, 109-2314-B-006-084-MY3, CMNCKU10806 & Headquarters of University Advancement, National Cheng Kung University, grant number: HUA 109-25-18-133.

Conflicts of Interest: The authors declare no conflict of interest.

References

1. McCormack, V.A.; Boffetta, P. Today's lifestyles, tomorrow's cancers: Trends in lifestyle risk factors for cancer in low- and middle-income countries. *Ann. Oncol.* **2011**, *22*, 2349–2357. [CrossRef] [PubMed]
2. Blackadar, C.B. Historical review of the causes of cancer. *World J. Clin. Oncol.* **2016**, *7*, 54–86. [CrossRef] [PubMed]
3. Bray, F.; Ferlay, J.; Soerjomataram, I.; Siegel, R.L.; Torre, L.A.; Jemal, A. Global cancer statistics 2018: GLOBOCAN estimates of incidence and mortality worldwide for 36 cancers in 185 countries. *CA Cancer J. Clin.* **2018**, *68*, 394–424. [CrossRef] [PubMed]
4. Arruebo, M.; Vilaboa, N.; Sáez-Gutierrez, B.; Lambea, J.; Tres, A.; Valladares, M.; González-Fernández, A. Assessment of the evolution of cancer treatment therapies. *Cancers* **2011**, *3*, 3279–3330. [CrossRef]
5. Suo, X.; Zhang, J.; Zhang, Y.; Liang, X.J.; Zhang, J.; Liu, D. A nano-based thermotherapy for cancer stem cell-targeted therapy. *J. Mater. Chem. B* **2020**, *8*, 3985–4001. [CrossRef]
6. Yin, P.T.; Shah, S.; Pasquale, N.J.; Garbuzenko, O.B.; Minko, T.; Lee, K.B. Stem cell-based gene therapy activated using magnetic hyperthermia to enhance the treatment of cancer. *Biomaterials* **2016**, *81*, 46–57. [CrossRef]
7. Spring, B.Q.; Rizvi, I.; Xu, N.; Hasan, T. The role of photodynamic therapy in overcoming cancer drug resistance. *Photochem. Photobiol. Sci.* **2015**, *14*, 1476–1491. [CrossRef]
8. Weiss, A.; Bonvin, D.; Berndsen, R.H.; Scherrer, E.; Wong, T.J.; Dyson, P.J.; Griffioen, A.W.; Nowak-Sliwinska, P. Angiostatic treatment prior to chemo- or photodynamic therapy improves anti-tumor efficacy. *Sci. Rep.* **2015**, *5*, 8990. [CrossRef]
9. Samant, R.S.; Shevde, L.A. Recent advances in anti-angiogenic therapy of cancer. *Oncotarget* **2011**, *2*, 122–134. [CrossRef]
10. Johnston, S.L. Biologic therapies: What and when? *J. Clin. Pathol.* **2007**, *60*, 8–17. [CrossRef]
11. Cairns, R.; Papandreou, I.; Denko, N. Overcoming physiologic barriers to cancer treatment by molecularly targeting the tumor microenvironment. *Mol. Cancer Res.* **2006**, *4*, 61–70. [CrossRef] [PubMed]

12. Debele, T.A.; Mekuria, S.L.; Tsai, H.C. Polysaccharide based nanogels in the drug delivery system: Application as the carrier of pharmaceutical agents. *Mater. Sci. Eng. C Mater. Biol. Appl.* **2016**, *68*, 964–981. [CrossRef] [PubMed]
13. Maeda, H. SMANCS and polymer-conjugated macromolecular drugs: Advantages in cancer chemotherapy. *Adv. Drug Deliv. Rev.* **2001**, *46*, 169–185. [CrossRef]
14. Leu, A.J.; Berk, D.A.; Lymboussaki, A.; Alitalo, K.; Jain, R.K. Absence of functional lymphatics within a murine sarcoma: A molecular and functional evaluation. *Cancer Res.* **2000**, *60*, 4324–4327.
15. Maeda, H. Tumor-Selective Delivery of Macromolecular Drugs via the EPR Effect: Background and Future Prospects. *Bioconjugate Chem.* **2010**, *21*, 797–802. [CrossRef]
16. Debele, T.A.; Peng, S.; Tsai, H.-C. Drug Carrier for Photodynamic Cancer Therapy. *Int. J. Mol. Sci.* **2015**, *16*, 22094–22136. [CrossRef]
17. Chidambaram, M.; Manavalan, R.; Kathiresan, K. Nanotherapeutics to overcome conventional cancer chemotherapy limitations. *J. Pharm. Pharm. Sci.* **2011**, *14*, 67–77. [CrossRef]
18. Nel, A.E.; Mädler, L.; Velegol, D.; Xia, T.; Hoek, E.M.V.; Somasundaran, P.; Klaessig, F.; Castranova, V.; Thompson, M. Understanding biophysicochemical interactions at the nano–bio interface. *Nat. Mater.* **2009**, *8*, 543–557. [CrossRef]
19. Behzadi, S.; Serpooshan, V.; Tao, W.; Hamaly, M.A.; Alkawareek, M.Y.; Dreaden, E.C.; Brown, D.; Alkilany, A.M.; Farokhzad, O.C.; Mahmoudi, M. Cellular uptake of nanoparticles: Journey inside the cell. *Chem. Soc. Rev.* **2017**, *46*, 4218–4244. [CrossRef]
20. Tenzer, S.; Docter, D.; Rosfa, S.; Wlodarski, A.; Kuharev, J.; Rekik, A.; Knauer, S.K.; Bantz, C.; Nawroth, T.; Bier, C.; et al. Nanoparticle size is a critical physicochemical determinant of the human blood plasma corona: A comprehensive quantitative proteomic analysis. *ACS Nano* **2011**, *5*, 7155–7167. [CrossRef]
21. Gao, S.; Yang, D.; Fang, Y.; Lin, X.; Jin, X.; Wang, Q.; Wang, X.; Ke, L.; Shi, K. Engineering Nanoparticles for Targeted Remodeling of the Tumor Microenvironment to Improve Cancer Immunotherapy. *Theranostics* **2019**, *9*, 126–151. [CrossRef]
22. Fröhlich, E. The role of surface charge in cellular uptake and cytotoxicity of medical nanoparticles. *Int. J. Nanomed.* **2012**, *7*, 5577–5591. [CrossRef] [PubMed]
23. He, C.; Hu, Y.; Yin, L.; Tang, C.; Yin, C. Effects of particle size and surface charge on cellular uptake and biodistribution of polymeric nanoparticles. *Biomaterials* **2010**, *31*, 3657–3666. [CrossRef] [PubMed]
24. Caracciolo, G.; Callipo, L.; De Sanctis, S.C.; Cavaliere, C.; Pozzi, D.; Laganà, A. Surface adsorption of protein corona controls the cell internalization mechanism of DC-Chol–DOPE/DNA lipoplexes in serum. *Biochim. Biophys. Acta (BBA) Biomembranes* **2010**, *1798*, 536–543. [CrossRef] [PubMed]
25. Sacchetti, C.; Motamedchaboki, K.; Magrini, A.; Palmieri, G.; Mattei, M.; Bernardini, S.; Rosato, N.; Bottini, N.; Bottini, M. Surface polyethylene glycol conformation influences the protein corona of polyethylene glycol-modified single-walled carbon nanotubes: Potential implications on biological performance. *ACS Nano* **2013**, *7*, 1974–1989. [CrossRef]
26. Pelaz, B.; del Pino, P.; Maffre, P.; Hartmann, R.; Gallego, M.; Rivera-Fernández, S.; de la Fuente, J.M.; Nienhaus, G.U.; Parak, W.J. Surface Functionalization of Nanoparticles with Polyethylene Glycol: Effects on Protein Adsorption and Cellular Uptake. *ACS Nano* **2015**, *9*, 6996–7008. [CrossRef]
27. Moore, A.; Marecos, E.; Bogdanov, A., Jr.; Weissleder, R. Tumoral distribution of long-circulating dextran-coated iron oxide nanoparticles in a rodent model. *Radiology* **2000**, *214*, 568–574. [CrossRef]
28. Ventola, C.L. Progress in Nanomedicine: Approved and Investigational Nanodrugs. *Pharm. Ther.* **2017**, *42*, 742–755.
29. Bobo, D.; Robinson, K.J.; Islam, J.; Thurecht, K.J.; Corrie, S.R. Nanoparticle-Based Medicines: A Review of FDA-Approved Materials and Clinical Trials to Date. *Pharm. Res.* **2016**, *33*, 2373–2387. [CrossRef]
30. Etheridge, M.L.; Campbell, S.A.; Erdman, A.G.; Haynes, C.L.; Wolf, S.M.; McCullough, J. The big picture on nanomedicine: The state of investigational and approved nanomedicine products. *Nanomedicine* **2013**, *9*, 1–14. [CrossRef]
31. Wang, Y.-X.J. Superparamagnetic iron oxide based MRI contrast agents: Current status of clinical application. *Quant. Imaging Med. Surg.* **2011**, *1*, 35–40. [CrossRef]
32. Kendall, M.; Lynch, I. Long-term monitoring for nanomedicine implants and drugs. *Nat. Nanotechnol.* **2016**, *11*, 206–210. [CrossRef] [PubMed]

33. Scott, A.M.; Wolchok, J.D.; Old, L.J. Antibody therapy of cancer. *Nat. Rev. Cancer* **2012**, *12*, 278–287. [CrossRef] [PubMed]
34. Havel, J.J.; Chowell, D.; Chan, T.A. The evolving landscape of biomarkers for checkpoint inhibitor immunotherapy. *Nat. Rev. Cancer* **2019**, *19*, 133–150. [CrossRef]
35. Dine, J.; Gordon, R.; Shames, Y.; Kasler, M.K.; Barton-Burke, M. Immune Checkpoint Inhibitors: An Innovation in Immunotherapy for the Treatment and Management of Patients with Cancer. *Asia Pac. J. Oncol. Nurs.* **2017**, *4*, 127–135. [CrossRef] [PubMed]
36. Sheng, W.Y.; Huang, L. Cancer immunotherapy and nanomedicine. *Pharm. Res.* **2011**, *28*, 200–214. [CrossRef] [PubMed]
37. Kim, J.; Gambhir, V.; Alatery, A.; Basta, S. Delivery of Exogenous Antigens to Induce Cytotoxic CD8+ T Lymphocyte Responses. *J. Biomed. Biotechnol.* **2010**, *2010*, 218752. [CrossRef]
38. Shresta, S.; Pham, C.T.; Thomas, D.A.; Graubert, T.A.; Ley, T.J. How do cytotoxic lymphocytes kill their targets? *Curr. Opin. Immunol.* **1998**, *10*, 581–587. [CrossRef]
39. Basta, S.; Alatery, A. The Cross-priming Pathway: A Portrait of an Intricate Immune System. *Scand. J. Immunol.* **2007**, *65*, 311–319. [CrossRef]
40. Bhat, P.; Leggatt, G.; Waterhouse, N.; Frazer, I.H. Interferon-γ derived from cytotoxic lymphocytes directly enhances their motility and cytotoxicity. *Cell Death Dis.* **2017**, *8*, e2836. [CrossRef]
41. Brinkmann, U.; Kontermann, R.E. The making of bispecific antibodies. *mAbs* **2017**, *9*, 182–212. [CrossRef] [PubMed]
42. Frankel, S.R.; Baeuerle, P.A. Targeting T cells to tumor cells using bispecific antibodies. *Curr. Opin. Chem. Biol.* **2013**, *17*, 385–392. [CrossRef] [PubMed]
43. Zhang, X.; Yang, Y.; Fan, D.; Xiong, D. The development of bispecific antibodies and their applications in tumor immune escape. *Exp. Hematol. Oncol.* **2017**, *6*, 12. [CrossRef] [PubMed]
44. Lindau, D.; Gielen, P.; Kroesen, M.; Wesseling, P.; Adema, G.J. The immunosuppressive tumour network: Myeloid-derived suppressor cells, regulatory T cells and natural killer T cells. *Immunology* **2013**, *138*, 105–115. [CrossRef] [PubMed]
45. Hanahan, D.; Weinberg, R.A. Hallmarks of cancer: The next generation. *Cell* **2011**, *144*, 646–674. [CrossRef]
46. Fujimura, T.; Kambayashi, Y.; Aiba, S. Crosstalk between regulatory T cells (Tregs) and myeloid derived suppressor cells (MDSCs) during melanoma growth. *Oncoimmunology* **2012**, *1*, 1433–1434. [CrossRef]
47. Fujimura, T.; Ring, S.; Umansky, V.; Mahnke, K.; Enk, A.H. Regulatory T cells stimulate B7-H1 expression in myeloid-derived suppressor cells in ret melanomas. *J. Investig. Dermatol.* **2012**, *132*, 1239–1246. [CrossRef]
48. Shimizu, J.; Yamazaki, S.; Sakaguchi, S. Induction of tumor immunity by removing CD25+CD4+ T cells: A common basis between tumor immunity and autoimmunity. *J. Immunol.* **1999**, *163*, 5211–5218.
49. Onizuka, S.; Tawara, I.; Shimizu, J.; Sakaguchi, S.; Fujita, T.; Nakayama, E. Tumor rejection by in vivo administration of anti-CD25 (interleukin-2 receptor alpha) monoclonal antibody. *Cancer Res.* **1999**, *59*, 3128–3133.
50. Yang, L.; Edwards, C.M.; Mundy, G.R. Gr-1+CD11b+ myeloid-derived suppressor cells: Formidable partners in tumor metastasis. *J. Bone Miner. Res.* **2010**, *25*, 1701–1706. [CrossRef]
51. Gabrilovich, D.I. Myeloid-Derived Suppressor Cells. *Cancer Immunol. Res.* **2017**, *5*, 3–8. [CrossRef]
52. Pucci, C.; Martinelli, C.; Ciofani, G. Innovative approaches for cancer treatment: Current perspectives and new challenges. *Ecancermedicalscience* **2019**, *13*, 961. [CrossRef] [PubMed]
53. Urruticoechea, A.; Alemany, R.; Balart, J.; Villanueva, A.; Viñals, F.; Capellá, G. Recent advances in cancer therapy: An overview. *Curr. Pharm. Des.* **2010**, *16*, 3–10. [CrossRef] [PubMed]
54. Dimberu, P.M.; Leonhardt, R.M. Cancer immunotherapy takes a multi-faceted approach to kick the immune system into gear. *Yale J. Biol. Med.* **2011**, *84*, 371–380. [PubMed]
55. Fang, L.; Lonsdorf, A.S.; Hwang, S.T. Immunotherapy for advanced melanoma. *J. Investig. Dermatol.* **2008**, *128*, 2596–2605. [CrossRef] [PubMed]
56. Kaufman, H.L.; Atkins, M.B.; Subedi, P.; Wu, J.; Chambers, J.; Joseph Mattingly, T.; Campbell, J.D.; Allen, J.; Ferris, A.E.; Schilsky, R.L.; et al. The promise of Immuno-oncology: Implications for defining the value of cancer treatment. *J. Immunother. Cancer* **2019**, *7*, 129. [CrossRef]
57. Patra, J.K.; Das, G.; Fraceto, L.F.; Campos, E.V.R.; Rodriguez-Torres, M.D.P.; Acosta-Torres, L.S.; Diaz-Torres, L.A.; Grillo, R.; Swamy, M.K.; Sharma, S.; et al. Nano based drug delivery systems: Recent developments and future prospects. *J. Nanobiotechnol.* **2018**, *16*, 71. [CrossRef]

58. Din, F.U.; Aman, W.; Ullah, I.; Qureshi, O.S.; Mustapha, O.; Shafique, S.; Zeb, A. Effective use of nanocarriers as drug delivery systems for the treatment of selected tumors. *Int. J. Nanomed.* **2017**, *12*, 7291–7309. [CrossRef]
59. Riley, R.S.; June, C.H.; Langer, R.; Mitchell, M.J. Delivery technologies for cancer immunotherapy. *Nat. Rev. Drug Discov.* **2019**, *18*, 175–196. [CrossRef]
60. Schmid, D.; Park, C.G.; Hartl, C.A.; Subedi, N.; Cartwright, A.N.; Puerto, R.B.; Zheng, Y.; Maiarana, J.; Freeman, G.J.; Wucherpfennig, K.W.; et al. T cell-targeting nanoparticles focus delivery of immunotherapy to improve antitumor immunity. *Nat. Commun.* **2017**, *8*, 1747. [CrossRef]
61. Mohan, T.; Verma, P.; Rao, D.N. Novel adjuvants & delivery vehicles for vaccines development: A road ahead. *Indian J. Med. Res.* **2013**, *138*, 779–795. [PubMed]
62. Trovato, M.; De Berardinis, P. Novel antigen delivery systems. *World J. Virol.* **2015**, *4*, 156–168. [CrossRef] [PubMed]
63. Grippin, A.J.; Sayour, E.J.; Mitchell, D.A. Translational nanoparticle engineering for cancer vaccines. *Oncoimmunology* **2017**, *6*, e1290036. [CrossRef] [PubMed]
64. Csaba, N.; Garcia-Fuentes, M.; Alonso, M.J. Nanoparticles for nasal vaccination. *Adv. Drug Deliv. Rev.* **2009**, *61*, 140–157. [CrossRef] [PubMed]
65. Hubbell, J.A.; Thomas, S.N.; Swartz, M.A. Materials engineering for immunomodulation. *Nature* **2009**, *462*, 449–460. [CrossRef]
66. Zhang, X.-Y.; Lu, W.-Y. Recent advances in lymphatic targeted drug delivery system for tumor metastasis. *Cancer Biol. Med.* **2014**, *11*, 247–254. [CrossRef]
67. McLennan, D.N.; Porter, C.J.H.; Charman, S.A. Subcutaneous drug delivery and the role of the lymphatics. *Drug Discov. Today Technol.* **2005**, *2*, 89–96. [CrossRef]
68. Moon, J.J.; Huang, B.; Irvine, D.J. Engineering nano- and microparticles to tune immunity. *Adv. Mater.* **2012**, *24*, 3724–3746. [CrossRef]
69. Liu, H.; Moynihan, K.D.; Zheng, Y.; Szeto, G.L.; Li, A.V.; Huang, B.; Van Egeren, D.S.; Park, C.; Irvine, D.J. Structure-based programming of lymph-node targeting in molecular vaccines. *Nature* **2014**, *507*, 519–522. [CrossRef]
70. Oussoren, C.; Storm, G. Liposomes to target the lymphatics by subcutaneous administration. *Adv. Drug Deliv. Rev.* **2001**, *50*, 143–156. [CrossRef]
71. Reddy, S.T.; van der Vlies, A.J.; Simeoni, E.; Angeli, V.; Randolph, G.J.; O'Neil, C.P.; Lee, L.K.; Swartz, M.A.; Hubbell, J.A. Exploiting lymphatic transport and complement activation in nanoparticle vaccines. *Nat. Biotechnol.* **2007**, *25*, 1159–1164. [CrossRef] [PubMed]
72. Fifis, T.; Gamvrellis, A.; Crimeen-Irwin, B.; Pietersz, G.A.; Li, J.; Mottram, P.L.; McKenzie, I.F.; Plebanski, M. Size-dependent immunogenicity: Therapeutic and protective properties of nano-vaccines against tumors. *J. Immunol.* **2004**, *173*, 3148–3154. [CrossRef]
73. Irvine, D.J.; Hanson, M.C.; Rakhra, K.; Tokatlian, T. Synthetic Nanoparticles for Vaccines and Immunotherapy. *Chem. Rev.* **2015**, *115*, 11109–11146. [CrossRef] [PubMed]
74. Kourtis, I.C.; Hirosue, S.; de Titta, A.; Kontos, S.; Stegmann, T.; Hubbell, J.A.; Swartz, M.A. Peripherally administered nanoparticles target monocytic myeloid cells, secondary lymphoid organs and tumors in mice. *PLoS ONE* **2013**, *8*, e61646. [CrossRef]
75. Mueller, S.N.; Tian, S.; DeSimone, J.M. Rapid and Persistent Delivery of Antigen by Lymph Node Targeting PRINT Nanoparticle Vaccine Carrier To Promote Humoral Immunity. *Mol. Pharm.* **2015**, *12*, 1356–1365. [CrossRef]
76. Zhan, X.; Tran, K.K.; Shen, H. Effect of the Poly(ethylene glycol) (PEG) Density on the Access and Uptake of Particles by Antigen-Presenting Cells (APCs) after Subcutaneous Administration. *Mol. Pharm.* **2012**, *9*, 3442–3451. [CrossRef]
77. Song, W.; Shen, L.; Wang, Y.; Liu, Q.; Goodwin, T.J.; Li, J.; Dorosheva, O.; Liu, T.; Liu, R.; Huang, L. Synergistic and low adverse effect cancer immunotherapy by immunogenic chemotherapy and locally expressed PD-L1 trap. *Nat. Commun.* **2018**, *9*, 2237. [CrossRef] [PubMed]
78. Gaudino, S.J.; Kumar, P. Cross-Talk Between Antigen Presenting Cells and T Cells Impacts Intestinal Homeostasis, Bacterial Infections, and Tumorigenesis. *Front. Immunol.* **2019**, *10*. [CrossRef] [PubMed]
79. Burgdorf, S.; Kautz, A.; Böhnert, V.; Knolle, P.A.; Kurts, C. Distinct pathways of antigen uptake and intracellular routing in CD4 and CD8 T cell activation. *Science* **2007**, *316*, 612–616. [CrossRef] [PubMed]

80. Swartz, M.A.; Hirosue, S.; Hubbell, J.A. Engineering approaches to immunotherapy. *Sci. Transl. Med.* **2012**, *4*, 148rv9. [CrossRef]
81. Shen, H.; Ackerman, A.L.; Cody, V.; Giodini, A.; Hinson, E.R.; Cresswell, P.; Edelson, R.L.; Saltzman, W.M.; Hanlon, D.J. Enhanced and prolonged cross-presentation following endosomal escape of exogenous antigens encapsulated in biodegradable nanoparticles. *Immunology* **2006**, *117*, 78–88. [CrossRef] [PubMed]
82. Kranz, L.M.; Diken, M.; Haas, H.; Kreiter, S.; Loquai, C.; Reuter, K.C.; Meng, M.; Fritz, D.; Vascotto, F.; Hefesha, H.; et al. Systemic RNA delivery to dendritic cells exploits antiviral defence for cancer immunotherapy. *Nature* **2016**, *534*, 396–401. [CrossRef] [PubMed]
83. Wille-Reece, U.; Flynn, B.J.; Loré, K.; Koup, R.A.; Kedl, R.M.; Mattapallil, J.J.; Weiss, W.R.; Roederer, M.; Seder, R.A. HIV Gag protein conjugated to a Toll-like receptor 7/8 agonist improves the magnitude and quality of Th1 and CD8[+] T cell responses in nonhuman primates. *Proc. Natl. Acad. Sci. USA* **2005**, *102*, 15190. [CrossRef] [PubMed]
84. Bandyopadhyay, A.; Fine, R.L.; Demento, S.; Bockenstedt, L.K.; Fahmy, T.M. The impact of nanoparticle ligand density on dendritic-cell targeted vaccines. *Biomaterials* **2011**, *32*, 3094–3105. [CrossRef]
85. Bonifaz, L.C.; Bonnyay, D.P.; Charalambous, A.; Darguste, D.I.; Fujii, S.; Soares, H.; Brimnes, M.K.; Moltedo, B.; Moran, T.M.; Steinman, R.M. In vivo targeting of antigens to maturing dendritic cells via the DEC-205 receptor improves T cell vaccination. *J. Exp. Med.* **2004**, *199*, 815–824. [CrossRef]
86. Bozzacco, L.; Trumpfheller, C.; Siegal, F.P.; Mehandru, S.; Markowitz, M.; Carrington, M.; Nussenzweig, M.C.; Piperno, A.G.; Steinman, R.M. DEC-205 receptor on dendritic cells mediates presentation of HIV gag protein to CD8[+] T cells in a spectrum of human MHC I haplotypes. *Proc. Natl. Acad. Sci. USA* **2007**, *104*, 1289. [CrossRef]
87. Cruz, L.J.; Rosalia, R.A.; Kleinovink, J.W.; Rueda, F.; Löwik, C.W.G.M.; Ossendorp, F. Targeting nanoparticles to CD40, DEC-205 or CD11c molecules on dendritic cells for efficient CD8+ T cell response: A comparative study. *J. Control. Release* **2014**, *192*, 209–218. [CrossRef]
88. Schlosser, E.; Mueller, M.; Fischer, S.; Basta, S.; Busch, D.H.; Gander, B.; Groettrup, M. TLR ligands and antigen need to be coencapsulated into the same biodegradable microsphere for the generation of potent cytotoxic T lymphocyte responses. *Vaccine* **2008**, *26*, 1626–1637. [CrossRef]
89. Chiang, C.L.; Kandalaft, L.E.; Coukos, G. Adjuvants for enhancing the immunogenicity of whole tumor cell vaccines. *Int. Rev. Immunol.* **2011**, *30*, 150–182. [CrossRef]
90. Soiffer, R.; Hodi, F.S.; Haluska, F.; Jung, K.; Gillessen, S.; Singer, S.; Tanabe, K.; Duda, R.; Mentzer, S.; Jaklitsch, M.; et al. Vaccination With Irradiated, Autologous Melanoma Cells Engineered to Secrete Granulocyte-Macrophage Colony-Stimulating Factor by Adenoviral-Mediated Gene Transfer Augments Antitumor Immunity in Patients With Metastatic Melanoma. *J. Clin. Oncol.* **2003**, *21*, 3343–3350. [CrossRef]
91. Zhu, G.; Zhang, F.; Ni, Q.; Niu, G.; Chen, X. Efficient Nanovaccine Delivery in Cancer Immunotherapy. *ACS Nano* **2017**, *11*, 2387–2392. [CrossRef] [PubMed]
92. Kuai, R.; Ochyl, L.J.; Bahjat, K.S.; Schwendeman, A.; Moon, J.J. Designer vaccine nanodiscs for personalized cancer immunotherapy. *Nat. Mater.* **2017**, *16*, 489–496. [CrossRef] [PubMed]
93. Liu, S.-Y.; Wei, W.; Yue, H.; Ni, D.-Z.; Yue, Z.-G.; Wang, S.; Fu, Q.; Wang, Y.-Q.; Ma, G.-H.; Su, Z.-G. Nanoparticles-based multi-adjuvant whole cell tumor vaccine for cancer immunotherapy. *Biomaterials* **2013**, *34*, 8291–8300. [CrossRef] [PubMed]
94. Balkwill, F.R.; Capasso, M.; Hagemann, T. The tumor microenvironment at a glance. *J. Cell Sci.* **2012**, *125*, 5591. [CrossRef]
95. Lechner, M.G.; Liebertz, D.J.; Epstein, A.L. Characterization of cytokine-induced myeloid-derived suppressor cells from normal human peripheral blood mononuclear cells. *J. Immunol.* **2010**, *185*, 2273–2284. [CrossRef]
96. Jayaraman, P.; Parikh, F.; Lopez-Rivera, E.; Hailemichael, Y.; Clark, A.; Ma, G.; Cannan, D.; Ramacher, M.; Kato, M.; Overwijk, W.W.; et al. Tumor-expressed inducible nitric oxide synthase controls induction of functional myeloid-derived suppressor cells through modulation of vascular endothelial growth factor release. *J. Immunol.* **2012**, *188*, 5365–5376. [CrossRef]
97. Mandapathil, M.; Szczepanski, M.J.; Szajnik, M.; Ren, J.; Jackson, E.K.; Johnson, J.T.; Gorelik, E.; Lang, S.; Whiteside, T.L. Adenosine and prostaglandin E2 cooperate in the suppression of immune responses mediated by adaptive regulatory T cells. *J. Biol. Chem.* **2010**, *285*, 27571–27580. [CrossRef]
98. Rodríguez, P.C.; Ochoa, A.C. Arginine regulation by myeloid derived suppressor cells and tolerance in cancer: Mechanisms and therapeutic perspectives. *Immunol. Rev.* **2008**, *222*, 180–191. [CrossRef]

99. Godin-Ethier, J.; Hanafi, L.A.; Piccirillo, C.A.; Lapointe, R. Indoleamine 2,3-dioxygenase expression in human cancers: Clinical and immunologic perspectives. *Clin. Cancer Res.* **2011**, *17*, 6985–6991. [CrossRef]
100. Platten, M.; Wick, W.; Van den Eynde, B.J. Tryptophan catabolism in cancer: Beyond IDO and tryptophan depletion. *Cancer Res.* **2012**, *72*, 5435–5440. [CrossRef]
101. De la Fuente, H.; Cibrián, D.; Sánchez-Madrid, F. Immunoregulatory molecules are master regulators of inflammation during the immune response. *FEBS Lett.* **2012**, *586*, 2897–2905. [CrossRef] [PubMed]
102. Su, T.; Yang, B.; Gao, T.; Liu, T.; Li, J. Polymer nanoparticle-assisted chemotherapy of pancreatic cancer. *Ther. Adv. Med. Oncol.* **2020**, *12*. [CrossRef] [PubMed]
103. Whiteside, T.L. The tumor microenvironment and its role in promoting tumor growth. *Oncogene* **2008**, *27*, 5904–5912. [CrossRef] [PubMed]
104. Estrella, V.; Chen, T.; Lloyd, M.; Wojtkowiak, J.; Cornnell, H.H.; Ibrahim-Hashim, A.; Bailey, K.; Balagurunathan, Y.; Rothberg, J.M.; Sloane, B.F.; et al. Acidity generated by the tumor microenvironment drives local invasion. *Cancer Res.* **2013**, *73*, 1524–1535. [CrossRef] [PubMed]
105. Sacchetti, C.; Rapini, N.; Magrini, A.; Cirelli, E.; Bellucci, S.; Mattei, M.; Rosato, N.; Bottini, N.; Bottini, M. In Vivo Targeting of Intratumor Regulatory T Cells Using PEG-Modified Single-Walled Carbon Nanotubes. *Bioconjugate Chem.* **2013**, *24*, 852–858. [CrossRef] [PubMed]
106. Zhu, S.; Niu, M.; O'Mary, H.; Cui, Z. Targeting of tumor-associated macrophages made possible by PEG-sheddable, mannose-modified nanoparticles. *Mol. Pharm.* **2013**, *10*, 3525–3530. [CrossRef] [PubMed]
107. Park, J.; Wrzesinski, S.H.; Stern, E.; Look, M.; Criscione, J.; Ragheb, R.; Jay, S.M.; Demento, S.L.; Agawu, A.; Licona Limon, P.; et al. Combination delivery of TGF-β inhibitor and IL-2 by nanoscale liposomal polymeric gels enhances tumour immunotherapy. *Nat. Mater.* **2012**, *11*, 895–905. [CrossRef] [PubMed]
108. Wei, S.C.; Duffy, C.R.; Allison, J.P. Fundamental Mechanisms of Immune Checkpoint Blockade Therapy. *Cancer Discov.* **2018**, *8*, 1069. [CrossRef]
109. Riva, A.; Chokshi, S. Immune checkpoint receptors: Homeostatic regulators of immunity. *Hepatol. Int.* **2018**, *12*, 223–236. [CrossRef]
110. Sharpe, A.H.; Wherry, E.J.; Ahmed, R.; Freeman, G.J. The function of programmed cell death 1 and its ligands in regulating autoimmunity and infection. *Nat. Immunol.* **2007**, *8*, 239–245. [CrossRef]
111. Nirschl, C.J.; Drake, C.G. Molecular pathways: Coexpression of immune checkpoint molecules: Signaling pathways and implications for cancer immunotherapy. *Clin. Cancer Res.* **2013**, *19*, 4917–4924. [CrossRef] [PubMed]
112. Zappasodi, R.; Merghoub, T.; Wolchok, J.D. Emerging Concepts for Immune Checkpoint Blockade-Based Combination Therapies. *Cancer Cell* **2018**, *33*, 581–598. [CrossRef] [PubMed]
113. Marin-Acevedo, J.A.; Dholaria, B.; Soyano, A.E.; Knutson, K.L.; Chumsri, S.; Lou, Y. Next generation of immune checkpoint therapy in cancer: New developments and challenges. *J. Hematol. Oncol.* **2018**, *11*, 39. [CrossRef] [PubMed]
114. Pardoll, D.M. The blockade of immune checkpoints in cancer immunotherapy. *Nat. Rev. Cancer* **2012**, *12*, 252–264. [CrossRef] [PubMed]
115. Altmann, D.M. A Nobel Prize-worthy pursuit: Cancer immunology and harnessing immunity to tumour neoantigens. *Immunology* **2018**, *155*, 283–284. [CrossRef] [PubMed]
116. Sharma, P.; Allison, J.P. The future of immune checkpoint therapy. *Science* **2015**, *348*, 56. [CrossRef]
117. Topalian, S.L.; Drake, C.G.; Pardoll, D.M. Immune checkpoint blockade: A common denominator approach to cancer therapy. *Cancer Cell* **2015**, *27*, 450–461. [CrossRef]
118. Leach, D.R.; Krummel, M.F.; Allison, J.P. Enhancement of antitumor immunity by CTLA-4 blockade. *Science* **1996**, *271*, 1734–1736. [CrossRef]
119. Chen, L. Co-inhibitory molecules of the B7-CD28 family in the control of T-cell immunity. *Nat. Rev. Immunol.* **2004**, *4*, 336–347. [CrossRef]
120. Keir, M.E.; Butte, M.J.; Freeman, G.J.; Sharpe, A.H. PD-1 and its ligands in tolerance and immunity. *Annu. Rev. Immunol.* **2008**, *26*, 677–704. [CrossRef]
121. Hodi, F.S.; O'Day, S.J.; McDermott, D.F.; Weber, R.W.; Sosman, J.A.; Haanen, J.B.; Gonzalez, R.; Robert, C.; Schadendorf, D.; Hassel, J.C.; et al. Improved Survival with Ipilimumab in Patients with Metastatic Melanoma. *N. Engl. J. Med.* **2010**, *363*, 711–723. [CrossRef] [PubMed]

122. Topalian, S.L.; Hodi, F.S.; Brahmer, J.R.; Gettinger, S.N.; Smith, D.C.; McDermott, D.F.; Powderly, J.D.; Carvajal, R.D.; Sosman, J.A.; Atkins, M.B.; et al. Safety, activity, and immune correlates of anti-PD-1 antibody in cancer. *N. Engl. J. Med.* **2012**, *366*, 2443–2454. [CrossRef] [PubMed]

123. Shih, K.; Arkenau, H.-T.; Infante, J.R. Clinical impact of checkpoint inhibitors as novel cancer therapies. *Drugs* **2014**, *74*, 1993–2013. [CrossRef] [PubMed]

124. Hui, E. Immune checkpoint inhibitors. *J. Cell Biol.* **2019**, *218*, 740–741. [CrossRef] [PubMed]

125. Vaddepally, R.K.; Kharel, P.; Pandey, R.; Garje, R.; Chandra, A.B. Review of Indications of FDA-Approved Immune Checkpoint Inhibitors per NCCN Guidelines with the Level of Evidence. *Cancers* **2020**, *12*, 738. [CrossRef] [PubMed]

126. Wang, C.; Ye, Y.; Hochu, G.M.; Sadeghifar, H.; Gu, Z. Enhanced Cancer Immunotherapy by Microneedle Patch-Assisted Delivery of Anti-PD1 Antibody. *Nano Lett.* **2016**, *16*, 2334–2340. [CrossRef]

127. Wang, C.; Sun, W.; Wright, G.; Wang, A.Z.; Gu, Z. Inflammation-Triggered Cancer Immunotherapy by Programmed Delivery of CpG and Anti-PD1 Antibody. *Adv. Mater.* **2017**, *29*. [CrossRef]

128. Zou, W.; Wolchok, J.D.; Chen, L. PD-L1 (B7-H1) and PD-1 pathway blockade for cancer therapy: Mechanisms, response biomarkers, and combinations. *Sci. Transl. Med.* **2016**, *8*, 283–291. [CrossRef]

129. Bai, R.; Chen, N.; Li, L.; Du, N.; Bai, L.; Lv, Z.; Tian, H.; Cui, J. Mechanisms of Cancer Resistance to Immunotherapy. *Front. Oncol.* **2020**, *10*, 1290. [CrossRef]

130. Feinberg, A.P.; Koldobskiy, M.A.; Göndör, A. Epigenetic modulators, modifiers and mediators in cancer aetiology and progression. *Nat. Rev. Genet.* **2016**, *17*, 284–299. [CrossRef]

131. Héninger, E.; Krueger, T.E.G.; Lang, J.M. Augmenting antitumor immune responses with epigenetic modifying agents. *Front. Immunol.* **2015**, *6*, 29. [CrossRef] [PubMed]

132. Ruan, H.; Hu, Q.; Wen, D.; Chen, Q.; Chen, G.; Lu, Y.; Wang, J.; Cheng, H.; Lu, W.; Gu, Z. A Dual-Bioresponsive Drug-Delivery Depot for Combination of Epigenetic Modulation and Immune Checkpoint Blockade. *Adv. Mater.* **2019**, *31*, e1806957. [CrossRef] [PubMed]

133. Min, Y.; Roche, K.C.; Tian, S.; Eblan, M.J.; McKinnon, K.P.; Caster, J.M.; Chai, S.; Herring, L.E.; Zhang, L.; Zhang, T.; et al. Antigen-capturing nanoparticles improve the abscopal effect and cancer immunotherapy. *Nat. Nanotechnol.* **2017**, *12*, 877–882. [CrossRef] [PubMed]

134. Palena, C.; Abrams, S.I.; Schlom, J.; Hodge, J.W. Cancer vaccines: Preclinical studies and novel strategies. *Adv. Cancer Res.* **2006**, *95*, 115–145. [CrossRef] [PubMed]

135. Ogi, C.; Aruga, A. Immunological monitoring of anticancer vaccines in clinical trials. *Oncoimmunology* **2013**, *2*, e26012. [CrossRef]

136. Kim, Y.; Kang, S.; Shin, H.; Kim, T.; Yu, B.; Kim, J.; Yoo, D.; Jon, S. Sequential and Timely Combination of a Cancer Nanovaccine with Immune Checkpoint Blockade Effectively Inhibits Tumor Growth and Relapse. *Angew. Chem. Int. Ed.* **2020**, *59*, 14628–14638. [CrossRef]

137. Fontana, F.; Fusciello, M.; Groeneveldt, C.; Capasso, C.; Chiaro, J.; Feola, S.; Liu, Z.; Mäkilä, E.M.; Salonen, J.J.; Hirvonen, J.T.; et al. Biohybrid Vaccines for Improved Treatment of Aggressive Melanoma with Checkpoint Inhibitor. *ACS Nano* **2019**, *13*, 6477–6490. [CrossRef]

138. Zhuang, J.; Holay, M.; Park, J.H.; Fang, R.H.; Zhang, J.; Zhang, L. Nanoparticle Delivery of Immunostimulatory Agents for Cancer Immunotherapy. *Theranostics* **2019**, *9*, 7826–7848. [CrossRef]

139. Sushnitha, M.; Evangelopoulos, M.; Tasciotti, E.; Taraballi, F. Cell Membrane-Based Biomimetic Nanoparticles and the Immune System: Immunomodulatory Interactions to Therapeutic Applications. *Front. Bioeng. Biotechnol.* **2020**, *8*. [CrossRef]

140. Getts, D.R.; Shea, L.D.; Miller, S.D.; King, N.J. Harnessing nanoparticles for immune modulation. *Trends Iimmunol.* **2015**, *36*, 419–427. [CrossRef]

141. Jiao, Q.; Li, L.; Mu, Q.; Zhang, Q. Immunomodulation of nanoparticles in nanomedicine applications. *BioMed Res. Int.* **2014**, *2014*, 426028. [CrossRef] [PubMed]

142. Liu, X.-Q.; Tang, R.-Z. Biological responses to nanomaterials: Understanding nano-bio effects on cell behaviors. *Drug Deliv.* **2017**, *24*, 1–15. [CrossRef] [PubMed]

143. Luo, Y.-H.; Chang, L.W.; Lin, P. Metal-Based Nanoparticles and the Immune System: Activation, Inflammation, and Potential Applications. *BioMed Res. Int.* **2015**, *2015*, 143720. [CrossRef] [PubMed]

144. Fadeel, B. Hide and Seek: Nanomaterial Interactions with the Immune System. *Front. Immunol.* **2019**, *10*, 133. [CrossRef] [PubMed]

145. Akira, S.; Takeda, K. Toll-like receptor signalling. *Nat. Rev. Immunol.* **2004**, *4*, 499–511. [CrossRef] [PubMed]

146. Chugh, H.; Sood, D.; Chandra, I.; Tomar, V.; Dhawan, G.; Chandra, R. Role of gold and silver nanoparticles in cancer nano-medicine. *Artif. Cells Nanomed. Biotechnol.* **2018**, *46*, 1210–1220. [CrossRef] [PubMed]
147. Yen, H.J.; Hsu, S.H.; Tsai, C.L. Cytotoxicity and immunological response of gold and silver nanoparticles of different sizes. *Small* **2009**, *5*, 1553–1561. [CrossRef]
148. Wolf-Grosse, S.; Mollnes, T.E.; Ali, S.; Stenvik, J.; Nilsen, A.M. Iron oxide nanoparticles enhance Toll-like receptor-induced cytokines in a particle size- and actin-dependent manner in human blood. *Nanomedicine* **2018**, *13*, 1773–1785. [CrossRef]
149. Vasilichin, V.A.; Tsymbal, S.A.; Fakhardo, A.F.; Anastasova, E.I.; Marchenko, A.S.; Shtil, A.A.; Vinogradov, V.V.; Koshel, E.I. Effects of Metal Oxide Nanoparticles on Toll-Like Receptor mRNAs in Human Monocytes. *Nanomaterials* **2020**, *10*, 127. [CrossRef]
150. Dykman, L.A.; Khlebtsov, N.G. Immunological properties of gold nanoparticles. *Chem. Sci.* **2017**, *8*, 1719–1735. [CrossRef]
151. Lee, J.Y.; Park, W.; Yi, D.K. Immunostimulatory effects of gold nanorod and silica-coated gold nanorod on RAW 264.7 mouse macrophages. *Toxicol. Lett.* **2012**, *209*, 51–57. [CrossRef] [PubMed]
152. Fallarini, S.; Paoletti, T.; Battaglini, C.O.; Ronchi, P.; Lay, L.; Bonomi, R.; Jha, S.; Mancin, F.; Scrimin, P.; Lombardi, G. Factors affecting T cell responses induced by fully synthetic glyco-gold-nanoparticles. *Nanoscale* **2013**, *5*, 390–400. [CrossRef] [PubMed]
153. Lin, A.Y.; Mattos Almeida, J.P.; Bear, A.; Liu, N.; Luo, L.; Foster, A.E.; Drezek, R.A. Gold Nanoparticle Delivery of Modified CpG Stimulates Macrophages and Inhibits Tumor Growth for Enhanced Immunotherapy. *PLoS ONE* **2013**, *8*, e63550. [CrossRef] [PubMed]
154. Ahn, S.; Lee, I.H.; Kang, S.; Kim, D.; Choi, M.; Saw, P.E.; Shin, E.C.; Jon, S. Gold nanoparticles displaying tumor-associated self-antigens as a potential vaccine for cancer immunotherapy. *Adv. Healthc. Mater.* **2014**, *3*, 1194–1199. [CrossRef] [PubMed]
155. Ninan, N.; Goswami, N.; Vasilev, K. The Impact of Engineered Silver Nanomaterials on the Immune System. *Nanomaterials* **2020**, *10*, 967. [CrossRef] [PubMed]
156. Elsabahy, M.; Wooley, K.L. Cytokines as biomarkers of nanoparticle immunotoxicity. *Chem. Soc. Rev.* **2013**, *42*, 5552–5576. [CrossRef] [PubMed]
157. Carlson, C.; Hussain, S.M.; Schrand, A.M.; Braydich-Stolle, L.K.; Hess, K.L.; Jones, R.L.; Schlager, J.J. Unique cellular interaction of silver nanoparticles: Size-dependent generation of reactive oxygen species. *J. Phys. Chem. B* **2008**, *112*, 13608–13619. [CrossRef]
158. Asgary, V.; Shoari, A.; Baghbani-Arani, F.; Sadat Shandiz, S.A.; Khosravy, M.S.; Janani, A.; Bigdeli, R.; Bashar, R.; Cohan, R.A. Green synthesis and evaluation of silver nanoparticles as adjuvant in rabies veterinary vaccine. *Int. J. Nanomed.* **2016**, *11*, 3597–3605. [CrossRef]
159. Liu, Y.; Balachandran, Y.L.; Li, D.; Shao, Y.; Jiang, X. Polyvinylpyrrolidone–Poly(ethylene glycol) Modified Silver Nanorods Can Be a Safe, Noncarrier Adjuvant for HIV Vaccine. *ACS Nano* **2016**, *10*, 3589–3596. [CrossRef]
160. Xu, Y.; Tang, H.; Liu, J.-H.; Wang, H.; Liu, Y. Evaluation of the adjuvant effect of silver nanoparticles both in vitro and in vivo. *Toxicol. Lett.* **2013**, *219*, 42–48. [CrossRef]
161. Kim, J.V.; Latouche, J.-B.; Rivière, I.; Sadelain, M. The ABCs of artificial antigen presentation. *Nat. Biotechnol.* **2004**, *22*, 403–410. [CrossRef] [PubMed]
162. Rhodes, K.R.; Green, J.J. Nanoscale artificial antigen presenting cells for cancer immunotherapy. *Mol. Immunol.* **2018**, *98*, 13–18. [CrossRef] [PubMed]
163. Mandal, S.; Eksteen-Akeroyd, Z.H.; Jacobs, M.J.; Hammink, R.; Koepf, M.; Lambeck, A.J.A.; van Hest, J.C.M.; Wilson, C.J.; Blank, K.; Figdor, C.G.; et al. Therapeutic nanoworms: Towards novel synthetic dendritic cells for immunotherapy. *Chem. Sci.* **2013**, *4*, 4168–4174. [CrossRef]
164. Kosmides, A.K.; Meyer, R.A.; Hickey, J.W.; Aje, K.; Cheung, K.N.; Green, J.J.; Schneck, J.P. Biomimetic biodegradable artificial antigen presenting cells synergize with PD-1 blockade to treat melanoma. *Biomaterials* **2017**, *118*, 16–26. [CrossRef] [PubMed]
165. Balar, A.V.; Weber, J.S. PD-1 and PD-L1 antibodies in cancer: Current status and future directions. *Cancer Immunol. Immunother.* **2017**, *66*, 551–564. [CrossRef] [PubMed]
166. Li, Y.; Li, F.; Jiang, F.; Lv, X.; Zhang, R.; Lu, A.; Zhang, G. A Mini-Review for Cancer Immunotherapy: Molecular Understanding of PD-1/PD-L1 Pathway & Translational Blockade of Immune Checkpoints. *Int. J. Mol. Sci.* **2016**, *17*, 1151. [CrossRef]

167. Wang, Q.; Wu, X. Primary and acquired resistance to PD-1/PD-L1 blockade in cancer treatment. *Int. Immunopharmacol.* **2017**, *46*, 210–219. [CrossRef]
168. Sun, L.; Zhang, L.; Yu, J.; Zhang, Y.; Pang, X.; Ma, C.; Shen, M.; Ruan, S.; Wasan, H.S.; Qiu, S. Clinical efficacy and safety of anti-PD-1/PD-L1 inhibitors for the treatment of advanced or metastatic cancer: A systematic review and meta-analysis. *Sci. Rep.* **2020**, *10*, 2083. [CrossRef]
169. Sui, X.; Ma, J.; Han, W.; Wang, X.; Fang, Y.; Li, D.; Pan, H.; Zhang, L. The anticancer immune response of anti-PD-1/PD-L1 and the genetic determinants of response to anti-PD-1/PD-L1 antibodies in cancer patients. *Oncotarget* **2015**, *6*, 19393–19404. [CrossRef]
170. Kroemer, G.; Galluzzi, L.; Kepp, O.; Zitvogel, L. Immunogenic Cell Death in Cancer Therapy. *Annu. Rev. Immunol.* **2013**, *31*, 51–72. [CrossRef]
171. Fucikova, J.; Kralikova, P.; Fialova, A.; Brtnicky, T.; Rob, L.; Bartunkova, J.; Spísek, R. Human tumor cells killed by anthracyclines induce a tumor-specific immune response. *Cancer Res.* **2011**, *71*, 4821–4833. [CrossRef] [PubMed]
172. Nam, J.; Son, S.; Park, K.S.; Zou, W.; Shea, L.D.; Moon, J.J. Cancer nanomedicine for combination cancer immunotherapy. *Nat. Rev. Mater.* **2019**, *4*, 398–414. [CrossRef]
173. Schmid, P.; Adams, S.; Rugo, H.S.; Schneeweiss, A.; Barrios, C.H.; Iwata, H.; Diéras, V.; Hegg, R.; Im, S.-A.; Shaw Wright, G.; et al. Atezolizumab and Nab-Paclitaxel in Advanced Triple-Negative Breast Cancer. *N. Engl. J. Med.* **2018**, *379*, 2108–2121. [CrossRef] [PubMed]
174. Kang, C.; Syed, Y.Y. Atezolizumab (in Combination with Nab-Paclitaxel): A Review in Advanced Triple-Negative Breast Cancer. *Drugs* **2020**, *80*, 601–607. [CrossRef]
175. Bonvalot, S.; Rutkowski, P.L.; Thariat, J.; Carrère, S.; Ducassou, A.; Sunyach, M.P.; Agoston, P.; Hong, A.; Mervoyer, A.; Rastrelli, M.; et al. NBTXR3, a first-in-class radioenhancer hafnium oxide nanoparticle, plus radiotherapy versus radiotherapy alone in patients with locally advanced soft-tissue sarcoma (Act.In.Sarc): A multicentre, phase 2-3, randomised, controlled trial. *Lancet Oncol.* **2019**, *20*, 1148–1159. [CrossRef]
176. Bonvalot, S.; Le Pechoux, C.; De Baere, T.; Kantor, G.; Buy, X.; Stoeckle, E.; Terrier, P.; Sargos, P.; Coindre, J.M.; Lassau, N.; et al. First-in-Human Study Testing a New Radioenhancer Using Nanoparticles (NBTXR3) Activated by Radiation Therapy in Patients with Locally Advanced Soft Tissue Sarcomas. *Clin. Cancer Res.* **2017**, *23*, 908–917. [CrossRef]
177. West, H.; McCleod, M.; Hussein, M.; Morabito, A.; Rittmeyer, A.; Conter, H.J.; Kopp, H.G.; Daniel, D.; McCune, S.; Mekhail, T.; et al. Atezolizumab in combination with carboplatin plus nab-paclitaxel chemotherapy compared with chemotherapy alone as first-line treatment for metastatic non-squamous non-small-cell lung cancer (IMpower130): A multicentre, randomised, open-label, phase 3 trial. *Lancet Oncol.* **2019**, *20*, 924–937. [CrossRef]
178. Pujade-Lauraine, E.; Fujiwara, K.; Dychter, S.S.; Devgan, G.; Monk, B.J. Avelumab (anti-PD-L1) in platinum-resistant/refractory ovarian cancer: JAVELIN Ovarian 200 Phase III study design. *Future Oncol.* **2018**, *14*, 2103–2113. [CrossRef]
179. Shi, Y. Clinical Translation of Nanomedicine and Biomaterials for Cancer Immunotherapy: Progress and Perspectives. *Adv. Ther.* **2020**, *3*, 1900215. [CrossRef]
180. Mikelez-Alonso, I.; Aires, A.; Cortajarena, A.L. Cancer Nano-Immunotherapy from the Injection to the Target: The Role of Protein Corona. *Int. J. Mol. Sci.* **2020**, *21*, 519. [CrossRef]
181. Yetisgin, A.A.; Cetinel, S.; Zuvin, M.; Kosar, A.; Kutlu, O. Therapeutic Nanoparticles and Their Targeted Delivery Applications. *Molecules* **2020**, *25*, 2193. [CrossRef] [PubMed]
182. Anselmo, A.C.; Mitragotri, S. Nanoparticles in the clinic: An update. *Bioeng. Transl. Med.* **2019**, *4*, e10143. [CrossRef] [PubMed]
183. Beg, M.S.; Brenner, A.J.; Sachdev, J.; Borad, M.; Kang, Y.K.; Stoudemire, J.; Smith, S.; Bader, A.G.; Kim, S.; Hong, D.S. Phase I study of MRX34, a liposomal miR-34a mimic, administered twice weekly in patients with advanced solid tumors. *Investig. New Drugs* **2017**, *35*, 180–188. [CrossRef] [PubMed]
184. Burris, H.A., III; Patel, M.R.; Cho, D.C.; Clarke, J.M.; Gutierrez, M.; Zaks, T.Z.; Frederick, J.; Hopson, K.; Mody, K.; Binanti-Berube, A.; et al. A phase 1, open-label, multicenter study to assess the safety, tolerability, and immunogenicity of mRNA-4157 alone in subjects with resected solid tumors and in combination with pembrolizumab in subjects with unresectable solid tumors (Keynote-603). *J. Glob. Oncol.* **2019**, *5*, 93. [CrossRef]

185. Zanganeh, S.; Hutter, G.; Spitler, R.; Lenkov, O.; Mahmoudi, M.; Shaw, A.; Pajarinen, J.S.; Nejadnik, H.; Goodman, S.; Moseley, M.; et al. Iron oxide nanoparticles inhibit tumour growth by inducing pro-inflammatory macrophage polarization in tumour tissues. *Nat. Nanotechnol.* **2016**, *11*, 986–994. [CrossRef]
186. Pfannenstiel, L.W.; Lam, S.S.; Emens, L.A.; Jaffee, E.M.; Armstrong, T.D. Paclitaxel enhances early dendritic cell maturation and function through TLR4 signaling in mice. *Cell. Immunol.* **2010**, *263*, 79–87. [CrossRef]
187. Graziani, S.R.; Vital, C.G.; Morikawa, A.T.; Van Eyll, B.M.; Fernandes Junior, H.J.; Kalil Filho, R.; Maranhão, R.C. Phase II study of paclitaxel associated with lipid core nanoparticles (LDE) as third-line treatment of patients with epithelial ovarian carcinoma. *Med. Oncol.* **2017**, *34*, 151. [CrossRef]
188. Shen, C.; Frakes, J.; Weiss, J.; Caudell, J.J.; Hackman, T.G.; Akulian, J.A.; El-Haddad, G.; Hu, Y.; Dixon, R.; Pearson, A.T.; et al. Phase I study of NBTXR3 activated by radiotherapy in patients with advanced cancers treated with an anti-PD-1 therapy. *J. Clin. Oncol.* **2020**, *38*, TPS3173. [CrossRef]

Publisher's Note: MDPI stays neutral with regard to jurisdictional claims in published maps and institutional affiliations.

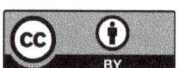

© 2020 by the authors. Licensee MDPI, Basel, Switzerland. This article is an open access article distributed under the terms and conditions of the Creative Commons Attribution (CC BY) license (http://creativecommons.org/licenses/by/4.0/).

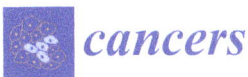

Review

Intercellular Mitochondrial Transfer in the Tumor Microenvironment

Hana Sahinbegovic [1,2,3,4], Tomas Jelinek [1,2], Matous Hrdinka [1,2], Juli R. Bago [1,2], Marcello Turi [1,3], Tereza Sevcikova [1,2,3], Amina Kurtovic-Kozaric [4], Roman Hajek [1,2] and Michal Simicek [1,2,3,*]

1. Department of Clinical Studies, Faculty of Medicine, University of Ostrava, 70300 Ostrava, Czech Republic; hana.sahinbegovic@fno.cz (H.S.); tomas.jelinek@fno.cz (T.J.); matous.hrdinka@fno.cz (M.H.); julio.rodriguez.bago@fno.cz (J.R.B.); marcello.turi@fno.cz (M.T.); tereza.sevcikova@fno.cz (T.S.); roman.hajek@fno.cz (R.H.)
2. Department of Hematooncology, University Hospital Ostrava, 70200 Ostrava, Czech Republic
3. Faculty of Science, University of Ostrava, 70800 Ostrava, Czech Republic
4. Faculty of Genetics and Bioengineering, International Burch University, 71210 Sarajevo, Bosnia and Herzegovina; amina.kurtovic@ibu.edu.ba
* Correspondence: michal.simicek@fno.cz

Received: 12 June 2020; Accepted: 2 July 2020; Published: 4 July 2020

Abstract: Cell-to-cell communication is a fundamental process in every multicellular organism. In addition to membrane-bound and released factors, the sharing of cytosolic components represents a new, poorly explored signaling route. An extraordinary example of this communication channel is the direct transport of mitochondria between cells. In this review, we discuss how intercellular mitochondrial transfer can be used by cancer cells to sustain their high metabolic requirements and promote drug resistance and describe relevant molecular players in the context of current and future cancer therapy.

Keywords: cancer; mitochondria; mitochondrial transfer; tunneling nanotubes; tumor microenvironment

1. Introduction

The majority of human cells use mitochondria as the main source of energy and metabolites. A typical cancer cell, however, tends to upregulate glycolysis, as postulated by Otto Warburg more than 100 years ago [1,2]. At first glance, this might seem counterproductive, as glycolysis produces fewer ATP molecules and causes constant acidification of the extracellular space by increased production of lactate [3]. On the other hand, an enhanced glycolytic rate contributes to the development of several cancer hallmarks, such as the ability to evade apoptosis by inhibition of oxidative phosphorylation (OXPHOS) [4] and the promotion of metastatic dissemination by the degradation of the extracellular matrix and tissue outgrowth [5]. Moreover, tumor cells often reside in a hypoxic environment that favors the use of anoxygenic production of energy. Therefore, the idea of forcing tumor cells to use OXPHOS instead of glycolysis has emerged as a promising therapeutic strategy [6,7].

Even though most cancers have impaired mitochondrial respiration, recent discoveries indicate that certain solid tumors, such as pancreatic ductal adenocarcinoma and endometrial carcinoma, and many hematological neoplasms rely heavily on OXPHOS and upregulated mitochondrial metabolism [8,9]. In line with these observations, a number of studies highlighted the importance of mitochondria-dependent metabolic reprogramming in boosting proliferation and in the development of drug resistance in several types of cancers [6,10]. Consequently, the clinical relevance of biological processes involving active and healthy mitochondria, initially meant to have a rather tumor suppressive role, is now being revised.

Historically, cancer research has been mostly done by using 2D in vitro models of established cell lines [11,12]. Although this is a powerful and valuable approach, it completely neglects the presence of neighboring non-tumor cells supporting or suppressing the cancer tissue. The influence of the microenvironment on tumor cells is very complex and often includes the direct involvement of tumor mitochondria. Cancer cells can release (e.g., upon necrosis) entire mitochondria or their components, such as mitochondrial DNA (mtDNA), ATP, cytochrome C, or formylated peptides, to the extracellular space [13]. These then serve as Damage-Associated Molecular Patterns (DAMPs) that activate the immune cells [14,15]. Resulting pro-inflammatory and immunosuppressive responses then either inhibit or stimulate the growth and/or metastatic capacity of the tumor [16,17].

The modulation of tumor mitochondria is an important mechanism that aids cancer cells to escape from the immune system control and develop drug resistance [6,10]. In addition to neoplastic and immune cells, the tumor microenvironment contains many different cell types that can control the state of the mitochondria in a tumor both directly, by cell–cell contacts [18], and indirectly, by secretion of soluble factors and a variety of extracellular vesicles [19]. Recently, a novel mechanism of intercellular communication based on a horizontal transfer of mitochondria between non-tumor and malignant cells was described [20–24]. This paradigm-breaking discovery has led to the question of whether the phenomenon of direct mitochondria sharing could also contribute to the aversion of malignant cells to existing drug combinations and possibly further promote tumor growth. We still know very little about this new, exciting way of sharing intracellular molecules and organelles. A deeper understanding of the underlying molecular mechanisms and consequences on cell physiology will likely explain many therapeutic failures and ultimately lead to novel, more efficient drug combinations.

In this review, we provide an overview of the current knowledge of intercellular mitochondrial transfer, with a particular focus on its relevance in cancer initiation, progression, and drug resistance. We present a summary of the known molecular players involved in sharing mitochondria and show examples of mitochondrial exchange in both solid and hematological tumors. Finally, we place all findings in the context of the current therapeutic strategies.

2. Means of Mitochondrial Transfer

The first observation of mitochondrial transfer in 2006 demonstrated that mitochondria from bone marrow stromal cells (BMSCs), but not free mitochondria or mtDNA from the medium, were able to relocate to mitochondria-deficient A549 lung cancer cells and rescue their aerobic respiration [18]. A follow-up study further supported the regulated directionality of the exchange as donor, non-irradiated PC12 cells with faulty mitochondria could not nourish recipient PC12 cells, leading them back to life [25]. Importantly, the transfer of mitochondria was also observed in vivo in mouse melanoma cells injected into mice expressing a fluorescently labelled mitochondrial protein [24].

Fundamental research on the physiological relevance of mitochondrial transfer suggested its importance in the regeneration of damaged or infected tissue [26,27]. The "mito-healing" theory was subsequently supported by additional studies in a variety of tissues, including vascular [28], brain [19], lung [29], cornea [30], and several other tissues. Transfer of mitochondria was also described in the immune system to combat bacterial infections [31]. The presence of pathogens inside immune cells is usually accompanied by a switch from glycolytic metabolism to OXPHOS as a means of triggering a fast anti-microbial response [32]. A striking example of infection-induced metabolic switch is seen in macrophages during acute respiratory distress syndrome, when macrophages are fed additional mitochondria by surrounding mesenchymal stem cells (MSCs), boosting their anti-inflammatory and phagocytic capacity [31]. Thus, the importance of mitochondria exchange in maintaining tissue homeostasis is clearly not disputable. However, the shuttling of mitochondria between cells could also have severe pathological consequences, particularly in cancer, where malignant cells tend to take advantage of the surrounding environment (Figure 1) [23,33,34].

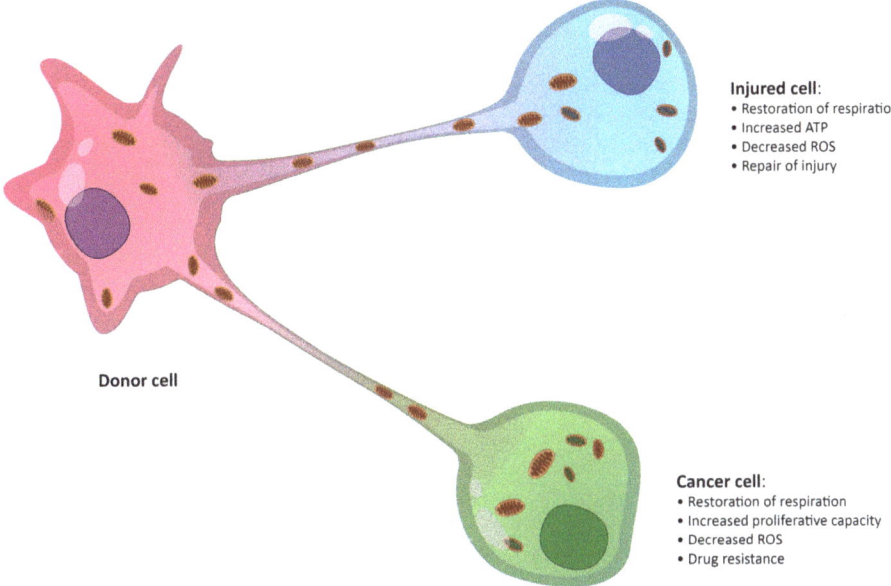

Figure 1. Putative effects of mitochondrial transfer on an injured cell and a cancer cell. ROS, reactive oxygen species.

The precise mechanism of mitochondrial transfer remains unknown, and so far, only a few crucial molecules involved in the process have been described. High OXPHOS demand and/or severe mitochondria damage are typical features of the recipient cells [23,35,36]. To initiate the transfer, the providing cells should not only possess non-damaged, healthy mitochondria [37] but also be specifically activated [22]. Metalloproteinase-1 (MMP-1), nestin, and proinflammatory cytokines have been identified as essential factors stimulating donor cells to dispatch mitochondria [22]. When cultured with leukemic cells, donor BMSCs exhibited increased levels of PGC1α, a master regulator of mitochondrial biogenesis necessary for efficient mitochondrial transfer [38]. The activation of donor functions often correlates with a rise in intracellular reactive oxygen species (ROS) [22,37] generated by the recipient cells [33]. The main trigger regulating the directional release of mitochondria is still unknown, but the signal is likely multifactorial and, at least partially, mediated by ROS.

3. Tunneling Nanotubes Are the Main Delivery Route for Mitochondria

Neighboring cells can share mitochondria through several mechanisms, including (i) the formation of extracellular vehicles (EVs), (ii) tunneling nanotubes (TNTs) formed at the sites of physical contact, (iii) mitochondrial ejection, or (iv) cytoplasmic fusion [39]. Multiple studies have shown that TNTs, ultrafine cytoplasmic bridges between cells, are the main delivery system for mitochondria in both healthy and tumor tissues (Figure 2) [23,33]. TNT-independent mitochondria sharing in certain tumors was also described [19,29,37]. However, there seems to be a rather scarce number of examples, and more investigation of the transfer mechanisms is needed.

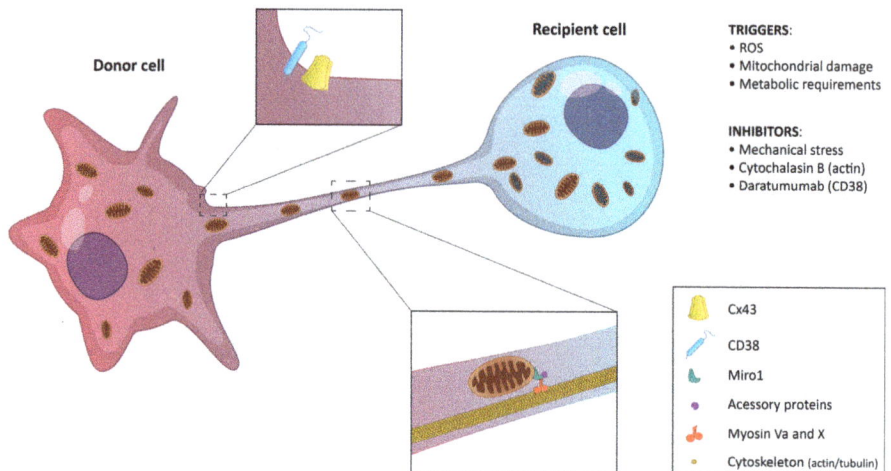

Figure 2. Schematic representation of mitochondrial transfer via tunneling nanotubes. The donor cell, usually a non-cancerous cell, sends mitochondria to the recipient cell. In certain cases, the transfer is possible in both directions. Key regulatory molecules and triggers are listed.

TNTs, discovered by Rustom et al. in 2004, serve as direct communication channels between neighboring cells to exchange a wide variety of molecules and organelles [40]. Their diameter ranges from 50 to 200 nm, and their length may reach up to 150 µm. TNTs are formed de novo in a matter of minutes and can connect multiple cells at once. Specific structural features or biomarkers unique to TNTs have not been identified. TNTs lack any attachment to the substrate, but their structure is enforced by actin [40] and microtubule filaments [25,41]. In experimental settings, the actin-disrupting drug cytochalasin B is often used as an efficient inhibitor of TNTs formation [23,33].

For the efficient transport of mitochondria, the presence of functional microtubules and associated molecular motors seems to be required [25]. Specifically, Myosin X and Myosin Va have been co-localized with mitochondria inside TNTs [40,42,43]. Some donor cells exhibit high expression of the small GTPase Miro1 localized on the outer mitochondrial membrane [44]. When Miro1 was depleted in MSCs cultured with LA-4 epithelial cells, mitochondrial transfer was ineffective, whereas Miro1 overexpression increased the ability of MSCs to donate mitochondria [45]. Mechanistically, Miro1 seems to co-ordinate mitochondrial movement along microtubules by promoting the assembly of a complex molecular motor machinery [46].

The role of TNT-localized actin in mitochondria exchange is less clear. It is known that filamentous actin impedes the passive transfer of soluble cytoplasmic molecules through TNTs [40] and serves as a scaffold that stabilizes TNT structure [47]. The actin-binding protein M-Sec has been shown to be important for the formation of TNTs and the intercellular propagation of calcium (Ca^{2+}) in macrophages [48,49]. Increased levels of Ca^{2+} activate mitochondria-localized Miro1 that further binds to microtubule-associated motor proteins [46].

Recently, CD38, an ectoenzyme involved in transmembrane signaling and cell adhesion, was identified as one of the key players in mitochondrial transfer [19,23]. In addition to its receptor function, CD38 modulates intracellular Ca^{2+} levels by generating cyclic ADP-ribose [50,51]. The Ca^{2+} regulatory role of CD38 seems important for mitochondrial delivery from BMSCs to myeloma cells [23] and from astrocytes to neurons in brain tissue damaged by stroke [19], even though the transfer occurs via a different mechanism (TNTs vs. EVs, respectively). Thus, an increase in intracellular Ca^{2+} might be a general mechanism priming mitochondria for transfer. However, it is unclear how CD38 enzymatic activity is initiated to raise cytosolic Ca^{2+} levels and further promote mitochondrial transfer. It is possible that an increase in extracellular NAD⁺, the substrate of CD38, induced by changes in the cellular redox state could play a role [52].

Interestingly, the presence of gap junction (GJ) proteins, especially connexin 43 [53], in TNTs has been confirmed [54]. Connexins are important for Ca^{2+} propagation between neighboring cells via TNTs [48,55,56]. Similarities in the composition of GJ and TNTs have also been pointed out [40]. In spite of this, GJ have been functionally distinguished from TNTs [55]. While GJ perform short-range cell-to-cell interactions and allow the transfer of molecules up to 1.2 kDa only [57,58], TNTs mediate long-range cell-to-cell interactions and allow the transfer of significantly bigger cargos [59,60]. More research will be needed to fully understand the contribution of GJ proteins to TNT formation and mitochondrial transfer.

4. Mitochondrial Transfer in Solid Cancers

The current knowledge on mitochondrial transfer in solid cancers is limited, and the results of various studies are often difficult to compare due to the use of different experimental systems (Table 1). Cells of mesenchymal origin or fibroblasts are the most commonly used mitochondria donors [18,21,36]. However, the tumor tissue is a complex environment composed of many different cell types, and competition between cells could have a significant effect on mitochondrial transfer [61]. Indeed, in the co-culture of BMSCs, endothelial cells, and MCF7 cells, the formation of TNTs between the three cell types was observed, but mitochondria were sent only from endothelial cells to MCF7 cells [21]. Recently, TNT-mediated mitochondrial transfer was also observed between natural killer T cells and breast cancer cells [62]. These studies indicate that the ability to donate mitochondria might be affected by the presence of a particular cell type in the tumor microenvironment. Therefore, results of mitochondrial transfer experiments using cells usually not present in the solid tumor microenvironment (e.g., BMSCs or umbilical cord Wharton's jelly cells) should be carefully interpreted. Nevertheless, the current data still provide interesting views of the general mechanisms of mitochondria shuttling.

Table 1. Mitochondrial transfer studies.

Donor Cells	Recipient Cells	Mechanism of Transport	Triggers	Cellular Effect	Reference
NON-TUMOR CELLS					
cardio-myocytes	cardio-fibroblasts	TNTs	ND	Transfer in both directions	[56]
MSCs	vascular smooth muscle cells	TNTs	ND	Stimulation of MSCs proliferation	[28]
BMSCs	alveolar epithelium	microvesicles	LPS-induced lung injury	Protection against acute lung injury	[29]
MSCs	HUVEC	TNTs	Hypoxia	Rescue of injured endothelial cells	[26]
MSCs	Epithelial cells	TNTs	Miro1 overexpression	ND	[45]
iPSC-MSCs	epithelial cells	TNTs	Cigarette smoke	Repair of damaged cells	[27]
PC12 cells	PC12 cells	TNTs	Damaged mitochondria in receiver cells	Rescue from apoptosis	[25]
astrocytes	neurons	microvesicles	Damage by stroke	Neuroprotection/recovery	[19]
MSCs	corneal epithelial cells	TNTs	OXPHOS inhibition	Protection from oxidative damage	[30]
BM-MSCs	macrophage	TNTs	Acute respiratory distress syndrome	Enhanced phagocytosis	[31]
iPSC-MSCs/BM-MSCs	cardio-myocytes	TNTs	Anthracycline	Increased mitochondrial transfer	[44]
BMSCs	hematopoietic stem cells	not specified	Bacterial infection-induced ROS	Granulocytes activation	[32]

Table 1. Cont.

Donor Cells	Recipient Cells	Mechanism of Transport	Triggers	Cellular Effect	Reference
SOLID TUMORS					
BMSCs	A549 cells	not specified	Non-functional mitochondria	Rescue of aerobic respiration	[18]
BMSCs	143B cells	not specified	Restrictive media	Rescue of mitochondria functions	[35]
MSCs/ epithelial cells	ovarian and breast cancer cells	TNTs	ND	Specific selection of donor cells	[21]
MSCs	lung adeno-carcinoma cells	TNTs	Miro1 increased mitochondrial donor capacity	ND	[45]
Wharton's jelly-derived MSCs	143B	not specified	Absence of mitochondria	Rescue of mitochondria functions	[36]
mouse tissue	melanoma cells	not specified	Absence of mitochondria	Rescue of mitochondria functions and tumor formation	[24]
Prostate cancer-associated fibroblasts	prostate cancer cell	TNTs	ND	Enhanced lactate metabolism and mitochondria motility	[63]
NKT cells	breast cancer cells	TNTs	ND	ND	[62]
HEMATOLOGICAL TUMORS					
BMSCs	AML	endocytosis	Chemotherapy agents	Increased viability	[37]
BMSCs	AML	TNTs	NOX2-derived ROS	ND	[33]
BMSCs	AML	TNTs	ND	ND	[38]
BMSCs	T-ALL	TNTs	ND	Chemoresistance	[64]
MSCs	ALL	TNTs	ROS	rescue from chemotheraphy	[22]
BMSCs	MM	TNTs	ND	Metabolic switch	[23]

ND: not defined; iPSC: induced pluripotent stem cell; BM-MSCs: bone marrow mesenchymal stem cells; NKT: natural killer T cell; AML: acute myeloid leukemia; T-ALL: T cell acute lymphoblastic leukemia; ALL: acute lymphoblastic leukemia; MM: multiple myeloma; TNTs: tunneling nanotubes; MSCs: mesenchymal stem cells; BMSCs: bone marrow stromal cells; OXPHOS: oxidative phosphorylation; ROS: reactive oxygen species.

Investigations of the mechanism of intercellular mitochondrial transfer in solid tumors point to TNTs as the main delivery route [21,45,63]. The very first mitochondrial transfer was seen between mesenchymal and lung cancer cells with severely damaged or completely missing mitochondria [18]. To promote mitochondrial transfer, many studies used inhibitors such as rotenone to block the electron transport in the respiratory chain [23,33,37,45,65]. Thus, the OXPHOS status in the recipient cells seems to be a crucial factor mediating mitochondrial transfer. However, no mitochondrial transfer occurred between BMSCs and osteosarcoma cells with pathogenic mutations in mtDNA, which encodes critical components of the OXPHOS system [35]. Moreover, BMSCs were shown to donate mitochondria to ovarian and breast cancer cells [21], lung adenocarcinoma cells [45], and prostate cancer cells [63] with no apparent mitochondrial damage. This suggests that not only the state of mitochondria but also specific metabolic requirements could play a role in promoting mitochondrial transfer.

5. Mitochondrial Transfer in Hematological Malignancies

The tumor microenvironment is critical for progression and drug resistance also in hematological cancers [11,59,60]. Acquiring new mitochondria in the bone marrow niche was recently suggested as a way by which leukemic cells can achieve drug resistance [22,23,37]. Up to date, mitochondrial transfer was observed in several types of hematological malignancies, where it seems to have a pro-tumor function [32,33,61].

6. Mitochondrial Transfer in Acute Lymphoblastic Leukemia

The cross-talk between acute lymphoblastic leukemia (ALL) cells and their niche proved that mitochondria are delivered via TNTs from MSCs to primary B-cell precursor ALL cells [22]. The presence of TNTs facilitated the signaling from ALL cells towards MSCs, affecting the release of cytokines and chemokines in the microenvironment, supporting the survival and chemoresistance of ALL cells [34]. In addition to B-cell ALL, transport of mitochondria from MSCs was later shown in T-cell ALL (T-ALL), where mitochondrial transfer was mediated by T-ALL cell/MSC adhesion and occurred through TNTs. However, in contrast to B-ALL cells, mitochondria were exported from malignant T-ALL cells to the surrounding MSCs, probably due to the preferential use of glycolysis in T-ALL cells [64]. This example provides a unique model that can help to uncover the signals and mechanisms driving the transfer directionality. Moreover, it would be interesting to see whether T-ALL cells could donate mitochondria to other cell types and whether the increase in mitochondria number in MSCs would directly support the tumoral properties of T-ALL cells.

7. Mitochondrial Transfer in Acute Myeloid Leukemia

Acute myeloid leukemia (AML) is a typical hematological malignancy highly dependent on OXPHOS [66]. Not surprisingly, AML cells are more prone to receive new mitochondria as compared to healthy CD34+ hematopoietic stem/progenitors or lymphoid CD3+ cells [37]. When co-cultured with human BMSCs, AML cells can gain additional mitochondria in a TNT-dependent process [33]. However, in other study, endocytic inhibitors blocked the mitochondria exchange between murine MS-5 BMSCs and human AML cells [37], suggesting a TNT-independent delivery.

Commonly used chemotherapeutics such as cytarabine [67], etoposide [68], and doxorubicin [69] are factors that promote mitochondrial uptake by AML cells [70]. Consequently, the treatment could have a pro-tumor effect by stimulating oxidative metabolism in resistant AML clones [12]. The surface molecule CD38 is another clinically relevant target in AML, critical for the transport of mitochondria from BMSCs to AML cells [71]. Daratumumab, a monoclonal anti-CD38 antibody approved for the treatment of multiple myeloma (MM) [72,73], was shown to block the delivery of mitochondria to AML cells under both in vitro and in vivo conditions, decrease the oxygen consumption rate (OCR), and inhibit the growth of leukemic cells [74,75]. These studies suggest a novel, previously unexpected anti-tumor mechanism of anti-CD38 therapy.

8. Mitochondrial Transfer in Multiple Myeloma

Aberrant myeloma cells reside in the hypoxic environment of the bone marrow [76]. Unexpectedly, primary multiple myeloma (MM) cells isolated from patients' biopsies were shown to have a higher basal OCR compared to long-term in vitro cultured MM cell lines [23]. Similarly, when established MM cell lines were injected into a mouse or co-cultured with BMSCs, their OCR and ATP production significantly increased [23]. Moreover, the presence of BMSCs enhanced mitochondrial metabolism and drug resistance in MM cells [23]. This suggests that the bone marrow microenvironment might stimulate aerobic respiration in MM cells. A deeper investigation of the responsible mechanism indicated the presence of TNT-mediated mitochondrial transfer from BMSCs to MM cells, and ROS-inducing compounds, including commonly used proteasome inhibitors, significantly potentiated this process [23,77].

CD38, a crucial player in mitochondrial transfer, is currently one of the most attractive molecules for targeted therapy in MM patients [74,78–80]. Treatment with an anti-CD38 antibody or genetic deletion of CD38 were shown to inhibit mitochondrial transfer from BMSCs to MM cells and induce tumor shrinkage in xenografts models [23]. Lower mitochondrial activity, particularly a drop in OXPHOS, was previously associated with increased sensitivity of MM cells to proteasome inhibitors [77]. In line with these observations are clinical data indicating high efficacy of a combinatory therapy using an anti-CD38 antibody and proteasome inhibitors [81]. On the other hand, proteasome inhibitors were shown to downregulate the expression of vascular cell adhesion molecule 1 (VCAM-1) on BMSCs [82], a major ligand for VLA-4 on MM cells, and thus impede the binding of BMSCs and MMs [83], that is required for efficient mitochondrial transfer.

9. Conclusions

The direct transfer of mitochondria from one cell to another has emerged as a thrilling mechanism, whose potential targeting offers great opportunities for both cancer therapy and tissue regeneration. The fact that mitochondrial transfer seems to be executed in a similar way in both solid and hematological cancers further multiplies the importance of this process. It also underlines the significance of tumor microenvironment and cellular plasticity in cancer progression and drug resistance. Furthermore, the involvement of mitochondrial transfer may offer an explanation for the yet unclear mechanisms of action of certain anti-cancer drugs. Although the entire signaling machinery driving mitochondrial transfer is still unknown, the discovery of key molecular players such as Miro1, connexin 43, and CD38 has already opened the doors for possible therapeutic targeting. Future research of the molecular processes governing mitochondria shuttling in both normal and pathological settings will likely bring many exciting discoveries and provide new therapeutic possibilities to improve tissue regeneration and cancer therapy.

Author Contributions: H.S. and M.S. wrote the original draft and designed the figures. M.T. prepared the figures. T.J.; M.H.; T.S.; A.K.-K., J.R.B. and R.H. reviewed and edited the manuscript. All authors have read and agreed to the published version of the manuscript.

Funding: This work was supported by The Czech Science Foundation (GA CR 19-25354Y), Institutional Development Plan of University of Ostrava (project no. IRP03_2018-2020), ERDF-Project ENOCH (No. CZ.02.1.01/0.0/0.0/16_019/0000868), and New Directions of Biomedical Research in the Ostrava Region (No. CZ.02.1.01/0.0/0.0/18_069/0010060), SGS03/LF/2019-2020, SGS03/PrF/2019-2020.

Conflicts of Interest: The authors declare no conflict of interest. The funders had no role in the design of the study; in the collection, analyses, or interpretation of data; in the writing of the manuscript, or in the decision to publish the results.

References

1. Warburg, O. On the Origin of Cancer Cells. *Am. Assoc. Adv. Sci.* **1956**, *123*, 309–314. [CrossRef] [PubMed]
2. Potter, M.; Newport, E.; Morten, K.J. The Warburg effect: 80 years on. *Biochem. Soc. Trans.* **2016**, *44*, 1499–1505. [CrossRef] [PubMed]
3. Moreno-Sanchez, R.; Rodriguez-Enriquez, S.; Saavedra, E.; Marin-Hernandez, A.; Gallardo-Perez, J.C. The bioenergetics of cancer: Is glycolysis the main ATP supplier in all tumor cells? *Biofactors* **2009**, *35*, 209–225. [CrossRef] [PubMed]
4. Michelakis, E.D.; Webster, L.; Mackey, J.R. Dichloroacetate (DCA) as a potential metabolic-targeting therapy for cancer. *Br. J. Cancer* **2008**, *99*, 989–994. [CrossRef]
5. Gatenby, R.A.; Gillies, R.J. Why do cancers have high aerobic glycolysis? *Nat. Rev. Cancer* **2004**, *4*, 891–899. [CrossRef]
6. Tsvetkov, P.; Detappe, A.; Cai, K.; Keys, H.R.; Brune, Z.; Ying, W.; Thiru, P.; Reidy, M.; Kugener, G.; Rossen, J.; et al. Mitochondrial metabolism promotes adaptation to proteotoxic stress. *Nat. Chem. Biol.* **2019**, *15*, 681–689. [CrossRef]
7. Kuntz, E.M.; Baquero, P.; Michie, A.M.; Dunn, K.; Tardito, S.; Holyoake, T.L.; Helgason, G.V.; Gottlieb, E. Targeting mitochondrial oxidative phosphorylation eradicates therapy-resistant chronic myeloid leukemia stem cells. *Nat. Med.* **2017**, *23*, 1234–1240. [CrossRef]
8. Moreno-Sanchez, R.; Rodriguez-Enriquez, S.; Marin-Hernandez, A.; Saavedra, E. Energy metabolism in tumor cells. *FEBS J.* **2007**, *274*, 1393–1418. [CrossRef]
9. Ashton, T.M.; McKenna, W.G.; Kunz-Schughart, L.A.; Higgins, G.S. Oxidative Phosphorylation as an Emerging Target in Cancer Therapy. *Clin. Cancer Res.* **2018**, *24*, 2482–2491. [CrossRef]

10. Song, I.S.; Kim, H.K.; Lee, S.R.; Jeong, S.H.; Kim, N.; Ko, K.S.; Rhee, B.D.; Han, J. Mitochondrial modulation decreases the bortezomib-resistance in multiple myeloma cells. *Int. J. Cancer* **2013**, *133*, 1357–1367. [CrossRef]
11. Chauncey, T.R. Drug resistance mechanisms in acute leukemia. *Curr. Opin. Oncol.* **2001**, *13*, 21–26. [CrossRef] [PubMed]
12. Zhan, J.; Gu, Y.; Chen, B. Mechanisms of drug resistance in acute myeloid leukemia. *OncoTargets Ther.* **2019**, *12*, 1937–1945. [CrossRef] [PubMed]
13. Roh, J.S.; Sohn, D.H. Damage-associated molecular patterns in inflammatory diseases. *Immune Netw.* **2018**, *18*, 1–14. [CrossRef]
14. Rubartelli, A.; Lotze, M.T. Inside, outside, upside down: Damage-associated molecular-pattern molecules (DAMPs) and redox. *Trends Immunol.* **2007**, *28*, 429–436. [CrossRef]
15. Zhang, Q.; Raoof, M.; Chen, Y.; Sumi, Y.; Sursal, T.; Junger, W.; Brohi, K.; Itagaki, K.; Hauser, C.J. Circulating mitochondrial DAMPs cause inflammatory responses to injury. *Nature* **2010**, *464*, 104–107. [CrossRef] [PubMed]
16. Hernandez, C.; Huebener, P.; Schwabe, R. Damage-associated molecular patterns in cancer: A double edged sword. *Oncogene* **2016**, *35*, 5931–5941. [CrossRef] [PubMed]
17. Krysko, O.; Aaes, T.L.; Bachert, C.; Vandenabeele, P.; Krysko, D.V. Many faces of DAMPs in cancer therapy. *Cell Death Dis.* **2013**, *4*, e631. [CrossRef]
18. Spees, J.L.; Olson, S.D.; Whitney, M.J.; Prockop, D.J. Mitochondrial transfer between cells can rescue aerobic respiration. *Proc. Natl. Acad. Sci. USA* **2006**, *103*, 1283–1288. [CrossRef]
19. Hayakawa, K.; Esposito, E.; Wang, X.; Terasaki, Y.; Liu, Y.; Xing, C.; Ji, X.; Lo, E.H. Transfer of mitochondria from astrocytes to neurons after stroke. *Nature* **2016**, *535*, 551–555. [CrossRef]
20. Lu, J.; Zheng, X.; Li, F.; Yu, Y.; Chen, Z.; Liu, Z.; Xu, H.; Yang, W. Tunneling nanotubes promote intercellular mitochondria transfer followed by increased invasiveness in bladder cancer cells. *Oncotarget* **2017**, *8*, 15539–15552. [CrossRef]
21. Pasquier, J.; Guerrouahen, B.S.; Al Thawadi, H.; Ghiabi, P.; Maleki, M.; Abu-Kaoud, N.; Jacob, A.; Mirshahi, M.; Galas, L.; Rafii, S.; et al. Preferential transfer of mitochondria from endothelial to cancer cells through tunneling nanotubes modulates chemoresistance. *J. Transl. Med.* **2013**, *11*, 1–14. [CrossRef] [PubMed]
22. Burt, R.; Dey, A.; Aref, S.; Aguiar, M.; Akarca, A.; Bailey, K.; Day, W.; Hooper, S.; Kirkwood, A.; Kirschner, K.; et al. Activated stromal cells transfer mitochondria to rescue acute lymphoblastic leukemia cells from oxidative stress. *Blood* **2019**, *134*, 1415–1429. [CrossRef] [PubMed]
23. Marlein, C.R.; Piddock, R.E.; Mistry, J.J.; Zaitseva, L.; Hellmich, C.; Horton, R.H.; Zhou, Z.; Auger, M.J.; Bowles, K.M.; Rushworth, S.A. CD38-driven mitochondrial trafficking promotes bioenergetic plasticity in multiple myeloma. *Cancer Res.* **2019**, *79*, 2285–2297. [CrossRef] [PubMed]
24. Dong, L.F.; Kovarova, J.; Bajzikova, M.; Bezawork-Geleta, A.; Svec, D.; Endaya, B.; Sachaphibulkij, K.; Coelho, A.R.; Sebkova, N.; Ruzickova, A.; et al. Horizontal transfer of whole mitochondria restores tumorigenic potential in mitochondrial DNA-deficient cancer cells. *eLife* **2017**, *6*, e22187. [CrossRef]
25. Wang, X.; Gerdes, H.H. Transfer of mitochondria via tunneling nanotubes rescues apoptotic PC12 cells. *Cell Death Differ.* **2015**, *22*, 1181–1191. [CrossRef]
26. Liu, K.; Ji, K.; Guo, L.; Wu, W.; Lu, H.; Shan, P.; Yan, C. Mesenchymal stem cells rescue injured endothelial cells in an in vitro ischemia-reperfusion model via tunneling nanotube like structure-mediated mitochondrial transfer. *Microvasc. Res.* **2014**, *92*, 10–18. [CrossRef]
27. Li, X.; Zhang, Y.; Yeung, S.C.; Liang, Y.; Liang, X.; Ding, Y.; Ip, M.S.M.; Tse, H.F.; Mak, J.C.W.; Lian, Q. Mitochondrial transfer of induced pluripotent stem cell-derived mesenchymal stem cells to airway epithelial cells attenuates cigarette smoke-induced damage. *Am. J. Respir. Cell Mol. Biol.* **2014**, *51*, 455–465. [CrossRef]
28. Vallabhaneni, K.C.; Haller, H.; Dumler, I. Vascular smooth muscle cells initiate proliferation of mesenchymal stem cells by mitochondrial transfer via tunneling nanotubes. *Stem Cells Dev.* **2012**, *21*, 3104–3113. [CrossRef]
29. Islam, M.N.; Das, S.R.; Emin, M.T.; Wei, M.; Sun, L.; Westphalen, K.; Rowlands, D.J.; Quadri, S.K.; Bhattacharya, S.; Bhattacharya, J. Mitochondrial transfer from bone-marrow-derived stromal cells to pulmonary alveoli protects against acute lung injury. *Nat. Med.* **2012**, *18*, 759–765. [CrossRef]
30. Jiang, D.; Gao, F.; Zhang, Y.; Wong, D.S.H.; Li, Q.; Tse, H.F.; Xu, G.; Yu, Z.; Lian, Q. Mitochondrial transfer of mesenchymal stem cells effectively protects corneal epithelial cells from mitochondrial damage. *Cell Death Dis.* **2016**, *7*, e2467. [CrossRef]

31. Jackson, M.V.; Morrison, T.J.; Doherty, D.F.; McAuley, D.F.; Matthay, M.A.; Kissenpfennig, A.; O'Kane, C.M.; Krasnodembskaya, A.D. Mitochondrial Transfer via Tunneling Nanotubes is an Important Mechanism by Which Mesenchymal Stem Cells Enhance Macrophage Phagocytosis in the in vitro and in vivo Models of ARDS. *Stem Cells* **2016**, *34*, 2210–2223. [CrossRef] [PubMed]
32. Mistry, J.J.; Marlein, C.R.; Moore, J.A.; Hellmich, C.; Wojtowicz, E.E.; Smith, J.G.W.; Macaulay, I.; Sun, Y.; Morfakis, A.; Patterson, A.; et al. ROS-mediated PI3K activation drives mitochondrial transfer from stromal cells to hematopoietic stem cells in response to infection. *Proc. Natl. Acad. Sci. USA* **2019**, *116*, 24610–24619. [CrossRef] [PubMed]
33. Marlein, C.R.; Zaitseva, L.; Piddock, R.E.; Robinson, S.D.; Edwards, D.R.; Shafat, M.S.; Zhou, Z.; Lawes, M.; Bowles, K.M.; Rushworth, S.A. NADPH oxidase-2 derived superoxide drives mitochondrial transfer from bone marrow stromal cells to leukemic blasts. *Blood* **2017**, *130*, 1649–1660. [CrossRef] [PubMed]
34. Polak, R.; Rooij, B.D.; Pieters, R.; Boer, M.L. Den B-cell precursor acute lymphoblastic leukemia cells use tunneling nanotubes to orchestrate their microenvironment. *Blood* **2015**, *126*, 2404–2414. [CrossRef] [PubMed]
35. Cho, Y.M.; Kim, J.H.; Kim, M.; Park, S.J.; Koh, S.H.; Ahn, H.S.; Kang, G.H.; Lee, J.-B.; Park, K.S.; Lee, H.K. Mesenchymal stem cells transfer mitochondria to the cells with virtually no mitochondrial function but not with pathogenic mtDNA mutations. *PLoS ONE* **2012**, *7*, e32778. [CrossRef] [PubMed]
36. Lin, H.; Liou, C.; Chen, S.; Hsu, T.; Chuang, J.; Wang, P.; Huang, S.; Tiao, M.; Chen, J.; Lin, T.; et al. Mitochondrial transfer from Wharton's jelly-derived mesenchymal stem cells to mitochondria-defective cells recaptures impaired mitochondrial function. *Mitochondrion* **2015**, *22*, 31–34. [CrossRef]
37. Moschoi, R.; Imbert, V.; Nebout, M.; Chiche, J.; Mary, D.; Prebet, T.; Saland, E.; Castellano, R.; Pouyet, L.; Collette, Y.; et al. Protective mitochondrial transfer from bone marrow stromal cells to acute myeloid leukemic cells during chemotherapy. *Blood* **2016**, *128*, 253–264. [CrossRef]
38. Marlein, C.R.; Zaitseva, L.; Piddok, R.; Schafat, M.; Collins, A.; Bowles, K.; Rushworth, S. PGC1α Driven Mitochondrial Biogenesis within the Bone Marrow Stromal Cells of the Acute Myeloid Leukemia Micro-Environment Is a Pre-Requisite for Mitochondrial Transfer to Leukemic Blasts. *Blood* **2017**, *130* (Suppl. 1), 3927.
39. Torralba, D.; Baixauli, F.; Sánchez-Madrid, F. Mitochondria know no boundaries: Mechanisms and functions of intercellular mitochondrial transfer. *Front. Cell Dev. Biol.* **2016**, *4*, 107. [CrossRef]
40. Rustom, A.; Saffrich, R.; Markovic, I.; Walther, P.; Gerdes, H.H. Nanotubular Highways for Intercellular Organelle Transport. *Science* **2004**, *303*, 1007–1010. [CrossRef]
41. Schapman, D.; Lebon, A.; Monterroso, B.; Bellenger, M.; Foll, F.L.; Pasquier, J.; Vaudry, H.; Vaudry, D.; Galas, L. Structural and functional analysis of tunneling nanotubes (TnTs) using g CW STED and g confocal approaches. *Biol. Cell* **2015**, *107*, 419–425. [CrossRef]
42. Gousset, K.; Marzo, L.; Commere, P.; Zurzolo, C. Myo10 is a key regulator of TNT formation in neuronal cells. *J. Cell Sci.* **2013**, *126*, 4424–4435. [CrossRef] [PubMed]
43. Tardivel, M.; Bégard, S.; Bousset, L.; Dujardin, S.; Coens, A.; Melki, R. Tunneling nanotube (TNT)-mediated neuron-to neuron transfer of pathological Tau protein assemblies. *Acta Neuropathol. Commun.* **2016**, *4*, 117. [CrossRef] [PubMed]
44. Zhang, Y.; Yu, Z.; Jiang, D.; Liang, X.; Liao, S.; Zhang, Z.; Yue, W.; Li, X.; Chiu, S.M.; Chai, Y.H.; et al. iPSC-MSCs with High Intrinsic MIRO1 and Sensitivity to TNF-α Yield Efficacious Mitochondrial Transfer to Rescue Anthracycline-Induced Cardiomyopathy. *Stem Cell Rep.* **2016**, *7*, 749–763. [CrossRef]
45. Ahmad, T.; Mukherjee, S.; Pattnaik, B.; Kumar, M.; Singh, S.; Rehman, R.; Tiwari, B.K.; Jha, K.A.; Barhanpurkar, A.P.; Wani, M.R.; et al. Miro1 regulates intercellular mitochondrial transport & enhances mesenchymal stem cell rescue efficacy. *EMBO J.* **2014**, *33*, 994–1010. [CrossRef]
46. López-Doménech, G.; Covill-Cooke, C.; Ivankovic, D.; Halff, E.F.; Sheehan, D.F.; Norkett, R.; Birsa, N.; Kittler, J.T. Miro proteins coordinate microtubule- and actin-dependent mitochondrial transport and distribution. *EMBO J.* **2018**, *37*, 321–336. [CrossRef]
47. Zhang, Y. Tunneling-nanotube. *Commun. Integr. Biol.* **2011**, *4*, 324–325. [CrossRef]
48. Hase, K.; Kimura, S.; Takatsu, H.; Ohmae, M.; Kawano, S.; Kitamura, H.; Ito, M.; Watarai, H.; Hazelett, C.; Yeaman, C.; et al. M-Sec promotes membrane nanotube formation by interacting with Ral and the exocyst complex. *Nat. Cell Biol.* **2009**, *12*, 1427–1432. [CrossRef]
49. Ohno, H.; Hase, K.; Kimura, S. M-Sec: Emerging secrets of tunneling nanotube formation. *Commun. Integr. Biol.* **2010**, *3*, 231–233. [CrossRef]

50. Aarhus, R.; Graeff, R.M.; Dickey, D.M.; Walseth, T.F.; Lee, H.C. ADP-ribosyl cyclase and CD38 catalyze the synthesis of a calcium-mobilizing metabolite from NADP. *J. Biol. Chem.* **1995**, *270*, 30327–30333. [CrossRef] [PubMed]
51. Lee, H.C. Physiologival functions of cyclic ADP-ribose and NAADP as calcium messangers. *Annu. Rev. Pharmacol. Toxicol.* **2001**, *41*, 317–345. [CrossRef] [PubMed]
52. Bruzzone, S.; Moreschi, I.; Guida, L.; Usai, C.; Zocchi, E.; De Flora, A. Extracellular NAD^+ regulates intracellular calcium levels and induces activation of human granulocytes. *Biochem. J.* **2006**, *393*, 697–704. [CrossRef]
53. Ariazi, J.; Benowitz, A.; De Biasi, V.; Den Boer, M.L.; Cherqui, S.; Cui, H.; Douillet, N.; Eugenin, E.A.; Favre, D.; Goodman, S.; et al. Tunneling Nanotubes and Gap Junctions—Their Role in Long-Range Intercellular Communication during Development, Health, and Disease Conditions. *Front. Mol. Neurosci.* **2017**, *10*, 333. [CrossRef] [PubMed]
54. Osswald, M.; Jung, E.; Sahm, F.; Solecki, G.; Venkataramani, V.; Blaes, J.; Weil, S.; Horstmann, H.; Wiestler, B.; Syed, M.; et al. Brain tumour cells interconnect to a functional and resistant network. *Nature* **2015**, *528*, 93–98. [CrossRef]
55. Wang, X.; Veruki, M.L.; Bukoreshtliev, N.V.; Hartveit, E.; Gerdes, H. Animal cells connected by nanotubes can be electrically coupled through interposed gap-junction channels. *Proc. Natl. Acad. Sci. USA* **2010**, *107*, 17194–17199. [CrossRef] [PubMed]
56. He, K.; Shi, X.; Zhang, X.; Dang, S.; Ma, X.; Liu, F.; Xu, M.; Lv, Z.; Han, D.; Fang, X.; et al. Long-distance intercellular connectivity between cardiomyocytes and cardiofibroblasts mediated by membrane nanotubes. *Cardiovasc. Res.* **2011**, *92*, 39–47. [CrossRef] [PubMed]
57. Eugenin, E.A. Role of Connexin/Pannexin containing channels in infectious diseases. *FEBS Lett.* **2014**, *588*, 1389–1395. [CrossRef] [PubMed]
58. Aasen, T. Connexins: Junctional and non-junctional modulators of proliferation. *Cell Tissue Res.* **2015**, *360*, 685–699. [CrossRef]
59. Gerdes, H.H.; Carvalho, R.N. Intercellular transfer mediated by tunneling nanotubes. *Curr. Opin. Cell Biol.* **2008**, *20*, 470–475. [CrossRef]
60. Gerdes, H.H.; Rustom, A.; Wang, X. Tunneling nanotubes, an emerging intercellular communication route in development. *Mech. Dev.* **2013**, *130*, 381–387. [CrossRef]
61. Whiteside, T. The tumor microenvironment and its role in promoting tumor growth. *Oncogene* **2008**, *27*, 5904–5912. [CrossRef] [PubMed]
62. Saha, T.; Dash, C.; Khiste, S.; Sengupta, S. A novel mechanism of immunosuppression via nanotube mediated mitochondrial trafficking between cancer cell and immune cell. *Cancer Res.* **2019**. [CrossRef]
63. Ippolito, L.; Morandi, A.; Taddei, M.L.; Parri, M.; Comito, G.; Iscaro, A.; Raspollini, M.R.; Magherini, F.; Rapizzi, E.; Masquelier, J.; et al. Cancer-associated fibroblasts promote prostate cancer malignancy via metabolic rewiring and mitochondrial transfer. *Oncogene* **2019**, *38*, 5339–5355. [CrossRef] [PubMed]
64. Wang, J.; Liu, X.; Qiu, Y.; Shi, Y.; Cai, J.; Wang, B.; Wei, X.; Ke, Q.; Sui, X.; Wang, Y.; et al. Cell adhesion-mediated mitochondria transfer contributes to mesenchymal stem cell-induced chemoresistance on T cell acute lymphoblastic leukemia cells. *J. Hematol. Oncol.* **2018**, *11*, 11. [CrossRef]
65. Poburko, D.; Santo-Domingo, J.; Demaurex, N. Dynamic regulation of the mitochondrial proton gradient during cytosolic calcium elevations. *J. Biol. Chem.* **2011**, *286*, 11672–11684. [CrossRef]
66. Basak, N.P.; Banerjee, S. Mitochondrial dependency in progression of acute myeloid leukemia. *Mitochondrion* **2015**, *21*, 41–48. [CrossRef]
67. Putten, W.V.; Sc, M.; Schouten, H.C.; Graux, C.; Ferrant, A.; Sonneveld, P.; Biemond, B.J.; Gratwohl, A.; Greef, G.E.D.; Verdonck, L.F.; et al. Cytarabine Dose for Acute Myeloid Leukemia. *N. Engl. J. Med.* **2011**, 1027–1036.
68. Greenberg, P.L.; Lee, S.J.; Advani, R.; Tallman, M.S.; Sikic, B.I.; Letendre, L.; Dugan, K.; Lum, B.; Chin, D.L.; Dewald, G.; et al. Mitoxantrone, Etoposide, and Cytarabine with or without Valspodar in Patients with Relapsed or Refractory Acute Myeloid Leukemia and High-Risk Myelodysplastic Syndrome: A Phase III Trial (E2995). *J. Clin. Oncol.* **2004**, *22*, 1078. [CrossRef]
69. Teuffel, O.; Leibundgut, K.; Lehrnbecher, T.; Alonzo, T.A.; Beyene, J.; Sung, L. Anthracyclines during induction therapy in acute myeloid leukaemia: A systematic review and meta-analysis. *Br. J. Haematol.* **2013**, *161*, 192–203. [CrossRef]

70. Hole, P.S.; Zabkiewicz, J.; Munje, C.; Newton, Z.; Pearn, L.; White, P.; Marquez, N.; Hills, R.K.; Burnett, A.K.; Tonks, A.; et al. Overproduction of NOX-derived ROS in AML promotes proliferation and is associated with defective oxidative stress signaling. *Blood* **2013**, *122*, 3322–3330. [CrossRef]
71. Naik, J.; Themeli, M.; de Jong-Korlaar, R.; Ruiter, R.W.J.; Poddighe, P.J.; Yuan, H.; de Bruijn, J.D.; Ossenkoppele, G.J.; Zweegman, S.; Smit, L.; et al. CD38 as a therapeutic target for adult acute myeloid leukemia and T-cell acute lymphoblastic leukemia Acute. *Haematologica* **2019**, *14*, 100–103. [CrossRef] [PubMed]
72. Abdallah, N.; Kumar, S.K. Daratumumab in untreated newly diagnosed multiple myeloma. *Ther. Adv. Hematol.* **2019**, *10*. [CrossRef]
73. Mateos, M.; Spencer, A.; Nooka, A.K.; Pour, L.; Weisel, K.; Cavo, M.; Laubach, J.P.; Cook, G. Daratumumab-based regimens are highly effective and well tolerated in relapsed or refractory multiple myeloma regardless of patient age: Subgroup analysis of the phase 3 CASTOR and POLLUX studies. *Haematologica* **2020**, *105*, 468–477. [CrossRef] [PubMed]
74. Mistry, J.; Hellmich, C.; Moore, J.A.; Marlein, C.; Pillinger, G.; Collings, A.; Bowles, K.; Rushworth, S. Daratumumab Inhibits AML Metabolic Capacity and Tumor Growth through Inhibition of CD38 Mediated Mitochondrial Transfer from Bone Marrow Stromal Cells to Blasts in the Leukemic Microenvironment. *Blood* **2019**. [CrossRef]
75. Farber, M.; Arnold, L.; Chen, Y.; Mollmann, M.; Duehrsen, U.; Hanoun, M. Inhibition of CD38 Shows Anti-Leukemic Activity in Acute Myeloid Leukemia. *Blood* **2018**, *132*, 1456. [CrossRef]
76. Saba, F.; Soleimani, M.; Abroun, S. New role of hypoxia in pathophysiology of multiple myeloma through miR-210. *EXCLI J.* **2018**, *17*, 647–662. [CrossRef]
77. Lipchick, B.; Fink, E.; Nikiforoc, M. Oxidative Stress and Proteasome Inhibitors in Multiple Myeloma. *Pharmacol. Res.* **2016**, *105*, 210–215. [CrossRef]
78. Krejcik, J.; Casneuf, T.; Nijhof, I.S.; Verbist, B.; Bald, J.; Plesner, T.; Syed, K.; Liu, K.; van de Donk, N.W.C.J.; Weiss, B.M.; et al. Daratumumab depletes CD38$^+$ immune regulatory cells, promotes T-cell expansion, and skews T-cell repertoire in multiple myeloma. *Blood* **2016**, *128*, 384–394. [CrossRef]
79. Moreno, A.L.; Perez, C.; Zabaleta, A.; Manrique, I.; Garate, S.; Jelinek, T.; Segura, V.; Moreno, C. The Mechanism of Action of The Anti-CD38 Monoclonal Antibody Isatuximab In Multiple Myeloma. *Clin. Cancer Res.* **2019**, *25*, 3176–3187. [CrossRef]
80. Martin, T.; Strickland, S.; Glenn, M.; Charpentier, E.; Guillemin, H.; Hsu, K.; Mikhael, J. Phase I trial of isatuximab monotherapy in the treatment of refractory multiple myeloma. *Blood Cancer J.* **2019**, *9*, 1–10. [CrossRef]
81. Spencer, A.; Lentzsch, S.; Weisel, K.; Avet-Loiseau, H.; Mark, T.M.; Spicka, I.; Masszi, T.; Lauri, B.; Levin, M.D.; Bosi, A.; et al. Daratumumab plus bortezomib and dexamethasone versus bortezomib and dexamethasone in relapsed or refractory multiple myeloma: Updated analysis of CASTOR. *Haematologica* **2018**, *103*, 2079–2087. [CrossRef] [PubMed]
82. Read, M.A.; Neish, A.S.; Luscinskas, F.W.; Palombella, V.J.; Yaniatis, T.; Collins, T. The Proteasome Pathway is Required for Cytokine-Induced Endothelial-Leukocyte Adhesion Molecule Expression. *Immunity* **1995**, *2*, 493–506. [CrossRef]
83. Chauhan, D.; Uchiyama, H.; Akbarali, Y.; Urashima, M.; Yamamoto, K.I.; Libermann, T.A.; Anderson, K.C. Multiple myeloma cell adhesion-induced interleukin-6 expression in bone marrow stromal cells involves activation of NF-κB. *Blood* **1996**, *87*, 1104–1112. [CrossRef] [PubMed]

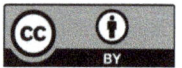

© 2020 by the authors. Licensee MDPI, Basel, Switzerland. This article is an open access article distributed under the terms and conditions of the Creative Commons Attribution (CC BY) license (http://creativecommons.org/licenses/by/4.0/).

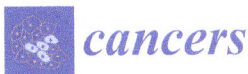

Review

Current Progresses and Challenges of Immunotherapy in Triple-Negative Breast Cancer

Karan Mediratta [1,2,3], Sara El-Sahli [1,2,3], Vanessa D'Costa [1,2,*] and Lisheng Wang [1,2,3,*]

1. Department of Biochemistry, Microbiology and Immunology, Faculty of Medicine, University of Ottawa, 451 Smyth Road, Ottawa, ON K1H 8M5, Canada; kmedi072@uottawa.ca (K.M.); selsa056@uottawa.ca (S.E.-S.)
2. Centre for Infection, Immunity and Inflammation, University of Ottawa, 451 Smyth Road, Ottawa, ON K1H 8M5, Canada
3. Ottawa Institute of Systems Biology, University of Ottawa, 451 Smyth Road, Ottawa, ON K1H 8M5, Canada
* Correspondence: vdcosta@uottawa.ca (V.D.); Lisheng.Wang@uottawa.ca (L.W.)

Received: 5 November 2020; Accepted: 24 November 2020; Published: 26 November 2020

Simple Summary: The breakthrough of immunotherapy in melanoma has generated a glimmer of hope for lethal triple negative breast cancer (TNBC). This review summarizes the recent advances, challenges and potential new approaches of immunotherapy in TNBC.

Abstract: With improved understanding of the immunogenicity of triple-negative breast cancer (TNBC), immunotherapy has emerged as a promising candidate to treat this lethal disease owing to the lack of specific targets and effective treatments. While immune checkpoint inhibition (ICI) has been effectively used in immunotherapy for several types of solid tumor, monotherapies targeting programmed death 1 (PD-1), its ligand PD-L1, or cytotoxic T lymphocyte-associated protein 4 (CTLA-4) have shown little efficacy for TNBC patients. Over the past few years, various therapeutic candidates have been reviewed, attempting to improve ICI efficacy on TNBC through combinatorial treatment. In this review, we describe the clinical limitations of ICI and illustrate candidates from an immunological, pharmacological, and metabolic perspective that may potentiate therapy to improve the outcomes of TNBC patients.

Keywords: triple-negative breast cancer; immunotherapy; immune checkpoint inhibitor; combination therapy; tumor microenvironment; cancer nanomedicine; tumor antigens; chimeric antigen receptor; cancer metabolism

---

1. Introduction

Breast cancer alone accounts for 30% of all female cancers and remains one of the leading causes of cancer-related deaths globally, with 626,679 deaths in 2018 alone [1,2]. Triple-negative breast cancer (TNBC) is the most refractory subtype, which accounts for 11.2% of new breast cancer cases, but disproportionately accounts for the majority of breast cancer-related deaths [3]. Chemotherapy remains the current mainstay treatment due to the lack of specific targets for TNBC. However, it is often associated with short-lived clinical responses [4], systemic toxicity [5] and enrichment of cancer stem cell (CSC) populations. CSCs are capable of self-renewal, differentiation, metastasis, and regeneration of a new tumor [6]. Moreover, CSCs possess an abundance of drug resistance mechanisms, including the expression of several ATP-binding cassette (ABC) transporters that contribute to the poor clinical outcomes associated with TNBC [7,8].

It is evident that effective treatment of TNBC would depend upon the elimination of CSC populations. In recent years, the emergence of immunotherapy (IT) has offered new perspectives in the treatment and management of TNBC. Despite the lack of targeted therapies for TNBC, recent studies suggest that TNBC is the most immunogenic breast cancer subtype [9–11]. In one study, TNBC was reported to have a higher expression of Programmed Death-Ligand 1 (PD-L1), an immune checkpoint molecule that contributes to immune evasion [12]. Through immunohistochemistry staining, TNBC tumors have been shown to exhibit higher numbers of intratumoral and stromal tumor-infiltrating lymphocytes (TILs) [13]. PD-L1 expression has been correlated with high levels of TILs, an association that has been considered as a favorable indicator for TNBC patients' prognosis [14,15]. Evaluating PD-L1 expression using immunohistochemistry assays such as VENTANA SP142 or Dako 22C3 has made it possible to identify patients who may benefit from immune checkpoint inhibition [16]. Other immune modulating receptors have also been identified as attractive targets for PD-L1$^-$ and/or TIL$^-$ tumors. Hallmarks of TNBC include dysregulated tumor vasculature, genomic instability, aberrant cell signaling, and deregulation of cellular energetics, each of which could be potential pharmacological targets for combination with immunotherapy. In this review, we discuss the progresses and challenges associated with the present modalities of immunotherapy with respect to TNBC and CSCs.

2. Immune Checkpoint Inhibition: Therapeutic Strategies

2.1. PD-1/PD-L1 Axis

Immune checkpoint inhibitors (ICIs) have been considered as viable candidates for the treatment of TNBC. Effector T-cells express the Programmed Death 1 (PD-1) cell surface receptor, which interacts with its ligand, PD-L1 (Figure 1). PD-L1 is normally expressed on the surfaces of dendritic cells and macrophages, and binding to PD-1 leads to the inhibition of cytotoxic T-cells [17]. By targeting tumors enriched with TILs that express PD-L1, T-cells within the tumor microenvironment (TME) can be activated [18]. Interestingly, higher rates of PD-L1 expression were found in TNBC patients than with other types of breast cancers [19]. Increased PD-L1 expression can occur via amplification of the PD-L1 gene at 9p24.1. While PD-L1 is normally amplified by 0.7% across most human cancers, this was elevated to 2.0% in TNBC and HER-2-positive breast cancers [20,21]. Sabatier et al. also demonstrated that higher PD-L1 expression resulted in a 50% pathological complete response (pCR), while normal PD-L1 expression resulted in a 21% pCR in response to neoadjuvant chemotherapy [22].

The anti-PD-L1 antibody Atezolizumab has been extensively studied and tested as first-line therapy in a phase I clinical trial (NCT01375842). Women with metastatic TNBC exhibited a median progression-free survival (PFS) of 4.0 months (95% CI, 1.6–10.1), a median overall survival (OS) of 17.6 months (95% CI, 10.2–N/A), and an incidence of treatment-related adverse events (trAEs) of 62% [23]. Contrarily, women who received Atezolizumab as second- or third-line therapy exhibited a median PFS of 1.8 months (95% CI, 1.4–2.3), a median OS of 7.3 months (95% CI, 6.1–10.8) and an incidence of trAEs of 43% [23]. The subsequent IMpassion130 phase III trial (NCT02425891) investigated whether Atezolizumab, combined with the chemotherapeutic agent nab-Paclitaxel, would generate improved clinical outcomes relative to chemotherapy alone. Blockade of PD-1/PD-L1 interactions in untreated metastatic TNBC patients significantly reduced tumor growth [24]. The median PFS prolongated to 7.2 months from 5.5 months (HR, 0.80; 95% CI, 0.69 to 0.92; $p = 0.002$) in the intention-to-treat population (with patients being randomized according to randomized treatment), and to 7.5 months from 5.0 months (HR, 0.62; 95% CI, 0.49 to 0.78; $p < 0.001$) among patients with PD-L1$^+$ tumors [24]. Furthermore, the median OS prolongated to 21.3 months from 17.6 months (HR, 0.84; 95% CI, 0.69 to 1.02; $p = 0.008$) in the intention-to-treat population, and to 25.0 months from 15.5 months (HR, 0.62; 95% CI, 0.45 to 0.86) among patients with PD-L1$^+$ tumors [24]. As such, Atezolizumab in combination with nab-Paclitaxel was FDA-approved for the treatment of locally advanced or metastatic PD-L1$^+$ TNBC in March 2019.

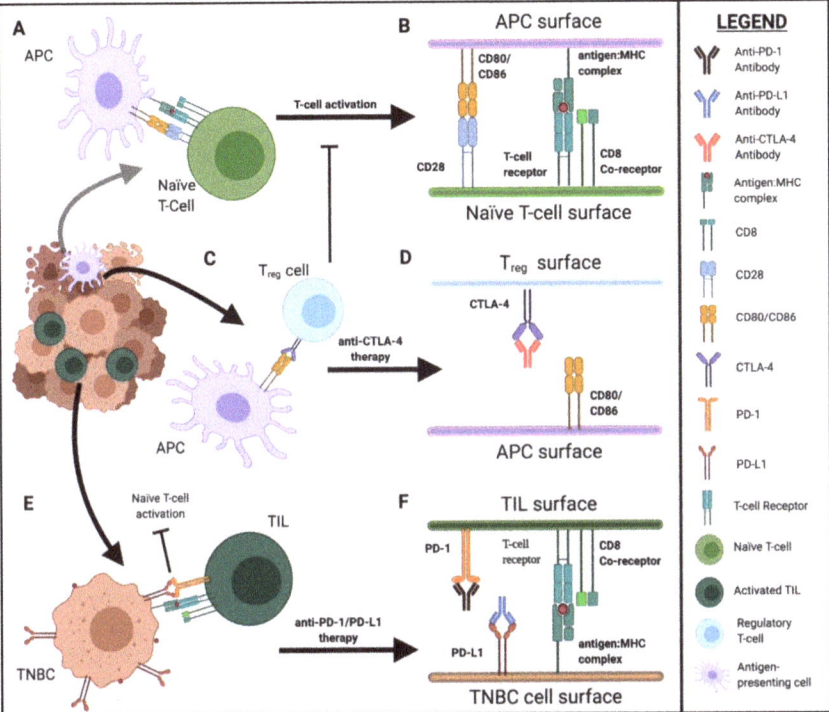

Figure 1. Possible mechanism of immune checkpoint inhibitors in triple-negative breast cancer (TNBC). Tumors consist of heterogenous cell populations including different types of immune infiltrating cells that undergo proliferation and apoptosis. (**A**) Tumor-infiltrating antigen-presenting cells (APCs) display tumor-associated antigens (TAAs) on their major histocompatibility complexes (MHC), which activate antigen-specific naïve T-cells. (**B**) Cluster of differentiation 80 (CD80) on the APC and cluster of differentiation 28 (CD28) are both co-signaling molecules necessary for T-cell activation and expansion. (**C**) CD80 molecules on tumor-infiltrating APCs preferentially bind to cytotoxic T lymphocyte protein-4 (CTLA-4), constitutively expressed on regulatory T cells (T_{reg}) that commonly recruit myeloid-derived suppressor cells (MDSCs) to the tumor microenvironment (TME) to inhibit T-cell activation. (**D**) Anti-CTLA-4 antibodies inhibit T_{reg} activation and enhance anti-tumor activity. (**E**) Tumor cells express programmed death ligand-1 (PD-L1) and tumor-infiltrating lymphocytes express its receptor, PD-1. The interaction between PD-1 and PD-L1 inactivates T-cell activation/expansion within the TME. (**F**) Anti-PD-1 or anti-PD-L1 antibodies prevent PD-1/PD-L1 engagement, thereby inhibiting the suppressive signals and promoting anti-tumor immunity. Figure created with BioRender.com.

Similarly, the anti-PD-1 antibody Pembrolizumab was assessed in the KEYNOTE-086 phase II trial (NCT02447003), administered as a monotherapy to cohorts of previously treated metastatic TNBC and untreated PD-L1+ metastatic TNBC [25]. The median PFS was 2.0 months (95% CI, 1.9 to 2.0) in the previously treated population and 2.1 months (95% CI, 2.0 to 2.2) for the patients with PD-L1+ tumors [25,26]. The median OS was 9.0 months (95% CI, 7.6 to 11.2) in the previously treated population and 18.0 months (95% CI, 12.9 to 23.0) for the patients with PD-L1+ tumors [25,26]. The incidence of trAEs was 60.6% in the previously treated population and 63.1% in the PD-L1+ population [25,26], comparable to anti-PD-L1 monotherapy. This study concluded that Pembrolizumab showed durable anti-tumor activity for patients with PD-L1+ metastatic TNBC and was followed by the KEYNOTE-335 phase III trial (NCT02819518). This study investigated whether Pembrolizumab, in combination with various chemotherapeutic agents, would provide improved clinical outcomes relative to chemotherapy with placebo. The results indicated that Pembrolizumab plus chemotherapy increased the median PFS from 5.6 months (95% CI, 5.3–7.5) to 9.7 months (95% CI, 7.6–11.3), relative to chemotherapy alone [27]. The objective response rate (ORR) increased from 40% (95% CI, 30%–50%, chemotherapy alone) to 53% (95% CI, 46–60) for the combinatorial treatment [27]. Fatal adverse events occurred in only 2.5% of patients receiving the combinatorial treatment, which was discontinued in 11% of patients due to trAEs [27]. As such, Pembrolizumab in combination with chemotherapy was granted accelerated FDA approval for patients with locally recurrent, unresectable, or metastatic TNBC in November 2020.

Conversely, several reports showed that anti-PD-1 or anti-PD-L1 antibodies did not exhibit better outcomes than chemotherapy in TNBC, while contributing to neurotoxicity [28,29]. Atezolizumab monotherapy demonstrated a low PFS of 1.9 months (95% CI, 1.4–2.5) and a high incidence of trAEs at 68% [23], leading to questions regarding its clinical efficacy. In the IMpassion130 trial, only a subset of patients with PD-L1$^+$ tumors benefited from the treatment compared to the intention-to-treat population (Table 1). Despite the importance of PD-L1 and TILs as predictive biomarkers, a clinical method for TIL assessment needs to be standardized, which may impact patient outcomes of ICIs [30]. Furthermore, the IMpassion130 trial failed to incorporate an Atezolizumab monotherapy arm, whereas the IMpower110 phase III clinical trial (NCT02409342) compared single-agent Atezolizumab to chemotherapy (Table 1). Preliminary results showed a modest increase in median OS from 14.1 months with chemotherapy to 17.5 months with Atezolizumab [31]. Results from the recent IMpassion131 phase III trial (NCT03125902) showed ineffectiveness in the combination of Atezolizumab and chemotherapy for the patients with metastatic TNBC. The median PFS increased insignificantly from 5.7 months (95% CI, 5.4–6.5) to 6.0 months (95% CI, 5.6–7.4), and the median OS increased slightly from 22.1 months (95% CI, 19.2–30.5) to 22.8 months (95% CI, 17.1–28.3) in the placebo plus Paclitaxel and Atezolizumab plus Paclitaxel treatment arms, respectively [32]. Another concern with the IMpassion130 trial is that patients previously treated with adjuvant chemotherapy and relapsed within 12 months were excluded from the trial. It is expected that this will be clarified in the IMpassion132 phase III trial (NCT03371017), which is studying an anti-PD-1 and chemotherapy combinatorial treatment [33]. With respect to Pembrolizumab, the KEYNOTE-119 phase III clinical trial compared single-agent Pembrolizumab to chemotherapy in metastatic TNBC patients (Table 1). The median PFS decreased from 3.3 months (95% CI, 2.7–4.0) with chemotherapy to 2.1 months (95% CI, 2.0–2.1) with Pembrolizumab monotherapy [34]. The median OS also decreased from 10.8 months (95% CI, 9.1–12.6) with chemotherapy to 9.9 months (95% CI, 8.3–11.4) with Pembrolizumab monotherapy, concluding that Pembrolizumab monotherapy did not provide clinical improvements relative to chemotherapy [34]. With conflicting trial results regarding the clinical efficacy of Pembrolizumab, further research is warranted. In addition, researchers have reported associations between ICI monotherapy and immune-mediated neurotoxicity due to potential molecular mimicry or hidden autoimmunity with neuronal antigens in the peripheral nervous system [29,35,36]. As such, improvements to PD-1/PD-L1 axis-associated immunotherapy in TNBC are needed.

Table 1. List of completed or ongoing clinical trials using PD-1/PD-L1 immune checkpoint inhibitors.

Trial (National Clinical Trial Identifier)	Phase	Condition	Interventions	Key Results	Reference
Atezolizumab Monotherapy (NCT01375842)	I	Locally advanced or metastatic solid tumors	(1) Atezolizumab (2) Placebo	Median PFS: 4.0 months for arm (1); 1.8 months for arm (2) Median OS: 17.6 months for arm (1); 7.3 months for arm (2) Incidence of trAEs: 62% for arm (1); 43% for arm (2)	[23]
IMpassion130 (NCT02425891)	III	Previously untreated metastatic TNBC	(1) Atezolizumab + Nab-Paclitaxel (2) Placebo + Nab-Paclitaxel	Median PFS: 7.2 months for arm (1); 5.5 months for arm (2) Median OS: 21.3 months for arm (1); 17.6 months for arm (2) Incidence of grade 3+ trAEs: 15.9% for arm (1); 8.2% for arm (2)	[24]
KEYNOTE-086 (NCT02447003)	II	Metastatic TNBC	(1) Pembrolizumab	Median PFS: 2.0 months for previously treated; 2.1 months for PD-L1$^+$ tumors Median OS: 9.0 months for previously treated; 18.0 months for PD-L1$^+$ tumors Incidence of trAEs: 60.6% for previously treated; 63.1% for PD-L1$^+$ tumors	[25,26]
KEYNOTE-335 (NCT02819518)	III	Previously untreated, locally recurrent, inoperable or metastatic TNBC	(1) Pembrolizumab + Chemotherapy (2) Placebo + Chemotherapy	Median PFS: 9.7 months for arm (1); 5.6 months for arm (2) ORR: 53% for arm (1); 40% for arm (2) Incidence of trAEs: 68.1% for arm (1); 66.9% for arm (2)	[27]
IMpower110 (NCT02409342)	III	Stage IV non-squamous or squamous non-small cell lung cancer	(1) Atezolizumab (2) (Carboplatin/Cisplatin) + (Pemetrexed/Gemcitabine)	Median OS: 17.5 months for arm (1); 14.1 months for arm (2) Incidence of trAEs: 60.5% (grade 3 +: 12.9%) for arm (1); 85.2% (grade 3 +: 44.1%) for arm (2)	[31]
IMpassion131 (NCT03125902)	III	Previously untreated, locally advanced or metastatic TNBC	(1) Atezolizumab + Paclitaxel (2) Placebo + Paclitaxel	Median PFS: 6.0 months for arm (1); 5.7 months for arm (2) Median OS: 22.8 months for arm (1); 22.1 months for arm (2)	[32]
KEYNOTE-119 (NCT02555657)	III	Metastatic TNBC	(1) Pembrolizumab (2) Chemotherapy	Median PFS: 2.1 months for arm (1); 3.3 months for arm (2) Median OS: 9.9 months for arm (1); 10.8 months for arm (2) Incidence of grade 3+ trAEs: 14% for arm (1); 36% for arm (2)	[34]

PFS: progression-free survival; OS: overall survival; ORR: objective response rate; trAEs: treatment-related adverse events.

2.2. CTLA-4 and Dual Checkpoint Inhibition

The cytotoxic T lymphocyte-associated protein 4 (CTLA-4) is an inhibitory receptor, constitutively expressed on regulatory T cells (T_{reg}) and upregulated on the surface of activated CD4$^+$ and CD8$^+$ T-cells [37,38]. CD-80/B7-1 and CD-86/B7-2 ligands expressed on antigen-presenting cells (APCs) can bind to CD-28 on T-cells to induce T-cell activation and cytokine secretion [39]. CTLA-4 competes with CD-28 to bind CD-80/B7-1 and CD-86/B7-2 ligands, and negatively regulates T-cell function [37–40]. CTLA-4 is essential for neutralizing potential naïve autoreactive T-cells in the secondary lymphoid organs [40]. The inhibition of CTLA-4 can prevent T-cell inhibition and enhance T-cell anti-tumor activity, making it an attractive target for antibody-based therapy (Figure 1). The anti-CTLA-4 antibody Ipilimumab, in combination with the anti-PD-1 antibody Nivolumab, has been FDA-approved for the treatment of melanoma, lung cancer, and renal cell carcinoma, among other cancers [41,42]. The CheckMate032 phase 1/2 trial (NCT01928394) showed modest improvements in ORR for non-small cell lung cancer, from 10% of patients receiving Nivolumab alone to 33% of patients receiving Nivolumab plus Ipilimumab in combination [43]. More recently, the CheckMate-9LA phase III trial

(NCT03215706) demonstrated the superior clinical effectiveness of Nivolumab and Ipilimumab in combination with chemotherapy for metastatic or recurrent non-small-cell lung cancer. Combinatorial treatment increased the median PFS from 5.0 months to 6.7 months, increased the median OS from 10.9 months to 15.6 months, and slightly increased the incidence of trAEs from 38% to 47% relative to chemotherapy alone [44].

Since anti-PD-1/PD-L1 monotherapy was shown to benefit only a subset of the population, additional clinical trials combining anti-CTLA-4 monotherapy have been performed in an effort to improve clinical outcomes but failed to do so. A randomized phase II trial (NCT02519322) testing the clinical efficacy of the Nivolumab as monotherapy in combination with the anti-CTLA-4 antibody Ipilimumab in patients with high-risk resectable melanoma was terminated early because of the high incidence of trAEs. Grade 3 trAEs were reported in 8% of patients in the Nivolumab monotherapy treatment arm and 73% of patients in the combinatorial treatment arm [45]. In a separate phase II clinical trial (NCT02536794), the anti-PD-1 antibody Durvalumab and anti-CTLA-4 antibody Tremelimumab were combined in a single treatment arm without comparison to monotherapy. The drugs were administered to estrogen receptor-positive (ER$^+$) breast cancer and TNBC patients. Preliminary data suggested that clinical benefit was derived in 71% of TNBC patients, but in none of the ER$^+$ breast cancer patients [46]. This trial was also discontinued due to ORRs not meeting the required criteria. The termination of both trials suggested that the risks associated with dual immune checkpoint inhibition may not exceed the benefits.

The use of anti-CTLA-4 antibodies in monotherapy and in combination with anti-PD-1/PD-L1 antibodies have been discredited, due to the lack of significant clinical response and high incidence of autoimmunity. Its ORR in combination with Nivolumab was modest relative to the results seen in the trial by inhibition of the PD-1/PD-L1 axis. Alternatively, anti-CTLA-4 antibodies may be complemented by the stimulator of interferon genes (STING) agonists that promote intratumoral T-cell infiltration and sensitize tumor cells to NK cell killing [47,48]. Harding et al. reported minimal tumor regression following anti-CTLA-4 therapy in B16 murine melanoma models with STING knockout [49]. However, CTLA-4 antibodies may lead to autoimmunity, due to its role in maintaining self-tolerance [50,51]. In a study by Tivol et al., CTLA-4 $^{-/-}$ mice demonstrated excessive proliferation of the lymph nodes, severely destructive myocarditis and pancreatitis, suggesting the role of CTLA-4 in deleting autoreactive T-cells in the periphery [52]. Consistent with this, a study by Gough et al. showed that polymorphisms within the human CTLA-4 gene are associated with autoimmune diseases [53]. This was also consistent with the CheckMate238 clinical trial (NCT02388906), in which grade 3 or 4 trAEs were reported among 45.9% of participants in the Ipilimumab group, followed by discontinued treatment for 42.6% of the patients [54,55]. Interestingly, the efficacy of immune checkpoint inhibition was found to depend on the composition of commensal bacteria. Introducing strains such as *Bacteroides fragilis* to germ-free or antibiotic-treated mice helped to overcome the poor response of CTLA-4 blockades and further induced polarization of T helper cell 1 (T$_{H1}$) [56]. As such, anti-CTLA-4 alone has not been considered as a viable front-line treatment option for TNBC to date.

2.3. Next Generation Immune Modulatory Targets

Many immune checkpoint molecules beyond PD-1/PD-L1 and CTLA-4 are currently under clinical investigation to identify additional drug targets for PD-L1$^-$ and TIL$^-$ patients or to enhance ICI monotherapy. The immunosuppressive protein sialic acid binding Ig-like lectin-15 (Siglec-15), normally expressed on myeloid cells, was shown to be upregulated in many human cancers [57]. With similar structural homology to PD-L1, Siglec-15 is targeted using the anti-Siglec-15 monoclonal antibody, NC318 [58]. In the phase I/II clinical trial (NCT03665285), NC318 was administered to patients with advanced or metastatic solid tumors, with results expected in 2021. T-cell Ig and ITIM domain (TIGIT) is another inhibitory receptor expressed on lymphocytes and upregulated upon activation [59]. Its ligands include CD112, CD113, and CD155, all of which are over-expressed in TNBC [60–62]. Interestingly, pre-clinical experiments on TIGIT$^{-/-}$ mice suggested higher safety and fewer trAEs than anti-PD1/PD-L1 or anti-CTLA-4 monotherapies [63]. Lymphocyte-activation gene 3 (LAG-3) and T-cell Ig and mucin domain-containing protein 3 (TIM-3) are also attractive immunosuppressive targets being actively investigated in breast cancer. Saleh et al. reported that the co-inhibition of PD-1 and PD-L1 further upregulated LAG-3 and TIM-3 in T-cells and T_{regs} when co-cultured with TNBC cells, but not with other breast cancer cell lines [64].

In contrast to co-inhibitory immune molecules, co-stimulatory molecules are equally attractive targets in immunotherapy. OX40 is a positive immune checkpoint molecule involved in T-cell proliferation following activation, and T_{reg} suppression [65]. Several clinical trials are investigating the efficacy of anti-OX40 antibodies in combination with ICI monotherapy for TNBC patients (NCT02528357, NCT03971409, NCT03241173). The inducible co-stimulatory receptor 4-1BB is expressed on activated T-cells and NK cells, and can be exploited to improve anti-tumor immunity [66,67]. However, the therapeutic value of 4-1BB in TNBC patients remains open to investigation. The glucocorticoid-induced TNFR-related (GITR) and inducible co-stimulator of T-cells (ICOS) are also attractive stimulatory targets. The ICOS monoclonal antibody, JTX-2011, was administered to TNBC patients in the phase I/II clinical trial (NCT02904226). Preliminary results reported a disease control rate of 25% with JTX-2011 monotherapy, and 29% in combination with Nivolumab (anti-PD-1) [68]. Notably, two grade 5 trAEs were observed among patients in the combinatorial treatment arm, potentially due to the simultaneous expression of ICOS on immunosuppressive T_{regs} [68]. In this regard, agonist antibodies in immunotherapy have been approached with caution and require additional research before implementation in the clinic.

3. Factors Affecting the Efficacy of Immune Checkpoint Inhibitors

Blockade of PD-1/PD-L1 and/or CTLA-4 has been demonstrated to be effective and durable in certain types of cancers. However, fewer than 10% of patients respond to single-agent treatments [69]. Co-administration of ICIs with chemotherapeutic agents, as described above, contributes to the enhanced immune priming [24,27,70]. Combinations with other therapies or factors may also increase efficacy, as described below.

3.1. Dysregulated Tumor Vasculature

Poor clinical outcomes associated with TNBC are partly attributed to the dysregulated angiogenesis that results in hypoxic conditions within the TME. As tumors expand over time, tumor cells within the tumor core become increasingly hypoxic, such that there is an upregulation of angiogenic growth factors associated with the expression of hypoxia-induced transcription factor (HIF-1) [71]. Angiogenic growth factors including vascular endothelial growth factor (VEGF), endothelial growth factor (EGF), and platelet-derived growth factor (PDGF) promote the migration of endothelial cells towards the tumor core, through which tumors acquire nutrients for growth and a route to metastasize into systemic circulation [71–73]. Under normal conditions, angiogenic growth factors are balanced by the metabolic demands of the surrounding tissue. However, the hypoxic conditions of the TME hijack this balance in favor of dysregulated angiogenesis [72,73].

Tumor-associated capillaries contribute to immunosuppression by reducing trafficking and activation of effector T-cells and restricting entry of cytotoxic drugs [74,75]. Tumor-associated endothelial cells may release interferon-γ (IFNγ) that upregulates PD-L1 expression to inhibit the anti-tumor activity of T-cells [76]. This is consistent with a study by Kammertoens et al., who showed that intratumoral injection of IFNγ caused rapid loss of tumor-associated vessels but also impeded anti-tumor activity of effector T-cells [77]. As IFNγ is mainly expressed by activated infiltrating T-cells, the IFNγ-mediated upregulation of PD-L1 can be exploited in a combinatorial therapy for non-responders to anti-PD-1 monotherapy [78]. Tian et al. reported an increase in pericyte coverage and a decrease in pulmonary metastasis (indicators of vasculature normalization) following immune checkpoint blockade in mice bearing TNBC 4T1 tumors [79,80].

To inhibit the growth and metastasis of TNBC and promote the anti-tumor activity of effector T-cells, a combination of immunotherapy with anti-angiogenic factors has been investigated. In the IMbrave150 phase III clinical trial (NCT03434379), the anti-PD-1 agent Atezolizumab was combined with anti-angiogenic agent Bevacizumab and compared with protein kinase inhibitor Sorafenib alone (Table 2). There was a clinically significant improvement in median PFS, which was 6.8 months (HR, 0.58; 95% CI, 5.7–8.3) in the Atezolizumab/Bevacizumab group and 4.3 months (HR, 0.59; 95% CI, 4.0–5.6) in the Sorafenib group [81]. Of note, grade 3 or 4 trAEs occurred in 56.5% of patients receiving Atezolizumab/Bevacizumab and 55.1% of patients receiving Sorafenib [81]. Furthermore, Huang et al. showed that lower doses of anti-VEGFR2 antibody improve tumor-associated vessel perfusion and reduce tumor hypoxia more effectively than the immunoglobulin-G (IgG) control and high-dose anti-VEGFR2 treatment groups [82]. This highlights the importance of further examining dosage and timing to optimize the combinatorial efficacy of anti-angiogenic and ICI treatments. The excessive use of anti-angiogenic agents may impede drug delivery and limit the infiltration of effector T-cells in the tumor [82,83]. Wu et al. proposed using angiopoietin-2 as a biomarker in addition to as a therapeutic target for predicting the clinical outcome of Bevacizumab monotherapy, due to its important role in treatment resistance [84]. Therefore, the combination of ICI with anti-angiogenesis therapy may represent a promising avenue for the future of TNBC treatment.

Table 2. List of completed or ongoing clinical trials using immune checkpoint inhibitors in combinatorial therapy.

Trial (National Clinical Trial Identifier)	Phase	Condition	Interventions	Key Results	Reference
IMbrave150 (NCT03434379)	III	Locally advanced or metastatic solid tumors	(1) Atezolizumab + Bevacizumab (2) Sorafenib	Median PFS: 6.8 months for arm (1); 4.3 months for arm (2) Median OS: 2 months: 67.2% for arm (1); 54.6% for arm (2) Incidence of grade 3+ trAEs: 56.5% for arm (1); 55.1% for arm (2)	[81]
(NCT02536469)	I	Advanced malignant solid tumors	(1) HuMax-IL-8	No objective tumor responses observed, 73% had stable disease at week 24 Serum IL-8 significantly reduced on day 3, relative to baseline ($p = 0.0004$) Incidence of trAEs: 33% (mostly grade 1)	[85]
MAGIC-8 (NCT03689699)	I/II	Hormone-sensitive prostate cancer	(1) Nivolumab (2) Nivolumab + BMS-986253	No preliminary data available, results expected in 2022	[86]
(NCT02754141)	I/II	Malignant solid tumors	(1) BMS-986179 (2) Nivolumab + BMS-986179	Incidence of trAEs: N/A for arm (1); 58% for arm (2) Incidence of grade 3 trAEs: N/A for arm (1); 15% for arm (2) Overall, both arms (1) and (2) are well-tolerated	[87]
(NCT01302405)	I	Advanced solid tumors	(1) PRI-724	Incidence of trAEs: 17% Incidence of grade 3+ trAEs: 11.1%PRI-724 has an acceptable toxicity profile	[88]
SYNERGY (NCT03616886)	I/II	Previously untreated, locally recurrent, inoperable or metastatic TNBC	(1) Paclitaxel + Carboplatin + Durvalumab + Oleclumab	No preliminary data available, results expected in 2023	[89]

PFS: progression-free survival; OS: overall survival; trAEs: treatment-related adverse events.

3.2. Interleukin-8 and CXCR1/CXCR2

Interleukin-8 (IL-8) is a chemokine responsible for the recruitment of neutrophils to areas of inflammation, infection, or injury [90]. IL-8 is secreted by macrophages, epithelial cells, airway smooth muscle cells, and endothelial cells [90,91]. IL-8 binds to CXCR1 and CXCR2 G-protein coupled receptors on granulocytes, monocytes, and endothelial cells [90–92]. Interestingly, breast cancer patients that highly expressed IL-8 were associated with poor relapse-free, overall, and distant metastasis-free survival [92]. Cheng et al. reported an overexpression of IL-8, CXCR1, and CXCR2 in breast, prostate, lung, and colon cancers [93]. The binding of IL-8 to CXCR1/CXCR2 was shown to induce the transition from an epithelial-like to mesenchymal-like status, thus promoting the migration, invasion, and reconstitution of a secondary tumor [94,95]. CXCR2 signaling also promotes the migration of human endothelial cells and angiogenesis, forming a positive feedback loop to further promote epithelial-to-mesenchymal transition (EMT) [96,97]. IL-8 inhibitors might play an important role as anti-angiogenic agents in combination with ICIs. In addition, IL-8 signaling directly promotes immunosuppression in the TME via the recruitment of myeloid-derived suppressor cells (MDSCs, Figure 2). MDSCs are capable of depleting nutrients such as L-arginine, L-tryptophan, and L-cysteine, all of which are essential for T-cell expansion [98,99]. MDSCs also inhibit anti-tumor activity by producing reactive oxygen species and peroxynitrite that can directly inactivate T-cell receptors [100], and by producing reactive nitrogen species that hinder the infiltration of cytotoxic T-cells into the tumor core [101]. Highfill et al. showed that early treatments with anti-PD-1 agents prevented tumor growth, but late treatments showed less benefit due to the presence of MDSCs in the TME [102]. They further showed that anti-CXCR2 monoclonal antibody therapy led to significant anti-tumor activity, even after delayed anti-PD1 treatment [102]. Sanmamed et al. also suggested using IL-8 as a prognostic biomarker to predict the clinical benefit of ICI therapy [103]. They observed that serum IL-8 levels decreased significantly among patients responding to anti-PD-1 checkpoint inhibition ($p < 0.001$) [103]. Serum IL-8 levels also increased significantly among non-responders to anti-PD-1 blockade ($p = 0.013$) [103]. Together, these results suggest that IL-8 inhibition may represent a potential candidate for combinatorial therapy with ICIs.

The anti-IL-8 antibody HuMax-IL8 (also known as BMS-986253) was developed for the successful depletion of tumor-secreted IL-8 and inhibition of CSC mesenchymal properties [85]. HuMax-IL8 also reduced the recruitment of polymorphonuclear MDSCs to the tumor core by preventing IL-8 from binding to CXCR2 receptors on the MDSCs [85]. The phase I trial for HuMax-IL8 (NCT02536469) concluded that serum IL-8 was significantly reduced after the third day of treatment relative to control ($p = 0.0004$) [86]. The incidence of trAEs was 33%, which was much lower than that of anti-angiogenic agents observed in clinical trials [86]. Additionally, the MAGIC-8 phase Ib/II clinical trial (NCT03689699) combined the anti-PD-1 agent Nivolumab with HuMax-IL8 for the treatment of hormone-sensitive prostate cancer [104]. The results of this study are expected in 2022. Thus, IL-8 inhibition may provide a benefit among non-responders of ICIs in TNBC patients, warranting further exploration.

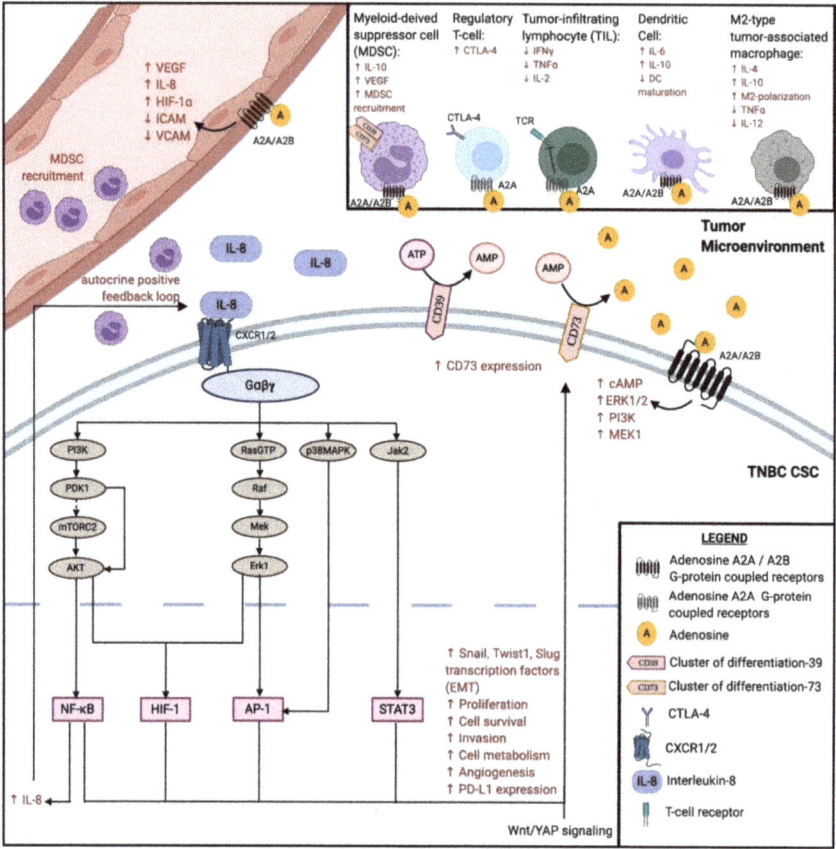

Figure 2. Various tumor-promoting mechanisms that can be exploited in combination with immune checkpoint inhibition. Overexpression of IL-8 and CXCR1/2 in TNBC generates an autocrine positive feedback loop that promotes EMT, HIF-1-mediated angiogenesis and endothelial migration, and recruitment of immunosuppressive MDSCs to the tumor microenvironment (TME). Transcription of NF-κB, HIF-1, AP-1, and STAT3, in combination with Wnt and YAP signaling, upregulates CD73 on TNBC cells. Immunogenic cell death in the TME releases ATP in abundance, which is subsequently converted to adenosine by CD39 and CD73. Excess adenosine in the TME bind to adenosine type 1 purinergic G-protein coupled receptors that further facilitate MDSC expansion, CTLA-4 upregulation, inhibition of TIL activation, inhibition of DC maturation, and M2-type TAM polarization. Activation of adenosine receptors on tumor-associated endothelial cells promotes angiogenesis via upregulation of VEGF and HIF-1α, along with a simultaneous downregulation of adhesion molecules essential for diapedesis. Finally, activation of adenosine receptors on the TNBC cell further upregulate cytosolic cyclic AMP (cAMP), Erk1/2, PI3K, and MEK1, all of which further enhance the IL-8 signaling pathway. Figure created with BioRender.com.

3.3. CD73 Expression

Cluster of differentiation 73 (CD73), normally expressed on T_{reg} cells, is an ectonucleotidase that dephosphorylates extracellular AMP to adenosine [105]. Its expression on bulk tumor cells and mesenchymal-like CSCs generates excess adenosine in the TME, which binds to the adenosine type 1 purinergic G-protein coupled receptor family (denoted A1, A2A, A2B, and A3), some of which are involved in inhibiting effector T-cell responses [106,107]. Adenosine acting on the A2A receptors has a suppressive effect on effector T-cells and an obligatory role in tumor immunomodulation [105,106,108]. In conjunction with IL-8 signaling, the excess adenosine levels facilitate MDSC expansion in the TME via the activation of A2B receptors to enhance immunosuppression [109]. Jin et al. showed that the knockdown of tumor CD73 and subsequent transfer of tumor-specific T-cells significantly enhanced tumor-free survival in tumor-bearing mice [108]. Hypoxic conditions within the tumor core, along with Wingless (Wnt) signaling, upregulate CD73 expression [110,111]. In addition to increasing immunosuppressive adenosine levels in the TME, CD73 modulates cell adhesion molecules within the endothelium, whereas upregulated CD73 promotes the attachment of lymphocytes and reduces their migration into the lymph nodes [112]. CD73 overexpression is also associated with poor prognosis in TNBC [113], highlighting the potential for targeting CD73 as part of a combinatorial treatment (Figure 2). In the phase I trial (NCT02754141), it was shown that the anti-CD73 agent BMS-986189 in combination with the anti-PD-1 antibody Nivolumab was well-tolerated in patients with advanced solid tumors [87]. TrAEs were observed in 58% of the patients receiving the combination, of which 15% were grade 3 in nature [87]. Alternatively, the SYNERGY phase I/II clinical trial (NCT03616886) compared the anti-CD73 agent Oleclumab with the anti-PD-1 agent Durvalumab, and chemotherapeutic agents, in single and combinatorial treatment arms (Table 2). The results of this study are expected in 2022.

3.4. Long Non-Coding RNAs and Microsatellite Instability

Long non-coding RNAs (lncRNAs) are ~200 nucleotides long and do not code for protein products [114]. Their role in disease regulation was only brought to light recently, when the lncRNA urothelial carcinoma-associated 1 (UCA1) was shown to contribute to resistance against tamoxifen therapy in ER$^+$ breast cancers [115]. The lncRNA ROR was associated with a decrease in the expression of E-cadherin, an epithelial marker, and an increase in the expression of the mesenchymal markers vimentin, zeb1, and zeb2 [116]. ROR promoted metastasis via the EMT process and contributed to tamoxifen therapy resistance [116]. LncRNAs (e.g., the nuclear-enriched autosomal transcript1 (NEAT1)) were also associated with immunosuppression. Yan et al. reported that NEAT1 inhibition suppressed CD8$^+$ T-cell apoptosis and enhanced anti-tumor activity [117]. Metastasis-associated lung adenocarcinoma transcript1 (MALAT1) is another lncRNA that was observed to upregulate the expression of PD-1 and CD-47 [118]. Wang et al. showed that knock-down of MALAT1 by shRNA decreased the expression of PD-1, and also suppressed the EMT process [119]. Despite the growing evidence regarding the potential role of lncRNAs in immunotherapy resistance, targeting them in the clinic remains a challenge. LncRNAs would be considered in combinatorial therapy, however, targeting them through RNAi-mediated gene silencing therapy, antisense oligonucleotide-based therapy, or small molecule inhibitors remains expensive and inconvenient, defies precision medicine, and may contribute to unforeseen systemic adverse events or trAEs [120,121]. Further research is therefore required before investigating their potential in the clinic.

Microsatellite instability (MSI) status has also been considered to impact efficacy of ICIs and is therefore used as a reliable biomarker. Microsatellites are short repetitive sequences scattered throughout the human genome as a result of aberrant DNA mismatch repair mechanisms [122]. Recent reports have suggested that a high MSI status, indicative of a hypermutation phenotype, may sensitize patients to ICIs [123,124]. Interestingly, 6.9% of TNBC cases showed a complete loss of relevant mismatch repair proteins, which were correlated with significantly greater PD-L1 expression [125]. Other contributors to MSI status may include tumor mutational burden, which is a measure of nonsynonymous mutations in tumor cells [126], and BRCA1 mutation status. BRCA1 expression modulates the silencing mechanisms in satellite DNA, such that BRCA1-mutated TNBC exhibit higher microsatellite instability than BRCA1-wildtype TNBC [127,128]. The phase II trial (NCT01876511) comparing Pembrolizumab efficacy in MSI-positive and MSI-negative colorectal cancer patients demonstrated an immune-related PFS of 78% among MSI-positive patients and 11% among MSI-negative patients [129]. Pembrolizumab was subsequently FDA-approved for unresectable or metastatic solid tumors with high MSI.

3.5. Wnt and YAP Signaling

Many components of the Wnt signaling pathway are involved in tumorigenesis via EMT and tumor regeneration [130–133]. Cytoplasmic stabilization and nuclear translocation of β-catenin into the nucleus allows for the expression of Wnt target genes [132]. The enrichment of β-catenin, nuclear translocation, and dysregulated Wnt signaling are all associated with poor clinical outcomes of TNBC [134]. The inhibition of Wnt signaling leads to the suppression of CSCs and bulk tumor cells in both TNBC cell lines and patient-derived xenograft (PDX) models [135]. Additionally, activation of β-catenin in tumor cells prevents spontaneous T-cell priming and infiltration of effector T-cells into the TME [136]. A mouse model for hepatocellular carcinoma also demonstrated the role of β-catenin in immune escape and resistance to anti-PD-1 monotherapy [137]. This was consistent with a study by Castagnoli et al., which reported a strong correlation between downstream Wnt signaling effector expression and PD-L1 expression in TNBC [138]. Furthermore, several studies have shown that Wnt inhibitors reduce PD-L1 expression and Wnt agonists enhance PD-L1 expression, suggesting Wnt inhibitors as possible adjuvants to anti-PD-1, anti-PD-L1, or anti-CTLA4 therapies [138,139]. In addition to modulating PD-L1 expression, Wnt/β-catenin signaling has been shown to inhibit T-cell maturation and activation and inhibit dendritic cells (DCs) from secreting chemokines essential for T-cell activation [140–142].

Yes-associated protein (YAP) signaling has also been shown to contribute to the EMT process. A study by Cordenonsi et al. demonstrated a strong correlation between YAP expression and mesenchymal-like CSC surface markers [143,144]. Moreover, YAP knockdown in TNBC cell lines led to a loss of cell proliferation and invasiveness [145]. Besides the role of YAP in modulating Wnt signaling via the β-catenin destruction complex [146], YAP was also shown to directly modulate PD-L1 expression in human TNBC [147]. Interestingly, recent studies have reported that the major transcription factor in YAP signaling, TEAD, has a binding site located close to the PD-L1 promoter. As such, YAP can bind directly to the enhancer region of PD-L1 [148,149]. YAP signaling has also been implicated in recruiting MDSCs to the TME, contributing to the suppression of anti-tumor activity in a similar manner to IL-8 [150]. Moreover, YAP signaling regulates the recruitment of tumor-associated macrophages (TAMs) to the TME. TAMs can differentiate into M1 and M2 phenotypes. M1-type TAMs secrete pro-inflammatory interleukin-1 (IL-1) and tumor necrosis factor-α (TNFα), which promote the expression of inducible nitric oxide synthase (iNOS) to enhance the antigen presentation process [151]. In contrast, M2-type TAMs secrete IL-10, IL-4, arginase-1, and other cytokines involved in resolving inflammation, wound-healing, and facilitating tumor growth [151]. High transcriptional levels of YAP have been reported to disproportionately promote the expression of M2-type TAMs in the TME to enhance tumor growth, drug resistance, and metastasis [152,153].

Wnt and YAP signaling might be important pharmacological targets for eliminating mesenchymal and epithelial CSC populations while simultaneously enhancing ICI immunotherapy outcomes. However, it remains unclear whether they can be implemented in combinatorial treatments, as molecular mechanisms remain unclear. Furthermore, the complexity of Wnt signaling and its broad involvement in normal stem cell self-renewal, differentiation, and organ homeostasis [154] suggest that inhibiting this pathway may be counterproductive and yield intolerable toxicity. However, a phase I clinical trial (NCT01302405) using the Wnt signaling inhibitor PRI-724 concluded an acceptable toxicity profile, with 11% of patients experiencing grade 3 trAEs [88]. Inhibition of YAP signaling poses its own challenges, as Ni et al. reported that YAP is essential for the differentiation of T_{reg} cells, which prevent autoimmune disease [155]. Our recent report suggested that dual inhibition of Wnt and YAP signaling, but neither alone, is required for suppressing both mesenchymal and epithelial CSC populations and diminishing Paclitaxel-induced CSC enrichment in immune-deficient mice [156]. Although combination therapies typically result in better drug responsiveness and synergism than single-agent monotherapies [157], further studies are needed to clarify the efficacy and toxicity of combination therapy with Wnt and/or YAP inhibitors and ICIs.

3.6. Nanoparticle Platforms as a Delivery System

Traditional ICIs are delivered systemically as monoclonal antibodies, which have the potential of activating self-reactive T-cells [158,159]. Immune-related adverse effects may be amplified in combinatorial ICI therapies and may be reduced or resolved by the use of corticosteroids. However, this can increase the risk of other complications and diminish the therapeutic potential of ICIs [158]. Nanoparticle platform-based therapies have revolutionized drug delivery owing to their ability to accumulate in solid tumors, reduce toxicity to vital organs, and increase the therapeutic index [160–162]. Studies have demonstrated the ability of nanoparticles (NPs) to deliver both hydrophobic and hydrophilic drugs, small molecule drugs, and antibodies to the TME, with minimal toxicity to surrounding tissues [160,163]. Studies have also demonstrated the ability of NPs to efficiently interact with and activate dendritic cells and macrophages within the TME [164]. For example, synthetic high-density lipoprotein (sHDL) nanodiscs loaded with Doxorubicin and combined with anti-PD-1 ICIs resulted in a seven-fold increase in IFNγ-positive $CD8^+$ T-cells in the TME, compared with Doxorubicin treatment alone [165]. Additional benefits of the sHDL nanodiscs included the complete regression of colon carcinoma tumors in 80–88% of the treated animals and no apparent cardiotoxicity post-treatment [165]. In another report, poly(lactic-co-glycolic acid) (PLGA) NPs co-loaded with Paclitaxel, combined with detoxified bacterial lipopolysaccharide, resulted in a significant increase in T_{H1} cells in B16F10 mouse models, in comparison to Paclitaxel treatment alone [166]. PLGA NP-treated mice exhibited a 40% lower tumor volume and a higher degree of retention in biological activities of both co-encapsulated drugs [166]. In a third study, nanoscale coordination of polymer (NCP) core-shell nanoparticles co-encapsulated with Oxaliplatin and pyrolipids for photodynamic therapy demonstrated synergism with anti-PD-1 ICI therapy in CT26 and HT29 mouse models [167]. This treatment also reduced tumor volume to 2.9% of their original size when combined with anti-PD-1 therapy, and to 39.1% of their original size in the absence of anti-PD-1 therapy [167]. Such synergy with anti-PD-1 therapy was also observed with peptide-based structure-transformable NPs [168], dendrimers used for siRNA delivery [169], and inorganic NPs composed of gold, titanium dioxide, or iron oxide [170,171]. It is evident that various NP platforms can be used to enhance tumor immunogenicity, favor ICI therapies, and promote the pharmacokinetics and pharmacodynamics of combinatorial treatments.

4. Cancer Cell Antigens: Potential Therapeutic Targets

Since ICI immunotherapy for TNBC benefits only a subset of patients, developing treatment strategies for TNBC patients with lower immunogenic tumors remains an unmet medical need. An ideal therapy would be one with target antigens expressed on bulk tumor cells and also overexpressed in CSC populations [172]. To effectively boost anti-tumor immunity, antigen expression should be evaluated on both CSCs and bulk tumor cells. Interestingly, cancer-testis antigens (CTAs) have been shown to be overexpressed in CSC populations [173]. CTAs are normally expressed in germ-line tissues such as the testis, placenta, and ovaries, but are also highly expressed across several cancer types [174]. In the following section, we will describe some CTAs and two other tumor antigens that have shown potential as biomarkers or immunotherapeutic targets in TNBC.

4.1. Cancer-Testis Antigens

The progression from primary tumor to metastasis is somewhat resembled in the gonads, where trophoblasts invade and burrow into the endometrium [175]. Placenta-specific protein 1 (Plac1) normally plays an important role in trophoblast invasion and migration but is also found to be expressed in a large range of human cancers [176,177]. As such, trophoblast-specific pathways could be reactivated, contributing to the activation of lymphocyte-mediated tumor growth [177]. It has been hypothesized that placental mammals have a certain degree of placental invasiveness that is positively correlated with the incidence of metastatic tumors [178]. Females with a lower degree of placental invasiveness in some species have evolved mechanisms to counter trophoblast invasion, and thus cancer metastasis [179]. Koslowski et al. showed that siRNA inhibition of Plac1 effectively suppressed tumor migration and invasion in breast cancer cell lines [180]. However, the correlation between Plac1 expression and clinical prognosis of TNBC remains unknown [180], and more research is required.

Another strong CTA candidate for TNBC immunotherapy is the New York esophageal squamous cell carcinoma 1 (NY-ESO-1). NY-ESO-1 is normally expressed in primary spermatocytes and rapidly declines in female oogonia [181]. NY-ESO-1 expression is believed to be involved in the proliferation of stem cells and epithelial CSC populations [182]. Ademuyiwa et al. reported NY-ESO-1 expression in 16% of TNBC patients, and antibody responses against NY-ESO-1 were observed in 73% of TNBC patients who were NY-ESO-1-positive [183]. It was also reported that NY-ESO-1-positive patients had higher $CD8^+$ T-cell infiltration in TNBC tumors [184]. NY-ESO-1-specific $CD8^+$ T-cells showed upregulated PD-1 expression, suppressing anti-tumor immunity [184]. As such, NY-ESO-1 may be an attractive candidate for a combinatorial therapy with anti-PD-1 ICI.

The MAGE-A family is also one of the CTAs that renders TNBC highly immunogenic. Raghavendra et al. reported MAGE-A expression in 47% of TNBC cases, and the majority of NY-ESO-1-positive TNBC tumors were also MAGE-A-positive [185]. MAGE-A is normally involved in chromosomal alignment and centrosome duplication [186]. In TNBC, the expression of MAGE-A, however, was positively correlated with the expression of mesenchymal-like CSC markers such as vimentin, but negatively correlated with the expression of epithelial-like CSC markers such as E-cadherin and β-catenin [187]. Targeting MAGE-A would likely enhance anti-tumor immunity by suppressing EMT. MAGE-A12 has been shown to enhance tumor cell proliferation and CSC maintenance [188]. Since targeting multiple CTAs would provide more benefit than targeting a single CTA in anti-tumor immunotherapy, clinical trials have looked at MAGE-A and NY-ESO-1-based vaccines. However, the MAGRIT phase III trial (NCT00480025, targeting MAGE-A3 in non-small cell lung cancer patients) was terminated due to the lack of clinical benefit [189]. Inter-tumoral heterogeneity could partially explain the extent to which certain CTAs are expressed in TNBC versus other tumors [190]. Further characterization of CTA expression in different types of tumor is essential for developing CTA-based therapies for a given tumor type. Although CTAs represent potential therapeutic targets, their expression remain elusive and appear limited to a small subset of patients [191,192].

4.2. Tumor Antigens, Cancer Vaccine, and Oncolytic Virus

The expression of tumor antigens susceptible to immunotherapies in CSC populations have been poorly characterized [186]. While conventional approaches to dendritic cell (DC) vaccines involve using bulk tumor cells as the antigen source, Ning et al. reported that DC vaccines loaded with the lysates of CSCs induced significantly better anti-tumor humoral and cellular immunity than those loaded with bulk tumor cells in mice [193]. Whole-tumor lysates, tumor-antigen-derived peptides, or antigen-encoding RNA/DNA have been used in cancer vaccines [194]. The resultant epitopes from vaccination were presented on major histocompatibility complexes (MHC) I or II by DCs for presentation to $CD8^+$ or $CD4^+$ T-cells, respectively [195].

Tumor-associated antigens (TAAs) have been considered as a possible solution for targeting CSCs, which are molecules expressed at high levels on cancer cells and low levels on healthy cells [196]. However, TAAs such as gp100 and tyrosinase have the potential for off-target toxicity, due to their systemic expression in normal tissues [196,197]. The challenge to select the appropriate antigen renders tumor vaccinations as a less favorable treatment option. One of the strategies used to overcome this challenge in the clinical setting is to use toll-like receptor (TLR) agonists, to potentiate the innate immune system [198]. In a phase II clinical trial (NCT00960752), the TLR-7/8 agonist Resiquimod was combined with gp100 and MAGE-3 peptide vaccines, with results expected later this year [199]. Other reports showed that TLR-7/8 agonists, among others, increase PD-L1 expression on DCs [200]. More studies will be needed to further consolidate the role of TAAs and CTAs in cancer vaccine and ICI immunotherapy for TNBC.

As an alternative approach to DC vaccinations, oncolytic viruses (OVs) have a well-characterized role in inducing anti-tumor immunity. OVs are naturally or genetically modified vectors that are able to selectively replicate in tumor cells, as tumor cells often have impaired antiviral defenses that make them susceptible to OV infections [201–208]. As OVs replicate in the tumor cells, they trigger an inflammatory response leading to immunogenic cell death (ICD) [204]. Following ICD, damage-associated molecular patterns (DAMPs) are released into the TME, which can be recognized by antigen-presenting cells that secrete cytokines including IFNα, IFNγ, TNFα, IL-6, and IL-12 to recruit innate immune cells [204,205]. Furthermore, ICD results in the release of TAAs and tumor-specific antigens (TSAs) into the TME, which activate antigen-specific CD4$^+$ and CD8$^+$ T-cells as part of adaptive immunity [206,207]. By stimulating both innate and adaptive immunity, OVs are able to maintain anti-tumor immunological memory to protect against tumor reconstitution. Similar to TLR agonists, a 2017 study revealed that the OV talimogene laherparepvec (T-VEC) increased PD-1 expression [208]. When T-VEC OV therapy was combined with the anti-PD-1 agent Pembrolizumab, the ORR increased by 62% [209]. In a phase I/II trial (NCT02779855), T-VEC OV therapy combined with neoadjuvant chemotherapy was compared with chemotherapy alone. Preliminary data showed an increase in pCR from 30% with chemotherapy alone to 55% in the combinatorial treatment for non-metastatic TNBC patients [210]. As OVs allow for the exploitation of DAMPs and tumor antigens, inflammation induced by the adenovirus primes the tumor for subsequent DC vaccination, which elicits an anti-tumor CD8$^+$ T-cell response in mice with lung cancer [211]. Furthermore, the Maraba MG1 rhabdovirus, boosted with adenovirus, led to MAGE-3-specific CD4$^+$ and CD8$^+$ T-cell expansion that persisted for several months in mice with MAGE-3-positive solid malignancies [212]. Despite some benefits of OVs in immunotherapy, the main challenge is the systemic antiviral mechanism, which has the potential to block OV replication and infection of tumor cells [212].

5. Chimeric Antigen Receptor T-Cell Therapy

Chimeric antigen receptor T-cell (CAR-T) therapy involves cytotoxic T-cells that are engineered to express fusion proteins that are capable of recognizing and binding to TAAs expressed by tumor cells. These fusion proteins commonly consist of an extracellular single chain variable fragment (scFv) domain for TAA recognition, a transmembrane domain, and an intracellular T-cell coactivation domain [213]. Engineered CAR-T cells offer personalized immunotherapy but are not subject to the same regulatory signaling as endogenous T-cells [214]. This may contribute to trAEs such as cytokine release syndrome, in which the rapid activation and proliferation of CAR-T cells contributes to the excess production of pro-inflammatory cytokines [215]. Zhou et al. showed that the TAB004 monoclonal antibody, capable of recognizing the tumor variant of mucin1 glycoprotein (tMUC1), can be used to make the scFv domain of their MUC28z CAR-T cells [216]. As tMUC1 is expressed in 95% of malignant tissues (including TNBC); IFNγ levels increased from 2.6 to 18.7 pg/mL among HCC70 cells upon the introduction of MUC28z CAR-T cells [216]. Tumor endothelial marker 8 (TEM8)-specific CAR-T cells have also shown to eliminate TEM8$^+$-TNBC tumor cells, and also target tumor-associated endothelial cells [217]. Selection of the right CAR scFv domain dictates the therapeutic potential of CAR-T cells against tumors.

Despite FDA approval, Singh et al. showed relatively poor results of CAR-T therapy against solid tumors, including TNBC, as they are unable to survive in the harsh TME [213]. This has not stopped research groups from exploring CAR-T therapy in TNBC. Based on reports of c-Met overexpression in 52% of TNBC tumors [218], a phase I trial (NCT01837602) demonstrated that c-Met-CAR T-cells did not induce cytokine release syndrome and exhibited on-target effects for c-Met-positive TNBC patients [219]. Previous reports also showed that various TNBC cells lines exhibit moderate to high levels of NKG2D ligand (NKG2DL) [220,221]. Accordingly, the use of the natural killer (NK) cell-activating receptor NKG2D CAR constructs in vivo led to significant MDA-MB-231 tumor regression in mice [220]. Furthermore, a phase I trial (NCT04107142) administered NKG2DL-targeting γ/δ CAR T-cells to patients of varying tumor types, including TNBC. The results for this study are expected in 2021. Similar to the strategies above, further CAR-T research may lead to novel therapeutic options for TNBC.

6. Immunotherapy and Metabolism

6.1. Metabolic Reprogramming in TNBC

It has long been established that tumor cells exhibit an altered cellular metabolism where they shift their metabolic reliance to sustain their proliferative and competitive needs. Metabolic reprogramming is now recognized as a hallmark of malignancy in various different cancers [222,223]. In a phenomenon called the Warburg effect, cancer cells tend to undergo aerobic glycolysis where they rely on glycolysis instead of oxidative phosphorylation, even in the presence of oxygen [223]. This dysregulated increase in glucose influx and glycolytic rate is thought to provide energy on a large scale while depleting the TME of nutrients other cells needed by other cells. While this "Warburg" phenotype is tumor-dependent, TNBC has been shown to be more dependent on glycolysis compared to other breast cancer subtypes, as they overexpress glycolytic components such as lactate dehydrogenase (LDHA), glucose transporter 1 (GLUT1), and monocarboxylate transporters (MCT1/4) [224–226]. Some TNBC tumors overexpressed the GTPase-activating protein USP6NL which is involved in regulating signal transduction and upregulation of GLUT1 via the Wnt/β-catenin pathway [227]. The knockdown of USP6NL has been shown to inhibit TNBC cell growth, motility, and EMT [228]. TNBC cells are also known to be reliant on an increase in fatty acid oxidation and glutamine metabolism as an alternative energy source and to sustain the increased rate of cell growth [229,230].

6.2. Aerobic Glycolysis and Immunosuppression

Perhaps, one of the most intriguing advantages for tumor cell metabolic redirection is its influence on immune cell infiltration, where an immunosuppressive environment is created within the TME. The increased efflux of lactate that is typical in a glycolytic phenotype, for example, results in the acidification of the TME, which has been shown to inhibit $CD8^+$ T-cell activity and TH_1 cell IFNγ production [231,232], while the depletion of glucose due to the increased competitive uptake by cancer cells leads to cytotoxic immune cell dysfunction. In TNBC, LDHA expression was shown to increase the number of T_{regs} and reduce the infiltration of $CD8^+$ T-cells [233]. In the same study, Haung et al. showed through a Kaplan–Meier survival analysis that co-expression of PD-L1 and LDHA in TNBC was linked to poor outcomes in patients with shorter OS and DFS [233]. Interestingly, they show that an over-expression of PD-L1 on TNBC cells results in an increase in LDHA and vice versa, identifying a therapeutic strategy to simultaneously inhibit metabolic and immunologic aspects of tumorigenesis by co-targeting LDHA and PD-L1 [233]. Feng et al. uncovered a role for TAZ, a YAP paralogous transcription cofactor and downstream effector of the Hippo pathway in the interplay between immunosuppression and aerobic glycolysis [234]. In their study, they show that a lactate-mediated increase in PD-L1 was dependent on TAZ in glycolytic cancer cells [234]. Furthermore, inhibiting the CSC-related Wnt pathway could aid in the decreased acidification of the TME and increased immune filtration [235]. The interplay of aerobic glycolysis and immunology in TNBC remains largely unexplored, with more players yet to be identified.

6.3. Glutamine Metabolism in Immunosuppression

Cancer cells also rely on glutamine metabolism for cell growth and anabolic processes. TNBC cells showed an increased reliance on glutamine uptake and metabolism where the glutamine transporters alanine, serine, cysteine-preferring transporter 2 (ASCT2), and L-type amino acid transporter 1 (LAT1) are over-expressed [236]. Once in the cell, glutamine is converted to glutamate and α-ketoglutarate, which could be converted to malate and then to pyruvate, effectively supplementing aerobic glycolysis and contributing to the Warburg phenotype. Lampa et al. reported that suppression of glutaminase synergized the inhibitory effect of mammalian target of rapamycin (mTOR) on the growth of TNBC cell lines [237]. However, a recent study by Leone et al. also used a novel glutaminase antagonist, JHU083, that inhibits glutamine-requiring enzymes [238]. They found that treatment with JHU083 reverted the Warburg effect and inhibited glycolysis, thus increasing the glucose and glutamine content in the tumor as well as increasing the infiltration of CD8$^+$ T-cells [238]. Metabolic analysis showed that the glutamine antagonist increased oxidative phosphorylation through an upregulation of mitochondrial proteins in T-cells but suppressed overall metabolism in cancer cells. While targeting glutamine uptake seems to be a plausible therapeutic strategy, it is limited by the fact that glutamine uptake is also essential for immune cell function [239]. However, combining JHU083 with immunotherapy led to a great response in vivo, where the mice treated with the glutamine antagonist and anti-PD-1 generated significant antitumor effects, with complete response rates close to 100% [238]. While the safety of the glutamine antagonist has yet to be determined, this work provides a glimmer of hope for simultaneously inhibiting metabolic reprogramming and activating the anti-tumor response as a means of therapy.

6.4. Lipid Metabolism in Immunosuppression

TNBC cells exhibit an increase in fatty acid oxidation (FAO) and a decrease in fatty acid synthesis (FAS) compared to other subtypes [239]. Specifically, FAO seems to be crucial in the maintenance of breast CSCs. Studies have reported a higher FAO rate in TNBC CSCs than non-CSCs [240,241]. Wang et al. found that FAO in breast CSCs is dependent on STAT3 signaling, identifying a possible avenue to target lipid metabolic rewiring through the inhibition of JAK/STAT3 [241]. Their work also establishes a link between chemoresistance and FAO levels, where blocking FAO re-sensitized cells to chemotherapy in vivo [241]. This was consolidated by Casciano et al., who reported a link between the highly amplified MYC transcription factor (which occurred in up to 50% of TNBC cases) and its role in promoting FAO [242]. While the role of MYC in TNBC metabolism remains largely unknown, it may be considered as a potential therapeutic avenue in the future.

Lipid metabolism also plays a role in immune cell development and activation. T_{reg} cells adapt to the nutrient depleted hypoxic TME by metabolically depending on fatty acids. T_{regs} relies on FAO for energy to proliferate and exert an immunosuppressive function [243], while T-cell activation is dependent on FAS [244]. Furthermore, increased lipid uptake upregulated PD-1 in CD8$^+$ T-cells, while PD-1 blockade activated these T-cells. Given that lipid metabolism is a crucial aspect of TNBC tumorigenicity and T_{reg} function, targeting enzymes involved with FAO could potentially lead to a reduction in TNBC tumor burden, CSC enrichment, and enhance anti-tumor immunity. While pharmacologically targeting FAO in TNBC has garnered preclinical success, more work is still required to decipher the effect on immune cell infiltration [245].

Emerging evidence points to cholesterol as another culprit in the interplay between immune evasion and metabolic reprogramming, as well as CSC enrichment. Cholesterol is a key component in the cell membrane and acts as an important signaling molecule essential to cell growth and survival [246]. Breast CSCs seem to rely heavily on cholesterol synthesis, possibly for the maintenance of the desired level of membrane fluidity. Reduced membrane cholesterol levels are associated with metastasis, whereas high membrane cholesterol levels and further changes in membrane biophysical properties are associated with increased chemoresistance in breast cancer cells [247]. Increased cholesterol synthesis was associated with shorter relapse-free survival, and a recent study showed that inhibition of cholesterol synthesis pathway reduced breast CSC enrichment [248]. Some reports have shown that the inhibition of cholesterol synthesis pathways using statins, or inhibition of its master regulator RAR-related orphan nuclear receptor γ (RORγ), induced TNBC tumor regression [249,250]. The cholesterol synthesis pathway also overlaps with CSC-related pathways, such as YAP signaling. The cholesterol-lowering drug Simvastatin is currently in clinical trials to treat breast cancer, which indirectly inhibits YAP through the inhibition of HMG-CoA-Reductase [251]. Proprotein convertase subtilisin/kexin 9 (PCSK9) monoclonal antibodies or vaccinations work to reduce cholesterol and have also been proposed to improve clinical outcomes in breast cancer patients [252]. Cholesterol metabolism also plays a role in immune cell activity, as they depend on their membrane to function [253]. A study by Ma et al. showed that cholesterol in the TME influences CD8$^+$ T-cells, leading to the expression of immune checkpoint molecules, such as PD-1 [254]. High levels of cholesterol were associated with low anti-tumor immunity, which was restored upon reducing cholesterol [255]. The effect of drugs such as Simvastatin on immune cell infiltration remain open to investigation.

6.5. Autophagy in TNBC

One of the major players in the immunometabolic landscape of TNBC may be autophagy. Autophagy is a process in which intracellular constituents are degraded or recycled to regulate metabolic pathways under nutrient deprivation to maintain cell survival [256]. A marker of autophagy, microtubule-associated protein 1 light chanin 3B (LC3B) is highly expressed in TNBC and associated with poor clinical outcomes [257]. Glycolysis or GLUT1 inhibitors have been shown to induce autophagy deficiency and eventual cell death in TNBC cells [258,259]. Interestingly, the anti-CD73 antibody 1D7 was shown to mediate autophagy and inhibit the motility of TNBC cells [260]. Wen et al. further demonstrated that the inhibition of autophagy sensitized TNBC cells to chemotherapeutic agents [261]. Glutamine antagonsists have also been discussed as potential therapeutic targets; however, glutaminase inhibition accelerates autophagy and upreuglates FAO as a means for tumor cell survival [262]. Autophagy directly promotes FAO by providing the mitochondria with free fatty acids, leading to the accumulation of lipid droplets [263]. Furthermore, autophagy has been shown to hinder T-cell-mediated anti-tumor activity against TNBC both in vitro and in vivo [264]. As such, the interplay between metabolic pathways and autophagy in TNBC requires further investigation.

6.6. Interplay of HIF-1α in Cancer Metabolism and Immunosurveillance

In addition to the previously described importance of HIF-1α in TNBC angiogenesis, its role in metabolic reprogramming provides another therapeutic avenue in breast cancer cells and CSCs. HIF-1α activity in response to hypoxia leads to the expression of glycolytic enzymes and contributes to the Warburg effect, which increases the acidification of the TME and decreases immune cell infiltration [255,265]. Work by Bharti et al. used high-resolution ^{1}H MRS (in vivo proton magnetic resonance spectroscopy) imaging in the aqueous and lipid phases of HIF-silenced tumors, after which the metabolic profiles were elucidated to determine the effect of HIF-1/2α inhibition [255]. They found that with HIF-1α silencing in TNBC, amino acids such as glutamine were decreased, along with lipid signals and droplets, suggesting that HIF-1α plays a role in TNBC metabolic adaptation [265]. Additionally, a study by Lee et al. discovered a strategy whereby silencing the oxidative stress master regulator NRF2 reduced HIF-1α accumulation and hindered HIF-1α induction of glycolysis-related genes [266]. In breast cancer cell lines, HIF-1α was found to increase the expression of adenosine receptor 2B (A2BR), which, as mentioned in earlier sections, plays a role in MDSC expansion and immunosuppression [267].

In breast cancer, HIF-1α also controls the expression of cluster of differentiation 47 (CD47), an integrin membrane protein expressed on many different cell types for the regulation of a wide range of cellular processes [268,269]. Specifically, cancer cells have been shown to overexpress CD47, where it forms a complex with signal-regulatory protein α (SRP- α) on phagocytes and inhibits macrophage-mediated phagocytosis of the TNBC cells [270]. CD47 expression is a well-known strategy by which tumor cells escape immunosurveillance. Researchers have explored blocking CD47 to induce a wide range of anti-tumor immune function [271–274]. High expression of CD47 in TNBC was associated with unfavorable prognosis, EMT signals, and metastasis [270]. Furthermore, a study by Kaur et al. showed that the blockade of CD47 was effective in TNBC CSC suppression and downregulation of stem-cell related pathways [274]. The preclinical success of targeting CD47 led to the therapy moving on to phase I clinical trials [275]. Interestingly, CD47 was recently shown to promote a Warburg phenotype by protecting the ubiquitin mediated degradation of ENO1, a glycolytic enzyme, providing another role of CD47 in cancer metabolic rewiring, in addition to its established role in immune evasion [276]. HIF-1α is also involved in decreasing the anti-tumor immune response via its control of the PD-1/PD-L1 in immune cells and tumor cells. The hypoxia-inducible element (HRE), where HIF-1α binds, was found in the PD-L1 proximal promoter [277]. Combined, the above information suggests that HIF-1α might serve as a therapeutic strategy to overcome both TNBC metabolic rewiring and immunosuppression.

7. Conclusions

Immune checkpoint inhibition has evolved significantly to reflect the immunogenic potential of TNBC, among other cancers. Despite some positive clinical outcomes with anti-PD-1/PD-L1 and anti-CTLA-4 antibodies, the monotherapy only provides benefit to a subset of the patients, warranting further studies. To date, a large number of clinical trials are looking at immune checkpoint inhibition as a treatment modality to complement chemotherapy. Since enrichment of CSCs and tumor reconstitution are often associated with chemotherapeutic agents, novel combination strategies include normalizing tumor-associated vasculature, modulating the TME, and targeting a multitude of receptors and transcription factors, which may lead to a more effective and durable response for TNBC treatment. In addition to active immunity, therapies that strengthen passive immunity or counter the metabolic reprogramming of tumors may be advantageous in future research. Although significant progress has been made, many challenges remain in the field when looking for a combinatorial immunotherapy to target TNBC.

Author Contributions: K.M., S.E.-S., V.D. and L.W. conceived of and wrote the manuscript. All authors have read and agreed to the published version of the manuscript.

Funding: This work was partially funded by operating grants from Cancer Research Society/University of Ottawa (24064) and Natural Sciences and Engineering Research Council RGPIN-2019-0522 to LW; New Frontiers in Research Fund NFRE-2019-00674 to V.D. and L.W.; Canadian Institutes of Health Research-The Canada Graduate Scholarship to SE.

Conflicts of Interest: All authors declare no conflict of interest.

References

1. Siegel, R.L.; Miller, K.D.; Jemal, A. Cancer statistics. *CA Cancer J. Clin.* **2020**, *70*, 7–30. [CrossRef] [PubMed]
2. Sharma, R. Breast cancer incidence, mortality and mortality-to-incidence ratio (MIR) are associated with human development, 1990–2016: Evidence from Global Burden of Disease Study 2016. *Breast Cancer* **2019**, *26*, 428–445. [CrossRef] [PubMed]
3. Dent, R.; Trudeau, M.; Pritchard, K.I.; Hanna, W.M.; Kahn, H.K.; Sawka, C.A.; Lickley, L.A.; Rawlinson, E.; Sun, P.; Narod, S.A. Triple-Negative breast cancer: Clinical features and patterns of recurrence. *Clin. Cancer Res.* **2007**, *13*, 4429–4434. [CrossRef] [PubMed]
4. Garrido-Castro, A.C.; Lin, N.U.; Polyak, K. Insights into molecular classifications of triple-negative breast cancer: Improving patient selection for treatment. *Cancer Discov.* **2019**, *9*, 176–198. [CrossRef]
5. Golan-Vered, Y.; Pud, D. Chemotherapy-Induced neuropathic pain and its relation to cluster symptoms in breast cancer patients treated with Paclitaxel. *Pain Pract.* **2013**, *13*, 46–52. [CrossRef]
6. Dean, M.; Fojo, T.; Bates, S. Tumour stem cells and drug resistance. *Nat. Rev. Cancer* **2005**, *5*, 275–284. [CrossRef]
7. Li, K.; Lai, H. TanshinoneIIA enhances the chemosensitivity of breast cancer cells to doxorubicin through down-regulating the expression of MDR-related ABC transporters. *Biomed. Pharm.* **2017**, *96*, 371–377. [CrossRef]
8. Han, J.; Lim, W.; You, D.; Jeong, Y.; Kim, S.; Lee, J.E.; Shin, T.H.; Lee, G.; Park, S. Chemoresistance in the human triple-negative breast cancer cell line MDA-MB-231 induced by doxorubicin gradient is associated with epigenetic alterations in histone deacetylase. *J. Oncol.* **2019**, *2019*, 1345026. [CrossRef]
9. Makhoul, I.; Atiq, M.; Alwbari, A.; Kieber-Emmons, T. Breast Cancer immunotherapy: An update. *Breast Cancer Basic Clin. Res.* **2018**, *12*, 1178223418774802. [CrossRef]

10. Kim, Y.-A.; Lee, H.J.; Heo, S.-H.; Park, H.S.; Park, S.Y.; Bang, W.; Song, I.H.; Park, I.A.; Gong, G. MxA expression is associated with tumor-infiltrating lymphocytes and is a prognostic factor in triple-negative breast cancer. *Breast Cancer Res. Treat.* **2016**, *156*, 597–606. [CrossRef] [PubMed]
11. Kitano, A.; Ono, M.; Yoshida, M.; Noguchi, E.; Shimomura, A.; Shimoi, T.; Kodaira, M.; Yunokawa, M.; Yonemori, K.; Shimizu, C.; et al. Tumour-infiltrating lymphocytes are correlated with higher expression levels of PD-1 and PD-L1 in early breast cancer. *ESMO Open* **2017**, *2*, e000150. [CrossRef] [PubMed]
12. Ali, H.R.; Glont, S.-E.; Blows, F.M.; Provenzano, E.; Dawson, S.-J.; Liu, B.; Hiller, L.; Dunn, J.; Poole, C.J.; Bowden, S.; et al. PD-L1 protein expression in breast cancer is rare, enriched in basal-like tumours and associated with infiltrating lymphocytes. *Ann. Oncol.* **2015**, *26*, 1488–1494. [CrossRef] [PubMed]
13. Vikas, P.; Borcherding, N.; Zhang, W. The clinical promise of immunotherapy in triple-negative breast cancer. *Cancer Manag. Res.* **2018**, *10*, 6823–6833. [CrossRef] [PubMed]
14. Mori, H.; Kubo, M.; Yamaguchi, R.; Nishimura, R.; Osako, T.; Arima, N.; Okumura, Y.; Okido, M.; Yamada, M.; Kai, M.; et al. The combination of PD-L1 expression and decreased tumor-infiltrating lymphocytes is associated with a poor prognosis in triple-negative breast cancer. *Oncotarget* **2017**, *8*, 15584–15592. [CrossRef]
15. Loi, S.; Michiels, S.; Salgado, R.; Sirtaine, N.; Jose, V.; Fumagalli, D.; Kellokumpu-Lehtinen, P.L.; Bono, P.; Kataja, V.; Desmedt, C.; et al. Tumour infiltrating lymphocytes are prognostic in triple negative breast cancer and predictive for trastuzumab benefit in early breast cancer: Results from the FinHER trail. *Ann. Oncol.* **2014**, *25*, 1544–1550. [CrossRef] [PubMed]
16. Lee, S.E.; Park, H.Y.; Lim, S.D.; Han, H.S.; Yoo, Y.B.; Kim, W.S. Concordance of programmed death-ligand 1 expression between SP142 and 22C3/SP263 assays in triple-negative breast cancer. *J. Breast Cancer* **2020**, *23*, 303–313. [CrossRef] [PubMed]
17. Bardhan, K.; Anagnostou, T.; Boussiotis, V.A. The PD1:PD-L1/2 pathway from discovery to clinical implementation. *Front. Immunol.* **2016**, *7*, 550. [CrossRef]
18. Lipson, E.J.; Forde, P.M.; Hammers, H.-J.; Emens, L.A.; Taube, J.M.; Topalian, S.L. Antagonists of PD-1 and PD-L1 in cancer treatment. *Semin. Oncol.* **2015**, *42*, 587–600. [CrossRef]
19. Mittendorf, E.A.; Philips, A.V.; Meric-Bernstam, F.; Qiao, N.; Wu, Y.; Harrington, S.; Su, X.; Wang, Y.; Gonzalez-Angulo, A.M.; Akcakanat, A.; et al. PD-L1 expression in triple-negative breast cancer. *Cancer Immunol. Res.* **2014**, *2*, 361–370. [CrossRef]
20. Goodman, A.M.; Piccioni, D.; Kato, S.; Boichard, A.; Wang, H.-Y.; Frampton, G.; Lippman, S.M.; Connelly, C.; Fabrizio, D.; Miller, V.; et al. Prevalence of PDL1 amplification and preliminary response to immune checkpoint blockade in solid tumors. *JAMA Oncol.* **2018**, *4*, 1237–1244. [CrossRef]
21. Barrett, M.T.; Anderson, K.S.; Lenkiewicz, E.; Andreozzi, M.; Cunliffe, H.E.; Klassen, C.L.; Dueck, A.C.; McCullough, A.E.; Reddy, S.K.; Ramanathan, R.K.; et al. Genomic amplification of 9p24.1 targeting JAK2, PD-L1 and PD-L2 is enriched in high-risk triple negative breast cancer. *Oncotarget* **2015**, *6*, 26483–26493. [CrossRef] [PubMed]
22. Sabatier, R.; Finetti, P.; Mamessier, E.; Adelaide, J.; Chaffanet, M.; Ali, H.R.; Viens, P.; Caldas, C.; Birnbaum, D.; Bertucci, F. Prognostic and predictive value of PDL1 expression in breast cancer. *Oncotarget* **2015**, *6*, 5449–5464. [CrossRef] [PubMed]
23. Emens, L.A.; Cruz, C.; Eder, J.P.; Braiteh, F.; Chung, C.; Tolaney, S.M.; Kuter, I.; Nanda, R.; Cassier, P.A.; Delord, J.P.; et al. Long-term clinical outcomes and biomarker analyses of atezolizumab therapy for patients with metastatic triple-negative breast cancer: A phase 1 study. *JAMA Oncol.* **2019**, *5*, 74–82. [CrossRef] [PubMed]
24. Schmid, P.; Adams, S.; Rugo, H.S.; Schneeweiss, A.; Barrios, C.H.; Iwata, H.; Diéras, V.; Hegg, R.; Im, S.A.; Wright, G.S.; et al. Atezolizumab and nab-paclitaxel in advanced triple-negative breast cancer. *N. Engl. J. Med.* **2018**, *379*, 2108–2121. [CrossRef] [PubMed]
25. Adams, S.; Schmid, P.; Rugo, H.; Winer, E.; Loirat, D.; Awada, A.; Cescon, D.; Iwata, H.; Campone, M.; Nanda, R.; et al. Pembrolizumab monotherapy for previously treated metastatic triple-negative breast cancer: Cohort A of the phase II KEYNOTE-086 study. *Ann. Oncol.* **2019**, *30*, 397–404. [CrossRef] [PubMed]
26. Adams, S.; Loi, S.; Toppmeyer, D.; Cescon, D.W.; De Laurentiis, M.D.; Nanda, R.; Winer, E.P.; Mukai, H.; Tamura, K.; Armstrong, A.; et al. Pembrolizumab monotherapy for previously untreated, PD-L1-positive, metastatic triple-negative breast cancer: Cohort B of the phase II KEYNOTE-086 study. *Ann. Oncol.* **2019**, *30*, 405–411. [CrossRef]

27. Schmid, P.; Cortes, J.; Pusztai, L.; McArthur, H.; Kümmel, S.; Bergh, J.; Denkert, C.; Park, Y.H.; Hui, R.; Harbeck, N.; et al. Pembrolizumab for early-triple negative breast cancer. *N. Engl. J. Med.* **2020**, *382*, 810–821. [CrossRef] [PubMed]
28. Vonderheide, R.H.; Domchek, S.M.; Clark, A.S. Immunotherapy for breast cancer: What are we missing? *Clin. Cancer Res.* **2017**, *23*, 2640–2646. [CrossRef]
29. Vilariño, N.; Bruna, J.; Kalofonou, F.; Anastopoulou, G.G.; Argyriou, A.A. Immune-Driven pathogenesis of neurotoxicity after exposure of cancer patients to immune checkpoint inhibitors. *Int. J. Mol. Sci.* **2020**, *21*, 5774. [CrossRef]
30. Hendry, S.; Salgado, R.; Gevaert, T.; Russell, P.A.; John, T.; Thapa, B.; Christie, M.; van de Vijver, K.; Estrada, V.M.; Gonzalez-Ericsson, P.I.; et al. Assessing tumor infiltrating lymphocytes in solid tumors: A practical review for pathologists and proposal for a standardized method from the International Immuno-Oncology Biomarkers Working Group Part 1: Assessing the host immune response, TILs in invasive breast carcinoma and ductal carcinoma in situ, metastatic tumor deposits and areas for further research. *Adv. Anat. Pathol.* **2017**, *24*, 235–251. [CrossRef]
31. Spigel, D.; Marinis, F.D.; Giaccone, G.; Reinmuth, N.; Vergnenegre, A.; Barrios, C.H.; Morise, M.; Felip, E.; Andric, Z.; Geatic, S.; et al. IMpower110: Interim overall survival (OS) analysis of a phase III study of atezolizumab (atezo) vs platinum-based chemotherapy (chemo) as first-line (1L) treatment (tx) in PD-L1-selected NSCLC. *Ann. Oncol.* **2019**, *30*, 915. [CrossRef]
32. Miles, D.W.; Gligorov, J.; André, F.; Cameron, D.; Schneeweiss, A.; Barrios, C.H.; Xu, B.; Wardley, A.M.; Kaen, D.; Andrade, L.; et al. LBA15–Primary results from IMpassion131, a double-blind placebo-controlled randomized phase III trial of first-line paclitaxel (PAC) ± atezolizumab (atezo) for unresectable locally advanced/metastatic triple-negative breast cancer (mTNBC). *Ann. Oncol.* **2020**, *31*, S1147. [CrossRef]
33. Kwa, M.J.; Adams, S. Checkpoint inhibitors in triple-negative breast cancer (TNBC): Where to go from here. *Cancer* **2018**, *124*, 2086–2103. [CrossRef] [PubMed]
34. Cortés, J.; Lipatov, O.; Im, S.-A.; Gonçalves, A.; Lee, K.; Schmid, P.; Tamura, K.; Testa, L.; Witzel, I.; Ohtani, S.; et al. KEYNOTE-119: Phase III study of pembrolizumab (pembro) versus single-agent chemotherapy (chemo) for metastatic triple negative breast cancer (mTNBC). *Ann. Oncol.* **2019**, *30*, v859–v860. [CrossRef]
35. Mirabile, A.; Brioschi, E.; Ducceschi, M.; Piva, S.; Lazzari, C.; Bulotta, A.; Viganò, M.G.; Petrella, G.; Gianni, L.; Gregorc, V. PD-1 inhibitors-related neurological toxicities in patients with non-small-cell lung cancer: A literature review. *Cancers* **2019**, *11*, 296. [CrossRef] [PubMed]
36. Fellner, A.; Makranz, C.; Lotem, M.; Bokstein, F.; Taliansky, A.; Rosenberg, S.; Blumenthal, D.; Mandel, J.; Fichman, S.; Kogan, E.; et al. Neurologic complications of immune checkpoint inhibitors. *J. Neuro-Oncol.* **2018**, *137*, 601–609. [CrossRef]
37. Nair, V.S.; Elkord, E. Immune checkpoint inhibitors in cancer therapy: A focus on T-regulatory cells. *Immunol. Cell Biol.* **2018**, *96*, 21–33. [CrossRef]
38. Walunas, T.L.; Lenschow, D.J.; Bakker, C.Y.; Linsley, P.S.; Freeman, G.J.; Green, J.M.; Thompson, C.B.; Bluestone, J.A. CTLA-4 can function as a negative regulator of T cell activation. *Immunity* **1994**, *1*, 405–413. [CrossRef]
39. Buchbinder, E.I.; Desai, A. CTLA-4 and PD-1 pathways: Similarities, differences, and implications of their inhibition. *Am. J. Clin. Oncol.* **2016**, *39*, 98–106. [CrossRef]
40. Krummey, S.M.; Hartigan, C.R.; Liu, D.; Ford, M.L. CD-28-Dependent CTLA-4 expression fine-tunes the activation of human Th17 cells. *iScience* **2020**, *23*, 100912. [CrossRef]
41. Larkin, J.; Chiarion-Sileni, V.; Gonzalez, R.; Grob, J.J.; Cowey, C.L.; Lao, C.D.; Schadendorf, D.; Dummer, R.; Smylie, M.; Rutkowski, P.; et al. Combined nivolumab and ipilimumab or monotherapy in previously untreated melanoma. *N. Engl. J. Med.* **2015**, *373*, 23–34. [CrossRef] [PubMed]
42. Kooshkaki, O.; Derakhshani, A.; Hosseinkhani, N.; Torabi, M.; Safaei, S.; Brunetti, O.; Racanelli, V.; Silvestris, N.; Baradaran, B. Combination of ipilimumab and nivolumab in cancers: From clinical practice to ongoing clinical trials. *Int. J. Mol. Sci.* **2020**, *21*, 4427. [CrossRef] [PubMed]
43. Antonia, S.J.; López-Martin, J.A.; Bendell, J.; Ott, P.A.; Taylor, M.; Eder, J.P.; Jäger, D.; Pietanza, M.C.; Le, D.T.; de Braud, F.; et al. Nivolumab alone and nivolumab plus ipilimumab in recurrent small-cell lung cancer (CheckMate 032): A multicenter, open-label, phase 1/2 trial. *Lancet Oncol.* **2016**, *17*, 883–895. [CrossRef]

44. Reck, M.; Ciuleanu, T.-E.; Dols, M.C.; Schenker, M.; Zurawski, B.; Menezes, J.; Richardet, E.; Bennouna, J.; Felip, E.; Juan-Vidal, O.; et al. Nivolumab (NIVO) + ipilimumab (IPI) + 2 cycles of platinum-doublet chemotherapy (chemo) vs 4 cycles chemo as first-line (1L) treatment (tx) for stage IV/recurrent non-small cell lung cancer (NSCLC): CheckMate 9LA. *J. Clin. Oncol.* **2020**, *38*, 9501. [CrossRef]

45. Amaria, R.N.; Reddy, S.M.; Tawbi, H.A.; Davies, M.A.; Ross, M.I.; Glitza, I.C.; Cormier, J.M.; Lewis, C.; Hwu, W.-J.; Hanna, E.; et al. Neoedjuvant immune checkpoint blockade in high-risk resectable melanoma. *Nat. Med.* **2018**, *24*, 1649–1654. [CrossRef]

46. Santa-Maria, C.A.; Kato, T.; Park, J.-H.; Flaum, L.E.; Jain, S.; Tellez, C.; Stein, R.M.; Shah, A.N.; Gross, L.; Uthe, R.; et al. Durvalumab and tremelimumab in metastatic breast cancer (MBC): Immunotherapy and immunopharmacogenomic dynamics. *J. Clin. Oncol.* **2017**, *35*, 3052. [CrossRef]

47. Ager, C.R.; Reilley, M.J.; Nicholas, C.; Bartkowiak, T.; Jaiswal, A.R.; Curran, M.A. Intratumoral STING activation with T-cell checkpoint modulation generates systemic antitumor immunity. *Cancer Immunol. Res.* **2017**, *5*, 676–684. [CrossRef]

48. Tan, Y.S.; Sansanaphongpricha, K.; Xie, Y.; Donnelly, C.R.; Luo, X.; Heath, B.R.; Zhao, X.; Bellile, E.L.; Hu, H.; Chen, H.; et al. Mitigating SOX2-potentiated immune escape of head and neck squamous cell carcinoma with a STING-inducing nanosatellite vaccine. *Clin. Cancer Res.* **2018**, *24*, 4242–4255. [CrossRef]

49. Harding, S.M.; Benci, J.L.; Irianto, J.; Discher, D.E.; Minn, A.J.; Greenberg, R.A. Mitotic progression following DNA damage enables pattern recognition within micronuclei. *Nature* **2017**, *548*, 466–470. [CrossRef]

50. Liu, Y.; Zheng, P. Preserving the CTLA-4 checkpoint for safer and more effective cancer immunotherapy. *Trends Pharmacol. Sci.* **2019**, *41*, 4–12. [CrossRef]

51. Zhang, Y.; Du, X.; Liu, M.; Tang, F.; Zhang, P.; Ai, C.; Fields, J.K.; Sundberg, E.J.; Latinovic, O.S.; Devenport, M.; et al. Hijacking antibody-induced CTLA-4 lysosomal degradation for safer and more effective cancer immunotherapy. *Cell Res.* **2019**, *29*, 609–627. [CrossRef] [PubMed]

52. Tivol, E.A.; Borriello, F.; Schweitzer, A.; Lynch, W.P.; Bluestone, J.A.; Sharpe, A.H. Loss of CTLA-4 leads to massive lymphoproliferation and fatal multiorgan tissue destruction, revealing a critical negative regulatory role of CTLA-4. *Immunity* **1995**, *3*, 541–547. [CrossRef]

53. Gough, S.C.L.; Walker, L.S.K.; Sansom, D.M. CTLA4 gene polymorphism and autoimmunity. *Immunol. Rev.* **2005**, *204*, 102–115. [CrossRef] [PubMed]

54. Weber, J.; Mandalà, M.; Del Vecchio, M.; Gogas, H.; Arance, A.M.; Cowey, C.L.; Dalle, S.; Schenker, M.; Chiarion-Sileni, V.; Marquez-Rodas, I.; et al. Adjuvant nivolumab versus ipilimumab in resected stage III or IV melanoma. *N. Engl. J. Med.* **2017**, *377*, 1824–1835. [CrossRef]

55. Calabrese, L.H.; Calabrese, C.; Cappelli, L.C. Rheumatic immune-related adverse events from cancer immunotherapy. *Nat. Rev. Rheumatol.* **2018**, *14*, 569–579. [CrossRef]

56. Vétizou, M.; Pitt, J.M.; Daillère, R.; Lepage, P.; Waldschmitt, N.; Flament, C.; Rusakiewicz, S.; Routy, B.; Roberti, M.P.; Duong, C.P.M.; et al. Anticancer immunotherapy by CTLA-4 blockade relies on the gut microbiota. *Science* **2015**, *350*, 1079–1084. [CrossRef]

57. Wang, J.; Sun, J.; Liu, L.N.; Flies, D.B.; Nie, X.; Toki, M.; Zhang, J.; Song, C.; Zarr, M.; Zhou, X.; et al. Siglec-15 as an immune suppressor and potential target for normalization cancer immunotherapy. *Nat. Med.* **2019**, *25*, 656–666. [CrossRef]

58. Cao, G.; Xiao, Z.; Yin, Z. Normalization cancer immunotherapy: Blocking Siglec-15! *Signal Tranduct. Target Ther.* **2019**, *4*, 10. [CrossRef]

59. Solomon, B.L.; Garrido-Laguna, I. TIGIT: A novel immunotherapy target moving from bench to bedside. *Cancer Immunol. Immunother.* **2018**, *67*, 1659–1667. [CrossRef]

60. Pandey, A.K.; Chauvin, J.M.; Brufsky, A.; Pagliano, O.; Ka, M.; Menna, C.; McAuliffe, P.; Zarour, H. Abstract P5-04-28: Targeting TIGIT and PD-1 in triple negative breast cancer. *Poster Sess. Abstr.* **2020**, *80*. [CrossRef]

61. Iguchi-Manaka, A.; Okumura, G.; Ichioka, E.; Kiyomatsu, H.; Ikeda, T.; Bando, H.; Shibuya, A.; Shibuya, K. High expression of soluble CD155 in estrogen receptor-negative breast cancer. *Breast Cancer* **2020**, *27*, 92–99. [CrossRef] [PubMed]

62. Sanchez-Correa, B.; Valhondo, I.; Hassouneh, F.; Lopez-Sejas, N.; Pera, A.; Bergua, J.M.; Arcos, M.J.; Bañas, H.; Casas-Avilés, I.; Durán, E.; et al. DNAM-1 and the TIGIT/PVRIG/TACTILE Axis: Novel immune checkpoints for natural killer cell-based cancer immunotherapy. *Cancers* **2019**, *11*, 877. [CrossRef] [PubMed]

63. Harjunpää, H.; Blake, S.J.; Ahern, E.; Allen, S.; Liu, J.; Yan, J.; Lutzky, V.; Takeda, K.; Aguilera, A.R.; Guillerey, C.; et al. Deficiency of host CD96 and PD-1 or TIGIT enhances tumor immunity without significantly compromising immune homeostasis. *OncoImmunology* **2018**, *7*, e1445949. [CrossRef] [PubMed]
64. Saleh, R.; Toor, S.M.; Khalaf, S.; Elkord, E. Toor breast cancer cells and PD-1/PD-L1 blockade upregulate the expression of PD-1, CTLA-4, TIM-3 and LAG-3 immune checkpoints in CD4+ T cells. *Vaccines* **2019**, *7*, 149. [CrossRef] [PubMed]
65. Piconese, S.; Valzasina, B.; Colombo, M.P. OX40 triggering blocks suppression by regulatory T cells and facilitates tumor rejection. *J. Exp. Med.* **2008**, *205*, 825–839. [CrossRef]
66. Chester, C.; Sanmamed, M.F.; Wang, J.; Melero, I. Immunotherapy targeting 4-1BB: Mechanistic rationale, clinical results, and future strategies. *Blood* **2018**, *131*, 49–57. [CrossRef]
67. Schrand, B.; Berezhnoy, A.; Brenneman, R.; Williams, A.; Levay, A.; Kong, L.-Y.; Rao, G.; Zhou, S.; Heimberger, A.B.; Gilboa, E. Targeting 4-1BB costimulation to the tumor stroma with bispecific aptamer conjugates enhances the therapeutic index of tumor immunotherapy. *Cancer Immunol. Res.* **2014**, *2*, 867–877. [CrossRef]
68. Yap, T.A.; Burris, H.A.; Kummar, S.; Falchook, G.S.; Pachynski, R.K.; Lorusso, P.; Tykodi, S.S.; Gibney, G.T.; Gainor, J.F.; Rahma, O.E.; et al. ICONIC: Biologic and clinical activity of first in class ICOS agonist antibody JTX-2011 +/- nivolumab (nivo) in patients (pts) with advanced cancers. *J. Clin. Oncol.* **2018**, *36*, 3000. [CrossRef]
69. Emens, L.A. Breast cancer immunotherapy: Facts and hopes. *Clin. Cancer Res.* **2018**, *24*, 511–520. [CrossRef]
70. Leisha, A.E.; Emens, L.A. Chemotherapy and tumor immunity: An unexpected collaboration. *Front. Biosci.* **2008**, *13*, 249–257. [CrossRef]
71. Bielenberg, D.R.; Zetter, B.R. The contribution of angiogenesis to the process of metastasis. *Cancer J.* **2015**, *21*, 267–273. [CrossRef] [PubMed]
72. Zimna, A.; Kurpisz, M. Hypoxia-Inducible factor-1 in physiological and pathophysiological angiogenesis: Applications and therapies. *BioMed Res. Int.* **2015**, *2015*, 549412. [CrossRef] [PubMed]
73. Liao, D.; Johnson, R.S. Hypoxia: A key regulator of angiogenesis in cancer. *Cancer Metastasis Rev.* **2007**, *26*, 281–290. [CrossRef] [PubMed]
74. Vishwanatha, J.K.; Castañeda-Gill, J.M. Antiangiogenic mechanisms and factors in breast cancer treatment. *J. Carcinog.* **2016**, *15*, 1. [CrossRef] [PubMed]
75. Fukumura, D.; Kloepper, J.; Amoozgar, Z.; Duda, D.G.; Jain, R.K. Enhancing cancer immunotherapy using antiangiogenics: Opportunities and challenges. *Nat. Rev. Clin. Oncol.* **2018**, *15*, 325–340. [CrossRef] [PubMed]
76. Schmittnaegel, M.; Rigamonti, N.; Kadioglu, E.; Cassará, A.; Rmili, C.W.; Kiialainen, A.; Kienast, Y.; Mueller, H.-J.; Ooi, C.-H.; Laoui, D.; et al. Dual angiopoietin-2 and VEGFA inhibition elicits antitumor activity that is enhanced by PD-1 checkpoint blockade. *Sci. Transl. Med.* **2017**, *9*, eaak9670. [CrossRef] [PubMed]
77. Kammertoens, T.; Friese, C.; Arina, A.; Idel, C.; Briesemeister, D.; Rothe, M.; Ivanov, A.; Szymborska, A.; Patone, G.; Kunz, S.; et al. Tumour ischaemia by interferon-γ resembles physiological blood vessel regression. *Nat. Cell Biol.* **2017**, *545*, 98–102. [CrossRef]
78. Allen, E.; Jabouille, A.; Rivera, L.B.; Lodewijckx, I.; Missiaen, R.; Steri, V.; Feyen, K.; Tawney, J.; Hanahan, D.; Michael, I.P.; et al. Combined antiangiogenic and anti-PD-L1 therapy stimulates tumor immunity through HEV formation. *Sci. Transl. Med.* **2017**, *9*, eaak9679. [CrossRef]
79. Tian, L.; Goldstein, A.; Wang, H.; Lo, H.C.; Kim, I.S.; Welte, T.; Sheng, K.; Dobrolecki, L.E.; Zhang, X.; Putluri, N.; et al. Mutual regulation of tumour vessel normalization and immunostimulatory reprogramming. *Nat. Cell Biol.* **2017**, *544*, 250–254. [CrossRef]
80. Zheng, X.; Fang, Z.; Liu, X.; Deng, S.; Zhou, P.; Wang, X.; Zhang, C.; Yin, R.; Hu, H.; Chen, X.; et al. Increased vessel perfusion predicts the efficacy of immune checkpoint blockade. *J. Clin. Investig.* **2018**, *128*, 2104–2115. [CrossRef]
81. Finn, R.S.; Qin, S.; Ikeda, M.; Galle, P.R.; Ducreux, M.; Kim, T.-Y.; Kudo, M.; Breder, V.; Merle, P.; Kaseb, A.O.; et al. Atezolizumab plus bevacizumab in unresectable hepatocellular carcinoma. *N. Engl. J. Med.* **2020**, *382*, 1894–1905. [CrossRef] [PubMed]

82. Huang, Y.; Yuan, J.; Righi, E.; Kamoun, W.S.; Ancukiewicz, M.; Nezivar, J.; Santosuosso, M.; Martin, J.D.; Martin, M.R.; Vianello, F.; et al. Vascular normalizing doses of antiangiogenic treatment reprogram the immunosuppressive tumor microenvironment and enhance immunotherapy. *Proc. Natl. Acad. Sci. USA* **2012**, *109*, 17561–17566. [CrossRef]
83. Rigamonti, N.; Kadioglu, E.; Keklikoglou, I.; Rmili, C.W.; Leow, C.C.; De Palma, M. Role of angiopoietin-2 in adaptive tumor resistance to VEGF signaling blockade. *Cell Rep.* **2014**, *8*, 696–706. [CrossRef] [PubMed]
84. Wu, X.; Giobbie-Hurder, A.; Liao, X.; Connelly, C.; Connolly, E.M.; Li, J.; Manos, M.P.; Lawrence, D.; McDermott, D.; Severgnini, M.; et al. Angiopoietin-2 as a biomarker and target for immune checkpoint therapy. *Cancer Immunol. Res.* **2017**, *5*, 17–28. [CrossRef] [PubMed]
85. Dominguez, C.; McCampbell, K.K.; David, J.M.; Palena, C. Neutralization of IL-8 decreases tumor PMN-MDSCs and reduces mesenchymalization of claudin-low triple-negative breast cancer. *JCI Insight* **2017**, *2*. [CrossRef] [PubMed]
86. Bilusic, M.; Heery, C.R.; Collins, J.M.; Donahue, R.N.; Palena, C.; Madan, R.A.; Karzai, F.; Marté, J.L.; Strauss, J.; Gatti-Mays, M.E.; et al. Phase I trial of HuMax-IL8 (BMS-986253), an anti-IL-8 monoclonal antibody, in patients with metastatic or unresectable solid tumors. *J. Immunother. Cancer* **2019**, *7*, 240. [CrossRef] [PubMed]
87. Siu, L.L.; Burris, H.; Le, D.T.; Hollebecque, A.; Steeghs, N.; Delord, J.P.; Hilton, J.; Barnhart, B.; Sega, E.; Sanghavi, K.; et al. Abstract CT180: Preliminary phase 1 profile of BMS-986179, an anti-CD73 antibody, in combination with nivolumab in patients with advanced solid tumors. *Cancer Res.* **2018**, *78*, 13. [CrossRef]
88. El-Khoueiry, A.B.; Ning, Y.; Yang, D.; Cole, S.; Kahn, M.; Berg, M.Z.; Fujimori, M.; Inada, T.; Kouji, H.; Lenz, H.J. A phase I first-in-human study of PRI-724 in patients (pts) with advanced solid tumors. *J. Clin. Oncol.* **2013**, *31*, 2501. [CrossRef]
89. Maurer, C.; Eiger, D.; Velghe, C.; Aftimos, P.; Maetens, M.; Gaye, J.; Paesmans, M.; Ignatiadis, M.; Piccart, M.; Buisseret, L. SYNERGY: Phase I and randomized phase II trial to investigate the addition of the anti-CD73 antibody oleclumab to durvalumab, paclitaxel and carboplatin for previously untreated, locally recurrent inoperable or metastatic triple-negative breast cancer (TNBC). *Ann. Oncol.* **2019**, *30*, iii47–iii64. [CrossRef]
90. Waugh, D.J.; Wilson, C. The interleukin-8 pathway in cancer. *Clin. Cancer Res.* **2008**, *14*, 6735–6741. [CrossRef]
91. Liu, Q.; Li, A.; Tian, Y.; Wu, J.D.; Liu, Y.; Li, T.; Chen, Y.; Han, X.; Wu, K. The CXCL8-CXCR1/2 pathways in cancer. *Cytokine Growth Factor Rev.* **2016**, *31*, 61–71. [CrossRef]
92. Kim, S.; You, D.; Jeong, Y.; Yu, J.; Kim, S.W.; Nam, S.J.; Lee, J.E. Berberine down-regulates IL-8 expression through inhibition of the EGFR/MEK/ERK pathway in triple-negative breast cancer cells. *Phytomedicine* **2018**, *50*, 43–49. [CrossRef] [PubMed]
93. Cheng, Y.; Ma, X.-L.; Wei, Y.-Q.; Wei, X. Potential roles and targeted therapy of the CXCLs/CXCR2 axis in cancer and inflammatory diseases. *Biochim. Biophys. Acta (BBA) Bioenergy* **2019**, *1871*, 289–312. [CrossRef] [PubMed]
94. Fernando, R.I.; Castillo, M.D.; Litzinger, M.; Hamilton, D.H.; Palena, C. IL-8 signaling plays a critical role in the epithelial-mesenchymal transition of human carcinoma cells. *Cancer Res.* **2011**, *71*, 5296–5306. [CrossRef] [PubMed]
95. Acosta, J.C.; O'Loghlen, A.; Banito, A.; Guijarro, M.V.; Augert, A.; Raguz, S.; Fumagalli, M.; Da Costa, M.; Brown, C.; Popov, N.; et al. Chemokine signaling via the CXCR2 receptor reinforces senescence. *Cell* **2008**, *133*, 1006–1018. [CrossRef] [PubMed]
96. Li, A.; Dubey, S.; Varney, M.L.; Dave, B.J.; Singh, R.K. IL-8 directly enhanced endothelial cell survival, proliferation, and matrix metalloproteinases production and regulated angiogenesis. *J. Immunol.* **2003**, *170*, 3369–3376. [CrossRef] [PubMed]
97. Shi, J.; Wei, P.-K. Interleukin-8: A potent promoter of angiogenesis in gastric cancer. *Oncol. Lett.* **2015**, *11*, 1043–1050. [CrossRef]
98. Yu, J.; Du, W.; Yan, F.; Wang, Y.; Li, H.; Cao, S.; Yu, W.; Shen, C.; Liu, J.; Ren, X. Myeloid-derived suppressor cells suppress antitumor immune responses through IDO expression and correlate with lymph node metastasis in patients with breast cancer. *J. Immunol.* **2013**, *190*, 3783–3797. [CrossRef]
99. Srivastava, M.K.; Sinha, P.; Clements, V.K.; Rodriguez, P.; Ostrand-Rosenberg, S. Myeloid-Derived suppressor cells inhibit T-cell activation by depleting cystine and cysteine. *Cancer Res.* **2010**, *70*, 68–77. [CrossRef]

100. Nagaraj, S.; Gupta, K.; Pisarev, V.; Kinarsky, L.; Sherman, S.; Kang, L.; Herber, D.; Schneck, J.; Gabrilovich, D.I. Altered recognition of antigen is a mechanism of CD8+ T cell tolerance in cancer. *Nat. Med.* **2007**, *13*, 828–835. [CrossRef]
101. Molon, B.; Ugel, S.; Del Pozzo, F.; Soldani, C.; Zilio, S.; Avella, D.; De Palma, A.; Mauri, P.; Monegal, A.; Rescigno, M.; et al. Chemokine nitration prevents intratumoral infiltration of antigen-specific T cells. *J. Exp. Med.* **2011**, *208*, 1949–1962. [CrossRef] [PubMed]
102. Highfill, S.L.; Cui, Y.; Giles, A.J.; Smith, J.P.; Zhang, H.; Morse, E.; Kaplan, R.N.; Mackall, C.L. Disruption of CXCR2-Mediated MDSC tumor trafficking enhances anti-PD1 efficacy. *Sci. Transl. Med.* **2014**, *6*, 237ra67. [CrossRef] [PubMed]
103. Sanmamed, M.F.; Perez-Gracia, J.L.; Schalper, K.A.; Fusco, J.P.; Gonzalez, A.; Rodriguez-Ruiz, M.E.; Oñate, C.; Perez, G.; Alfaro, C.; Martín-Algarra, S.; et al. Changes in serum interleukin-8 (IL-8) levels reflect and predict response to anti-PD-1 treatment in melanoma and non-small-cell lung cancer patients. *Ann. Oncol.* **2017**, *28*, 1988–1995. [CrossRef] [PubMed]
104. Dallos, M.; Aggen, D.H.; Hawley, J.; Lim, E.A.; Stein, M.N.; Kelly, W.K.; Nanus, D.M.; Drake, C.G. A randomized phase Ib/II study of nivolumab with or without BMS-986253 in combination with a short course of ADT in men with castration-sensitive prostate cancer (MAGIC-8). *J. Clin. Oncol.* **2019**, *37*, TPS329. [CrossRef]
105. Deaglio, S.; Dwyer, K.M.; Gao, W.; Friedman, D.; Usheva, A.; Erat, A.; Chen, J.F.; Enjyoji, K.; Linden, J.; Oukka, M.; et al. Adenosine generation catalyzed by CD39 and CD73 expressed on regulatory T cells mediates immune suppression. *J. Exp. Med.* **2007**, *204*, 1257–1265. [CrossRef]
106. He, P.; Zhou, W.; Liu, M.; Chen, Y. Recent advances of small molecular regulators targeting G protein-coupled receptors family for oncology immunotherapy. *Curr. Top. Med. Chem.* **2019**, *19*, 1464–1483. [CrossRef]
107. Sciarra, A.; Monteiro, I.; Ménétrier-Caux, C.; Caux, C.; Gilbert, B.; Halkic, N.; Rosa, S.L.; Romero, P.; Sempoux, C.; Leval, L.D. CD73 expression in normal and pathological human hepatobiliopancreatic tissues. *Cancer Immunol. Immunother.* **2019**, *68*, 467–478. [CrossRef]
108. Jin, D.; Fan, J.; Wang, L.; Thompson, L.F.; Liu, A.; Daniel, B.J.; Shin, T.; Curiel, T.J.; Zhang, B. CD73 on Tumor cells impairs antitumor T-cell responses: A novel mechanism of tumor-induced immune suppression. *Cancer Res.* **2010**, *70*, 2245–2255. [CrossRef]
109. Ryzhov, S.; Novitskiy, S.V.; Goldstein, A.E.; Biktasova, A.; Blackburn, M.R.; Biaggioni, I.; Dikov, M.M.; Foektistov, I. Adenosinergic regulation of the expansion and immunosuppressive activity of CD11b+Gr1+ cells. *J. Immunol.* **2011**, *187*, 6120–6129. [CrossRef]
110. Synnestvedt, K.; Furuta, G.T.; Comerford, K.M.; Louis, N.; Karhausen, J.; Eltzschig, H.K.; Hansen, K.R.; Thompson, L.F.; Colgan, S.P. Ecto-5′-nucleotidase (CD73) regulation by hypoxia-inducible factor-1 mediates permeability changes in intestinal epithelia. *J. Clin. Investig.* **2002**, *110*, 993–1002. [CrossRef]
111. Adzic, M.; Nedeljkovic, N. Unveiling the role of Ecto-5′-Nucleotidase/CD73 in astrocyte migration by using pharmacological tools. *Front. Pharmacol.* **2018**, *9*, 153. [CrossRef] [PubMed]
112. Takedachi, M.; Qu, D.; Ebisuno, Y.; Oohara, H.; Joachims, M.L.; McGee, S.T.; Maeda, E.; McEver, R.P.; Tanaka, T.; Miyasaka, M.; et al. CD73-generated adenosine restricts lymphocyte migration into draining lymph nodes. *J. Immunol.* **2008**, *180*, 6288–6296. [CrossRef] [PubMed]
113. Loi, S.; Pommey, S.; Haibe-Kains, B.; Beavis, P.A.; Darcy, P.K.; Smyth, M.J.; Stagg, J. CD73 promotes anthracycline resistance and poor prognosis in triple negative breast cancer. *Proc. Natl. Acad. Sci. USA* **2013**, *110*, 11091–11096. [CrossRef] [PubMed]
114. Kung, J.T.Y.; Colognori, D.; Lee, J.T. Long noncoding RNAs: Past, present, and future. *Genetics* **2013**, *193*, 651–669. [CrossRef]
115. Wang, C.J.; Zhu, C.C.; Xu, J.; Wang, M.; Zhao, W.Y.; Liu, Q.; Zhao, G.; Zhang, Z.Z. The lncRNA UCA1 promotes proliferation, migration, immune escape and inhibits apoptosis in gastric cancer by sponging anti-tumor miRNAs. *Mol. Cancer* **2019**, *18*, 115. [CrossRef] [PubMed]
116. Campos-Parra, A.D.; López-Urrutia, E.; Moreno, L.T.O.; López-Camarillo, C.; Meza-Menchaca, T.; González, G.F.; Montes, L.P.B.; Pérez-Plasencia, C. Long non-coding RNAs as new master regulators of resistance to systemic treatments in breast cancer. *Int. J. Mol. Sci.* **2018**, *19*, 2711. [CrossRef]
117. Yan, K.; Fu, Y.; Zhu, N.; Wang, Z.; Hong, J.-L.; Li, Y.; Li, W.-J.; Zhang, H.-B.; Song, J.-H. Repression of lncRNA NEAT1 enhances the antitumor activity of CD8+T cells against hepatocellular carcinoma via regulating miR-155/Tim-3. *Int. J. Biochem. Cell Biol.* **2019**, *110*, 1–8. [CrossRef]

118. Xiping, Z.; Bo, C.; Shifeng, Y.; Feijiang, Y.; Hongjian, Y.; Qihui, C.; Binbin, T. Roles of MALAT1 in development and migration of triple negative and Her-2 positive breast cancer. *Oncotarget* **2018**, *9*, 2255–2267. [CrossRef]
119. Wang, Q.-M.; Lian, G.-Y.; Song, Y.; Huang, Y.-F.; Gong, Y. LncRNA MALAT1 promotes tumorigenesis and immune escape of diffuse large B cell lymphoma by sponging miR-195. *Life Sci.* **2019**, *231*, 116335. [CrossRef]
120. Lu, T.; Wang, Y.; Chen, D.; Liu, J.; Jiao, W. Potential clinical application of lncRNAs in non-small cell lung cancer. *OncoTargets Ther.* **2018**, *11*, 8045–8052. [CrossRef]
121. Wu, T.; Du, Y. LncRNAs: From basic research to medical application. *Int. J. Biol. Sci.* **2017**, *13*, 295–307. [CrossRef] [PubMed]
122. Cortes-Ciriano, I.; Lee, S.; Park, W.-Y.; Kim, T.-M.; Park, P.J. A molecular portrait of microsatellite instability across multiple cancers. *Nat. Commun.* **2017**, *8*, 15180. [CrossRef] [PubMed]
123. Le, D.T.; Durham, J.N.; Smith, K.N.; Wang, H.; Barlett, B.R.; Aulakh, L.K.; Lu, S.; Kemberling, H.; Wilt, C.; Luber, B.S.; et al. Mismatch repair deficiency predicts response of solid tumors to PD-1 blockade. *Science* **2017**, *357*, 409–413. [CrossRef] [PubMed]
124. Horimoto, Y.; Hlaing, M.T.; Saeki, H.; Kitano, S.; Nakai, K.; Sasaki, R.; Kurisaki-Arakawa, A.; Arakawa, A.; Otsuji, N.; Matsuoka, S.; et al. Microsatellite instability and mismatch repair protein expressions in lymphocyte-predominant breast cancer. *Cancer Sci.* **2020**, *111*, 2647–2654. [CrossRef] [PubMed]
125. Hou, Y.; Nitta, H.; Parwani, A.V.; Li, Z. PD-L1 and CD8 are associated with deficient mismatch repair status in triple-negative and HER2-positive breast cancers. *Hum. Pathol.* **2019**, *86*, 108–114. [CrossRef] [PubMed]
126. Mei, P.; Freitag, C.E.; Wei, L.; Zhang, Y.; Parwani, A.V.; Li, Z. High tumor mutation burden is associated with DNA damage repair gene mutation in breast carcinomas. *Diagn. Pathol.* **2020**, *15*, 1–7. [CrossRef]
127. Zhu, Q.; Pao, G.M.; Huynh, A.M.; Suh, H.; Tonnu, N.; Nederlof, P.M.; Gage, F.H.; Verma, I.M. BRCA1 tumour suppression occurs via heterochromatin-mediated silencing. *Nat. Cell Biol.* **2011**, *477*, 179–184. [CrossRef]
128. Nolan, E.; Savas, P.; Policheni, A.N.; Darcy, P.K.; Vaillant, F.; Mintoff, C.P.; Dushyanthen, S.; Mansour, M.; Pang, J.-M.B.; Fox, S.B.; et al. Combined immune checkpoint blockade as a therapeutic strategy forBRCA1-mutated breast cancer. *Sci. Transl. Med.* **2017**, *9*, eaal4922. [CrossRef]
129. Le, D.T.; Uram, J.N.; Wang, H.; Bartlett, B.R.; Kemberling, H.; Eyring, A.D.; Skora, A.D.; Luber, B.S.; Azad, N.S.; Laheru, D.; et al. PD-1 Blockade in tumors with mismatch-repair deficiency. *N. Engl. J. Med.* **2015**, *372*, 2509–2520. [CrossRef]
130. Kahlert, U.D.; Maciaczyk, D.; Doostkam, S.; Orr, B.A.; Simons, B.; Bogiel, T.; Reithmeier, T.; Prinz, M.; Schubert, J.; Niedermann, G.; et al. Activation of canonical WNT/β-catenin signaling enhances in vitro motility of glioblastoma cells by activation of ZEB1 and other activators of epithelial-to-mesenchymal transition. *Cancer Lett.* **2012**, *325*, 42–53. [CrossRef]
131. Vincan, E.; Barker, N. The upstream components of the Wnt signalling pathway in the dynamic EMT and MET associated with colorectal cancer progression. *Clin. Exp. Metastasis* **2008**, *25*, 657–663. [CrossRef] [PubMed]
132. Loh, N.Y.; Hedditch, E.L.; Baker, A.L.; Jary, E.; Ward, R.L.; Ford, C.E. The Wnt signalling pathway is upregulated in an in vitro model of acquired tamoxifen resistant breast cancer. *BMC Cancer* **2013**, *13*, 174. [CrossRef] [PubMed]
133. Green, J.L.; La, J.; Yum, K.W.; Desai, P.; Rodewald, L.-W.; Zhang, X.; Leblanc, M.; Nusse, R.; Lewis, M.T.; Wahl, G.M. Paracrine Wnt signaling both promotes and inhibits human breast tumor growth. *Proc. Natl. Acad. Sci. USA* **2013**, *110*, 6991–6996. [CrossRef] [PubMed]
134. Xu, J.; Prosperi, J.R.; Choudhury, N.; Olopade, O.I.; Goss, K.H. B-Catenin is required for the tumorigenic potential of triple-negative breast cancer cells. *PLoS ONE* **2015**, *10*, e0117097. [CrossRef]
135. Pohl, S.-G.; Brook, N.; Agostino, M.; Arfuso, F.; Kumar, A.P.; Dharmarajan, A. Wnt signaling in triple-negative breast cancer. *Oncogenesis* **2017**, *6*, e310. [CrossRef]
136. Spranger, S.; Bao, R.; Gajewski, T.F. Melanoma-intrinsic B-catenin signalling prevents anti-tumour immunity. *Nat. Cell Biol.* **2015**, *523*, 231–235. [CrossRef]
137. De Galarreta, M.R.; Bresnahan, E.; Molina-Sánchez, P.; Lindblad, K.E.; Maier, B.; Sia, D.; Puigvehí, M.; Miguela, V.; Casanova-Acebes, M.; Dhainaut, M.; et al. B-Catenin activation promotes immune escape and resistance to Anti-PD-1 therapy in hepatocellular carcinoma. *Cancer Discov.* **2019**, *9*, 1124–1141. [CrossRef]

138. Castagnoli, L.; Cancila, V.; Cordoba-Romero, S.L.; Faraci, S.; Talarico, G.; Belmonte, B.; Iorio, M.V.; Milani, M.; Volpari, T.; Chiodoni, C.; et al. WNT signaling modulates PD-L1 expression in the stem cell compartment of triple-negative breast cancer. *Oncogene* **2019**, *38*, 4047–4060. [CrossRef]
139. Wang, B.; Tian, T.; Kalland, K.-H.; Ke, X.; Qu, Y. Targeting Wnt/B-Catenin signaling for cancer immunotherapy. *Trends Pharmacol. Sci.* **2018**, *39*, 648–658. [CrossRef]
140. Driessens, G.; Zheng, Y.; Locke, F.; Cannon, J.L.; Gounari, F.; Gajewski, T.F. Beta-catenin inhibits T cell activation by selective interference with linker for activation of T cells-phospholipase C-y1phosphorylation. *J. Immunol.* **2010**, *186*, 784–790. [CrossRef]
141. Kerdidani, D.; Chouvardas, P.; Arjo, A.R.; Giopanou, I.; Ntaliarda, G.; Guo, Y.A.; Tsikitis, M.; Kazamias, G.; Potaris, K.; Stathopoulos, G.T.; et al. Wnt1 silences chemokine genes in dendritic cells and induces adaptive immune resistance in lung adenocarcinoma. *Nat. Commun.* **2019**, *10*, 1405. [CrossRef] [PubMed]
142. Bilir, B.; Kucuk, O.; Moreno, C.S. Wnt signaling blockage inhibits cell proliferation and migration, and induces apoptosis in triple-negative breast cancer cells. *J. Transl. Med.* **2013**, *11*, 280. [CrossRef] [PubMed]
143. Cordenonsi, M.; Zanconato, F.; Azzolin, L.; Forcato, M.; Rosato, A.; Frasson, C.; Inui, M.; Montagner, M.; Parenti, A.R.; Poletti, A.; et al. The hippo transducer TAZ confers cancer stem cell-related traits on breast cancer cells. *Cell* **2011**, *147*, 759–772. [CrossRef] [PubMed]
144. Hiemer, S.E.; Szymaniak, A.D.; Varelas, X. The transcriptional regulators TAZ and YAP direct transforming growth factor &beta-induced tumorigenic phenotypes in breast cancer cells. *J. Biol. Chem.* **2014**, *289*, 13461–13474. [CrossRef]
145. Chang, S.-S.; Yamaguchi, H.; Xia, W.; Lim, S.-O.; Khotskaya, Y.; Wu, Y.; Chang, W.-C.; Liu, Q.; Hung, M.-C. Aurora A kinase activates YAP signaling in triple-negative breast cancer. *Oncogene* **2017**, *36*, 1265–1275. [CrossRef] [PubMed]
146. Azzolin, L.; Panciera, T.; Soligo, S.; Enzo, E.; Bicciato, S.; Dupont, S.; Bresolin, S.; Frasson, C.; Basso, G.; Guzzardo, V.; et al. YAP/TAZ incorporation in the B-Catenin destruction complex orchestrates the Wnt response. *Cell* **2014**, *158*, 157–170. [CrossRef] [PubMed]
147. Maeda, T.; Hiraki, M.; Jin, C.; Rajabi, H.; Tagde, A.; Alam, M.; Bouillez, A.; Hu, X.; Suzuki, Y.; Miyo, M.; et al. MUC1-C induces PD-L1 and immune evasion in triple-negative breast cancer. *Cancer Res.* **2017**, *78*, 205–215. [CrossRef]
148. Kim, M.H.; Kim, C.G.; Kim, S.-K.; Shin, S.J.; Choe, E.A.; Park, S.H.; Shin, E.-C.; Kim, J. YAP-Induced PD-L1 expression drives immune evasion in BRAFi-Resistant melanoma. *Cancer Immunol. Res.* **2018**, *6*, 255–266. [CrossRef]
149. Miao, J.; Hsu, P.-C.; Yang, Y.-L.; Xu, Z.; Dai, Y.; Wang, Y.; Chan, G.; Huang, Z.; Hu, B.; Li, H.; et al. YAP regulates PD-L1 expression in human NSCLC cells. *Oncotarget* **2017**, *8*, 114576–114587. [CrossRef]
150. Wang, G.; Lu, X.; Dey, P.; Deng, P.; Wu, C.C.; Jiang, S.; Fang, Z.; Zhao, K.; Konaparthi, R.; Hua, S.; et al. Targeting YAP-Dependent MSDC infiltration impairs tumor progression. *Cancer Discov.* **2016**, *6*, 80–95. [CrossRef]
151. Locati, M.; Mantovani, A.; Sica, A. Macrophage activation and polarization as an adaptive component of innate immunity. *Adv. Immunol.* **2013**, *120*, 163–184. [CrossRef] [PubMed]
152. Yang, M.; Liu, J.; Shao, J.; Qin, Y.; Ji, Q.; Zhang, X.; Du, J. Cathepsin S-mediated autophagic flux in tumor-associated macrophages accelerate tumor development by promoting M2 polarization. *Mol. Cancer* **2014**, *13*, 43. [CrossRef] [PubMed]
153. Yang, W.; Yang, S.; Zhang, F.; Cheng, F.; Wang, X.; Rao, J. Influence of the Hippo-YAP signalling pathway on tumor associated macrophages (TAMs) and its implications on cancer immunosuppressive microenvironment. *Ann. Transl. Med.* **2020**, *8*, 399. [CrossRef] [PubMed]
154. Nusse, R.; Clevers, H. Wnt/B-Catenin signaling, disease, and emerging therapeutic modalities. *Cell* **2017**, *169*, 985–999. [CrossRef] [PubMed]
155. Ni, X.; Tao, J.; Barbi, J.; Chen, Q.; Park, B.V.; Li, Z.; Zhang, N.; Lebid, A.; Ramaswamy, A.; Wei, P.; et al. YAP is essential for treg-mediated suppression of antitumor immunity. *Cancer Discov.* **2018**, *8*, 1026–1043. [CrossRef] [PubMed]
156. Sulaiman, A.; McGarry, S.; Li, L.; Jia, D.; Ooi, S.; Addison, C.; Dimitroulakos, J.; Arnaout, A.; Nessim, C.; Yao, Z.; et al. Dual inhibition of Wnt and Yes-associated protein signaling retards the growth of triple-negative breast cancer in both mesenchymal and epithelial states. *Mol. Oncol.* **2018**, *12*, 423–440. [CrossRef]

157. Saputra, E.C.; Huang, L.; Chen, Y.; Tucker-Kellogg, L. Combination therapy and the evolution of resistance: The theoretical merits of synergism and antagonism in cancer. *Cancer Res.* **2018**, *78*, 2419–2431. [CrossRef]
158. Friedman, C.F.; Proverbs-Singh, T.A.; Postow, M.A. Treatment of the immune-related adverse effects of immune checkpoint inhibitors: A review. *JAMA Oncol.* **2016**, *2*, 1346–1353. [CrossRef]
159. Postow, M.A.; Sidlow, R.; Hellmann, M.D. Immune-Related adverse events associated with immune checkpoint blockade. *N. Engl. J. Med.* **2018**, *378*, 158–168. [CrossRef]
160. Gurunathan, S.; Kang, M.-H.; Qasim, M.; Kim, J.-H. Nanoparticle-Mediated combination therapy: Two-in-one approach for cancer. *Int. J. Mol. Sci.* **2018**, *19*, 3264. [CrossRef]
161. Shi, J.; Kantoff, P.W.; Wooster, R.; Farokhzad, O.C. Cancer nanomedicine: Progress, challenges, and opportunities. *Nat. Rev. Cancer* **2017**, *17*, 20–37. [CrossRef] [PubMed]
162. Peer, D.; Karp, J.M.; Hong, S.; Farokhzad, O.C.; Margalit, R.; Langer, R. Nanocarriers as an emerging platform for cancer therapy. *Nat. Nanotechnol.* **2007**, *2*, 751–760. [CrossRef] [PubMed]
163. Sercombe, L.; Veerati, T.; Moheimani, F.; Wu, S.Y.; Sood, A.K.; Hua, S. Advances and challenges of liposome assisted drug delivery. *Front. Pharmacol.* **2015**, *6*, 286. [CrossRef] [PubMed]
164. Wang, J.; Chen, H.-J.; Hang, T.; Yu, T.; Liu, G.; He, G.; Xiao, S.; Yang, B.R.; Yang, C.; Liu, F.; et al. Physical activation of innate immunity by spiky particles. *Nat. Nanotechnol.* **2018**, *13*, 1078–1086. [CrossRef]
165. Kuai, R.; Yuan, W.; Son, S.; Nam, J.; Xu, Y.; Fan, Y.; Schwendeman, A.; Moon, J.J. Elimination of established tumors with nanodisc-based combination chemoimmunotherapy. *Sci. Adv.* **2018**, *4*, eaao1736. [CrossRef]
166. Roy, A.; Singh, M.S.; Upadhyay, P.; Bhaskar, S. Nanoparticle mediated co-delivery of paclitaxel and a TLR-4 agonist results in tumor regression and enhanced immune response in the tumor microenvironment of a mouse model. *Int. J. Pharm.* **2013**, *445*, 171–180. [CrossRef]
167. He, C.; Duan, X.; Guo, N.; Chan, C.; Poon, C.; Weichselbaum, N.G.R.R.; Lin, W. Core-shell nanoscale coordination polymers combine chemotherapy and photodynamic therapy to potentiate checkpoint blockade cancer immunotherapy. *Nat. Commun.* **2016**, *7*, 12499. [CrossRef]
168. Xu, C.; Yu, Y.; Sun, Y.; Kong, L.; Yang, C.; Hu, M.; Yang, T.; Zhang, J.; Hu, Q.; Zhang, Z. Transformable nanoparticle-enabled synergistic elicitation and promotion of immunogenic cell death for triple-negative breast cancer immunotherapy. *Adv. Funct. Mater.* **2019**, *29*, 1905213. [CrossRef]
169. Wang, P.; Zhao, X.-H.; Wang, Z.; Meng, M.; Li, X.; Ning, Q. Generation 4 polyamidoamine dendrimers is a novel candidate of nano-carrier for gene delivery agents in breast cancer treatment. *Cancer Lett.* **2010**, *298*, 34–49. [CrossRef]
170. Retif, P.; Pinel, S.; Toussaint, M.; Frochot, C.; Chouikrat, R.; Bastogne, T.; Barberi-Heyob, M. Nanoparticles for Radiation Therapy Enhancement: The Key Parameters. *Theranostics* **2015**, *5*, 1030–1044. [CrossRef]
171. Ngwa, W.; Dougan, S.; Kumar, R. Combining nanoparticle-aided radiation therapy with immunotherapy to enhance local and metastatic tumor cell kill during pancreatic cancer treatment. *Int. J. Radiat. Oncol.* **2017**, *99*, E611–E612. [CrossRef]
172. Ruiu, R.; Tarone, L.; Rolih, V.; Barutello, G.; Bolli, E.; Riccardo, F.; Cavallo, F.; Conti, L. Cancer stem cell immunology and immunotherapy: Harnessing the immune system against cancer's source. *Prog. Mol. Biol. Transl. Sci.* **2019**, *164*, 119–188. [CrossRef] [PubMed]
173. Yamada, R.; Takahashi, A.; Torigoe, T.; Morita, R.; Tamura, Y.; Tsukahara, T.; Kanaseki, T.; Kubo, T.; Watarai, K.; Kondo, T.; et al. Preferential expression of cancer/testis genes in cancer stem-like cells: Proposal of a novel sub-category, cancer/testis/stem gene. *Tissue Antigens* **2013**, *81*, 428–434. [CrossRef] [PubMed]
174. Simpson, A.J.G.; Caballero, O.L.; Jungbluth, A.; Chen, Y.-T.; Old, L.J. Cancer/testis antigens, gametogenesis and cancer. *Nat. Rev. Cancer* **2005**, *5*, 615–625. [CrossRef] [PubMed]
175. Li, Y.; Li, J.; Wang, Y.; Zhang, Y.; Chu, J.; Sun, C.; Fu, Z.; Huang, Y.; Zhang, H.; Yuan, H.; et al. Roles of cancer/testis antigens (CTAs) in breast cancer. *Cancer Lett.* **2017**, *399*, 64–73. [CrossRef]
176. Wei, X.; Chen, F.; Xin, K.; Wang, Q.; Yu, L.; Liu, B.; Liu, Q. Cancer-Testis antigen peptide vaccine for cancer immunotherapy: Progress and prospects. *Transl. Oncol.* **2019**, *12*, 733–738. [CrossRef]
177. Li, Y.; Chu, J.; Li, J.; Feng, W.; Yang, F.; Wang, Y.; Zhang, Y.; Sun, C.; Yang, M.; Vasilatos, S.N.; et al. Cancer/testis antigen-Plac1 promotes invasion and metastasis of breast cancer through Furin/NICD/PTEN signaling pathway. *Mol. Oncol.* **2018**, *12*, 1233–1248. [CrossRef]
178. Costanzo, V.; Bardelli, A.; Siena, S.; Abrignani, S. Exploring the links between cancer and placenta development. *Open Biol.* **2018**, *8*, 180081. [CrossRef]

179. D'Souza, A.W.; Wagner, G.P. Malignant cancer and invasive placentation: A case for positive pleiotropy between endometrial and malignancy phenotypes. *Evol. Med. Public Health* **2014**, *2014*, 136–145. [CrossRef]
180. Koslowski, M.; Sahin, U.; Mitnacht-Kraus, R.; Seitz, G.; Huber, C.; Türeci, Ö. A placenta-specific gene ectopically activated in many human cancers is essentially involved in malignant cell processes. *Cancer Res.* **2007**, *67*, 9528–9534. [CrossRef]
181. Satie, A.-P.; Meyts, E.R.-D.; Spagnoli, G.C.; Henno, S.; Olivo, L.; Jacobsen, G.K.; Rioux-Leclercq, N.; Jégou, B.; Samson, M. The cancer-testis gene, NY-ESO-1, is expressed in normal fetal and adult testes and in spermatocytic seminomas and testicular carcinoma in situ. *Lab. Investig.* **2002**, *82*, 775–780. [CrossRef]
182. Cronwright, G.; Blanc, K.L.; Götherström, C.; Darcy, P.; Ehnman, M.; Brodin, B. Cancer/testis antigen expression in human mesenchymal stem cells: Down-regulation of SSX impairs cell migration and matrix metalloproteinase 2 expression. *Cancer Res.* **2005**, *65*, 2207–2215. [CrossRef]
183. Ademuyiwa, F.O.; Bshara, W.; Attwood, K.; Morrison, C.; Edge, S.B.; Karpf, A.R.; James, S.A.; Ambrosone, C.B.; O'Connor, T.L.; Levine, E.G.; et al. NY-ESO-1 cancer testis antigen demonstrates high immunogenicity in triple negative breast cancer. *PLoS ONE* **2012**, *7*, e38783. [CrossRef]
184. Fourcade, J.; Kudela, P.; Sun, Z.; Shen, H.; Land, S.R.; Lenzner, D.; Guillaume, P.; Luescher, I.F.; Sander, C.; Ferrone, S.; et al. PD-1 is a regulator of NY-ESO-1-specific CD8+ T cell expansion in melanoma patients. *J. Immunol.* **2009**, *182*, 5240–5249. [CrossRef]
185. Raghavendra, A.; Croft, P.K.; Vargas, A.C.; Smart, C.E.; Simpson, P.T.; Saunus, J.M.; Lakhani, S.R. Expression of MAGE-A and NY-ESO-1 cancer/testis antigens is enriched in triple-negative invasive breast cancers. *Histopathology* **2018**, *73*, 68–80. [CrossRef]
186. Wang, X.; Qi, Y.; Kong, X.; Zhai, J.; Li, Y.; Song, Y.; Wang, J.; Feng, X.; Fang, Y. Immunological therapy: A novel thriving area for triple-negative breast cancer treatment. *Cancer Lett.* **2019**, *442*, 409–428. [CrossRef]
187. Wang, H.; Sang, M.; Geng, C.; Liu, F.; Gu, L.; Shan, B. MAGE-A is frequently expressed in triple negative breast cancer and associated with epithelial-mesenchymal transition. *Neoplasma* **2016**, *63*, 44–56. [CrossRef]
188. Zajac, P.; Schultz-Thater, E.; Tornillo, L.; Sadowski, C.; Trella, E.; Mengus, C.; Iezzi, G.; Spagnoli, G.C. MAGE-A antigens and cancer immunotherapy. *Front. Med.* **2017**, *4*, 18. [CrossRef]
189. Vansteenkiste, J.; Cho, B.C.; Vanakesa, T.; De Pas, T.; Zielinski, M.; Kim, M.S.; Jassem, J.; Yoshimura, M.; Dahabreh, J.; Nakayama, H.; et al. Efficacy of the MAGE-A3 cancer immunotherapeutic as adjuvant therapy in patients with resected MAGE-A3-positive non-small-cell lung cancer (MAGRIT): A randomised, double-blind, placebo-controlled, phase 3 trial. *Lancet Oncol.* **2016**, *17*, 822–835. [CrossRef]
190. Thomas, R.; Al-Khadairi, G.; Roelands, J.; Hendrickx, W.; Dermime, S.; Bedognetti, D.; Decock, J. NY-ESO-1 based immunotherapy of cancer: Current perspectives. *Front. Immunol.* **2018**, *9*, 947. [CrossRef]
191. Chomez, P.; De Backer, O.; Bertrand, M.; De Plaen, E.; Boon, T.; Lucas, S. An overview of the MAGE gene family with the identification of all human members of the family. *Cancer Res.* **2001**, *61*, 5544–5551. [PubMed]
192. Fennemann, F.L.; De Vries, I.J.M.; Figdor, C.G.; Verdoes, M. Attacking tumors from all sides: Personalized multiplex vaccines to tackle intratumor heterogeneity. *Front. Immunol.* **2019**, *10*, 824. [CrossRef] [PubMed]
193. Ning, N.; Pan, Q.; Zheng, F.; Teitz-Tennenbaum, S.; Egenti, M.; Yet, J.; Li, M.; Ginestier, C.; Wicha, M.S.; Moyer, J.S.; et al. Cancer stem cell vaccination confers significant antitumor immunity. *Cancer Res.* **2012**, *72*, 1853–1864. [CrossRef] [PubMed]
194. Constantino, J.; Gomes, C.; Falcão, A.; Neves, B.M.; Cruz, M.T. Dendritic cell-based immunotherapy: A basic review and recent advances. *Immunol. Res.* **2017**, *65*, 798–810. [CrossRef] [PubMed]
195. Boudreau, J.E.; Bonehill, A.; Thielemans, K.; Wan, Y. Engineering dendritic cells to enhance cancer immunotherapy. *Mol. Ther.* **2011**, *19*, 841–853. [CrossRef]
196. Tagliamonte, M.; Petrizzo, A.; Tornesello, M.L.; Buonaguro, F.M.; Buonaguro, L. Antigen-specific vaccines for cancer treatment. *Hum. Vaccines Immunother.* **2014**, *10*, 3332–3346. [CrossRef]
197. Stanton, S.E.; Gad, E.; Corulli, L.R.; Lu, H.; Disis, M.L. Tumor-associated antigens identified early in mouse mammary tumor development can be effective vaccine targets. *Vaccine* **2019**, *37*, 3552–3561. [CrossRef]
198. Jarnicki, A.G.; Conroy, H.; Brereton, C.; Donnelly, G.; Toomey, D.; Walsh, K.; Sweeney, C.; Leavy, O.; Fletcher, J.; Lavelle, E.C.; et al. Attenuating regulatory T cell induction by TLR agonists through inhibition of p38 MAPK signaling in dendritic cells enhances their efficacy as vaccine adjuvants and cancer immunotherapeutics. *J. Immunol.* **2008**, *180*, 3797–3806. [CrossRef]
199. Goutagny, N.; Estornes, Y.; Hasan, U.; Lebecque, S.; Caux, C. Targeting pattern recognition receptors in cancer immunotherapy. *Target. Oncol.* **2012**, *7*, 29–54. [CrossRef]

200. Wölfle, S.J.; Strebovsky, J.; Bartz, H.; Sähr, A.; Arnold, C.; Kaiser, C.; Dalpke, A.H.; Heeg, K. PD-L1 expression n tolerogenic APCs is controlled by STAT-3. *Eur. J. Immunol.* **2011**, *41*, 413–424. [CrossRef]
201. Fend, L.; Yamazaki, T.; Remy, C.; Fahrner, C.; Gantzer, M.; Nourtier, V.; Préville, X.; Quéméneur, E.; Kepp, O.; Adam, J.; et al. Immune checkpoint blockade, immunogenic chemotherapy or IFN-α blockade boost the local and abscopal effects of oncolytic virotherapy. *Cancer Res.* **2017**, *77*, 4146–4157. [CrossRef]
202. Lichty, B.D.; Breitbach, C.J.; Stojdl, D.F.; Bell, J.C. Going viral with cancer immunotherapy. *Nat. Rev. Cancer* **2014**, *14*, 559–567. [CrossRef] [PubMed]
203. Qureshy, Z.; Johnson, D.E.; Grandis, J.R. Targeting the JAK/STAT pathway in solid tumors. *J. Cancer Metastasis Treat.* **2020**, *6*, 27. [CrossRef]
204. Marelli, G.; Howells, A.; Lemoine, N.R.; Wang, Y. Oncolytic viral therapy and the immune system: A double-edged sword against cancer. *Front. Immunol.* **2018**, *9*, 866. [CrossRef] [PubMed]
205. Felt, S.A.; Moerdyk-Schauwecker, M.J.; Grdzelishvili, V.Z. Induction of apoptosis in pancreatic cancer cells by vesicular stomatitis virus. *Virology* **2015**, *474*, 163–173. [CrossRef] [PubMed]
206. Kanerva, A.; Nokisalmi, P.; Diaconu, I.; Koski, A.; Cerullo, V.; Liikanen, I.; Tähtinen, S.; Oksanen, M.; Heiskanen, R.; Pesonen, S.; et al. Antiviral and antitumor T-cell immunity in patients treated with GM-CSF-coding oncolytic adenovirus. *Clin. Cancer Res.* **2013**, *19*, 2734–2744. [CrossRef] [PubMed]
207. Angelova, A.L.; Grekova, S.P.; Heller, A.; Kuhlmann, O.; Soyka, E.; Giese, T.; Aprahamian, M.; Bour, G.; Rüffer, S.; Cziepluch, C.; et al. Complementary induction of immunogenic cell death by oncolytic parvovirus H-1PV and gemcitabine in pancreatic cancer. *J. Virol.* **2014**, *88*, 5263–5276. [CrossRef]
208. Shi, T.; Song, X.; Wang, Y.; Liu, F.; Wei, J. Combining oncolytic viruses with cancer immunotherapy: Establishing a new generation of cancer treatment. *Front. Immunol.* **2020**, *11*, 683. [CrossRef]
209. Ribas, A.; Dummer, R.; Puzanov, I.; VanderWalde, A.; Andtbacka, R.H.I.; Michielin, O.; Olszanski, A.J.; Malvehy, J.; Cebon, J.; Fernandez, E.; et al. Oncolytic virotherapy promotes intratumoral T cell infiltration and improves Anti-PD-1 immunotherapy. *Cell* **2017**, *170*, 1109–1119. [CrossRef]
210. Soliman, H.; Hogue, D.; Han, H.; Mooney, B.; Costa, R.; Lee, M.C.; Niell, B.; Khakapour, N.; Weinfurtner, R.J.; Hoover, S.; et al. Abstract CT040: A phase I trial of talimogene laherparepvec combined with neoadjuvant chemotherapy for non-metastatic triple negative breast cancer. *Clinical Trials* **2019**, *79*, CT040. [CrossRef]
211. Woller, N.; Knocke, S.; Mundt, B.; Gürlevik, E.; Strüver, N.; Kloos, A.; Boozari, B.; Schache, P.; Manns, M.P.; Malek, N.P.; et al. Virus-induced tumor inflammation facilitates effective DC cancer immunotherapy in a Treg-dependent manner in mice. *J. Clin. Investig.* **2011**, *121*, 2570–2582. [CrossRef] [PubMed]
212. Pol, J.G.; Acuna, S.A.; Yadollahi, B.; Tang, N.; Stephenson, K.B.; Atherton, M.J.; Hanwell, D.; El-Warrak, A.; Goldstein, A.; Moloo, B.; et al. Preclinical evaluation of a MAGE-A3 vaccination utilizing the oncolytic Maraba virus currently in first-in-human trials. *OncoImmunology* **2019**, *8*, e1512329. [CrossRef] [PubMed]
213. Singh, N.; June, C.H. Boosting engineered T cells. *Science* **2019**, *365*, 119–120. [CrossRef] [PubMed]
214. Ma, L.; Dichwalkar, T.; Chang, J.Y.; Cossette, B.; Garafola, D.; Zhang, A.Q.; Fichter, M.; Wang, C.; Liang, S.; Silva, M.; et al. Enhanced CAR-T cell activity against solid tumors by vaccine boosting through the chimeric receptor. *Science* **2019**, *365*, 162–168.
215. Giavridis, T.; Stegen, S.J.C.V.D.; Eyquem, J.; Hamieh, M.; Piersigilli, A.; Sadelain, M. CAR T cell-induced cytokine release syndrome is mediated by macrophages and ablated by IL-1 blockade. *Nat. Med.* **2018**, *24*, 731–738. [CrossRef]
216. Zhou, R.; Yazdanifar, M.; Das Roy, L.; Whilding, L.M.; Gavrill, A.; Maher, J.; Mukherjee, P. CAR T cells targeting the tumor MUC1 glycoprotein reduce triple-negative breast cancer growth. *Front. Immunol.* **2019**, *10*, 1149. [CrossRef]
217. Byrd, T.T.; Fousek, K.; Pignata, A.; Szot, C.; Samaha, H.; Seaman, S.; Dobrolecki, L.; Salsman, V.S.; Oo, H.Z.; Bielamowicz, K.; et al. TEM8/ANTXR1-Specific CAR T cells as a targeted therapy for triple-negative breast cancer. *Cancer Res.* **2018**, *78*, 489–500. [CrossRef]
218. Zhao, X.; Qu, J.; Hui, Y.; Zhang, H.; Sun, Y.; Liu, X.; Zhao, X.; Zhao, Z.; Yang, Q.; Wang, F.; et al. Clinicopathological and prognostic significance of c-Met overexpression in breast cancer. *Oncotarget* **2017**, *8*, 56758–56767. [CrossRef]
219. Tchou, J.; Zhao, Y.; Levine, B.L.; Zhang, P.J.; Davis, M.M.; Melenhorst, J.J.; Kulikovskaya, I.; Brennan, A.L.; Liu, X.; Lacey, S.F.; et al. Safety and efficacy of intratumoral injections of chimeric antigen receptor (CAR) T cells in metastatic breast cancer. *Cancer Immunol. Res.* **2017**, *5*, 1152–1161. [CrossRef]

220. Han, Y.; Xie, W.; Song, D.-G.; Powell, D.J., Jr. Control of triple-negative breast cancer using ex vivo self-enriched, costimulated NKG2D CAR T cells. *J. Hematol. Oncol.* **2018**, *11*, 92. [CrossRef]
221. Abdel-Latif, M.; Youness, R.A. Why natural killer cells in triple negative breast cancer? *World J. Clin. Oncol.* **2020**, *11*, 464–476. [CrossRef] [PubMed]
222. Dupuy, F.; Tabariès, S.; Andrzejewski, S.; Dong, Z.; Blagih, J.; Annis, M.G.; Omeroglu, A.; Gao, D.; Leung, S.; Amir, E.; et al. PDK1-Dependent metabolic reprogramming dictates metastatic potential in breast cancer. *Cell Metab.* **2015**, *22*, 577–589. [CrossRef] [PubMed]
223. Vanhove, K.; Graulus, G.-J.; Mesotten, L.; Thomeer, M.; Derveaux, E.; Noben, J.-P.; Guedens, W.; Adriaensens, P. The metabolic landscape of lung cancer: New insights in a disturbed glucose metabolism. *Front. Oncol.* **2019**, *9*, 1215. [CrossRef] [PubMed]
224. Lanning, N.J.; Castle, J.P.; Singh, S.J.; Leon, A.N.; Tovar, E.A.; Sanghera, A.; MacKeigan, J.P.; Filipp, F.V.; Graveel, C.R. Metabolic profiling of triple-negative breast cancer cells reveals metabolic vulnerabilities. *Cancer Metab.* **2017**, *5*, 6. [CrossRef] [PubMed]
225. Choi, J.; Jung, W.-H.; Koo, J.S. Metabolism-Related proteins are differentially expressed according to the molecular subtype of invasive breast cancer defined by surrogate immunohistochemistry. *Pathobiology* **2013**, *80*, 41–52. [CrossRef]
226. Romero-Cordoba, S.L.; Rodriguez-Cuevas, S.; Bautista-Pina, V.; Maffuz-Aziz, A.; D'Ippolito, E.; Cosentino, G.; Baroni, S.; Iorio, M.V.; Hidalgo-Miranda, A. Loss of function of miR-342-3p results in MCT1 over-expression and contributes to oncogenic metabolic reprogramming in triple negative breast cancer. *Sci. Rep.* **2018**, *8*, 12252. [CrossRef]
227. Avanzato, D.; Pupo, E.; Ducano, N.; Isella, C.; Bertalot, G.; Luise, C.; Pece, S.; Bruna, A.; Rueda, O.M.; Caldas, C.; et al. High USP6NL levels in breast cancer sustain chronic AKT phosphorylation and GLUT1 stability fueling aerobic glycolysis. *Cancer Res.* **2018**, *78*, 3432–3444. [CrossRef]
228. Ma, T.; Liu, H.; Liu, Y.; Liu, T.; Wang, H.; Qiao, F.; Song, L.; Zhang, L. USP6NL mediated by LINC00689/miR-142-3p promotes the development of triple-negative breast cancer. *BMC Cancer* **2020**, *20*, 998. [CrossRef]
229. Shen, L.; O'Shea, J.M.; Kaadige, M.R.; Cunha, S.; Wilde, B.R.; Cohen, A.L.; Welm, A.L.; Ayer, D.E. Metabolic reprogramming in triple-negative breast cancer through Myc suppression of TXNIP. *Proc. Natl. Acad. Sci. USA* **2018**, *112*, 5425–5430. [CrossRef]
230. Park, J.H.; Vithayathil, S.; Kumar, S.; Sung, P.-L.; Dobrolecki, L.E.; Putluri, V.; Bhat, V.B.; Bhowmik, S.K.; Gupta, V.; Arora, K.; et al. Fatty acid oxidation-driven Src links mitochondrial energy reprogramming and oncogenic properties in triple-negative breast cancer. *Cell Rep.* **2016**, *14*, 2154–2165. [CrossRef]
231. Bellone, M.; Calcinotto, A.; Filipazzi, P.; De Milito, A.; Fais, S.; Rivoltini, L. The acidity of the tumor microenvironment is a mechanism of immune escape that can be overcome by proton pump inhibitors. *OncoImmunology* **2013**, *2*, e22058. [CrossRef] [PubMed]
232. Díaz, F.E.; Dantas, E.; Geffner, J. Unravelling the interplay between extracellular acidosis and immune cells. *Mediat. Inflamm.* **2018**, *2018*, 1–11. [CrossRef] [PubMed]
233. Huang, X.; Xie, X.; Wang, H.; Xiao, X.; Yang, L.; Tian, Z.; Guo, X.; Zhang, L.; Tang, H.; Xie, X. PDL1 and LDHA act as ceRNAs in triple negative breast cancer by regulating miR-34a. *J. Exp. Clin. Cancer Res.* **2017**, *36*, 129. [CrossRef]
234. Feng, J.; Yang, H.; Zhang, Y.; Wei, H.; Zhu, Z.; Zhu, B.; Yang, M.; Cao, W.; Wang, L.; Wu, Z. Tumor cell-derived lactate induces TAZ-dependent upregulation of PD-L1 through GPR81 in human lung cancer cells. *Oncogene* **2017**, *36*, 5829–5839. [CrossRef] [PubMed]
235. Sprowl-Tanio, S.; Habowski, A.N.; Pate, K.T.; McQuade, M.M.; Wang, K.; Edwards, R.A.; Grun, F.; Lyou, Y.; Waterman, M.L. Lactate/pyruvate transporter MCT-1 is a direct Wnt target that confers sensitivity to 3-bromopyruvate in colon cancer. *Cancer Metab.* **2016**, *4*, 20. [CrossRef]
236. Van Geldermalsen, M.; Wang, Q.; Nagarajah, R.; Marshall, A.D.; Thoeng, A.; Gao, D.; Ritchie, W.; Feng, Y.; Bailey, C.G.; Deng, N.; et al. ASCT2/SLC1A5 controls glutamine uptake and tumour growth in triple-negative basal-like breast cancer. *Oncogene* **2016**, *35*, 3201–3208. [CrossRef]
237. Lampa, M.; Arlt, H.; Christopher, W.; Ospina, B.; Reeves, J.; Zhang, B.; Murtie, J.; Deng, G.; Barberis, C.; Hoffmann, D.; et al. Glutaminase is essential for the growth of triple-negative breast cancer cells with a deregulated glutamine metabolism pathway and its suppression synergizes with mTOR inhibition. *PLoS ONE* **2017**, *12*, e0185092. [CrossRef]

238. Leone, R.D.; Zhao, L.; Englert, J.M.; Sun, I.-M.; Oh, M.-H.; Arwood, M.L.; Bettencourt, I.A.; Patel, C.H.; Wen, J.; Tam, A.; et al. Glutamine blockade induces divergent metabolic programs to overcome tumor immune evasion. *Science* **2019**, *366*, 1013–1021. [CrossRef]
239. Ogrodzinski, M.P.; Bernard, J.J.; Lunt, S.Y. Deciphering metabolic rewiring in breast cancer subtypes. *Transl. Res.* **2017**, *189*, 105–122. [CrossRef]
240. Han, S.; Wei, R.; Zhang, X.; Jiang, N.; Fan, M.; Huang, J.H.; Xie, B.; Zhang, L.; Miao, W.; Butler, A.C.-P.; et al. CPT1A/2-Mediated FAO enhancement—A metabolic target in radioresistant breast cancer. *Front. Oncol.* **2019**, *9*, 1201. [CrossRef]
241. Wang, T.; Fahrmann, J.F.; Lee, H.; Li, Y.J.; Tripathi, S.C.; Yue, C.; Zhang, C.; Lifshitz, V.; Song, J.; Yuan, Y.; et al. JAK/STAT3-Regulated fatty acid β-oxidation is critical for breast cancer stem cell self-renewal and chemoresistance. *Cell Metab.* **2018**, *27*, 136–150. [CrossRef] [PubMed]
242. Casciano, J.C.; Perry, C.; Cohen-Nowak, A.J.; Miller, K.D.; Voorde, J.V.; Zhang, Q.; Chalmers, S.; Sandison, M.E.; Liu, Q.; Hedley, A.; et al. MYC regulates fatty acid metabolism through a multigenic program in claudin-low triple negative breast cancer. *Br. J. Cancer* **2020**, *122*, 868–884. [CrossRef] [PubMed]
243. Miska, J.; Lee-Chang, C.; Rashidi, A.; Muroski, M.E.; Chang, A.L.; Lopez-Rosas, A.; Zhang, P.; Panek, W.K.; Cordero, A.; Han, Y.; et al. HIF-1α is a metabolic switch between glycolytic-driven migration and oxidative phosphorylation-driven immunosuppression of Tregs in Glioblastoma. *Cell Rep.* **2019**, *27*, 226–237.e4. [CrossRef] [PubMed]
244. Xu, T.; Stewart, K.M.; Wang, X.; Liu, K.; Xie, M.; Ryu, J.K.; Li, K.; Ma, T.; Wang, H.; Ni, L.; et al. Metabolic control of Th17 and induced Treg cell balance by an epigenetic mechanism. *Nature* **2017**, *548*, 228–233. [CrossRef]
245. Camarda, R.; Zhou, A.Y.; Kohnz, R.A.; Balakrishnan, S.; Mahieu, C.; Anderton, B.; Eyob, H.; Kajimura, S.; Tward, A.; Krings, G.; et al. Inhibition of fatty acid oxidation as a therapy for MYC-overexpressing triple-negative breast cancer. *Nat. Med.* **2016**, *22*, 427–432. [CrossRef]
246. Kuzu, O.F.; Noory, M.A.; Robertson, G.P. The role of cholesterol in cancer. *Cancer Res.* **2018**, *76*, 2063–2070. [CrossRef]
247. Szlasa, W.; Zendran, I.; ZalesiŃska, A.; Tarek, M.; Kulbacka, J. Lipid composition of the cancer cell membrane. *J. Bioenerg. Biomembr.* **2020**, *52*, 321–342. [CrossRef]
248. Ehmsen, S.; Pedersen, M.H.; Wang, G.; Terp, M.G.; Arslanagic, A.; Hood, B.L.; Conrads, T.P.; Leth-Larsen, R.; Ditzel, H.J. Increased cholesterol biosynthesis is a key characteristic of breast cancer stem cells influencing patient outcome. *Cell Rep.* **2019**, *27*, 3927–3938.e6. [CrossRef]
249. Cai, D.; Zhang, X.; Chen, H.-W. A master regulator of cholesterol biosynthesis constitutes a therapeutic liability of triple negative breast cancer. *Mol. Cell. Oncol.* **2020**, *7*, 1701362. [CrossRef]
250. Shaitelman, S.F.; Stauder, M.C.; Allen, P.; Reddy, S.; Lakoski, S.; Atkinson, B.; Reddy, J.P.; Amaya, D.; Guerra, W.; Ueno, N.; et al. Impact of statin use on outcomes in triple negative breast cancer. *J. Cancer* **2017**, *8*, 2026–2032. [CrossRef]
251. Sorrentino, G.; Ruggeri, N.; Specchia, V.; Cordenonsi, M.; Mano, M.; Dupont, S.; Manfrin, A.; Ingallina, E.; Sommaggio, R.; Piazza, S.; et al. Metabolic control of YAP and TAZ by the mevalonate pathway. *Nat. Cell Biol.* **2014**, *16*, 357–366. [CrossRef] [PubMed]
252. Momtazi-Borojeni, A.A.; Nik, M.E.; Jaafari, M.R.; Banach, M.; Sahebkar, A. Effects of immunization against PCSK9 in an experimental model of breast cancer. *Arch. Med. Sci.* **2019**, *15*, 570–579. [CrossRef] [PubMed]
253. Bietz, A.; Zhu, H.; Xue, M.; Xu, C. Cholesterol metabolism in T Cells. *Front. Immunol.* **2017**, *8*, 1664. [CrossRef] [PubMed]
254. Ma, X.; Bi, E.; Lu, Y.; Su, P.; Huang, C.; Liu, L.; Wang, Q.; Yang, M.; Kalady, M.F.; Qian, J.; et al. Cholesterol induces CD8+ T cell exhaustion in the tumor microenvironment. *Cell Metab.* **2019**, *30*, 143–156.e5. [CrossRef]
255. Bharti, S.K.; Mironchik, Y.; Wildes, F.; Penet, M.-F.; Goggins, E.; Krishnamachary, B.; Bhujwalla, Z.M. Metabolic consequences of HIF silencing in a triple negative human breast cancer xenograft. *Oncotarget* **2018**, *9*, 15326–15339. [CrossRef]
256. Pérez-Hernández, M.; Arias, A.; Martínez-García, D.; Pérez-Tomás, R.; Quesada, R.; Soto-Cerrato, V. Targeting autophagy for cancer treatment and tumor chemosensitization. *Cancers* **2019**, *11*, 1599. [CrossRef]
257. Zhao, H.; Yang, M.; Zhao, J.; Wang, J.; Zhang, Y.; Zhang, Q. High expression of LC3B is associated with progression and poor outcome in triple-negative breast cancer. *Med. Oncol.* **2013**, *30*, 475. [CrossRef]

258. Zhang, Q.; Zhang, Y.; Zhang, P.; Chao, Z.; Xia, F.; Jiang, C.C.; Zhang, X.D.; Jiang, Z.; Liu, H. Hexokinase II inhibitor, 3-BrPA induced autophagy by stimulating ROS formation in human breast cancer cells. *Genes Cancer* **2014**, *5*, 100–112. [CrossRef]
259. Li, M.; Liu, J.; Li, S.; Feng, Y.; Yi, F.; Wang, L.; Wei, S.; Cao, L. Autophagy-related 7 modulates tumor progression in triple-negative breast cancer. *Lab. Investig.* **2019**, *99*, 1266–1274. [CrossRef]
260. Qiao, Z.; Li, X.; Kang, N.; Yang, Y.; Chen, C.; Wu, T.; Zhao, M.; Liu, Y.; Ji, X. A novel specific Anti-CD73 antibody inhibits triple-negative breast cancer cell motility by regulating autophagy. *Int. J. Mol. Sci.* **2019**, *20*, 1057. [CrossRef]
261. Wen, J.; Yeo, S.; Wang, C.; Chen, S.; Sun, S.; Haas, M.A.; Tu, W.; Jin, F.; Guan, J.-L. Autophagy inhibition re-sensitizes pulse stimulation-selected paclitaxel-resistant triple negative breast cancer cells to chemotherapy-induced apoptosis. *Breast Cancer Res. Treat.* **2015**, *149*, 619–629. [CrossRef]
262. Halama, A.; Kulinski, M.; Dib, S.S.; Zaghlool, S.B.; Siveen, K.S.; Iskandarani, A.; Zierer, J.; Prabhu, K.S.; Satheesh, N.J.; Bhagwat, A.M.; et al. Accelerated lipid catabolism and autophagy are cancer survival mechanisms under inhibited glutaminolysis. *Cancer Lett.* **2018**, *430*, 133–147. [CrossRef] [PubMed]
263. Bosc, C.; Broin, N.; Fanjul, M.; Saland, E.; Farge, T.; Courdy, C.; Batut, A.; Masoud, R.; Larrue, C.; Skuli, S.; et al. Autophagy regulates fatty acid availability for oxidative phosphorylation through mitochondria-endoplasmic reticulum contact sites. *Nat. Commun.* **2020**, *11*, 4056. [CrossRef] [PubMed]
264. Li, Z.-L.; Zhang, H.-L.; Huang, Y.; Huang, J.-H.; Sun, P.; Zhou, N.-N.; Chen, Y.-H.; Mai, J.; Wang, Y.; Yu, Y.; et al. Autophagy deficiency promotes triple-negative breast cancer resistance to T cell-mediated cytotoxicity by blocking tenascin-C degradation. *Nat. Commun.* **2020**, *11*, 3806. [CrossRef] [PubMed]
265. Du, Y.; Wei, N.; Ma, R.; Jiang, S.; Song, D. A miR-210-3p regulon that controls the warburg effect by modulating HIF-1α and p53 activity in triple-negative breast cancer. *Cell Death Dis.* **2020**, *11*, 731. [CrossRef]
266. Lee, S.; Hallis, S.P.; Jung, K.-A.; Ryu, D.; Kwak, M.-K. Impairment of HIF-1α-mediated metabolic adaption by NRF2-silencing in breast cancer cells. *Redox Biol.* **2019**, *24*, 101210. [CrossRef] [PubMed]
267. Lan, J.; Lu, H.; Samanta, D.; Salman, S.; Lu, Y.; Semenza, G.L. Hypoxia-inducible factor 1-dependent expression of adenosine receptor 2B promotes breast cancer stem cell enrichment. *Proc. Natl. Acad. Sci. USA* **2018**, *115*, E9640–E9648. [CrossRef]
268. Zhang, H.; Lu, H.; Xiang, L.; Bullen, J.W.; Zhang, C.; Samanta, D.; Gilkes, D.M.; He, J.; Semenza, G.L. HIF-1 regulates CD47 expression in breast cancer cells to promote evasion of phagocytosis and maintenance of cancer stem cells. *Proc. Natl. Acad. Sci. USA* **2015**, *112*, E6215–E6223. [CrossRef]
269. Liu, X.; Kwon, H.; Li, Z.; Fu, Y.-X. Is CD47 an innate immune checkpoint for tumor evasion? *J. Hematol. Oncol.* **2017**, *10*, 12. [CrossRef]
270. Yuan, J.; Shi, X.; Chen, C.; He, H.; Liu, L.; Wu, J.; Yan, H. High expression of CD47 in triple negative breast cancer is associated with epithelial-mesenchymal transition and poor prognosis. *Oncol. Lett.* **2019**, *18*, 3249–3255. [CrossRef]
271. Zhang, W.; Huang, Q.; Xiao, W.; Zhao, Y.; Pi, J.; Xu, H.; Zhao, H.; Xu, J.; Evans, C.; Jin, H. Advances in anti-tumor treatments targeting the CD47/SIRPα axis. *Front. Immunol.* **2020**, *11*, 18. [CrossRef] [PubMed]
272. Gu, S.; Ni, T.; Wang, J.; Liu, Y.; Fan, Q.; Wang, Y.; Huang, T.; Chu, Y.; Sun, X.; Wang, Y. CD47 blockade inhibits tumor progression through promoting phagocytosis of tumor cells by M2 polarized macrophages in endometrial cancer. *J. Immunol. Res.* **2018**, *2018*, 6156757. [CrossRef] [PubMed]
273. Ingram, J.R.; Blomberg, O.S.; Sockolosky, J.T.; Ali, L.; Schmidt, F.I.; Pishesha, N.; Espinosa, C.; Dougan, S.K.; Garcia, K.C.; Ploegh, H.L.; et al. Localized CD47 blockade enhances immunotherapy for murine melanoma. *Proc. Natl. Acad. Sci. USA* **2017**, *114*, 10184–10189. [CrossRef] [PubMed]
274. Kaur, S.; Elkahloun, A.G.; Singh, S.P.; Chen, Q.-R.; Meerzaman, D.M.; Song, T.; Manu, N.; Wu, W.; Mannan, P.; Garfield, S.H.; et al. A function-blocking CD47 antibody suppresses stem cell and EGF signaling in triple-negative breast cancer. *Oncotarget* **2016**, *7*, 10133–10152. [CrossRef]
275. Sikic, B.I.; Lakhani, N.; Patnaik, A.; Shah, S.A.; Chandana, S.R.; Rasco, D.; Colevas, A.D.; O'Rourke, T.; Narayanan, S.; Papadopoulos, K.; et al. First-in-Human, first-in-class phase I trial of the anti-CD47 antibody Hu5F9-G4 in patients with advanced cancers. *J. Clin. Oncol.* **2019**, *37*, 946–953. [CrossRef]

276. Hu, T.; Liu, H.; Liang, Z.; Wang, F.; Zhou, C.; Zheng, X.; Zhang, Y.; Song, Y.; Hu, J.; He, X.; et al. Tumor-intrinsic CD47 signal regulates glycolysis and promotes colorectal cancer cell growth and metastasis. *Theranostics* **2020**, *10*, 4056–4072. [CrossRef]
277. Noman, M.Z.; DeSantis, G.; Janji, B.; Hasmim, M.; Karray, S.; Dessen, P.; Bronte, V.; Chouaib, S. PD-L1 is a novel direct target of HIF-1α, and its blockade under hypoxia enhanced MDSC-mediated T cell activation. *J. Exp. Med.* **2014**, *211*, 781–790. [CrossRef]

Publisher's Note: MDPI stays neutral with regard to jurisdictional claims in published maps and institutional affiliations.

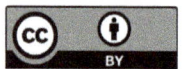

© 2020 by the authors. Licensee MDPI, Basel, Switzerland. This article is an open access article distributed under the terms and conditions of the Creative Commons Attribution (CC BY) license (http://creativecommons.org/licenses/by/4.0/).

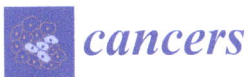

Review

Immunotherapy: A Challenge of Breast Cancer Treatment

Marilina García-Aranda [1,2,3,4] and Maximino Redondo [1,2,3,4,*]

1. Research Unit, Hospital Costa del Sol, Autovía A-7, km 187, 29603 Marbella, Spain; marilina@hcs.es
2. Research Network in Health Services in Chronic Diseases (Red de Investigación en Servicios de Salud en Enfermedades Crónicas, REDISSEC), Carlos III Health Institute (Instituto de Salud Carlos III). Av. de Monforte de Lemos, 5. 28029 Madrid, Spain
3. Malaga Biomedical Research Institute (Instituto de Investigación Biomédica de Málaga, IBIMA), Calle Doctor Miguel Díaz Recio, 28. 29010 Málaga, Spain
4. Surgery, Biochemistry and Immunology Department, School of Medicine, University of Malaga, 29010 Málaga, Spain
* Correspondence: mredondo@hcs.es

Received: 30 October 2019; Accepted: 18 November 2019; Published: 20 November 2019

Abstract: Breast cancer is the most commonly diagnosed cancer in women and is a leading cause of cancer death in women worldwide. Despite the significant benefit of the use of conventional chemotherapy and monoclonal antibodies in the prognosis of breast cancer patients and although the recent approval of the anti-PD-L1 antibody atezolizumab in combination with chemotherapy has been a milestone for the treatment of patients with metastatic triple-negative breast cancer, immunologic treatment of breast tumors remains a great challenge. In this review, we summarize current breast cancer classification and standard of care, the main obstacles that hinder the success of immunotherapies in breast cancer patients, as well as different approaches that could be useful to enhance the response of breast tumors to immunotherapies.

Keywords: immunotherapy; breast cancer; resistance; checkpoint; targeted treatment; personalized medicine

1. Introduction

1.1. Breast Cancer

According to the last Global Cancer Statistics (GLOBOCAN 2018), breast cancer represented 11.6% of all cancers, which places this disease as the second most commonly diagnosed cancer after lung cancer, and caused 6.6% of the total cancer deaths in 2018 [1]. Among women, incidence rates for breast cancer significantly exceeded those for other cancers in both transitioned and transitioning countries, remaining as the most frequently diagnosed cancer and the leading cause of cancer death in women worldwide [1].

Although for the majority of breast cancer patients it is not possible to identify a specific risk factor [2], these are diverse and well documented and include obesity, physical inactivity, alcohol consumption, use of hormone therapy, high breast density, and hereditary susceptibility due to mutations in autosomal dominant genes [3], which represents between 5–10% of all breast cancer cases in women [3]. Among these genetic alterations, mutations affecting *BRCA1* and *BRCA2* genes, which control DNA repair and transcriptional regulation in response to DNA damage, can lead to the accumulation of genetic alterations and greatly increase lifetime risk to develop different types of malignancies, including breast cancer [4]. Indeed, mutations in BRCA1 and BRCA2 genes are associated with an increased risk of inherited breast and ovarian cancer, representing the strongest susceptibility markers that have been identified for breast cancer worldwide, with an estimated 45–80% lifetime risk of breast cancer for BRCA1-BRCA2 mutation carriers [4]. In a similar manner, mutations affecting *TP53* are also related to triple negative breast cancer [3].

As with other types of cancer, early diagnosis greatly increases the chances for successful treatment, allowing for a 20% reduction in overall mortality rates [5]. In this regard, despite reported handicaps of screening programs like high overdiagnosis rates and costs, risks that are derived from ionizing radiation, or false positive biopsy recommendations, both mammography, breast self-examinations, clinical breast examinations, digital breast tomosynthesis, ultrasonography, magnetic resonance imaging, and oncogene identification represent the main tools for early diagnosis, sorting out, and prevention of risk factors as well as timely treatment to lessen breast cancer morbidity [5].

Besides screening programs, adjuvant chemotherapy has also had a significant impact on the prognosis of breast cancer patients, having significantly improved their overall survival, disease-free survival [6], and death rates related to breast-cancer since the early 1990s [7]. In this respect, breast cancer has traditionally been classified into three subtypes with different prognoses and treatment responses [8,9] (Table 1).

Table 1. Breast cancer classification and standard of care.

Subtype	Overview	Standard of Care
HR+: Luminal-A, Luminal-B	This subtype accounts for up to 75% of breast cancer tumor cases [10] and is characterized by being hormone receptor positive. Luminal A breast tumors, which represent 50–60% of all breast cancers, are defined as ER+ and/or PR+, HER2-, and low Ki67 (<14%) [9,10]. These tumors usually exhibit low histological grade, low mitotic activity, and good prognosis [10]. Luminal B tumors, which represent 15–20% of breast cancers, are defined as ER+ and/or PR+/- (PR<20% + Ki67≥14%) with HER2- as well as ER+ and/or PR+/- (any PR+ and any Ki67) and HER2+ [9,11]. These tumors are generally characterized by a more aggressive phenotype with a higher histological grade and proliferative index than Luminal A tumors [10]. Indeed, although Luminal B tumors respond better to neoadjuvant chemotherapy, they usually present worse prognoses [10].	Sensitive to hormone-targeted treatments, with a response rate of approximately 50–60%. Tamoxifen (TMX, Novaldex®) and aromatase inhibitors are the most common drugs that are used in clinical practice as first-line treatments. However, natural or acquired resistance to treatment along with long-term toxicities limit the effectiveness of the treatment [8].
HER2-Enriched	Constitutively activated in 20–30% of breast cancers, being responsible for dysregulated cell proliferation [12] and aggressive biological and clinical behavior [10]. These tumors are defined as ER-, PR-, and HER2+ [11].	Humanized monoclonal antibodies against HER2 extracellular domain and small kinase inhibitors [8]. Acquired resistance to treatment is a recurrent problem for HER2-enriched breast cancer patients.
Basal-Like	TNBC tumors, which constitute approximately 80% of the basal-like tumors and account for 10–15% of breast carcinomas [8], are defined as ER-, PR-, HER2-, CK5/6+, and/or EGFR+ [11].	Chemotherapy is the current standard of care for advanced TNBC despite limited efficacy and poor survival outcomes [13]. Different targeted treatments for TNBC are under pre-clinical or clinical development [13,14].

HR+: Positive for Hormone Receptors. ER+: Expressing Estrogen Receptors. PR+: Expressing Progesterone Receptors. HER2: Positive for Human Epidermal Growth Factor Receptor 2 (Receptor tyrosine-protein kinase ERBB2, CD340). TNBC: Triple Negative Breast Cancer. CK5/6+: Expressing cytokeratin 5/6. EGFR+: Expressing Epidermal Growth Factor Receptor.

Even though most breast cancer patients are diagnosed early enough to be successfully treated with surgery, chemotherapy, radiotherapy, or a combination thereof [8], nearly 30% of women that are initially diagnosed with early-stage disease will eventually develop a metastatic disease [7], which ultimately leads to patient death. In this scenario, and given their high efficacy and selectivity, the development of cancer immunotherapies and other treatment strategies targeting tumor cells have positioned themselves as promising options to win the battle against breast cancer in opposition to conventional treatments that lack tumor selectivity and cause more side effects.

1.2. Immunotherapy as an Option for Cancer Treatment

According to the cancer immunoediting model [15], the relation between tumor cells and the immune system is a dynamic process which consists of three main phases (Figure 1):

1. Elimination: During this phase, cancer cells are successfully recognized and destroyed by the body's immune system [16]. The success of the immune system to eliminate tumor cells depends on the ability of the antigen to trigger the immune response, or immunogenicity, which can be summarized as follows:

    - Genetic abnormalities lead to the production of new antigens by tumor cells, which are processed and presented as antigen-derived peptides on the cell surface in association with Human Leukocyte Antigen class I (HLA-I).
    - Neoantigens that are present in tumor microenvironment are recognized, processed, and presented on the surface of Antigen Presenting Cells (APCs) as antigen-derived peptides in association with Human Leukocyte Antigen class-II (HLA-II), which can be recognized by helper T-cell receptors and leads to B-cell and cytotoxic T-cell stimulation and maturation.
    - After T-cell activation by co-stimulatory signals provided by APCs, T-cells recognize neoantigens presented by HLA-I and attack the targeted tumor cell by the secretion of cytotoxic granules and/or via Fas cell surface death receptor (FAS) and caspase activation.

2. Equilibrium: During this phase, transformed cells with a resistant or non-immunogenic phenotype escape the elimination phase and proliferate, although the immune system is able to control the tumor growth [16].

3. Escape: The selective pressure caused by anti-cancer treatments or immune-surveillance promotes the uncontrolled proliferation of cells with a resistant or a non-immunogenic phenotype, leading to tumor progression and metastasis.

One of the characteristics of advanced tumors is their capability to evade adaptive immune responses [17], which would explain the direct relationship between tumor growth and immune evasion [18]. Since mechanisms leading to tumor evasion are diverse [19] (Table 2), a significant effort has been made in recent years to develop new strategies to trigger tumor cell death by stimulating the patient's natural defenses to recognize and destroy tumor cells.

Table 2. Immune system mechanisms of tumor evasion.

Target	Mechanism	Overview
Alterations in APCs	Inhibition of APC maturation and activation which impedes the appropriate co-stimulatory and cytokine signals to T cells and triggers the generation of regulatory T cells [20].	Different factors present in the tumor microenvironment such as IL-6, M-CSF, IL-10, VEGF, and TGF-β negatively regulate antigen-presenting cell functions [21].
	Selective increase in regulatory APCs that prevent immune responses by secreting TGF-β and stimulating the proliferation of regulatory T-cells [20].	Tumor microenvironment can induce a selective increase in the number of regulatory APCs, which can induce T-cell unresponsiveness by controlling T-cell polarity [20].

Table 2. Cont.

Target	Mechanism	Overview
Dysfunction of effector cells	Enhanced proliferation of regulatory T-cells that suppress inflammation and regulate immune system activity.	Tumor microenvironment induces the proliferation of regulatory T-cells, which are able to inhibit T-cell proliferation and cytokine production, leading to immune suppression, which favors the immune escape of tumor cells [20].
	Induction of effector T-cells apoptosis through tumor-generated CD95L and activation of the T-cell CD95 receptor.	CD95 and CD95L are critical survival factors for cancer cells that protect and promote cancer stem cells [22]. Apart from suppressing the immune response, CD95L promotes tumor growth and invasiveness and triggers the acquisition of cancer stem cell phenotypes [22].
	Alterations in T-cell signal transduction after antigen stimulation which leads to a decreased response.	Alterations such as the decreased expression of CD3ζ, p56^{lck}, and JAK-3, decreased mobilization of calcium signaling, inability to translocate NF-kB-p65, or decreased production of IL2 are frequently found in cancer patients [19].
Changes in tumor cells	Selection of tumor cells that are resistant to apoptosis, one of the hallmarks of cancer [17].	The pressure of immune surveillance or chemotherapeutic drugs enhances the selection and proliferation of cancer cells with mutations or alterations affecting one or various pathways controlling apoptosis.
	Alterations in HLA I expression.	Since the initiation of adaptive immune response occurs after T-cell receptor binding to antigen-loaded HLA-I presented by tumor cells, alterations in HLA-I expression, which is found in approximately 40–90% of human tumors derived from HLA-I positive tissues [23], impedes T-cell activation or causes loss of recognition.
	Alterations in the immune checkpoints.	After recognition of peptide antigen associated with the HLA-I, T-cell activation is controlled by co-stimulatory and co-inhibitory receptors and their ligands (immune-checkpoints). The over-expression of co-inhibitory molecules or the absence of co-stimulatory molecules typically leads to a T-cell exhausted phenotype.

CD95: Fas/APO-1. CD95L: CD95 ligand. APC: Antigen Presenting Cell/Dendritic Cell. HLA: Human Leukocyte Antigen. IL: Interleukin. JAK-3: Janus kinase 3. M-CSF: Macrophage Colony-Stimulating Factor. NF-kB: Nuclear Factor-kappa-B transcription complex. TGF: Transforming Growth Factor. VEGF: Vascular Endothelial Growth Factor.

These findings have been the basis for the development of different modalities of anticancer immunotherapy, including tumor-targeting immunotherapies, oncolytic viruses, anticancer vaccines, or adoptive cell immunotherapies [24] that are designed to target tumor cells and work with the immune system at different levels (Figure 2). As a result of the great success achieved in different studies and trials that demonstrate the efficacy of immunotherapies not only against primary tumors, but also preventing metastasis and recurrence [25], cancer immunotherapy has become the fourth pillar of cancer care, complementing surgery, cytotoxic therapy, and radiotherapy [26].

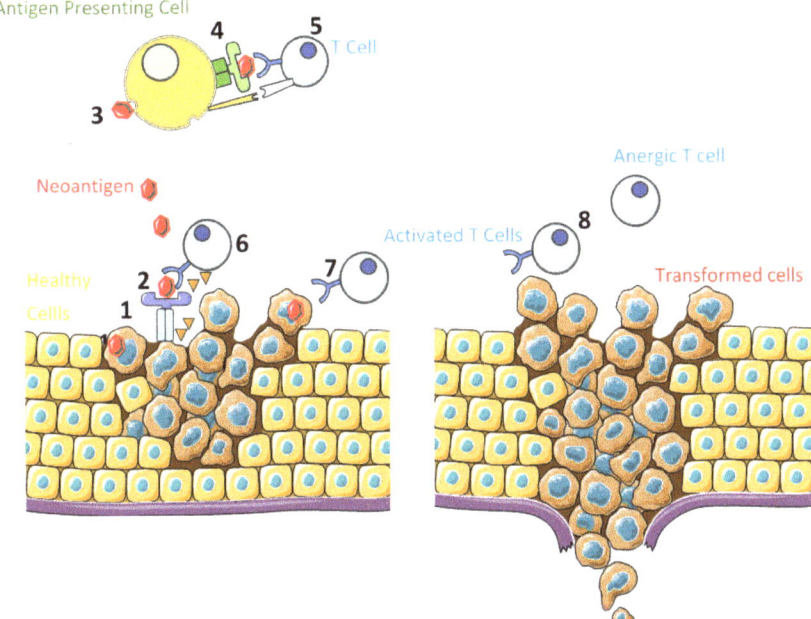

Figure 1. Cancer Immunoediting. ELIMINATION: (1) Neoantigen production by transformed cells. (2) Neoantigen presentation on the surface of transformed cells, associated with HLA-I. (3) Neoantigen recognition and processing by antigen presenting cells. (4) Neoantigen presentation on the surface of antigen presenting cells, associated with HLA-II. (5) T-cell activation in the presence of co-stimulatory signals. (6) Transformed cell recognition by activated T cells and elimination. EQUILIBRIUM: (7) Transformed cells with a resistant or non-immunogenic phenotype escape elimination and proliferate, although the immune system is still able to control the tumor growth. ESCAPE: (8) Uncontrolled proliferation of cells with a resistant or a non-immunogenic phenotype, leading to tumor progression and metastasis.

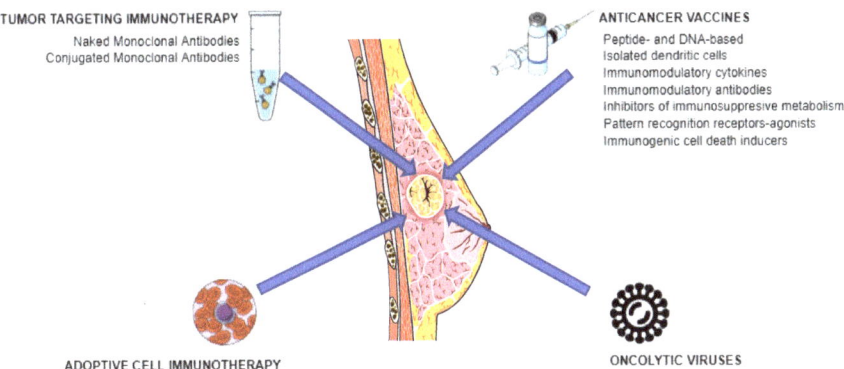

Figure 2. Modalities of cancer immunotherapy.

In this regard, the recent approval of treatments based on the use of checkpoint inhibitors has been a turning point for the treatment of patients with different tumors including melanoma, non-small cell lung cancer, renal cell carcinoma, Hodgkin's lymphoma, bladder cancer, head and neck squamous cell carcinoma, Merkel-cell carcinoma, microsatellite instability high, or mismatch repair deficient solid tumors [27], since they have demonstrated that they significantly increase survival rates when compared to standard therapy among different tumor types [23]. The impact of the basic studies allowed the development of checkpoint inhibitor therapies, which is the reason that James P. Allison and Tasuku Honjo won the Nobel Prize in Physiology and Medicine in 2018.

1.3. Checkpoint Inhibitors

Provided that activated $CD8^+$ (cytotoxic T lymphocytes or T-cells) recognize and destroy pathogen-infected or aberrant cells like cancer cells, they are considered the main effectors of cell-mediated immunity. On the other hand, since T cells also increase antibody responses through the action of CD4 (T-helper cells) and the enhancement of antibody production by B cells, their activation represents a critical step for the initiation and regulation of the immune response [28].

In accordance with the two-signal model of lymphocyte activation, both co-stimulatory signals and antigen-specific signals mediating the engagement of T-cell receptor (TCR) to HLA-II expressed on the surface of antigen-presenting cells participate in T-cell activation and maturation [29]. The subsequent response is regulated by a balance between co-stimulatory and inhibitory signals, or immune-checkpoints [30], at multiple steps during the immune response [31], which limits tissue damage and allows for the maintenance of self-tolerance. Given their immunosuppressive functions, dysregulated expression of inhibitory signals implies a major advantage in the tumor microenvironment, leading to immune evasion (Table 2).

Nowadays, and due to their association with the inhibition of lymphocyte activity and subsequent anergy, different immune checkpoint receptor-ligand combinations are the subject of intense study as tools for cancer treatment by restoring immune system function either as mono or in combination therapies [30,32]. Among these, and because of their central role during the immune response and peripheral tolerance, both Cytotoxic T-Lymphocyte-Associated Antigen 4 (CTLA4, CD152) and Programmed Cell Death Protein 1 (PD-1, CD279)/Programmed Cell Death Protein 1 Ligand (PD-L1, CD274) pathways have proved to be valid targets for the development of new cancer treatments and have allowed for the clinical approval of a number of CTLA and PD-1/PD-L1 checkpoint inhibitors (Table 3).

Table 3. Approved checkpoint inhibitors for cancer treatment.

Immune Checkpoint Target	Overview	Approved Drugs
CTLA4 (CD152)	One of the co-inhibitory proteins constitutively expressed on the surface of regulatory T cells (Tregs) and frequently upregulated in other types of T cells, like $CD4^+$ T, cells upon activation, and exhausted T cells, among other inhibitory receptors [33]. CTLA-4 blockade prevents interaction with CD80/86 resulting in up-regulation of T-cell activity.	Yervoy® (ipilimumab, Bristol Myers Squibb) was first approved by the FDA in 2011 and is classified as monotherapy for the treatment of advanced melanoma [34]. In combination with nivolumab (Opdivo®), ipilimumab is also classified as a first-line treatment for adult patients with intermediate/poor-risk advanced renal cell carcinoma, patients with nonresectable or metastatic melanoma across BRAF status, and previously treated MSI-H or dMMR metastatic colorectal cancer [35].
PD-1 (CD279)	PD-1 is one of the co-inhibitory membrane receptors of which its expression can be induced in active T cells upon stimulation of T-cell receptor complex or exposition to different cytokines [33]. Since PD-1 binding to its ligands, PD-L1 and PD-L2, leads to T-cell inactivation, PD-1 blockade enhances T cell-mediated immune responses.	Opdivo® (nivolumab, Bristol-Myers Squibb) is a PD-1 blocking antibody that, after first being approved by the FDA in 2014, is recommended for the treatment of advanced melanoma, advanced non-small cell lung cancer, advanced small cell lung cancer, advanced renal cell carcinoma, classical Hodgkin lymphoma, advanced squamous cell carcinoma of the head and neck, urothelial carcinoma, MSI-H or dMMR metastatic colorectal cancer, and hepatocellular carcinoma [36]. A combined regimen with ipilumumab increases progression-free survival and overall survival only in patients with low tumor PD-L1 expression [37].

Table 3. *Cont.*

Immune Checkpoint Target	Overview	Approved Drugs
PD-L1 (CD274)	One of the immune inhibitory receptor ligands expressed by hematopoietic, non-hematopoietic cells such as T-cells and B-cells and different types of tumor cells.	Keytruda® (pembrolizumab, Merck KGaA) is a human PD-1-blocking antibody that was first approved by the FDA in 2014 and is recommended for the treatment of advanced melanoma, non-small cell lung cancer, head and neck cancer squamous cell carcinoma, classical Hodgkin lymphoma, primary mediastinal large B-cell lymphoma, urothelial carcinoma, MSI-H cancer, gastric cancer, cervical cancer, hepatocellular carcinoma, Merkel cell carcinoma, and renal cell carcinoma [38].
		Libtayo® (cemiplimab-rwlc, Sanofi S.A.) is a PD-1 blocking antibody that was first approved by the FDA in 2018 and is indicated for the treatment of patients with metastatic cutaneous squamous cell carcinoma [39].
		Tecentriq® (atezolizumab, Genentech Inc.) is a PD-L1 blocking antibody that was first approved by the FDA in 2016 and is recommended for the treatment of advanced urothelial carcinoma, metastatic non-small cell lung cancer, and extensive-stage small cell lung cancer for use in combination with Abraxane® for the treatment of metastatic triple-negative breast cancer [38].
		Bavencio® (avelumab, Merck EMD Serono) is a PD-L1 blocking antibody that was first approved by the FDA in 2017 and is used for the treatment of patients with metastatic Merkel cell carcinoma, advanced or metastatic urothelial carcinoma, and in combination with axitinib for patients with advanced renal cell carcinoma [40].
		Imfizi® (durvalumab, AstraZeneca plc) is an anti PD-L1 human monoclonal antibody that was first approved by the FDA in 2017 and is used for the treatment of patients with unresectable non-small cell lung cancer that has not progressed after chemoradiation [41].

CTLA4: Cytotoxic T-lymphocyte associated protein 4; PD-1: Programmed Cell Death Protein 1; PD-L1: Programmed Cell Death Protein 1-Ligand; MSI-H: Microsatellite instability high; dMMR: Mismatch repair deficient.

As previously mentioned, apart from T-cell receptor interaction with HLA-II, T-cell activation is controlled by further antigen-independent costimulatory signals such as CD28 (Cluster of Differentiation 28) and CTLA-4. In this respect, and contrary to CD28 signals, which are required for T-cell activation and cytokine secretion, CTLA-4 signaling inhibits T-cell activation, which is especially important in lymph nodes where CTLA4 neutralizes potentially autoreactive T-cells at the initial stage of naïve CD4 and CD8 cell activation [31]. Both CD28 and CTLA-4 can be stimulated by CD80 (B7-1) and CD86 (B7-2) ligands that are expressed on activated APCs, leading to T-cell proliferation and differentiation through the production of growth cytokines when there is an elevated CD28:CD80/CD86 ratio [42] or to dephosphorylation of T-cell receptor signaling proteins by tyrosine phosphatases [43], leading to T-cell inactivation and anergy, in the case of an increased CTLA-4:CD80/CD86 ratio [42].

Since CTLA-4 binds to CD80/86 with very high affinity, this receptor mediates immunosuppression by competing for CD28 and also by inducing CD80/86 removal from antigen presenting cells' surface [33]. For this reason, by blocking the interaction between CTLA-4 and CD80/86 ligands, CTLA-4 inhibitors can prevent T-cells exhaustion and boost the antitumor T-cell response [44]. Despite the demonstrated survival benefit of ipilimumab in patients with advanced melanoma, severe immune-mediated adverse effects, high cost, and modest response rates (ranging between 4% and 16% when used in monotherapy) [44] remain as the main impediments for its use.

On the other hand, PD-1 predominantly regulates previously activated T-cells at the later stages of an immune response [31], mainly within tissue and tumors [30,31]. The expression of this membrane receptor, which can be temporarily induced in activated CD8 T-cells, natural killer T-cells, or myeloid cells following the activation and stimulation of T-cell receptor by cytokines and interleukin, is constitutive in T-cells exhibiting the exhausted phenotype [23]. PD-1 binding to its ligand, PD-L1, promotes the dephosphorylation of T-cell receptor proximal signal components and leads to the inhibition of signaling pathways commanded by protein kinases including PI3K/AKT (phosphoinositide 3-kinase/Protein Kinase B), PTEN (phosphatase and tensin homolog), CK2 (casein kinase 2) [37], and RAS/MEK/ERK (mitogen-activated protein kinase MAPK/extracellular-signal-regulated-kinase), which decreases T-cell proliferation, survival, cytokine production, and other effector functions [23]. Thus, by interrupting the interaction between PD-1 and PD-L1, checkpoint inhibitors can restore antitumor immune responses and promote immune-mediated elimination of tumor cells [32]. Although nivolumab alone or combined with ipilimumab significantly improves the overall and complete response rates compared with ipilimumab alone in patients with metastatic melanoma [45], response rates to PD-1/PD-L1 blocking therapies only ranges between 20–38% among different tumor types [23], which implies that the majority of advanced stage patients cannot benefit from these therapies.

Despite the low response rates and immune-related adverse events in some cancer patients, both CTLA4 and PD-1/PD-L1 inhibitors have broadly demonstrated their value to boost potent and durable anti-tumor responses and to increase the average life expectancy for metastatic cancer patients [23].

2. Breast Cancer Immunotherapy

2.1. First Approaches

The first cancer immunotherapy treatments were based on the use of humanized monoclonal antibodies with the ability to bind and neutralize a targeted altered molecule expressed by cancer cells and on which their survival and proliferation depends. The approval in September 1998 of trastuzumab (Herceptin®, Genentech, Inc., South San Francisco, CA, United States) represented the release of the first antibody for the treatment of metastatic breast cancer patients with HER2 (Receptor tyrosine-protein kinase ERBB2, CD340) overexpression and/or gene amplification, which represented a milestone in the treatment of breast cancer. After trastuzumab, other different anti-HER2 monoclonal antibodies including lapatinib (Tykerb®, GlaxoSmithKline, Brentford, United Kingdom), neratinib (Nerlynx®, Puma Biotechnology, Los Angeles, CA, United States), gefitinib (Iressa®, AstraZeneca, Cambridge, United Kingdom), or afatinib (Giotrif®, Boehringer Ingelheim Pharmaceuticals, Inc., Ingelheim am Rhein, Germany) [8] as monotherapy or in combination with conventional treatments have contributed to increasing the number of therapeutic options for breast cancer patients.

Although the use of monoclonal antibodies targeting altered proteins has definitely improved the outcome of cancer patients, modest response rates (Table 4) and resistance development [46] remain as the major impediments for treatment success and require the search for new approaches apart from combined therapies, among which antibody-drug conjugates (ADC) such as the recently FDA approved ado-trastuzumab emtansine (Kadcyla®, Genentech, Inc., South San Francisco, CA, United States) [47] and T cell bispecific antibodies stand out among the most promising strategies for breast cancer patients [48].

Table 4. Approved humanized monoclonal antibodies for breast cancer treatment.

Monoclonal Antibody	Response Rates (Monotherapy)	Most Common Treatment-Related Adverse Events
Trastuzumab	35% (95% CI, 24.4% to 44.7%) and none in patients with 3+ and 2+ HER2 overexpression by immunohistochemistry, respectively [49]. Further, 34% (95% CI, 23.9% to 45.7%) and 7% (95% CI, 0.8% to 22.8%) in patients with and without HER2 gene amplification by fluorescence in situ hybridization analysis, respectively [49]. Approximately 15% of patients relapse after therapy [50].	Chills (25%), asthenia (23%), fever (22%), pain (18%), nausea (14%), cardiac dysfunction (2%) [49].

Table 4. *Cont.*

Monoclonal Antibody	Response Rates (Monotherapy)	Most Common Treatment-Related Adverse Events
Pertuzumab	3% to 7.6% complete response and 16.7% partial response in previously trastuzumab-treated breast cancer patients [51,52].	Diarrhea (48.3%), Nausea (34.5%), vomiting (24%), fatigue (17%), asthenia (17%), back pain (10%) [51].
Lapatinib	24% in trastuzumab-naïve and less than 10% in trastuzumab-refractory breast tumors [53]. Partial response in 39% (95% CI, 30% to 48%) of patients with relapsed or refractory HER2-positive inflammatory breast cancer [54].	Diarrhea (59%), fatigue (20%), nausea (20%), rash (18%), anorexia (16%), dyspnoea (14%), vomiting (13%), back pain (11%) [54].
Neratinib	Pathological complete response in 56% of HER2-positive but HR- breast cancer patients compared to 33% in the control group. Further, 84% response rate in HER2-positive and hormone receptor-positive compared to a 59% response rate in HER2+ and hormone receptor-negative [55].	Diarrhea (83.9%), nausea (37.9%), abdominal pain (28.4%) [55].
Gefitinib	No complete or partial responses observed in previously treated patients with advanced breast cancer [56].	Diarrhea (45.2%), skin rash (12%) [56].
Afatinib	Partial response in 10% and progressive disease in 39% of extensively pretreated HER2-positive patients metastatic breast cancer progressing after trastuzumab. No complete response observed [57].	Diarrhea (24.4%), skin rash (9.8%) [57].

As a result of the latest studies in this field and in line with the encouraging long-term success of checkpoint inhibitors in the treatment of different tumors, distinct research groups have focused their efforts in developing analog treatments for breast cancer patients. In fact, as a result of the findings from the Phase III double-blind IMpassion130 trial (ClinicalTrials.gov ID NCT02425891), which reported a 40% reduced risk of disease progression or death in patients receiving atezolizumab plus nab-placlitaxel or placebo [58–60], in March 2019, the FDA approved the first checkpoint inhibitor immunotherapy drug, the anti-PD-L1 antibody atezolizumab (Tecentriq ®), in combination with chemotherapy (Abraxane®) for the treatment of triple-negative, metastatic breast cancer patients with positive PD-L1 protein expression [61]. However, despite this great milestone, modest complete response rates (7.1%, 95% CI, 4.9–9.9 and 10.3%, 95% CI, 6.3–15.6 in PD-L1 positive subgroup) and immune-mediated serious adverse events such as pneumonitis, hepatitis, colitis, and endocrinopathies that can cause treatment discontinuation [59] remain as notable impediments for the success of this treatment and justify the search of new therapeutic strategies.

2.2. Mechanisms of Immune Evasion in Breast Cancer

As stated above, tumor immune evasion can occur as a result of defective tumor-directed T-cell activation, deficient activated T-cell infiltration into the tumor microenvironment, or because of the tumor cell resistance to cytotoxic action of the immune cells [62].

2.2.1. Breast Tumor Microenvironment

Immunogenicity is defined as the ability to induce a humoral and/or cell-mediated adaptive immune response. In fact, both the burden of tumor mutations and the load of neo-epitopes represent two of the factors that are linked to response to checkpoint inhibitors in different malignancies like melanoma or lung cancer [63]. However, although tumor neoantigens that are produced as a result of breast cancer cells' genomic instability can be recognized by the immune system and induce T-cell responses and antitumor immunity [62,64], the immunogenicity of breast cancer can be rather heterogeneous, depending to a large extent on the specific subtype of breast cancer [65].

In the particular case of HER2-positive breast tumors, gene profiling studies have shown that highly suspicious calcifications are associated with decreased immune system activity and *ERBB2* overexpression [66]. For this reason, breast calcifications would be useful not only in the radiological assessment of breast lesions [67], but also in the management of breast cancer patient candidates for immunotherapy. On the other hand, although estrogen receptor-negative and HER2-positive have shown evidence of immunogenicity [65], these types of inflammatory breast tumors are rare (1–5% of cases) [68] when compared to triple negative breast tumors, which are unique among breast cancer subtypes in having strong antigen expression [69] and high stromal and tumor-infiltrating lymphocytes, parameters with a strong prognostic and predictive significance to immunotherapy and chemotherapy [62,63,70,71]. Accordingly, triple negative breast tumors with high infiltration of tumor-associated macrophages have been found to have a higher risk of metastasis and lower rates of disease-free survival and overall survival, having been proposed as potentially useful prognostic markers for triple negative breast cancer patients [72,73].

Except for these immunogenic subtypes, breast tumors have historically been classified as immunologically silent [62] or "cold" tumors, characterized by the presence of low mutation and neoantigen burden and few effector tumor infiltrating lymphocytes, factors proposed as prognostic markers [62], and metastasis to lymph nodes correlation [74].

Since non-inflamed tumors represent a significant impediment to the success of T-cell-based immunotherapies, different studies have aimed their efforts towards developing new strategies to increase the presence of immune infiltrates and hence, to improve patient prognosis. Among these, in addition to directly causing cell damage [75], the use of local tumor hyperthermia has proven to be a valuable tool as an immunotherapy strategy for cancer [76] by boosting immune cell activation and increasing the sensitivity of tumor cells to anti-tumor immune responses by different mechanisms, including:

- Enhancing the expression of tumor surface HLA class I polypeptide-related sequence A (MICA) and HLA type I, which promote tumor cell sensitivity to lysis by NK cells and CD8$^+$ cells, respectively [75].
- Increasing the release of heat shock proteins, which leads to NK cells activation as well as to APCs activation and antigen presentation to CD8$^+$ cells [75].
- Increasing the release of tumor cells exosomes, which apart from containing chemokines, transfer potential tumor antigens to APCs and subsequent CD8$^+$ activation [75].
- Promoting changes in the tumor vasculature, which facilitates better trafficking of immune cells between the tumor and draining lymph nodes [75].

In this context, different studies are reporting promising results for hyperthermia as complementary treatment to surgery, chemo, radio, and immunotherapy in breast cancer patients [75,77–79]. However, convincing data about the benefit of the combination of hyperthermia with checkpoint inhibitors for breast cancer treatment should be provided by multicenter clinical trials in which related side-effects are also evaluated [79]. Likewise, radiation has also shown to increase mutational load of tumors, optimize antigen presentation, and decrease immune suppressors in the tumor microenvironment, priming the tumor for immunotherapy [71], which justifies additional studies in these fields.

Besides the presence of high tumor infiltrating lymphocytes, recognition of tumor cells is a critical step for the success of the immune response. In this regard, although estrogen has an immunoenhancing impact on the immune system [80] with an apparent effect in all major innate and adaptive immune cells [81], high levels of estrogens may interfere with HLA-II expression and IFN-γ signaling, with significant implications for tumor immune escape [82]. Estrogens are also well known to be a risk factor for breast cancer by enhancing the expression of genes involved in tumor cell survival and proliferation as well as growth factors including vascular endothelial growth factor (VEGF) [83], epidermal growth factor (EGF), insulin growth factor (IGF), fibroblast growth factor (FGF) [69,84], and their receptors [8]. Since estrogen presence in tumor microenvironment can also play a significant immunosuppressive role by promoting tolerance of weakly immunogenic tumor cells [69], the use of antiestrogen therapies in combination with aromatase inhibitors could be a rational strategy to enhance the response to immunotherapies. However, although adjuvant hormonal therapy combined with HER2-targeted agents in hormone receptor-positive and HER2-positive breast cancer patients already represents a standard treatment, recent studies have shown that estrogen deprivation promotes transcriptional programs that favor immune evasion and increases PD-L1 expression in metastasis arising from breast cancer patients receiving adjuvant hormonal therapy for their local disease [85]. For this reason, the use of hormone-therapies in combination with PD-1/PD-L1 blocking immunotherapies should be thoroughly investigated. On the other hand, and for the reasons mentioned above, the application of conventional monoclonal antibodies targeting one or more growth factors would be a useful adjuvant to enhance the efficacy of breast cancer immunotherapy by improving APCs function [86,87].

2.2.2. Changes in Breast Tumor Cells

Instead of loss of the targeted protein, resistance to cancer immunotherapies, such as monoclonal antibodies, is frequently due to the activation of alternate pathways [53] like immunosuppressive checkpoint pathways.

Among these, and largely due to the FDA approval of atezolizumab, blockade of the PD-1/PD-L1 pathway constitutes one of the most promising strategies for breast cancer immunotherapy. Despite this important addition to the number of therapeutic options available for metastatic breast cancer patients, it is important to note that the objective response rate achieved by atezolizumab was 53% versus 33% for the placebo group [88] and that to date, it has been approved for the treatment of the triple-negative subtype, which only constitutes 10–15% of breast carcinomas [89], with positive PD-L1 protein expression, which occurs in approximately 20% of breast cancers (mainly HER2-positive and triple negative) [62].

Similarly to the PD-L1 pathway, different randomized clinical trials are currently evaluating the effect of PD-1 inhibitors as monotherapy or in combination with conventional and non-conventional treatments [62,65] in breast cancer patients with results that although modest, are encouraging. In this respect, even though PD-L1 status remains the core predictor for anti-PD-1/PD-L1 therapies and patient selection [23], the validity of PD-L1 expression as a prognostic marker remains controversial [62] and justifies the need to develop new immunotherapy biomarker panels as well as new strategies to improve response rates.

Another major impediment to immunotherapy success in breast cancer patients is the selection of apoptosis-resistant cells, which constitutes one of the hallmarks of cancer [17]. Since both chemo- and immunotherapies directly or indirectly activate the cellular apoptosis machinery, tumor sensitivity to anti-cancer treatments will significantly depend on the level of expression of anti-apoptotic proteins [24] in general and, more specifically, on the existence of a pro-survival profile characterized by an increased ratio between anti-/pro-apoptotic proteins [24,90,91].

Provided that antiapoptotic proteins such as clusterin (APO-J) [91,92], BCL-2, BMF [24] as well as different pro-survival kinases [8] are frequently altered in metastatic breast cancer, the use of profiling techniques or systematic mapping of anti-apoptotic gene dependencies would be justified in order to effectively select those patients that could better benefit from combined treatments of protein inhibitors and immunotherapy. In this regard, different studies have already evidenced the need to use therapies with a combination of inhibitors targeting different anti-apoptotic proteins in order to achieve better clinical benefits and avoid the activation of alternate pro-survival pathways [8,23,24].

HLA-I expression on the surface of breast tumor cells, which is positively correlated with tumor-infiltrating lymphocytes, is essential for an effective cytotoxic response [93] and the subsequent success of T-cell mediated immunotherapies. For this reason, loss or changes in HLA-I expression, which is another of the hallmarks of cancer [17], also represent a significant impediment for breast cancer immunotherapy.

Total loss of HLA-I is found in 37% of in situ breast carcinomas, 43% of the primary tumors, and 70% of the lymph node metastases [94]. Since HLA-I expression in these tumors is related with a pro-death phenotype characterized by an increased proapoptotic *BAX*/antiapoptotic *BCL2* ratio [94], preliminary studies for patients' selection would be justified in order to ensure the success of immunotherapies in breast cancer patients.

In the case of triple negative breast tumors, HLA-I expression is variable, contributing when altered to the development of an immunosuppressive tumor microenvironment and immune escape [69]. However, since the activation of the HLA-II presentation pathway occurs in approximately 30% of triple negative breast cancer patients [95], associated with the presence of tumor infiltrating lymphocytes and improved prognosis [95,96], the expression of both receptors are factors that must be taken into consideration prior to the application of immunotherapy treatment.

With respect to HER2 overexpressing tumors, although this receptor-tyrosine kinase represents a valuable target for T-cell based immunotherapies, these tumors may escape cytotoxic T lymphocyte-mediated lysis by downregulating HLA-I, since the expression of both receptors is inversely correlated with breast cancer cells [69,97]. Similarly, in normal and cancerous breast tissues, HLA-I expression is inversely correlated with the expression of estrogen receptors, which may be related to the low level of tumor-infiltrating lymphocytes [93], and hence, with the failure of the T-cell cytotoxic response. It is worth emphasizing at this point that provided that agents targeting different protein kinases such as Mitogen Activated Protein Kinase (MAPK) or HER2 may increase HLA-I expression in breast cancer cells [97,98], the use of kinase inhibitors would be a valuable strategy to increase the antitumor effects of T-cell based immunotherapies. Similarly, strategies aimed at inducing HLA-II expression in tumor cells may be valuable tools to increase patient response and prognosis to such therapies [96].

3. Conclusions

Where to go

The improvement of the response rates for immunotherapies remains a great challenge for cancer treatment in general and for breast cancer in particular. Considering the relatively limited T-cell infiltration in most breast cancers, the development of novel strategies that are aimed to enable sufficient lymphocyte infiltration as well as to generate de novo T-cell responses that overlap the immunosuppressive tumor environment may be key to the success of this kind of therapy in breast cancer patients [63].

Among the different approaches that are currently being considered and despite their limited efficacy when delivered as a monotherapy [99], oncolytic viruses have demonstrated their safety [100] and ability in targeting and killing cancer cells as well as in stimulating immunotherapeutic effects in patients [101], positioning themselves as a promising strategy to increase treatment efficacy when used in combination therapy [99–101] and as a unique platform for personalized treatment of patients with advanced breast cancer [101].

Recent evidence on the role of tumor-associated macrophages in breast tumor growth, progression, treatment resistance, and metastasis has paved the way for the development of novel macrophage-targeted breast treatment strategies, such as the inhibition of macrophage recruitment, repolarization of tumor-associated macrophages to an antitumor phenotype, and the enhancement of macrophage-mediated tumor cell killing or phagocytosis, which are currently being evaluated in clinical trials [102]. Despite the promising results of preclinical studies, these therapies have proved limited clinical efficacy, therefore the development of new strategies that improve the effectiveness of such treatments is necessary.

On the other hand, results of adoptive cell immunotherapies, which includes Chimeric Antigen Receptor (CAR) T cell therapy and Tumor-Infiltrating Lymphocyte (TIL) therapy, based on the isolation of antitumor T cells from the primary tumor, further ex vivo expansion and activation, and subsequent reinfusion of such cells into the patient [65], are also proving valuable in both preclinical and clinical studies for the treatment of patients with breast cancer in general and HER2 positive tumors in particular [65,103]. In a similar line, next-generation sequencing and bioinformatic technologies have become a fundamental tool to facilitate neoantigen identification and the consequent improvement of personalized neoantigen-based translational immunotherapy studies [104], as well as to develop neoantigen vaccines to induce neoantigen-specific T-cell responses through the activation of antigen-presenting cells [105,106].

Results obtained with nanoparticles are no less important, having been postulated as the great asset to overcome the limitations of existing immunotherapy, being able to improve overall anti-cancer immune responses with minimal systemic side effects [107]. However, although nanoparticles in different in vitro and in vivo breast cancer models [108] have already proven their efficacy in defeating the immune-suppressive effect of tumor microenvironment [107] and drug resistance [108], as well as in delivering neoantigens and adjuvants to tumor cells [107], reducing the side effects of anticancer drugs [109], certain nanoparticles like titanium dioxide, silica, and gold complexes can lead to the formation of micrometer-size gaps in the blood vessel's endothelial walls and the intravasation of surviving cancer cells into the surrounding vasculature, which increases the risk of metastasis [110].

Another main drawback of immunotherapies, especially within a combined regimen, is the occurrence of immune-related side-effects affecting different organs such as the skin (rash, pruritus) or gastrointestinal tract (diarrhea, colitis) (Table 4). Although the severity of these immune-related adverse events are generally mild, life-threatening complications may also occur [111] and would end up, in many cases, in a reduction of the optimal treatment dose or medication discontinuation. For this reason, there is still a strong need for further research in order to develop biomarker panels that allow for patient selection and predict the response to immunotherapies and immune-related adverse events.

Author Contributions: M.G.-A. contributed to the conceptualization, writing and review and M.R. contributed to the supervision and review of the manuscript.

Funding: This research was partially supported by grants from Consejería de Salud de la Junta de Andalucía (PI 16/0298) and the European Regional Development Fund.

Acknowledgments: The authors wish to thank Adolfo Reque for his helpful advice during the preparation of this work.

Conflicts of Interest: The authors declare no conflict of interest.

References

1. Bray, F.; Ferlay, J.; Soerjomataram, I.; Siegel, R.L.; Torre, L.A.; Jemal, A. Global cancer statistics 2018: GLOBOCAN estimates of incidence and mortality worldwide for 36 cancers in 185 countries. *CA Cancer J. Clin.* **2018**, *68*, 394–424. [CrossRef] [PubMed]
2. World Health Organization. Breast Cancer: Prevention and Control. Available online: https://www.who.int/cancer/detection/breastcancer/en/index2.html (accessed on 25 April 2019).
3. Sheikh, A.; Hussain, S.A.; Ghori, Q.; Naeem, N.; Fazil, A.; Giri, S.; Sathian, B.; Mainali, P.; Al Tamimi, D.M. The spectrum of genetic mutations in breast cancer. *Asian Pac. J. Cancer Prev.* **2015**, *16*, 2177–2185. [CrossRef] [PubMed]
4. Paul, A.; Paul, S. The breast cancer susceptibility genes (BRCA) in breast and ovarian cancers. *Front. Biosci. (Landmark Ed.)* **2014**, *19*, 605–618. [CrossRef] [PubMed]
5. Shah, T.A.; Guraya, S.S. Breast cancer screening programs: Review of merits, demerits, and recent recommendations practiced across the world. *J. Microsc. Ultrastruct.* **2017**, *5*, 59–69. [CrossRef] [PubMed]
6. Rossi, L.; Stevens, D.; Pierga, J.Y.; Lerebours, F.; Reyal, F.; Robain, M.; Asselain, B.; Rouzier, R. Impact of Adjuvant Chemotherapy on Breast Cancer Survival: A Real-World Population. *PLoS ONE* **2015**, *10*, e0132853. [CrossRef]
7. Redig, A.J.; McAllister, S.S. Breast cancer as a systemic disease: A view of metastasis. *J. Intern. Med.* **2013**, *274*, 113–126. [CrossRef]

8. Garcia-Aranda, M.; Redondo, M. Protein Kinase Targets in Breast Cancer. *Int. J. Mol. Sci.* **2017**, *18*, 2543. [CrossRef]
9. Fragomeni, S.M.; Sciallis, A.; Jeruss, J.S. Molecular Subtypes and Local-Regional Control of Breast Cancer. *Surg. Oncol. Clin. N. Am.* **2018**, *27*, 95–120. [CrossRef]
10. Yersal, O.; Barutca, S. Biological subtypes of breast cancer: Prognostic and therapeutic implications. *World J. Clin. Oncol.* **2014**, *5*, 412–424. [CrossRef]
11. Kondov, B.; Milenkovikj, Z.; Kondov, G.; Petrushevska, G.; Basheska, N.; Bogdanovska-Todorovska, M.; Tolevska, N.; Ivkovski, L. Presentation of the Molecular Subtypes of Breast Cancer Detected By Immunohistochemistry in Surgically Treated Patients. *Open Access Maced. J. Med. Sci.* **2018**, *6*, 961–967. [CrossRef]
12. Mohit, E.; Hashemi, A.; Allahyari, M. Breast cancer immunotherapy: Monoclonal antibodies and peptide-based vaccines. *Expert Rev. Clin. Immunol.* **2014**, *10*, 927–961. [CrossRef] [PubMed]
13. Vidula, N.; Bardia, A. Targeted therapy for metastatic triple negative breast cancer: The next frontier in precision oncology. *Oncotarget* **2017**, *8*, 106167–106168. [CrossRef] [PubMed]
14. Ahmed, K.; Koval, A.; Xu, J.; Bodmer, A.; Katanaev, V.L. Towards the first targeted therapy for triple-negative breast cancer: Repositioning of clofazimine as a chemotherapy-compatible selective Wnt pathway inhibitor. *Cancer Lett.* **2019**, *449*, 45–55. [CrossRef] [PubMed]
15. Dunn, G.P.; Bruce, A.T.; Ikeda, H.; Old, L.J.; Schreiber, R.D. Cancer immunoediting: From immunosurveillance to tumor escape. *Nat. Immunol.* **2002**, *3*, 991–998. [CrossRef]
16. Bhatia, A.; Kumar, Y. Cancer-immune equilibrium: Questions unanswered. *Cancer Microenviron.* **2011**, *4*, 209–217. [CrossRef]
17. Hanahan, D.; Weinberg, R.A. Hallmarks of cancer: The next generation. *Cell* **2011**, *144*, 646–674. [CrossRef]
18. Nicolini, A.; Ferrari, P.; Rossi, G.; Carpi, A. Tumour growth and immune evasion as targets for a new strategy in advanced cancer. *Endocr. Relat. Cancer* **2018**, *1*, R577–R604. [CrossRef]
19. Campoli, M.; Ferrone, S.; Zea, A.H.; Rodriguez, P.C.; Ochoa, A.C. Mechanisms of tumor evasion. In *Tumor Immunology and Cancer Vaccines*; Springer: Berlin, Germany, 2005; pp. 61–88.
20. Ma, Y.; Shurin, G.V.; Gutkin, D.W.; Shurin, M.R. Tumor associated regulatory dendritic cells. *Semin. Cancer Biol.* **2012**, *22*, 298–306. [CrossRef]
21. Fu, C.; Jiang, A. Dendritic Cells and CD8 T Cell Immunity in Tumor Microenvironment. *Front. Immunol.* **2018**, *9*, 3059. [CrossRef]
22. Peter, M.E.; Hadji, A.; Murmann, A.E.; Brockway, S.; Putzbach, W.; Pattanayak, A.; Ceppi, P. The role of CD95 and CD95 ligand in cancer. *Cell Death Differ.* **2015**, *22*, 549. [CrossRef]
23. Garcia-Aranda, M.; Redondo, M. Targeting Protein Kinases to Enhance the Response 2 to anti-PD-1/PD-L1 immunotherapy. *Int. J. Mol. Sci.* **2019**, *20*, 2296. [CrossRef] [PubMed]
24. García-Aranda, M.; Pérez-Ruiz, E.; Redondo, M. Bcl-2 inhibition to overcome resistance to chemo-and immunotherapy. *Int. J. Mol. Sci.* **2018**, *19*, 3950. [CrossRef] [PubMed]
25. Kroemer, G.; Zitvogel, L. Cancer immunotherapy in 2017: The breakthrough of the microbiota. *Nat. Rev. Immunol.* **2018**, *18*, 87–88. [CrossRef] [PubMed]
26. Emens, L.A.; Ascierto, P.A.; Darcy, P.K.; Demaria, S.; Eggermont, A.M.M.; Redmond, W.L.; Seliger, B.; Marincola, F.M. Cancer immunotherapy: Opportunities and challenges in the rapidly evolving clinical landscape. *Eur. J. Cancer* **2017**, *81*, 116–129. [CrossRef]
27. Sun, C.; Mezzadra, R.; Schumacher, T.N. Regulation and Function of the PD-L1 Checkpoint. *Immunity* **2018**, *48*, 434–452. [CrossRef]
28. Pross, S. T-Cell Activation. In *xPharm: The Comprehensive Pharmacology Reference*; Enna, S.J., Bylund, D.B., Eds.; Elsevier: New York, NY, USA, 2007; pp. 1–7. [CrossRef]
29. Fontana, M.F.; Vance, R.E. Two signal models in innate immunity. *Immunol. Rev.* **2011**, *243*, 26–39. [CrossRef]
30. Pardoll, D.M. The blockade of immune checkpoints in cancer immunotherapy. *Nat. Rev. Cancer* **2012**, *12*, 252. [CrossRef]
31. Buchbinder, E.I.; Desai, A. CTLA-4 and PD-1 Pathways: Similarities, Differences, and Implications of Their Inhibition. *Am. J. Clin. Oncol.* **2016**, *39*, 98–106. [CrossRef]
32. Darvin, P.; Toor, S.M.; Sasidharan Nair, V.; Elkord, E. Immune checkpoint inhibitors: Recent progress and potential biomarkers. *Exp. Mol. Med.* **2018**, *50*, 165. [CrossRef]

33. Seidel, J.A.; Otsuka, A.; Kabashima, K. Anti-PD-1 and Anti-CTLA-4 Therapies in Cancer: Mechanisms of Action, Efficacy, and Limitations. *Front. Oncol.* **2018**, *8*, 86. [CrossRef]
34. FDA. Ipilimumab. Application Number: 125377Orig1s000. Available online: https://www.accessdata.fda.gov/drugsatfda_docs/nda/2011/125377Orig1s000SumR.pdf (accessed on 29 May 2019).
35. FDA. Yervoy Approval History. Available online: https://www.drugs.com/history/yervoy.html (accessed on 30 May 2019).
36. FDA. Opdivo Approval History. Available online: https://www.drugs.com/history/opdivo.html (accessed on 30 May 2019).
37. European Medicines Agency (EMA). Yervoy (ipilimimab). Available online: https://www.ema.europa.eu/en/medicines/human/EPAR/yervoy (accessed on 19 November 2019).
38. FDA. Keytruda Approval History. Available online: https://www.drugs.com/history/keytruda.html (accessed on 20 May 2019).
39. FDA. Libtayo Approval History. Available online: https://www.drugs.com/history/libtayo.html (accessed on 30 May 2019).
40. FDA. Bavencio Approval History. Available online: https://www.drugs.com/history/bavencio.html (accessed on 4 June 2019).
41. FDA. Imfizi Approval History. Available online: https://www.drugs.com/history/imfinzi.html (accessed on 4 June 2019).
42. Bell, R.B.; Feng, Z.; Bifulco, C.B.; Leidner, R.; Weinberg, A.; Fox, B.A. 15—Immunotherapy. In *Oral, Head and Neck Oncology and Reconstructive Surgery*; Bell, R.B., Fernandes, R.P., Andersen, P.E., Eds.; Elsevier: New York, NY, USA, 2018; pp. 314–340. [CrossRef]
43. Guntermann, C.; Alexander, D.R. CTLA-4 suppresses proximal TCR signaling in resting human CD4+ T cells by inhibiting ZAP-70 Tyr319 phosphorylation: A potential role for tyrosine phosphatases. *J. Immunol.* **2002**, *168*, 4420–4429. [CrossRef] [PubMed]
44. Fellner, C. Ipilimumab (yervoy) prolongs survival in advanced melanoma: Serious side effects and a hefty price tag may limit its use. *Pharm. Ther.* **2012**, *37*, 503–530.
45. Menshawy, A.; Eltonob, A.A.; Barkat, S.A.; Ghanem, A.; Mniesy, M.M.; Mohamed, I.; Abdel-Maboud, M.; Mattar, O.M.; Elfil, M.; Bahbah, E.I.; et al. Nivolumab monotherapy or in combination with ipilimumab for metastatic melanoma: Systematic review and meta-analysis of randomized-controlled trials. *Melanoma Res.* **2018**, *28*, 371–379. [CrossRef] [PubMed]
46. Shuptrine, C.W.; Surana, R.; Weiner, L.M. Monoclonal antibodies for the treatment of cancer. *Semin. Cancer Biol.* **2012**, *22*, 3–13. [CrossRef]
47. FDA. FDA Approves Ado-Trastuzumab Emtansine for Early Breast Cancer. Available online: https://www.fda.gov/drugs/resources-information-approved-drugs/fda-approves-ado-trastuzumab-emtansine-early-breast-cancer (accessed on 12 September 2019).
48. Nejadmoghaddam, M.R.; Minai-Tehrani, A.; Ghahremanzadeh, R.; Mahmoudi, M.; Dinarvand, R.; Zarnani, A.H. Antibody-Drug Conjugates: Possibilities and Challenges. *Avicenna J. Med. Biotechnol.* **2019**, *11*, 3–23.
49. Vogel, C.L.; Cobleigh, M.A.; Tripathy, D.; Gutheil, J.C.; Harris, L.N.; Fehrenbacher, L.; Slamon, D.J.; Murphy, M.; Novotny, W.F.; Burchmore, M. Efficacy and safety of trastuzumab as a single agent in first-line treatment of HER2-overexpressing metastatic breast cancer. *J. Clin. Oncol.* **2002**, *20*, 719–726. [CrossRef]
50. Tolaney, S.M.; Krop, I.E. Mechanisms of trastuzumab resistance in breast cancer. *Anticancer Agents Med. Chem.* **2009**, *9*, 348–355. [CrossRef]
51. Cortés, J.; Fumoleau, P.; Bianchi, G.V.; Petrella, T.M.; Gelmon, K.; Pivot, X.; Verma, S.; Albanell, J.; Conte, P.; Lluch, A. Pertuzumab monotherapy after trastuzumab-based treatment and subsequent reintroduction of trastuzumab: Activity and tolerability in patients with advanced human epidermal growth factor receptor 2-positive breast cancer. *J. Clin. Oncol.* **2012**, *30*, 1594–1600. [CrossRef]
52. Baselga, J.; Gelmon, K.A.; Verma, S.; Wardley, A.; Conte, P.; Miles, D.; Bianchi, G.; Cortes, J.; McNally, V.A.; Ross, G.A. Phase II trial of pertuzumab and trastuzumab in patients with human epidermal growth factor receptor 2–positive metastatic breast cancer that progressed during prior trastuzumab therapy. *J. Clin. Oncol.* **2010**, *28*, 1138. [CrossRef]
53. Peddi, P.F.; Hurvitz, S.A. Trastuzumab emtansine: The first targeted chemotherapy for treatment of breast cancer. *Future Oncol.* **2013**, *9*, 319–326. [CrossRef]

54. Kaufman, B.; Trudeau, M.; Awada, A.; Blackwell, K.; Bachelot, T.; Salazar, V.; DeSilvio, M.; Westlund, R.; Zaks, T.; Spector, N.; et al. Lapatinib monotherapy in patients with HER2-overexpressing relapsed or refractory inflammatory breast cancer: Final results and survival of the expanded HER2+ cohort in EGF103009, a phase II study. *Lancet Oncol.* **2009**, *10*, 581–588. [CrossRef]
55. Tao, Z.; Li, S.X.; Shen, K.; Zhao, Y.; Zeng, H.; Ma, X. Safety and Efficacy Profile of Neratinib: A Systematic Review and Meta-Analysis of 23 Prospective Clinical Trials. *Clin. Drug Investig.* **2019**, *39*, 27–43. [CrossRef] [PubMed]
56. Baselga, J.; Albanell, J.; Ruiz, A.; Lluch, A.; Gascon, P.; Guillem, V.; Gonzalez, S.; Sauleda, S.; Marimon, I.; Tabernero, J.M.; et al. Phase II and tumor pharmacodynamic study of gefitinib in patients with advanced breast cancer. *J. Clin. Oncol.* **2005**, *23*, 5323–5333. [CrossRef] [PubMed]
57. Lin, N.U.; Winer, E.P.; Wheatley, D.; Carey, L.A.; Houston, S.; Mendelson, D.; Munster, P.; Frakes, L.; Kelly, S.; Garcia, A.A.; et al. A phase II study of afatinib (BIBW 2992), an irreversible ErbB family blocker, in patients with HER2-positive metastatic breast cancer progressing after trastuzumab. *Breast Cancer Res. Treat.* **2012**, *133*, 1057–1065. [CrossRef] [PubMed]
58. FDA. FDA Grants Genentech's Tecentriq in Combination with Abraxane Accelerated Approval for People with PD-L1-Positive, Metastatic Triple-Negative Breast Cancer. Available online: https://www.drugs.com/newdrugs/fda-grants-genentech-s-tecentriq-combination-abraxane-accelerated-approval-pd-l1-positive-4927.html (accessed on 28 October 2019).
59. Atezolizumab, T. IMpassion130 Efficacy Results in First-Line PD-L1+ Metastatic Triple-Negative Breast Cancer. Available online: https://www.tecentriq-hcp.com/tnbc/clinical-data-efficacy/study-efficacy.html (accessed on 29 October 2019).
60. Schmid, P.; Adams, S.; Rugo, H.S.; Schneeweiss, A.; Barrios, C.H.; Iwata, H.; Dieras, V.; Hegg, R.; Im, S.A.; Shaw Wright, G.; et al. Atezolizumab and Nab-Paclitaxel in Advanced Triple-Negative Breast Cancer. *N. Engl. J. Med.* **2018**, *379*, 2108–2121. [CrossRef]
61. FDA. Tecentriq Approval History. Available online: https://www.drugs.com/history/tecentriq.html (accessed on 28 October 2019).
62. Swoboda, A.; Nanda, R. Immune Checkpoint Blockade for Breast Cancer. *Cancer Treat. Res.* **2018**, *173*, 155–165. [CrossRef]
63. Vonderheide, R.H.; Domchek, S.M.; Clark, A.S. Immunotherapy for Breast Cancer: What Are We Missing? *Clin. Cancer Res. Off. J. Am. Assoc. Cancer Res.* **2017**, *23*, 2640–2646. [CrossRef]
64. Zhang, X.; Kim, S.; Hundal, J.; Herndon, J.M.; Li, S.; Petti, A.A.; Soysal, S.D.; Li, L.; McLellan, M.D.; Hoog, J. Breast cancer neoantigens can induce CD8+ T-cell responses and antitumor immunity. *Cancer Immunol. Res.* **2017**, *5*, 516–523. [CrossRef]
65. Ayoub, N.M.; Al-Shami, K.M.; Yaghan, R.J. Immunotherapy for HER2-positive breast cancer: Recent advances and combination therapeutic approaches. *Breast Cancer Targets Ther.* **2019**, *11*, 53–69. [CrossRef]
66. Shin, S.U.; Lee, J.; Kim, J.H.; Kim, W.H.; Song, S.E.; Chu, A.; Kim, H.S.; Han, W.; Ryu, H.S.; Moon, W.K. Gene expression profiling of calcifications in breast cancer. *Sci. Rep.* **2017**, *7*, 11427. [CrossRef]
67. Tse, G.M.; Tan, P.H.; Cheung, H.S.; Chu, W.C.; Lam, W.W. Intermediate to highly suspicious calcification in breast lesions: A radio-pathologic correlation. *Breast Cancer Res. Treat.* **2008**, *110*, 1–7. [CrossRef] [PubMed]
68. Dirix, L.Y.; Vermeulen, P.B. Inflammatory HER2-positive breast cancer. *Lancet Oncol.* **2012**, *13*, 324–326. [CrossRef]
69. Makhoul, I.; Atiq, M.; Alwbari, A.; Kieber-Emmons, T. Breast Cancer Immunotherapy: An Update. *Breast Cancer Basic Clin. Res.* **2018**, *12*, 1178223418774802. [CrossRef] [PubMed]
70. Bonaventura, P.; Shekarian, T.; Alcazer, V.; Valladeau-Guilemond, J.; Valsesia-Wittmann, S.; Amigorena, S.; Caux, C.; Depil, S. Cold Tumors: A Therapeutic Challenge for Immunotherapy. *Front. Immunol.* **2019**, *10*, 168. [CrossRef]
71. Vikas, P.; Borcherding, N.; Zhang, W. The clinical promise of immunotherapy in triple-negative breast cancer. *Cancer Manag. Res.* **2018**, *10*, 6823–6833. [CrossRef]
72. Yuan, Z.Y.; Luo, R.Z.; Peng, R.J.; Wang, S.S.; Xue, C. High infiltration of tumor-associated macrophages in triple-negative breast cancer is associated with a higher risk of distant metastasis. *OncoTargets Ther.* **2014**, *7*, 1475. [CrossRef]

73. Ni, C.; Yang, L.; Xu, Q.; Yuan, H.; Wang, W.; Xia, W.; Gong, D.; Zhang, W.; Yu, K. CD68- and CD163-positive tumor infiltrating macrophages in non-metastatic breast cancer: A retrospective study and meta-analysis. *J. Cancer* **2019**, *10*, 4463–4472. [CrossRef]
74. Wang, Z.; Liu, W.; Chen, C.; Yang, X.; Luo, Y.; Zhang, B. Low mutation and neoantigen burden and fewer effector tumor infiltrating lymphocytes correlate with breast cancer metastasization to lymph nodes. *Sci. Rep.* **2019**, *9*, 253. [CrossRef]
75. Toraya-Brown, S.; Fiering, S. Local tumour hyperthermia as immunotherapy for metastatic cancer. *Int. J. Hyperth.* **2014**, *30*, 531–539. [CrossRef]
76. Skitzki, J.J.; Repasky, E.A.; Evans, S.S. Hyperthermia as an immunotherapy strategy for cancer. *Curr. Opin. Investig. Drugs* **2009**, *10*, 550–558.
77. Zagar, T.M.; Oleson, J.R.; Vujaskovic, Z.; Dewhirst, M.W.; Craciunescu, O.I.; Blackwell, K.L.; Prosnitz, L.R.; Jones, E.L. Hyperthermia for locally advanced breast cancer. *Int. J. Hyperth.* **2010**, *26*, 618–624. [CrossRef] [PubMed]
78. Rethfeldt, E.; Becker, M.; Koldovsky, P. Whole-body hyperthermia in the treatment of breast cancer. *Breast Cancer Res.* **2001**, *3*, A51. [CrossRef]
79. Yagawa, Y.; Tanigawa, K.; Kobayashi, Y.; Yamamoto, M. Cancer immunity and therapy using hyperthermia with immunotherapy, radiotherapy, chemotherapy, and surgery. *J. Cancer Metastasis Treat.* **2017**, *3*, 219. [CrossRef]
80. Taneja, V. Sex Hormones Determine Immune Response. *Front. Immunol.* **2018**, *9*, 1931. [CrossRef]
81. Khan, D.; Ansar Ahmed, S. The Immune System Is a Natural Target for Estrogen Action: Opposing Effects of Estrogen in Two Prototypical Autoimmune Diseases. *Front. Immunol.* **2016**, *6*. [CrossRef]
82. Mostafa, A.A.; Codner, D.; Hirasawa, K.; Komatsu, Y.; Young, M.N.; Steimle, V.; Drover, S. Activation of ERα signaling differentially modulates IFN-γ induced HLA-class II expression in breast cancer cells. *PLoS ONE* **2014**, *9*, e87377. [CrossRef]
83. Pietras, R.J. Interactions between estrogen and growth factor receptors in human breast cancers and the tumor-associated vasculature. *Breast J.* **2003**, *9*, 361–373. [CrossRef]
84. Rothenberger, N.J.; Somasundaram, A.; Stabile, L.P. The Role of the Estrogen Pathway in the Tumor Microenvironment. *Int. J. Mol. Sci.* **2018**, *19*, 611. [CrossRef]
85. Hühn, D.; Martí-Rodrigo, P.; Mouron, S.; Hansel, C.; Tschapalda, K.; Häggblad, M.; Lidemalm, L.; Quintela-Fandino, M.A.; Carreras-Puigvert, J.; Fernandez-Capetillo, O. Estrogen deprivation triggers an immunosuppressive phenotype in breast cancer cells. *bioRxiv* **2019**, 715136. [CrossRef]
86. Gabrilovich, D.I.; Ishida, T.; Nadaf, S.; Ohm, J.E.; Carbone, D.P. Antibodies to vascular endothelial growth factor enhance the efficacy of cancer immunotherapy by improving endogenous dendritic cell function. *Clin. Cancer Res.* **1999**, *5*, 2963–2970.
87. Hahn, T.; Akporiaye, E.T. Targeting transforming growth factor beta to enhance cancer immunotherapy. *Curr. Oncol.* **2006**, *13*, 141–143. [PubMed]
88. FDA. FDA Approves Atezolizumab for PD-L1 Positive Unresectable Locally Advanced or Metastatic Triple-Negative Breast Cancer. Available online: https://www.fda.gov/drugs/drug-approvals-and-databases/fda-approves-atezolizumab-pd-l1-positive-unresectable-locally-advanced-or-metastatic-triple-negative (accessed on 28 October 2019).
89. Dawood, S. Triple-negative breast cancer. *Drugs* **2010**, *70*, 2247–2258. [CrossRef] [PubMed]
90. Garcia-Aranda, M.; Serrano, A.; Redondo, M. Regulation of Clusterin Gene Expression. *Curr. Protein Pept. Sci.* **2018**, *19*, 612–622. [CrossRef] [PubMed]
91. Garcia-Aranda, M.; Tellez, T.; Munoz, M.; Redondo, M. Clusterin inhibition mediates sensitivity to chemotherapy and radiotherapy in human cancer. *Anticancer Drugs* **2017**, *28*, 702–716. [CrossRef] [PubMed]
92. Tellez, T.; Garcia-Aranda, M.; Redondo, M. The role of clusterin in carcinogenesis and its potential utility as therapeutic target. *Curr. Med. Chem.* **2016**, *23*, 4297–4308. [CrossRef]
93. Lee, H.J.; Song, I.H.; Park, I.A.; Heo, S.H.; Kim, Y.A.; Ahn, J.H.; Gong, G. Differential expression of major histocompatibility complex class I in subtypes of breast cancer is associated with estrogen receptor and interferon signaling. *Oncotarget* **2016**, *7*, 30119–30132. [CrossRef]
94. Redondo, M.; Garcia, J.; Villar, E.; Rodrigo, I.; Perea-Milla, E.; Serrano, A.; Morell, M. Major histocompatibility complex status in breast carcinogenesis and relationship to apoptosis. *Hum. Pathol.* **2003**, *34*, 1283–1289. [CrossRef]

95. Axelrod, M.L.; Cook, R.S.; Johnson, D.B.; Balko, J.M. Biological Consequences of MHC-II Expression by Tumor Cells in Cancer. *Clin. Cancer Res.* **2019**, *25*, 2392–2402. [CrossRef]
96. Forero, A.; Li, Y.; Chen, D.; Grizzle, W.E.; Updike, K.L.; Merz, N.D.; Downs-Kelly, E.; Burwell, T.C.; Vaklavas, C.; Buchsbaum, D.J.; et al. Expression of the MHC Class II Pathway in Triple-Negative Breast Cancer Tumor Cells Is Associated with a Good Prognosis and Infiltrating Lymphocytes. *Cancer Immunol. Res.* **2016**, *4*, 390–399. [CrossRef]
97. Inoue, M.; Mimura, K.; Izawa, S.; Shiraishi, K.; Inoue, A.; Shiba, S.; Watanabe, M.; Maruyama, T.; Kawaguchi, Y.; Inoue, S.; et al. Expression of MHC Class I on breast cancer cells correlates inversely with HER2 expression. *Oncoimmunology* **2012**, *1*, 1104–1110. [CrossRef]
98. Chaganty, B.K.R.; Lu, Y.; Qiu, S.; Somanchi, S.S.; Lee, D.A.; Fan, Z. Trastuzumab upregulates expression of HLA-ABC and T cell costimulatory molecules through engagement of natural killer cells and stimulation of IFNγ secretion. *Oncoimmunology* **2015**, *5*, e1100790. [CrossRef] [PubMed]
99. Tai, C.J.; Liu, C.H.; Pan, Y.C.; Wong, S.H.; Tai, C.J.; Richardson, C.D.; Lin, L.T. Chemovirotherapeutic Treatment Using Camptothecin Enhances Oncolytic Measles Virus-Mediated Killing of Breast Cancer Cells. *Sci. Rep.* **2019**, *9*, 6767. [CrossRef] [PubMed]
100. Eissa, I.R.; Bustos-Villalobos, I.; Ichinose, T.; Matsumura, S.; Naoe, Y.; Miyajima, N.; Morimoto, D.; Mukoyama, N.; Zhiwen, W.; Tanaka, M.; et al. The Current Status and Future Prospects of Oncolytic Viruses in Clinical Trials against Melanoma, Glioma, Pancreatic, and Breast Cancers. *Cancers* **2018**, *10*, 356. [CrossRef] [PubMed]
101. O'Bryan, S.M.; Mathis, J.M. Oncolytic Virotherapy for Breast Cancer Treatment. *Curr. Gene Ther.* **2018**, *18*, 192–205. [CrossRef]
102. Qiu, S.Q.; Waaijer, S.J.H.; Zwager, M.C.; de Vries, E.G.E.; van der Vegt, B.; Schroder, C.P. Tumor-associated macrophages in breast cancer: Innocent bystander or important player? *Cancer Treat. Rev.* **2018**, *70*, 178–189. [CrossRef]
103. Wang, Z.X.; Cao, J.X.; Wang, M.; Li, D.; Cui, Y.X.; Zhang, X.Y.; Liu, J.L.; Li, J.L. Adoptive cellular immunotherapy for the treatment of patients with breast cancer: A meta-analysis. *Cytotherapy* **2014**, *16*, 934–945. [CrossRef]
104. Chen, F.; Zou, Z.; Du, J.; Su, S.; Shao, J.; Meng, F.; Yang, J.; Xu, Q.; Ding, N.; Yang, Y.; et al. Neoantigen identification strategies enable personalized immunotherapy in refractory solid tumors. *J. Clin. Investig.* **2019**, *129*, 2056–2070. [CrossRef]
105. Criscitiello, C.; Viale, G.; Curigliano, G. Peptide vaccines in early breast cancer. *Breast* **2019**, *44*, 128–134. [CrossRef]
106. Castle, J.C.; Uduman, M.; Pabla, S.; Stein, R.B.; Buell, J.S. Mutation-Derived Neoantigens for Cancer Immunotherapy. *Front. Immunol.* **2019**, *10*, 1856. [CrossRef]
107. Park, W.; Heo, Y.J.; Han, D.K. New opportunities for nanoparticles in cancer immunotherapy. *Biomater. Res.* **2018**, *22*, 24. [CrossRef]
108. Thoidingjam, S.; Tiku, A.B. New developments in breast cancer therapy: Role of iron oxide nanoparticles. *Adv. Nat. Sci. Nanosci. Nanotechnol.* **2017**, *8*, 023002. [CrossRef]
109. Hussain, Z.; Khan, J.A.; Murtaza, S. Nanotechnology: An Emerging Therapeutic Option for Breast Cancer. *Crit. Rev. ™ Eukaryot. Gene Expr.* **2018**, *28*, 163–175. [CrossRef] [PubMed]
110. Peng, F.; Setyawati, M.I.; Tee, J.K.; Ding, X.; Wang, J.; Nga, M.E.; Ho, H.K.; Leong, D.T. Nanoparticles promote in vivo breast cancer cell intravasation and extravasation by inducing endothelial leakiness. *Nat. Nanotechnol.* **2019**, *14*, 279–286. [CrossRef] [PubMed]
111. Liu, R.; Fernandez-Penas, P.; Sebaratnam, D.F. Management of adverse events related to new cancer immunotherapy (immune checkpoint inhibitors). *Med. J. Aust.* **2017**, *206*, 412. [CrossRef] [PubMed]

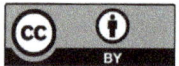

© 2019 by the authors. Licensee MDPI, Basel, Switzerland. This article is an open access article distributed under the terms and conditions of the Creative Commons Attribution (CC BY) license (http://creativecommons.org/licenses/by/4.0/).

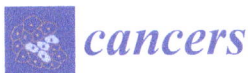

Review

Immunotherapy in Pediatric Solid Tumors—A Systematic Review

Raoud Marayati [†], Colin H. Quinn [†] and Elizabeth A. Beierle *

Division of Pediatric Surgery, Department of Surgery, University of Alabama at Birmingham, Birmingham, AL 35294, USA; rmarayati@uabmc.edu (R.M.); chquinn@uab.edu (C.H.Q.)
* Correspondence: elizabeth.beierle@childrensal.org
† These authors contributed equally to this work.

Received: 16 November 2019; Accepted: 12 December 2019; Published: 14 December 2019

Abstract: Despite advances in the treatment of many pediatric solid tumors, children with aggressive and high-risk disease continue to have a dismal prognosis. For those presenting with metastatic or recurrent disease, multiple rounds of intensified chemotherapy and radiation are the typical course of action, but more often than not, this fails to control the progression of the disease. Thus, new therapeutics are desperately needed to improve the outcomes for these children. Recent advances in our understanding of both the immune system's biology and its interaction with tumors have led to the development of novel immunotherapeutics as alternative treatment options for these aggressive malignancies. Immunotherapeutic approaches have shown promising results for pediatric solid tumors in early clinical trials, but challenges remain concerning safety and anti-tumor efficacy. In this review, we aim to discuss and summarize the main classes of immunotherapeutics used to treat pediatric solid tumors.

Keywords: pediatric solid tumors; immunotherapy; chimeric antigen receptors; cancer vaccines; oncolytic viral therapy; immune checkpoint inhibitors; immunomodulation

1. Introduction

Immunotherapy is being popularized as an approach to target pediatric cancer. This treatment modality has proven effective in pediatric hematological malignancies such as acute lymphocytic leukemia (ALL), but there remains much to be learned before we can harness the potential of immunotherapy in the treatment of solid tumors. Here, we examine two broad immunotherapy approaches that may be utilized for the treatment of pediatric solid tumors: direct utilization of the immune system properties and immune system modulation. Within each of these categories, we discuss the benefits and challenges of each therapy for solid tumors and specifically highlight the effects on pediatric populations. The overarching objective of this review is to discuss immunotherapies that are currently in use as well as those with potential future use in the treatment of pediatric solid tumors.

2. Direct Utilization of the Immune System

2.1. Oncolytic Virus-Based Therapy

Oncolytic virus-based therapy is an emerging approach designed to target a variety of cancers. The concept for utilizing oncolytic virotherapy in cancer treatment originated from observations that patients with Hodgkin's lymphoma temporarily improved following a hepatitis infection [1]. Oncolytic viruses are constructed by altering the genetic profile of a viral vector to render the virus apathogenic while maintaining its ability to infect, replicate, and spread amongst host cells. Oncolytic viruses are also often engineered with specific receptors for cancer cells, rendering them target-specific and potentially more efficacious [2]. The cancer cells will then behave as hosts and will be subjected to the oncolytic effects of the virus.

The benefit of oncolytic viral therapy is twofold: (1) it harnesses a virus's innate ability to lyse cancer cells and (2) it has the potential to trigger a cytotoxic immune response. In cancer cells, the upregulation of DNA replication assists in the production of viral progeny. The buildup of progeny results in lysis of the cells and infection of neighboring cancer cells [3]. This approach is effective for solid tumors, as viral delivery may be accomplished through direct intratumoral injections, resulting in direct killing of the malignant cells without producing severe systemic side effects or unwanted hepatic degradation of the virus, which may occur with systemic injection [4]. As a result of viral-mediated tumor cell lysis, pathogen-associated molecular patterns (PAMPs), damage-associated molecular patterns (DAMPs), and tumor-associated antigens (TAA) are released. These molecular signals initiate an immune response directed at the tumor even if this tumor has previously and successfully evaded the immune system [5]. These molecular signaling molecules allow for an intact immune system to utilize natural killer (NK) cells, dendritic cells (DCs), and other antigen-presenting cells (APCs) to directly target the cancer cells [6].

A variety of replicating viruses have been studied as cancer therapeutics, including adenoviruses, herpesviruses, paramyxoviruses, picornaviruses, poxviruses, reoviruses, rhabdoviruses, and togaviruses [7]. In pediatrics, variants of oncolytic Herpes simplex virus (oHSV) have been shown effective in a variety of solid tumors, such as glioblastoma, neuroblastoma, and sarcoma [8]. oHSVs have been genetically engineered to allow for selective uptake or replication of the virus by tumor cells but not healthy tissue [9,10]. Additionally, particular oHSVs have been engineered to produce chemokines or increased amounts of TAA, which stimulates and bolsters the immune system response directed toward the tumor [6,11].

There is great potential to use the immune response to target tumors through oHSV. NK cells are the first line of defense and will destroy the cancer cells or use cytokines to recruit other immune cells. Following this innate immune response, an adaptive response may ensue [12,13]. Such a reaction could potentially lead to immune memory, negating the need for retreatment and theoretically, tumor relapse. This built-in defense mechanism could then take over for the destruction of most of the tumor. Barriers to this response, especially in solid tumors, include complete viral clearance, dense fibrosis surrounding the tumor, and the tumor microenvironment (TME) [5]. Combination therapy provides a means to overcome these barriers. In melanoma, combining T-VEC, a modified herpes simplex virus, with a MEK inhibitor (trametinib) produced an increased infiltration of CD8+ T cells into the tumor and a decreased tumor size in vivo [14]. A pre-clinical investigation of the TME in sarcoma showed that modulation of tumor-associated macrophages (TAMs) could potentiate an immune response. This study focused on Ewing sarcoma and oHSV. The investigators demonstrated that by targeting the TME with trabectedin, a currently approved chemotherapeutic, the M2 macrophage population was decreased, allowing for uninhibited viral infection by the rRp450 virus. They also showed that combining rRp450 with trabectedin in an in vivo xenograft model of Ewing sarcoma significantly decreased tumor volume and increased animal survival [15]. Such studies provide an avenue for future investigations in viral therapy.

Currently, there are no commercially available viral therapies that are routinely used for extracranial solid tumors in pediatric patients. T-VEC is a viral therapy available for the treatment of melanoma in adults, but studies have not specifically tested its use in a pediatric-only population [16]. There are only four clinical trials listed on www.clinicaltrials.gov that are actively recruiting for viral therapy in pediatric cancers: oHSV in cerebellar tumors (NCT03911388), oHSV in supratentorial brain tumors (NCT02457845), adenovirus in gliomas (NCT03178032), and an oncolytic poliovirus in gliomas (NCT03043391). Considering there are 28 actively recruiting clinical trials listed for adults, there is obvious room for expansion of this therapeutic approach for pediatric solid tumors.

2.2. Antigen-Targeting Therapy

Tumor antigen-targeting therapy, initially based on antibody–drug conjugates (ADC), utilizes specific monoclonal antibodies (mAbs) as an approach to target cancer cells and cause antibody-dependent cell-mediated toxicity (ADCC). Initially, these mAbs were used to assist in more direct drug delivery of chemotherapeutics [17]. In pediatrics, this model has been employed to target a tumor-specific antigen, GD2, which is a di-ganglioside expressed on neuroblastoma and osteosarcoma. In these tumors, a specific antibody targeting GD2 has been developed and is used in clinical treatment [18,19]. Additionally, a newer target for neuroblastoma treatment is anaplastic lymphoma kinase (ALK). An mAb targeting the ALK surface receptor, mAb30/49, led to decreased tumor cell proliferation and viability in vitro [20].

In order to increase the efficacy of these antibodies, researchers are examining techniques to evoke the activity of immune cells, such as NK cells, to involve them in tumor cell lysis. Investigators have demonstrated this concept using an anti-GD2 antibody, hu14.18K322A, combined with IL-15. This combination resulted in decreased tumor cell viability in vitro and growth in vivo, as well as in an increase in mature NK cells in the TME [21].

To take advantage of the immune system, antibodies have been developed in combination with proteins designed to elicit an immune-stimulating response. FDA-approved drugs, such as dinutuximab (Ch14.18, murine/human chimeric antibody to GD2) and naxitamab (hu3F8, a humanized mAB to GD2), are administered in combination with granulocyte-macrophage colony stimulating factor (GM-CSF) to boost the immune response [22]. A phase I clinical trial studied naxitamab with GM-CSF and its effects on resistant neuroblastoma (NCT012757626). A total of 31 children had evaluable disease. Of those, 14 (45%) had a complete or partial tumor response, 5 (16%) had stable disease, and 11 (35%) had progressive disease [23]. To study the role of the immune system in more depth, researchers have utilized dinutuximab in a patient-derived xenograft (PDX) model. Investigators have shown that following surgical resection of neuroblastoma in a PDX model, increased animal survival and decreased tumor invasiveness were achieved with the administration of dinutuximab and activated NK cells [24]. For the mAb to achieve such an immune reaction independently, a different technology must be applied.

Bispecific antibodies, unlike normal antibodies, elicit a cytotoxic T cell response against a specific tumor target. The Bispecific T Engager (BiTE) technology activates a T cell response by binding to CD3 on T cells [25]. The molecule combines the CD3 binding site with a second site that is tumor-specific. BiTE directly targets the cancer and limits damage to non-malignant tissue (Figure 1). The direct activation of cytotoxic T cells limits the need for other anti-cancer interventions. Currently, clinical trials with BiTE antibodies are limited to just two TAA: CD19 and EpCAM [26]. Of the two, only anti-CD19 (blinatumomab) has been investigated in children and it has been limited to hematologic malignancies. Blinatumomab was administered to children with relapsed/refractory ALL. In this phase I/II study, 39% of the children that received the determined dosage and treatment plan achieved a minimal residual disease response [27]. Elitzur and colleagues reported 11 pediatric patients with ALL who were treated with blinatumomab as a bridge to further therapy after suffering from severe chemotherapy toxicities. All 11 children went on to resume standard chemotherapy with an overall survival of 80% [28]. Further preclinical studies and clinical trials with other TAA for BiTE antibodies will be required before this promising technology may be translated for clinical use in the treatment of pediatric solid tumors.

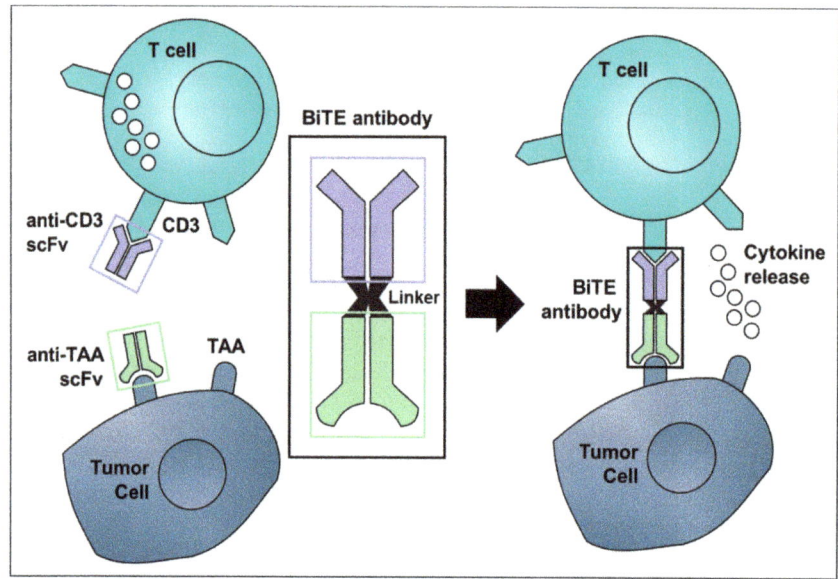

Figure 1. A schematic representation of the Bispecific T-cell Engager (BiTE) technology. The BiTE antibody connects the CD3 binding site on T cells with a tumor-associated antigen (TAA) specific to tumor cells. This triggers T cell activation and cytokine release, ultimately resulting in an anti-tumor response. The anti-CD3 single-chain variable fragment (scFv, shown in purple) is shared by all BiTE antibodies. The target antigen-specific scFv (in light green) is different for each BiTE antibody and can recognize targets such as CD19 or EpCAM.

2.3. Immune Checkpoint Inhibitors

Cytotoxic T-lymphocyte-associated antigen-4 (CTLA-4), the first immune-checkpoint receptor to be targeted clinically, is expressed on the surface of activated T cells and transmits an inhibitory signal to T cells. Normal T cell activation requires the engagement of the T cell receptor (TCR)/CD3 complex and the CD28 co-stimulatory signal, which then leads to increased expression of the co-inhibitory signal, CTLA-4. CTLA-4 binds to B7 molecules (CD80 and CD86) with greater affinity, thus out-competes CD28 for their shared ligands, preventing T cell activation. CTLA-4 signaling is utilized by some tumor cells to evade T cell anti-tumor activity. Thus, CTLA-4 blockade potentiates effective immune responses against tumor cells [29]. CTLA-4 is also found in regulatory T cells (Tregs) and contributes to their inhibitory function. CTLA-4 blockade in Tregs results in their decreased immunosuppression [30].

Preclinical data suggest that pediatric solid tumors have high expression of CTLA-4. In a panel of 34 adult and pediatric tumor cell lines, including osteosarcoma, rhabdomyosarcoma, and neuroblastoma, CTLA-4 expression was found at different densities on 88% of the cell lines examined, with higher intensity of staining in osteosarcoma [31]. In addition, 20 pediatric patients, 11 with osteosarcoma and 9 with Ewing sarcoma, had significantly increased expression of CTLA-4 on both CD4+ and CD8+ T cells obtained from peripheral blood samples compared to healthy controls [32]. These findings indicate that targeting CTLA-4 may be useful in these pediatric tumor types.

Ipilimumab is a mAb directed toward CTLA-4 signaling. Ipilimumab is FDA-approved for the treatment of adults and children with unresectable or metastatic melanoma. Recently, a phase I clinical trial (NCT01445379) included a total of 33 patients aged 2–21 years with recurrent or refractory solid tumors treated with CTLA-4 blockade. In this study, ipilimumab was well tolerated and resulted in increased activation of cytotoxic T lymphocyte without increased infiltration of Tregs; however, no objective tumor regression was observed [33].

Programmed cell death receptor 1 (PD-1) and its ligands (PD-L1 and PD-L2) are also part of the immune checkpoint pathway. PD-1 plays a role in downregulating T cell activation, which leads to tumor tolerance, while PD-Ls inhibit cytokine production and anti-tumor lymphocytes in the TME [34]. PD-1 is also highly expressed on Tregs and, when engaged by its ligand, is thought to enhance the activity and proliferation of these cells [35].

Several preclinical studies examined the expression of PD-1 and PD-L1 in pediatric cancer subtypes, with conflicting results. Only 9% of 451 pediatric tumors expressed PD-L1 in at least 1% of tumor cells, with the highest expressors being Burkitt lymphoma (80%), glioblastoma multiforme (36%), and neuroblastoma (14%) [36]. Conversely, in another study of children with advanced melanoma, relapsed or refractory solid tumors, or lymphoma, 33% of 689 screened tumors were positive for PD-L1 expression [37]. Of note, PD-L1 staining was associated with inferior survival among neuroblastoma patients [36], and higher expression of PD-1 correlated with disease progression in patients with osteosarcoma [38].

Pembrolizumab, an anti-PD-1 antibody, is FDA-approved for the treatment of both adults and children with refractory Hodgkin's lymphoma. Nivolumab, another anti-PD-1 antibody, has shown responses in adult solid tumors [39,40]. In pediatric solid tumors, these therapies remain under investigation. In five children aged 3–7 years with brain tumors treated with pembrolizumab, all progressed, and the median survival was 3.2 months [41]. In a retrospective review of 10 children with recurrent or refractory brain tumors treated with nivolumab, 9 patients had radiographic disease progression. Three patients had partial response at the primary tumor site, of whom two had progression of metastatic disease [42]. In other small studies of nivolumab treatment in pediatric brain tumor patients, results were mixed. [43,44]. Currently, a phase I/II trial (NCT03585465) is assessing nivolumab in combination with chemotherapy in pediatric patients with refractory/relapsing solid tumors or lymphoma. Two other trials are evaluating nivolumab alone: NCT02992964 is a pilot study of nivolumab in pediatric patients with refractory/recurrent hypermutated malignancies, and NCT02901145 is evaluating nivolumab in progressive/relapsed pediatric solid tumors, including osteosarcoma, Ewing sarcoma, neuroblastoma, and rhabdomyosarcoma.

Dual checkpoint blockade is hypothesized to prevent immune escape and may be promising in the treatment of pediatric solid tumors. Combinations of CTLA-4 and PD-1 antibodies are currently being investigated [45]. In an implantable murine model of metastatic osteosarcoma, treatment with anti-PD-L1 antibody resulted in downregulation of PD-L1 expression and upregulation of CD80/CD86 expression on tumor cells, as well as upregulation of CTLA-4 on tumor infiltrating CD8+ T cells [46]. Furthermore, combination therapy of PD-1/CTLA-4 signaling blockade resulted in complete protection from metastasis in 50% of treated mice as well as in T cell memory protection against future tumor inoculation [46]. Currently, NCT02304458 is an ongoing phase I/II trial evaluating PD-1/CTLA-4 signaling blockade combination therapy in pediatric patients with relapsed/refractory solid tumors.

3. Modulation of the Immune System

3.1. Tumor Microenvironment: Cancer-Associated Fibroblasts, Tumor-Associated Macrophages, and Myeloid-Derived Suppressor Cells

Many non-tumor cells including macrophages and fibroblasts are present in the TME and affect the malignant potential of tumor cells. Cancer-associated fibroblasts (CAFs) and TAMs are two of the primary infiltrating stromal cells.

CAFs are activated fibroblasts that play an important role in promoting tumor growth, invasion, and angiogenesis [47]. In a study of 60 primary neuroblastoma tumors, increased CAFs were associated with significantly higher microvascular proliferation and Schwannian stroma-poor histopathology, both poor prognostic factors [48]. In addition, blocking CAF-derived prostaglandin E2 (PGE2) production with a small molecule inhibitor was shown to reduce neuroblastoma cell growth, impair angiogenesis, and reduce tumor growth in vivo [49]. Further, in a genetically modified murine lung carcinoma model, depletion of CAFs resulted in significant inhibition of tumor growth and enhanced anti-tumor immunity [50]. While CAFs could be a potential therapeutic target in pediatric solid tumors, there are currently no methods suitable for clinical translation, and further studies are needed to guide the development of such stroma-directed therapy.

TAMs, which most closely resemble M2 macrophages, are major contributors to the TME. Whether TAMs promote or impede tumor growth is tissue-dependent. High infiltration of TAMs was first described in neuroblastoma and shown to be associated with worse prognosis [51,52]. On the contrary, TAMs play a beneficial role in medulloblastoma and induced tumor growth suppression in vitro as well as in various mouse models [53]. Furthermore, the presence of TAMs, detected by genome-wide mRNA profiling and immunohistochemistry, was shown to be associated with suppression of metastasis and improved overall survival in patients with high-grade osteosarcoma [54], thus providing a rationale for the use of macrophage-activating agents such as liposomal muramyl tripeptide phosphatidylethanolamine (L-MTP-PE). L-MTP-PE is a synthetic analog of a bacterial wall component that induces the activation of monocytes and macrophages in the TME, thereby promoting their anti-tumor activity [55]. Conflicting results exist regarding the utility of L-MTP-PE [56]. A report from the Children's Oncology Group (COG) analyzed whether the addition of L-MTP-PE would improve outcomes in patients with osteosarcoma and found a statistically significant improvement of the overall survival from 70 to 78% [57]. However, 91 patients with metastatic osteosarcoma were separately analyzed, with no significant survival difference seen with the administration of L-MTP-PE [58].

Cancer cells also recruit myeloid-derived suppressor cells (MDSCs) to the TME as a mechanism to successfully evade the immune system. MDSCs are a population of tumor-infiltrating cells with immune-suppressive and tumor-promoting activity. MDSCs suppress both adaptive and innate arms of immunity through direct inhibition of the cytotoxic functions of T cells and NK cells [59]. Inhibition of MDSCs in three different immunocompetent mouse models of neuroblastoma resulted in the inhibition of tumor growth [60]. Thus, immunotherapies aimed at eliminating this suppressor cell subset could be advantageous in targeting the TME by counteracting the tumor escape mechanism and resuscitating the immune system. There are currently no known such therapies for pediatric solid tumors.

3.2. Cytokines and Growth Factors

Cytokines and growth factors that influence immune cells' proliferation, phenotype, or function remain under investigation with respect to treatment of pediatric solid tumors.

An example of anti-tumor cytokine therapy involves interleukin 2 (IL-2). IL-2 is a gamma-c cytokine produced by T helper 1 cells that functions to activate T cell proliferation and facilitate the maintenance of NK cells [61]. Currently, IL-2 is FDA-approved for treating adults with renal cell carcinoma (RCC) and malignant melanoma [62]. In children with large refractory sarcoma or neuroblastoma, several phase I and II trials utilizing IL-2 as monotherapy have shown no measurable anti-tumor effects, and relapses occurred despite immune activation [63–65]. Of note, one of five children with RCC had a complete response which was consistent with the 10–20% response rate observed in adults [64]. However, IL-2 administered with alternating cycles of GM-CSF plus the mAb ch14.18 (dinutuximab) resulted in higher rates of event-free (66% versus 46%) and overall (86% versus 75%) survival after 2 years compared to standard therapy alone in children with high-risk neuroblastoma [18].

Alpha-interferon (IFN-α) is another cytokine known to activate cytotoxic T lymphocytes and NK cells [66]. IFN-α is FDA-approved for use in adults to treat malignant melanoma, chronic myelogenous leukemia (CML), hairy cell leukemia, and acquired immunodeficiency syndrome (AIDS)-related Kaposi sarcoma. A limited number of studies have evaluated the use of IFN therapy to treat pediatric solid tumors. High-dose IFN-α administered for 4 weeks followed by a lower maintenance dose for 48 weeks was feasible in children with resected stage III melanoma and was associated with less toxicity than in adults treated with the same regimen [67]. However, 2 out of 15 patients were taken off that study for recurrent disease during maintenance therapy [67]. A phase II study (NCT00041145) of pegylated

IFN-α in 32 children with diffuse intrinsic pontine glioma (DIPG) reported prolonged median time to progression without significant improvement of the two-year survival rate [68], concluding that monotherapy with pegylated IFN-α may not be adequate, and further evaluation for use in combination studies is needed. Recently, a phase II trial (NCT00678951) explored the effect of IFN-α in children with unresectable plexiform neurofibromas and found both clinical and radiographic improvements; weekly injections of IFN-α resulted in at least doubling of the time to progression [69]. Currently, a combination of pegylated IFN-α, chemotherapy, and surgery is being tested in a phase III COG trial to treat patients, including children over the age of 5, with high-grade osteosarcoma (NCT00134030).

The cytokine receptor activator of nuclear factor-κB ligand (RANKL) is a member of the tumor necrosis factor (TNF) family that, in addition to being expressed on the surface of osteoblasts, is released by activated T lymphocytes [70]. RANKL regulates bone metabolism and plays a role in the pathophysiology of bone metastasis. RANKL induces osteoclast activation, which then mediates bone resorption and release of growth factors, resulting in a cycle of bone destruction and tumor proliferation [71]. Denosumab, a RANKL antibody, inhibits this osteoclast-mediated bone destruction. It has been used in phase II clinical trials in adults with multiple myeloma and metastatic breast and prostate cancer where it suppressed bone resorption [72]. In a study of 40 patients including 14 children, RANKL was expressed in 75% of high-grade osteosarcomas, and its expression correlated with a more aggressive clinical course, poor response to neoadjuvant chemotherapy, and poor event-free survival [73]. Denosumab may thus have a utility in the treatment of osteosarcoma and is currently being evaluated in a phase II clinical trial (NCT02470091) in children with recurrent or refractory osteosarcoma.

TNF, a peptide produced by macrophages and lymphocytes, has cytostatic and cytolytic effects on tumor cells in vitro [74] as well as stimulates necrosis and tumor regression in vivo [75]. Therapies incorporating recombinant TNF have been limited by the development of systemic toxicities, including hypotension, hemorrhagic gastritis, hyperbilirubinemia, and elevated creatinine [76]. Recombinant TNF has been studied in combination with dactinomycin in a phase I trial in 21 patients with refractory malignancies, including sarcoma and Wilms tumor. Evidence of anti-tumor activity was observed in only three patients, including one with Wilms tumor. Based on the anti-tumor activity observed in that patient with Wilms tumor, a phase II trial evaluated the combination of TNF and dactinomycin in patients with relapsed or refractory Wilms tumor. The combination was well tolerated and resulted in complete response in 16% and stable disease in 26% of patients [77].

Tumor necrosis factor-related apoptosis-inducing ligand (TRAIL) is another member of the TNF superfamily. TRAIL activates death receptors expressed on tumor cells, such as TRAIL-R1 and TRAIL-R2, inducing apoptosis [78]. Osteosarcoma, Ewing sarcoma, and rhabdomyosarcoma cell lines that express TRAIL death receptor were found to be sensitive to TRAIL-mediated apoptosis [79,80]. Lexatumumab, an agonistic human mAB against TRAIL-R2, binds and activates TRAIL-R2. Lexatumumab was evaluated in a phase I trial (NCT00428272) in pediatric patients with recurrent or progressive solid tumors, including osteosarcoma, Ewing sarcoma, rhabdomyosarcoma, soft tissue sarcoma, hepatoblastoma, and nephroblastoma [81]. While no patients experienced either a complete or a partial response, several showed evidence of anti-tumor activity. A patient with osteosarcoma demonstrated resolution of the clinical symptoms and positron emission tomography activity, ongoing for more than 1 year off therapy, while a patient with hepatoblastoma showed a dramatic biomarker response [81].

GM-CSF is a myeloid growth factor that stimulates hematopoietic stem cells to make granulocytes and monocytes. In acute myeloid leukemia (AML), GM-CSF led to sensitization of leukemic cells and enhanced the cytotoxicity effects of chemotherapy [82]. Inhaled GM-CSF was evaluated in three adolescents with pulmonary metastases from osteosarcoma and Ewing sarcoma (NCT00673179). There were virtually no toxicities, and a patient with Ewing sarcoma demonstrated a complete response [83].

Other cytokines studied include IFN-γ, which is produced by NK cells and T cells in response to viral and intracellular bacterial infections as well as during anti-tumor responses. IFN-γ is currently FDA-approved for the treatment of children with osteopetrosis and chronic granulomatous disease. In addition, INF-γ has shown activity against Ewing sarcoma in combination with a TRAIL agonist in preclinical models [84] and has potential for clinical translation.

3.3. Chimeric Antigen Receptor T Cell Therapy

Chimeric antigen receptor (CAR) T cell therapy has been rapidly expanding in pediatric cancer therapeutics. In this approach, autologous T cells are collected from the patient, expanded, and subsequently engineered to express CARs, which are designed to redirect T cells to a selected tumor antigen. This non-physiologic T cell activation bypasses the need for tumor antigen presentation to major histocompatibility complex (MHC) Class I molecules, which are often downregulated in cancer, and allows antigen-expressing malignant cells to be recognized and destroyed by the CAR-redirected T cells. Different generations of CAR T cells exist. The first generations carry a single-chain fragment variable region (scFv) or activation domain against a TAA [85], while the second and third generations involve the addition of one or two co-stimulatory molecules, such as CD28, CD137 (4-1 BB), and/or CD134 (OX-40), and show improved T cell proliferation and survival and anti-tumor effects [86–88].

The majority of studies involving CAR T cells in the pediatric population were aimed at hematological malignancies, with fewer designed for malignant solid tumors [89]. Neuroblastoma was the first pediatric solid tumor on which CAR T cells have been tested in clinical trials [90,91]. In a phase I trial using first-generation CAR T cells targeting GD2 in refractory neuroblastoma, there was a 45% response rate in patients with active disease. Three of 11 (27%) patients achieved complete remission, with 2 achieving sustained remission for more than 5 years [90]. Currently, third-generation anti-GD2 CAR T cells which integrate the CD28 and OX-40 costimulatory domains are undergoing a phase I study (NCT01822652) for patients with refractory neuroblastoma [92]. The development of CAR T cells targeting ALK has also been suggested. Although no clinical trials have yet been initiated, human anti-ALK CAR T cells were shown to eradicate ALK-positive neuroblastoma tumors in a xenogeneic immunodeficient murine model [93]. However, the efficacy of these CAR T cells was dependent on both target tumor antigen and CAR receptor density [93].

HER2/Neu, which is highly expressed in medulloblastoma, osteosarcoma, and nephroblastoma, has also been incorporated into CAR T cells [94,95]. HER2-specific CAR T cells efficiently recognize and eliminate tumor cells even with modest levels of HER2 expression [96,97] and have been tested in a preclinical model of osteosarcoma [98]. In a phase I clinical trial utilizing anti-HER2 CAR T cells in 19 patients with advanced pediatric sarcoma (NCT00902044), 4 had stable disease for 3 to 14 months, and the median overall survival was 10.3 months [99].

Other CAR T cells being evaluated in clinical trials include those targeting interleukin 13 receptor alpha (IL-13Rα), which is shown to be overexpressed in gliomas and other pediatric brain tumors [100,101]. IL13Rα2-specific CAR T cells targeted and killed high-grade glioma cells and glioma stem-like initiating cells in vitro [102], as well as caused the regression of established human glioblastoma orthotopic xenografts [103]. Currently, no trials utilizing IL13Rα2-specific CAR T cells are actively enrolling pediatric patients.

While dramatic clinical responses were seen in clinical trials, significant potential toxicities were associated with the use of CAR T cell therapy. Cytokine release syndrome (CRS) has been the most commonly described severe toxicity and is characterized by fever, tachycardia, hypotension, and hypoxia. Reports of CRS ranged from mild flu-like symptoms to life-threatening multi-organ system failure [104]. This constellation of inflammatory symptoms results from the release of cytokines from the CAR T cells and other immune cells. A variety of neurotoxicities have also been reported with CAR T cell therapy, ranging from somnolence, tremors, and seizures to cerebral edema and death [104]. Models utilizing serum cytokine levels after CAR T cell infusion are being developed to predict those at risk for severe CRS or neurotoxicity and may guide future interventions with immunosuppression or cytokine-directed therapy [105]. Approaches to ameliorate CRS or neurotoxicity while maintaining treatment efficacy include directly targeting specific cytokines, such as IL6 blockade by tocilizumab [106], as well as the use of an inducible caspase suicide safety switch that may be activated, leading to programmed cell death to prevent unanticipated toxicities [107]. The latter has been tested in a clinical trial for pediatric patients and led to the elimination of 90% of CAR T cells within 30 minutes of the infusion [108]. Another type of toxicity associated with CAR T cell therapy is agammaglobulinemia, which may be corrected with gammaglobulin replacement.

3.4. Natural Killer Cell-Based Immunotherapy

NK cells have been investigated as potential immunotherapeutics due to their anti-tumor effects, through either direct cytotoxicity or antibody-dependent cellular toxicity. A major component of NK cell target recognition depends on the surveillance of human leukocyte antigen (HLA) class I molecules by killer immunoglobulin-like receptors (KIRs) [109]. KIRs are expressed on the surface of NK cells and transmit immune inhibitory signals to maintain tolerance to NK cells. Cancer cells without an inhibitory HLA ligand may trigger NK cell activation.

The potential for the therapeutic application of NK cells was primarily tested in hematologic malignancies, such as AML and ALL [110]. In these studies, reduced risk of relapse and improved survival were observed after allogeneic hematopoietic stem cell transplantation (HSCT) when HLA ligands against the inhibitory KIRs present in the donor were absent in the recipient. HSCT has also been proposed as a potential curative alternative in children with refractory solid tumors, such as Ewing sarcoma [111], neuroblastoma [112], melanoma [113], and hepatoblastoma [114]. Perez-Martinez et al. suggested that the clinically beneficial graft-versus-tumor (GVT) effect seen after HSCT may be mediated by donor–recipient inhibitory KIR–HLA mismatched NK cells [115]. That study examined three children with refractory solid tumors and observed a clinical response in the two patients with a KIR–HLA mismatched donor during the time when NK cells were the major lymphocyte population. In addition, the degree of tumor response appeared to correlate with the number of KIR-activating receptors [115].

A few ongoing early clinical trials are investigating the role of autologous and allogeneic NK cells in pediatric solid tumors. NCT01875601 is employing ex vivo activated and expanded autologous NK cells with recombinant human IL-15 in children with brain tumors, sarcoma, Wilms tumor, and rhabdomyosarcoma after lympho-depleting chemotherapy. Two trials (NCT01576692 and NCT01857934) are exploring the safety and feasibility of allogenic NK cell infusions from haploidentical donors in children with high-risk neuroblastoma in combination with the humanized anti-GD2 antibody (hu14.18K322A) and standard chemotherapy. NCT01287104 is assessing the feasibility and toxicity of infusing escalating doses of donor-derived activated NK cell donor lymphocyte infusions (NK-DLI) following HLA-matched T cell-depleted (TCD) peripheral blood stem cell transplant (PBSCT) in patients with metastatic or recurrent pediatric solid tumors. NCT00640796 was recently completed. This phase I study was designed to determine the safety of infusing expanded NK cells, obtained from a patient's family member with partial HLA mismatch, into pediatric patients with Ewing sarcoma family of tumors (ESFT) and rhabdomyosarcoma. The results of this trial are not yet available.

The efficacy of NK cell-based immunotherapy may be reduced by numerous factors such as limited in vivo proliferation and the immunosuppressive milieu of the TME. Furthermore, tumor cells develop various strategies to evade NK cell attack or to impair the activity and function of NK cell therapy. For example, tumor cells often upregulate the expression of KIR ligands, such as HLA-G [116]. HLA-G may inhibit the proliferation and cytotoxicity of NK cells [117]. Ectopic HLA-G expression on Ewing sarcoma suppressed the activity of GD2-specific CAR-expressing NK cells [118]. In addition, blocking of HLA-G on tumor cells in patients with chronic lymphocytic leukemia (CLL) increased their susceptibility to NK cell-mediated cytotoxicity [119]. Strategies to augment the anti-tumor efficacy of NK cells, prolong their survival and persistence in vivo, and restore their functions from exhaustion in the TME will maximize the effects of this novel therapy. Furthermore, NK cells have not been associated with significant off-target effects, graft-versus-host disease, or CRS [120], making this therapy an attractive modality to explore.

3.5. Cancer Vaccines

Vaccines are some of the oldest means for modulating the immune response. The idea behind this therapy is that an exposure to a pathogen will allow for the generation of an adaptive immune response toward future re-exposure to that pathogen. For cancer, this same idea has also been explored in hopes of generating an anti-tumor response and cell-mediated immunity [5]. In comparison to other immunotherapies, this manipulation of the immune system shows promise specifically for pediatric solid tumors but has had limited study.

Anti-cancer vaccines typically exploit DCs. These antigen-presenting cells serve an important role as a bridge between the adaptive and the innate immune response, allowing for both an active and a passive attack on the tumor [121,122]. Different mechanisms used to stimulate T cell responses from DCs include mRNA strands, cell surface receptors, and lysed intracellular proteins. Researchers proved this point by pulsing DCs with sarcoma cell lysate and priming with cytokines. These DCs were administered to mice for immunization. They found these cells adept at producing a primary T cell response as well as significantly decreased pulmonary metastasis of the sarcoma tumor cells [123]. In pediatrics, a rhabdomyosarcoma cell line known as M3-9-M was grown in vivo and tested similarly with a vaccine. The authors were able to demonstrate a decrease in tumor growth in vivo, and upon depletion of CD4+ and CD8+ T cells, a lack of tumor cell response, indicating the necessity of a T cell response for anti-tumor effects [124].

In clinical trials, vaccines have been an area of focus for the treatment of gliomas, neuroblastoma, sarcoma, and Wilms tumor. In one clinical trial, dendritic vaccines were administered to pediatric patients with solid tumors, with one patient achieving a significant decrease in tumor size, and two patients showing undetectable disease. The tumor lysates were tested for immune response. Compared to pre-vaccine samples, the post-vaccine tumor lysates had a significantly higher level of IFN-γ, thus indicating the effectiveness of this vaccine at producing an immune response [125]. This study also demonstrated that dendritic cell-based vaccines could be administered in the outpatient setting and were not associated with significant toxicities in children [125]. Many of the future directions of the use of dendritic cell-based vaccines are toward improving efficacy through further immunomodulation [121]. Other clinical trials are studying the combination of vaccines with chemotherapeutics. A phase I/II trial for relapsed or refractory neuroblastoma and sarcoma used decitabine and DC/MAGE-A1, MAGE-A3, and NY-ESO-1 peptide vaccines (NCT01241162). Using CD137 as a T cell marker, 6 out of the 10 patients given the vaccine had a T cell response. Of those six patients, one had a complete tumor response, while one remains disease-free two years after the trial [126,127]. Such trials are the groundbreaking work that is needed to further implement these therapies and determine what is most effective in the pediatric population.

4. Conclusions

Immunotherapeutics with either direct utilization or modulation of the immune system provide novel treatment approaches for the treatment of children with solid tumors (Table 1). Although these therapies have shown promising clinical results, they are currently utilized in a limited number of pediatric cancer diagnoses. A more generalized pediatric use will require further studies to firmly establish the safety and treatment efficacy of these approaches and identify ways to integrate them with current conventional treatment regimens for a greater impact in pediatric solid tumors.

Table 1. Immunotherapy clinical trials for pediatric solid tumors discussed in this review.

Immunotherapy Approach	Disease	Target	Agent/Compound	NCT #	Phase of Study
Viral therapy	Cerebellar Brain Tumor	N/A	G207 (HSV)	03911388	Phase I (recruiting)
Viral therapy	Supratentorial Brain Tumor	N/A	G207 (HSV) +/− radiation	02457845	Phase I (recruiting)
Viral therapy	DIPG	N/A	DNX-2401 (adenovirus)	03178032	Phase I (recruiting)
Viral therapy	Glioma	N/A	Recombinant Polio/Rhinovirus	03043391	Phase I (recruiting)
Antigen-targeting and growth factor therapy	Neuroblastoma	GD2	hu3F8 (mAB against GD2) and GM-CSF	01757626	Phase I/II (recruiting)
Immune checkpoint inhibitor	Solid tumors	CTLA-4	Ipilimumab	01445379	Phase I (completed)
Immune checkpoint inhibitor	Solid tumors or lymphoma	PD-1	Nivolumab with chemotherapy	03585465	Phase I/II (recruiting)
Immune checkpoint inhibitor	Hypermutated malignancies	PD-1	Nivolumab	02992964	Phase I/II (recruiting)
Immune checkpoint inhibitor	Solid tumors	PD-1	Nivolumab	02901145	Phase I/II (not yet recruiting)
Immune checkpoint inhibitor	Solid tumors or sarcoma	PD-1/CTLA-4	Nivolumab +/− ipilimumab	02304458	Phase I/II (recruiting)
Cytokine therapy	DIPG	N/A	Pegylated IFN-α2b	00041145	Phase II (completed)
Cytokine therapy	Plexiform neurofibroma	N/A	Pegylated IFN-α2b	00678951	Phase II (completed)
Cytokine therapy	Osteosarcoma	N/A	Pegylated IFN-α2b	00134030	Phase III (active, not recruiting)
Cytokine targeted therapy	Osteosarcoma	RANKL	Denosumab (mAB against RANKL)	02470091	Phase II (active, not recruiting)
Cytokine targeted therapy	Solid tumors	TRAIL-R2	Lexatumumab (mAB against TRAIL-R2)	00428272	Phase I (terminated)
Growth factor therapy	Osteosarcoma, Ewing sarcoma	N/A	Inhaled GM-CSF (Sargramostim)	00673179	Phase I (terminated)
CAR T cells	Neuroblastoma	GD2	Anti-GD2 CAR T cells	01822652	Phase I (active, not recruiting)
CAR T cells	Sarcoma	HER2	Anti-HER2 CAR T cells	00902044	Phase I (recruiting)
NK cells with cytokine therapy	Brain tumors, sarcoma, Wilms tumor, RMS	N/A	NK cells +/− rhIL-15 after lympho-depletion	01875601	Phase I (completed)
NK cells with antigen targeted therapy	Neuroblastoma	GD2	hu14.18K322A (anti-GD2), NK cells	01576692	Phase I (completed)
NK cells with antigen targeted therapy	Neuroblastoma	GD2	hu14.18K322A (anti-GD2), NK cells	01857934	Phase II (active, not recruiting)
NK cells	Solid tumors	N/A	NK cells	01287104	Phase I (completed)
NK cells	Ewing sarcoma, RMS	N/A	NK cells	00640796	Phase I (completed)
Cancer Vaccine	Neuroblastoma, sarcoma, RMS	Cancer testes antigen	Decitabine and DC vaccine + adjuvant	01241162	Phase I (Completed)

#, number; HSV, Herpes simplex Virus; DIPG, diffuse intrinsic pontine glioma; NK, natural killer; hu3F8, humanized 3F8; mAB, monoclonal antibody; GM-CSF, granulocyte-macrophage colony stimulating factor; CTLA-4, cytotoxic T-lymphocyte-associated antigen-4; PD-1, programmed cell death receptor 1; IFN, interferon; RANKL, receptor activator of nuclear factor-κB ligand; TRAIL-R, tumor necrosis factor-related apoptosis-inducing ligand receptor; CAR, chimeric antigen receptor; RMS, rhabdomyosarcoma; rhIL-15, recombinant human interleukin 15; DC, dendritic cell.

Author Contributions: Writing the manuscript, R.M. and C.H.Q.; Review and editing, E.A.B.

Funding: All work was performed at the University of Alabama at Birmingham. This work was funded, in part, by National Institutes of Health T32 CA229102 (R.M.), and T35 HL007473 (C.H.Q.).

Conflicts of Interest: The authors declare that there are no conflicts of interest regarding the publication of this paper.

References

1. Kelly, E.; Russell, S.J. History of oncolytic viruses: Genesis to genetic engineering. *Mol. Ther.* **2007**, *15*, 651–659. [CrossRef] [PubMed]
2. Sze, D.Y.; Reid, T.R.; Rose, S.C. Oncolytic virotherapy. *J. Vasc. Interv. Radiol.* **2013**, *24*, 1115–1122. [CrossRef] [PubMed]
3. Coffey, M.C.; Strong, J.E.; Forsyth, P.A.; Lee, P.W. Reovirus therapy of tumors with activated Ras pathway. *Science* **1998**, *282*, 1332–1334. [CrossRef] [PubMed]
4. Sanchala, D.S.; Bhatt, L.K.; Prabhavalkar, K.S. Oncolytic Herpes Simplex Viral Therapy: A Stride toward Selective Targeting of Cancer Cells. *Front. Pharmacol.* **2017**, *8*, 270. [CrossRef] [PubMed]
5. Wedekind, M.F.; Denton, N.L.; Chen, C.Y.; Cripe, T.P. Pediatric Cancer Immunotherapy: Opportunities and Challenges. *Paediatr Drugs* **2018**, *20*, 395–408. [CrossRef] [PubMed]
6. Yin, J.; Markert, J.M.; Leavenworth, J.W. Modulation of the Intratumoral Immune Landscape by Oncolytic Herpes Simplex Virus Virotherapy. *Front. Oncol.* **2017**, *7*, 136. [CrossRef]
7. Pol, J.G.; Levesque, S.; Workenhe, S.T.; Gujar, S.; Le Boeuf, F.; Clements, D.R.; Fahrner, J.E.; Fend, L.; Bell, J.C.; Mossman, K.L.; et al. Trial Watch: Oncolytic viro-immunotherapy of hematologic and solid tumors. *Oncoimmunology* **2018**, *7*, e1503032. [CrossRef]
8. Waters, A.M.; Friedman, G.K.; Ring, E.K.; Beierle, E.A. Oncolytic virotherapy for pediatric malignancies: Future prospects. *Oncolytic Virother.* **2016**, *5*, 73–80. [CrossRef]
9. Tong, Y.; Qian, W. Targeting cancer stem cells with oncolytic virus. *Stem. Cell Investig.* **2014**, *1*, 20. [CrossRef]
10. Foreman, P.M.; Friedman, G.K.; Cassady, K.A.; Markert, J.M. Oncolytic Virotherapy for the Treatment of Malignant Glioma. *Neurotherapeutics* **2017**, *14*, 333–344. [CrossRef]
11. Bridle, B.W.; Stephenson, K.B.; Boudreau, J.E.; Koshy, S.; Kazdhan, N.; Pullenayegum, E.; Brunelliere, J.; Bramson, J.L.; Lichty, B.D.; Wan, Y. Potentiating cancer immunotherapy using an oncolytic virus. *Mol. Ther.* **2010**, *18*, 1430–1439. [CrossRef] [PubMed]
12. Cantoni, C.; Grauwet, K.; Pietra, G.; Parodi, M.; Mingari, M.C.; Maria, A.D.; Favoreel, H.; Vitale, M. Role of NK cells in immunotherapy and virotherapy of solid tumors. *Immunotherapy* **2015**, *7*, 861–882. [CrossRef] [PubMed]
13. Li, Y.; Yin, J.; Li, T.; Huang, S.; Yan, H.; Leavenworth, J.; Wang, X. NK cell-based cancer immunotherapy: From basic biology to clinical application. *Sci. China Life Sci.* **2015**, *58*, 1233–1245. [CrossRef]
14. Bommareddy, P.K.; Aspromonte, S.; Zloza, A.; Rabkin, S.D.; Kaufman, H.L. MEK inhibition enhances oncolytic virus immunotherapy through increased tumor cell killing and T cell activation. *Sci. Transl. Med.* **2018**, *10*. [CrossRef]
15. Denton, N.L.; Chen, C.Y.; Hutzen, B.; Currier, M.A.; Scott, T.; Nartker, B.; Leddon, J.L.; Wang, P.Y.; Srinivas, R.; Cassady, K.A.; et al. Myelolytic Treatments Enhance Oncolytic Herpes Virotherapy in Models of Ewing Sarcoma by Modulating the Immune Microenvironment. *Mol. Ther. Oncolytics* **2018**, *11*, 62–74. [CrossRef]
16. Rehman, H.; Silk, A.W.; Kane, M.P.; Kaufman, H.L. Into the clinic: Talimogene laherparepvec (T-VEC), a first-in-class intratumoral oncolytic viral therapy. *J. Immunother. Cancer* **2016**, *4*, 53. [CrossRef]
17. Vedi, A.; Ziegler, D.S. Antibody therapy for pediatric leukemia. *Front. Oncol.* **2014**, *4*, 82. [CrossRef]
18. Yu, A.L.; Gilman, A.L.; Ozkaynak, M.F.; London, W.B.; Kreissman, S.G.; Chen, H.X.; Smith, M.; Anderson, B.; Villablanca, J.G.; Matthay, K.K.; et al. Anti-GD2 antibody with GM-CSF, interleukin-2, and isotretinoin for neuroblastoma. *N. Engl. J. Med.* **2010**, *363*, 1324–1334. [CrossRef]
19. Heiner, J.P.; Miraldi, F.; Kallick, S.; Makley, J.; Neely, J.; Smith-Mensah, W.H.; Cheung, N.K. Localization of GD2-specific monoclonal antibody 3F8 in human osteosarcoma. *Cancer Res.* **1987**, *47*, 5377–5381.
20. Carpenter, E.L.; Haglund, E.A.; Mace, E.M.; Deng, D.; Martinez, D.; Wood, A.C.; Chow, A.K.; Weiser, D.A.; Belcastro, L.T.; Winter, C.; et al. Antibody targeting of anaplastic lymphoma kinase induces cytotoxicity of human neuroblastoma. *Oncogene* **2012**, *31*, 4859–4867. [CrossRef]

21. Nguyen, R.; Moustaki, A.; Norrie, J.L.; Brown, S.; Akers, W.J.; Shirinifard, A.; Dyer, M.A. Interleukin-15 Enhances Anti-GD2 Antibody-Mediated Cytotoxicity in an Orthotopic PDX Model of Neuroblastoma. *Clin. Cancer Res.* **2019**. [CrossRef] [PubMed]
22. Ploessl, C.; Pan, A.; Maples, K.T.; Lowe, D.K. Dinutuximab: An Anti-GD2 Monoclonal Antibody for High-Risk Neuroblastoma. *Ann. Pharmacother.* **2016**, *50*, 416–422. [CrossRef] [PubMed]
23. Kushner, B.H.; Cheung, I.Y.; Modak, S.; Basu, E.M.; Roberts, S.S.; Cheung, N.K. Humanized 3F8 Anti-GD2 Monoclonal Antibody Dosing With Granulocyte-Macrophage Colony-Stimulating Factor in Patients With Resistant Neuroblastoma: A Phase 1 Clinical Trial. *JAMA Oncol.* **2018**, *4*, 1729–1735. [CrossRef] [PubMed]
24. Barry, W.E.; Jackson, J.R.; Asuelime, G.E.; Wu, H.W.; Sun, J.; Wan, Z.; Malvar, J.; Sheard, M.A.; Wang, L.; Seeger, R.C.; et al. Activated Natural Killer Cells in Combination with Anti-GD2 Antibody Dinutuximab Improve Survival of Mice after Surgical Resection of Primary Neuroblastoma. *Clin. Cancer Res.* **2019**, *25*, 325–333. [CrossRef]
25. Baeuerle, P.A.; Reinhardt, C. Bispecific T-cell engaging antibodies for cancer therapy. *Cancer Res.* **2009**, *69*, 4941–4944. [CrossRef]
26. Hoffman, L.M.; Gore, L. Blinatumomab, a Bi-Specific Anti-CD19/CD3 BiTE((R)) Antibody for the Treatment of Acute Lymphoblastic Leukemia: Perspectives and Current Pediatric Applications. *Front. Oncol.* **2014**, *4*, 63. [CrossRef]
27. von Stackelberg, A.; Locatelli, F.; Zugmaier, G.; Handgretinger, R.; Trippett, T.M.; Rizzari, C.; Bader, P.; O'Brien, M.M.; Brethon, B.; Bhojwani, D.; et al. Phase I/Phase II Study of Blinatumomab in Pediatric Patients With Relapsed/Refractory Acute Lymphoblastic Leukemia. *J. Clin. Oncol.* **2016**, *34*, 4381–4389. [CrossRef]
28. Elitzur, S.; Arad-Cohen, N.; Barzilai-Birenboim, S.; Ben-Harush, M.; Bielorai, B.; Elhasid, R.; Feuerstein, T.; Gilad, G.; Gural, A.; Kharit, M.; et al. Blinatumomab as a bridge to further therapy in cases of overwhelming toxicity in pediatric B-cell precursor acute lymphoblastic leukemia: Report from the Israeli Study Group of Childhood Leukemia. *Pediatr. Blood Cancer* **2019**, *66*, e27898. [CrossRef]
29. Leach, D.R.; Krummel, M.F.; Allison, J.P. Enhancement of antitumor immunity by CTLA-4 blockade. *Science* **1996**, *271*, 1734–1736. [CrossRef]
30. Walker, L.S. Treg and CTLA-4: Two intertwining pathways to immune tolerance. *J. Autoimmun.* **2013**, *45*, 49–57. [CrossRef]
31. Contardi, E.; Palmisano, G.L.; Tazzari, P.L.; Martelli, A.M.; Fala, F.; Fabbi, M.; Kato, T.; Lucarelli, E.; Donati, D.; Polito, L.; et al. CTLA-4 is constitutively expressed on tumor cells and can trigger apoptosis upon ligand interaction. *Int. J. Cancer* **2005**, *117*, 538–550. [CrossRef] [PubMed]
32. Hingorani, P.; Maas, M.L.; Gustafson, M.P.; Dickman, P.; Adams, R.H.; Watanabe, M.; Eshun, F.; Williams, J.; Seidel, M.J.; Dietz, A.B. Increased CTLA-4(+) T cells and an increased ratio of monocytes with loss of class II (CD14(+) HLA-DR(lo/neg)) found in aggressive pediatric sarcoma patients. *J. Immunother. Cancer* **2015**, *3*, 35. [CrossRef] [PubMed]
33. Merchant, M.S.; Wright, M.; Baird, K.; Wexler, L.H.; Rodriguez-Galindo, C.; Bernstein, D.; Delbrook, C.; Lodish, M.; Bishop, R.; Wolchok, J.D.; et al. Phase I Clinical Trial of Ipilimumab in Pediatric Patients with Advanced Solid Tumors. *Clin. Cancer Res.* **2016**, *22*, 1364–1370. [CrossRef] [PubMed]
34. Brahmer, J.R.; Tykodi, S.S.; Chow, L.Q.; Hwu, W.J.; Topalian, S.L.; Hwu, P.; Drake, C.G.; Camacho, L.H.; Kauh, J.; Odunsi, K.; et al. Safety and activity of anti-PD-L1 antibody in patients with advanced cancer. *N. Engl. J. Med.* **2012**, *366*, 2455–2465. [CrossRef]
35. Pardoll, D.M. The blockade of immune checkpoints in cancer immunotherapy. *Nat. Rev. Cancer* **2012**, *12*, 252–264. [CrossRef]
36. Majzner, R.G.; Simon, J.S.; Grosso, J.F.; Martinez, D.; Pawel, B.R.; Santi, M.; Merchant, M.S.; Geoerger, B.; Hezam, I.; Marty, V.; et al. Assessment of programmed death-ligand 1 expression and tumor-associated immune cells in pediatric cancer tissues. *Cancer* **2017**, *123*, 3807–3815. [CrossRef]
37. Geoerger, B.; Kang, H.J.; Yalon-Oren, M.; Marshall, L.V.; Vezina, C.; Pappo, A.S.; Laetsch, T.W.; Petrilli, A.S.; Ebinger, M.; Toporski, J.; et al. KEYNOTE-051: An update on the phase 2 results of pembrolizumab (pembro) in pediatric patients (pts) with advanced melanoma or a PD-L1–positive advanced, relapsed or refractory solid tumor or lymphoma. *J. Clin. Oncol.* **2018**, *36*, 10525. [CrossRef]
38. Zheng, W.; Xiao, H.; Liu, H.; Zhou, Y. Expression of programmed death 1 is correlated with progression of osteosarcoma. *APMIS* **2015**, *123*, 102–107. [CrossRef]

39. Robert, C.; Schachter, J.; Long, G.V.; Arance, A.; Grob, J.J.; Mortier, L.; Daud, A.; Carlino, M.S.; McNeil, C.; Lotem, M.; et al. Pembrolizumab versus Ipilimumab in Advanced Melanoma. *N. Engl. J. Med.* **2015**, *372*, 2521–2532. [CrossRef]
40. Topalian, S.L.; Hodi, F.S.; Brahmer, J.R.; Gettinger, S.N.; Smith, D.C.; McDermott, D.F.; Powderly, J.D.; Carvajal, R.D.; Sosman, J.A.; Atkins, M.B.; et al. Safety, activity, and immune correlates of anti-PD-1 antibody in cancer. *N. Engl. J. Med.* **2012**, *366*, 2443–2454. [CrossRef]
41. Blumenthal, D.T.; Yalon, M.; Vainer, G.W.; Lossos, A.; Yust, S.; Tzach, L.; Cagnano, E.; Limon, D.; Bokstein, F. Pembrolizumab: First experience with recurrent primary central nervous system (CNS) tumors. *J. Neurooncol.* **2016**, *129*, 453–460. [CrossRef]
42. Gorsi, H.S.; Malicki, D.M.; Barsan, V.; Tumblin, M.; Yeh-Nayre, L.; Milburn, M.; Elster, J.D.; Crawford, J.R. Nivolumab in the Treatment of Recurrent or Refractory Pediatric Brain Tumors: A Single Institutional Experience. *J. Pediatr. Hematol. Oncol.* **2019**, *41*, e235–e241. [CrossRef] [PubMed]
43. Bouffet, E.; Larouche, V.; Campbell, B.B.; Merico, D.; de Borja, R.; Aronson, M.; Durno, C.; Krueger, J.; Cabric, V.; Ramaswamy, V.; et al. Immune Checkpoint Inhibition for Hypermutant Glioblastoma Multiforme Resulting From Germline Biallelic Mismatch Repair Deficiency. *J. Clin. Oncol.* **2016**, *34*, 2206–2211. [CrossRef] [PubMed]
44. Zhu, X.; McDowell, M.M.; Newman, W.C.; Mason, G.E.; Greene, S.; Tamber, M.S. Severe cerebral edema following nivolumab treatment for pediatric glioblastoma: Case report. *J. Neurosurg. Pediatr.* **2017**, *19*, 249–253. [CrossRef] [PubMed]
45. Twyman-Saint Victor, C.; Rech, A.J.; Maity, A.; Rengan, R.; Pauken, K.E.; Stelekati, E.; Benci, J.L.; Xu, B.; Dada, H.; Odorizzi, P.M.; et al. Radiation and dual checkpoint blockade activate non-redundant immune mechanisms in cancer. *Nature* **2015**, *520*, 373–377. [CrossRef]
46. Lussier, D.M.; Johnson, J.L.; Hingorani, P.; Blattman, J.N. Combination immunotherapy with alpha-CTLA-4 and alpha-PD-L1 antibody blockade prevents immune escape and leads to complete control of metastatic osteosarcoma. *J. Immunother. Cancer* **2015**, *3*, 21. [CrossRef]
47. Sounni, N.E.; Noel, A. Targeting the tumor microenvironment for cancer therapy. *Clin. Chem.* **2013**, *59*, 85–93. [CrossRef]
48. Zeine, R.; Salwen, H.R.; Peddinti, R.; Tian, Y.; Guerrero, L.; Yang, Q.; Chlenski, A.; Cohn, S.L. Presence of cancer-associated fibroblasts inversely correlates with Schwannian stroma in neuroblastoma tumors. *Mod. Pathol.* **2009**, *22*, 950–958. [CrossRef]
49. Kock, A.; Larsson, K.; Bergqvist, F.; Eissler, N.; Elfman, L.H.M.; Raouf, J.; Korotkova, M.; Johnsen, J.I.; Jakobsson, P.J.; Kogner, P. Inhibition of Microsomal Prostaglandin E Synthese-1 in Cancer-Associated Fibroblasts Suppresses Neuroblastoma Tumor Growth. *EBioMedicine* **2018**, *32*, 84–92. [CrossRef]
50. Kraman, M.; Bambrough, P.J.; Arnold, J.N.; Roberts, E.W.; Magiera, L.; Jones, J.O.; Gopinathan, A.; Tuveson, D.A.; Fearon, D.T. Suppression of antitumor immunity by stromal cells expressing fibroblast activation protein-alpha. *Science* **2010**, *330*, 827–830. [CrossRef]
51. Asgharzadeh, S.; Salo, J.A.; Ji, L.; Oberthuer, A.; Fischer, M.; Berthold, F.; Hadjidaniel, M.; Liu, C.W.; Metelitsa, L.S.; Pique-Regi, R.; et al. Clinical significance of tumor-associated inflammatory cells in metastatic neuroblastoma. *J. Clin. Oncol.* **2012**, *30*, 3525–3532. [CrossRef] [PubMed]
52. Song, L.; Asgharzadeh, S.; Salo, J.; Engell, K.; Wu, H.W.; Sposto, R.; Ara, T.; Silverman, A.M.; DeClerck, Y.A.; Seeger, R.C.; et al. Valpha24-invariant NKT cells mediate antitumor activity via killing of tumor-associated macrophages. *J. Clin. Investig.* **2009**, *119*, 1524–1536. [CrossRef] [PubMed]
53. Maximov, V.; Chen, Z.; Wei, Y.; Robinson, M.H.; Herting, C.J.; Shanmugam, N.S.; Rudneva, V.A.; Goldsmith, K.C.; MacDonald, T.J.; Northcott, P.A.; et al. Tumour-associated macrophages exhibit anti-tumoural properties in Sonic Hedgehog medulloblastoma. *Nat. Commun.* **2019**, *10*, 2410. [CrossRef] [PubMed]
54. Buddingh, E.P.; Kuijjer, M.L.; Duim, R.A.; Burger, H.; Agelopoulos, K.; Myklebost, O.; Serra, M.; Mertens, F.; Hogendoorn, P.C.; Lankester, A.C.; et al. Tumor-infiltrating macrophages are associated with metastasis suppression in high-grade osteosarcoma: A rationale for treatment with macrophage activating agents. *Clin. Cancer Res.* **2011**, *17*, 2110–2119. [CrossRef]
55. Mori, K.; Ando, K.; Heymann, D. Liposomal muramyl tripeptide phosphatidyl ethanolamine: A safe and effective agent against osteosarcoma pulmonary metastases. *Expert. Rev. Anticancer. Ther.* **2008**, *8*, 151–159. [CrossRef]

56. Kager, L.; Potschger, U.; Bielack, S. Review of mifamurtide in the treatment of patients with osteosarcoma. *Ther. Clin. Risk. Manag.* **2010**, *6*, 279–286. [CrossRef]
57. Meyers, P.A.; Schwartz, C.L.; Krailo, M.D.; Healey, J.H.; Bernstein, M.L.; Betcher, D.; Ferguson, W.S.; Gebhardt, M.C.; Goorin, A.M.; Harris, M.; et al. Osteosarcoma: The addition of muramyl tripeptide to chemotherapy improves overall survival–a report from the Children's Oncology Group. *J. Clin. Oncol.* **2008**, *26*, 633–638. [CrossRef]
58. Chou, A.J.; Kleinerman, E.S.; Krailo, M.D.; Chen, Z.; Betcher, D.L.; Healey, J.H.; Conrad, E.U., 3rd; Nieder, M.L.; Weiner, M.A.; Wells, R.J.; et al. Addition of muramyl tripeptide to chemotherapy for patients with newly diagnosed metastatic osteosarcoma: A report from the Children's Oncology Group. *Cancer* **2009**, *115*, 5339–5348. [CrossRef]
59. Gabrilovich, D.I.; Nagaraj, S. Myeloid-derived suppressor cells as regulators of the immune system. *Nat. Rev. Immunol.* **2009**, *9*, 162–174. [CrossRef]
60. Santilli, G.; Piotrowska, I.; Cantilena, S.; Chayka, O.; D'Alicarnasso, M.; Morgenstern, D.A.; Himoudi, N.; Pearson, K.; Anderson, J.; Thrasher, A.J.; et al. Polyphenon [corrected] E enhances the antitumor immune response in neuroblastoma by inactivating myeloid suppressor cells. *Clin Cancer Res.* **2013**, *19*, 1116–1125. [CrossRef]
61. Liao, W.; Lin, J.X.; Leonard, W.J. Interleukin-2 at the crossroads of effector responses, tolerance, and immunotherapy. *Immunity* **2013**, *38*, 13–25. [CrossRef] [PubMed]
62. Konjevic, G.; Mirjacic Martinovic, K.; Vuletic, A.; Babovic, N. In-vitro IL-2 or IFN-alpha-induced NKG2D and CD161 NK cell receptor expression indicates novel aspects of NK cell activation in metastatic melanoma patients. *Melanoma Res.* **2010**, *20*, 459–467. [CrossRef] [PubMed]
63. Roper, M.; Smith, M.A.; Sondel, P.M.; Gillespie, A.; Reaman, G.H.; Hammond, G.D.; Levitt, D.; Rosolen, A.; Colamonici, O.R.; Neckers, L.M.; et al. A phase I study of interleukin-2 in children with cancer. *Am. J. Pediatr. Hematol. Oncol.* **1992**, *14*, 305–311. [CrossRef] [PubMed]
64. Bauer, M.; Reaman, G.H.; Hank, J.A.; Cairo, M.S.; Anderson, P.; Blazar, B.R.; Frierdich, S.; Sondel, P.M. A phase II trial of human recombinant interleukin-2 administered as a 4-day continuous infusion for children with refractory neuroblastoma, non-Hodgkin's lymphoma, sarcoma, renal cell carcinoma, and malignant melanoma. A childrens cancer group study. *Cancer* **1995**, *75*, 2959–2965. [CrossRef]
65. Kalwak, K.; Ussowicz, M.; Gorczynska, E.; Turkiewicz, D.; Toporski, J.; Dobaczewski, G.; Latos-Grazynska, E.; Ryczan, R.; Noworolska-Sauren, D.; Chybicka, A. Immunologic effects of intermediate-dose IL-2 i.v. after autologous hematopoietic cell transplantation in pediatric solid tumors. *J. Interferon Cytokine Res.* **2003**, *23*, 173–181. [CrossRef]
66. Hakanson, A.; Gustafsson, B.; Krysander, L.; Hakansson, L. Tumour-infiltrating lymphocytes in metastatic malignant melanoma and response to interferon alpha treatment. *Br. J. Cancer* **1996**, *74*, 670–676. [CrossRef]
67. Navid, F.; Furman, W.L.; Fleming, M.; Rao, B.N.; Kovach, S.; Billups, C.A.; Cain, A.M.; Amonette, R.; Jenkins, J.J.; Pappo, A.S. The feasibility of adjuvant interferon alpha-2b in children with high-risk melanoma. *Cancer* **2005**, *103*, 780–787. [CrossRef]
68. Warren, K.; Bent, R.; Wolters, P.L.; Prager, A.; Hanson, R.; Packer, R.; Shih, J.; Camphausen, K. A phase 2 study of pegylated interferon alpha-2b (PEG-Intron((R))) in children with diffuse intrinsic pontine glioma. *Cancer* **2012**, *118*, 3607–3613. [CrossRef]
69. Jakacki, R.I.; Dombi, E.; Steinberg, S.M.; Goldman, S.; Kieran, M.W.; Ullrich, N.J.; Pollack, I.F.; Goodwin, A.; Manley, P.E.; Fangusaro, J.; et al. Phase II trial of pegylated interferon alfa-2b in young patients with neurofibromatosis type 1 and unresectable plexiform neurofibromas. *Neuro Oncol.* **2017**, *19*, 289–297. [CrossRef]
70. Kohli, S.S.; Kohli, V.S. Role of RANKL-RANK/osteoprotegerin molecular complex in bone remodeling and its immunopathologic implications. *Indian J. Endocrinol Metab.* **2011**, *15*, 175–181. [CrossRef]
71. Roodman, G.D. Mechanisms of bone metastasis. *N. Engl. J. Med.* **2004**, *350*, 1655–1664. [CrossRef] [PubMed]
72. Fizazi, K.; Lipton, A.; Mariette, X.; Body, J.J.; Rahim, Y.; Gralow, J.R.; Gao, G.; Wu, L.; Sohn, W.; Jun, S. Randomized phase II trial of denosumab in patients with bone metastases from prostate cancer, breast cancer, or other neoplasms after intravenous bisphosphonates. *J. Clin. Oncol.* **2009**, *27*, 1564–1571. [CrossRef] [PubMed]
73. Lee, J.A.; Jung, J.S.; Kim, D.H.; Lim, J.S.; Kim, M.S.; Kong, C.B.; Song, W.S.; Cho, W.H.; Jeon, D.G.; Lee, S.Y.; et al. RANKL expression is related to treatment outcome of patients with localized, high-grade osteosarcoma. *Pediatr. Blood Cancer* **2011**, *56*, 738–743. [CrossRef]

74. Nakano, K.; Abe, S.; Sohmura, Y. Recombinant human tumor necrosis factor–I. Cytotoxic activity in vitro. *Int. J. Immunopharmacol.* **1986**, *8*, 347–355. [CrossRef]
75. Lejeune, F.J.; Lienard, D.; Matter, M.; Ruegg, C. Efficiency of recombinant human TNF in human cancer therapy. *Cancer Immunol.* **2006**, *6*, 6.
76. Seibel, N.L.; Dinndorf, P.A.; Bauer, M.; Sondel, P.M.; Hammond, G.D.; Reaman, G.H. Phase I study of tumor necrosis factor-alpha and actinomycin D in pediatric patients with cancer: A Children's Cancer Group study. *J. Immunother. Emphasis Tumor Immunol.* **1994**, *16*, 125–131. [CrossRef]
77. Meany, H.J.; Seibel, N.L.; Sun, J.; Finklestein, J.Z.; Sato, J.; Kelleher, J.; Sondel, P.; Reaman, G. Phase 2 trial of recombinant tumor necrosis factor-alpha in combination with dactinomycin in children with recurrent Wilms tumor. *J. Immunother.* **2008**, *31*, 679–683. [CrossRef]
78. Daniels, R.A.; Turley, H.; Kimberley, F.C.; Liu, X.S.; Mongkolsapaya, J.; Ch'En, P.; Xu, X.N.; Jin, B.Q.; Pezzella, F.; Screaton, G.R. Expression of TRAIL and TRAIL receptors in normal and malignant tissues. *Cell Res.* **2005**, *15*, 430–438. [CrossRef]
79. Picarda, G.; Lamoureux, F.; Geffroy, L.; Delepine, P.; Montier, T.; Laud, K.; Tirode, F.; Delattre, O.; Heymann, D.; Redini, F. Preclinical evidence that use of TRAIL in Ewing's sarcoma and osteosarcoma therapy inhibits tumor growth, prevents osteolysis, and increases animal survival. *Clin. Cancer Res.* **2010**, *16*, 2363–2374. [CrossRef]
80. Petak, I.; Douglas, L.; Tillman, D.M.; Vernes, R.; Houghton, J.A. Pediatric rhabdomyosarcoma cell lines are resistant to Fas-induced apoptosis and highly sensitive to TRAIL-induced apoptosis. *Clin. Cancer Res.* **2000**, *6*, 4119–4127.
81. Merchant, M.S.; Geller, J.I.; Baird, K.; Chou, A.J.; Galli, S.; Charles, A.; Amaoko, M.; Rhee, E.H.; Price, A.; Wexler, L.H.; et al. Phase I trial and pharmacokinetic study of lexatumumab in pediatric patients with solid tumors. *J. Clin. Oncol.* **2012**, *30*, 4141–4147. [CrossRef] [PubMed]
82. Baek, J.H.; Sohn, S.K.; Kim, D.H.; Kim, J.G.; Yang, D.H.; Kim, Y.K.; Lee, J.J.; Kim, H.J. Pilot remission induction therapy with idarubicin, plus an intensified dose of ara-C and priming with granulocyte colony-stimulating factor for acute myeloid leukemia. *Acta Haematol.* **2007**, *117*, 109–114. [CrossRef] [PubMed]
83. Anderson, P.M.; Markovic, S.N.; Sloan, J.A.; Clawson, M.L.; Wylam, M.; Arndt, C.A.; Smithson, W.A.; Burch, P.; Gornet, M.; Rahman, E. Aerosol granulocyte macrophage-colony stimulating factor: A low toxicity, lung-specific biological therapy in patients with lung metastases. *Clin. Cancer Res.* **1999**, *5*, 2316–2323. [PubMed]
84. Merchant, M.S.; Yang, X.; Melchionda, F.; Romero, M.; Klein, R.; Thiele, C.J.; Tsokos, M.; Kontny, H.U.; Mackall, C.L. Interferon gamma enhances the effectiveness of tumor necrosis factor-related apoptosis-inducing ligand receptor agonists in a xenograft model of Ewing's sarcoma. *Cancer Res.* **2004**, *64*, 8349–8356. [CrossRef] [PubMed]
85. Cartellieri, M.; Bachmann, M.; Feldmann, A.; Bippes, C.; Stamova, S.; Wehner, R.; Temme, A.; Schmitz, M. Chimeric antigen receptor-engineered T cells for immunotherapy of cancer. *J. Biomed. Biotechnol.* **2010**, *2010*, 956304. [CrossRef] [PubMed]
86. Hombach, A.; Wieczarkowiecz, A.; Marquardt, T.; Heuser, C.; Usai, L.; Pohl, C.; Seliger, B.; Abken, H. Tumor-specific T cell activation by recombinant immunoreceptors: CD3 zeta signaling and CD28 costimulation are simultaneously required for efficient IL-2 secretion and can be integrated into one combined CD28/CD3 zeta signaling receptor molecule. *J. Immunol.* **2001**, *167*, 6123–6131. [CrossRef]
87. Pule, M.A.; Straathof, K.C.; Dotti, G.; Heslop, H.E.; Rooney, C.M.; Brenner, M.K. A chimeric T cell antigen receptor that augments cytokine release and supports clonal expansion of primary human T cells. *Mol. Ther.* **2005**, *12*, 933–941. [CrossRef]
88. Zhong, X.S.; Matsushita, M.; Plotkin, J.; Riviere, I.; Sadelain, M. Chimeric antigen receptors combining 4-1BB and CD28 signaling domains augment PI3kinase/AKT/Bcl-XL activation and CD8+ T cell-mediated tumor eradication. *Mol. Ther.* **2010**, *18*, 413–420. [CrossRef]
89. Huang, M.A.; Krishnadas, D.K.; Lucas, K.G. Cellular and Antibody Based Approaches for Pediatric Cancer Immunotherapy. *J. Immunol. Res.* **2015**, *2015*, 675269. [CrossRef]
90. Louis, C.U.; Savoldo, B.; Dotti, G.; Pule, M.; Yvon, E.; Myers, G.D.; Rossig, C.; Russell, H.V.; Diouf, O.; Liu, E.; et al. Antitumor activity and long-term fate of chimeric antigen receptor-positive T cells in patients with neuroblastoma. *Blood* **2011**, *118*, 6050–6056. [CrossRef]

91. Pule, M.A.; Savoldo, B.; Myers, G.D.; Rossig, C.; Russell, H.V.; Dotti, G.; Huls, M.H.; Liu, E.; Gee, A.P.; Mei, Z.; et al. Virus-specific T cells engineered to coexpress tumor-specific receptors: Persistence and antitumor activity in individuals with neuroblastoma. *Nat. Med.* **2008**, *14*, 1264–1270. [CrossRef] [PubMed]
92. Heczey, A.; Louis, C.U. Advances in chimeric antigen receptor immunotherapy for neuroblastoma. *Discov. Med.* **2013**, *16*, 287–294. [PubMed]
93. Walker, A.J.; Majzner, R.G.; Zhang, L.; Wanhainen, K.; Long, A.H.; Nguyen, S.M.; Lopomo, P.; Vigny, M.; Fry, T.J.; Orentas, R.J.; et al. Tumor Antigen and Receptor Densities Regulate Efficacy of a Chimeric Antigen Receptor Targeting Anaplastic Lymphoma Kinase. *Mol. Ther.* **2017**, *25*, 2189–2201. [CrossRef] [PubMed]
94. Orentas, R.J.; Lee, D.W.; Mackall, C. Immunotherapy targets in pediatric cancer. *Front. Oncol.* **2012**, *2*, 3. [CrossRef]
95. Ragab, S.M.; Samaka, R.M.; Shams, T.M. HER2/neu expression: A predictor for differentiation and survival in children with Wilms tumor. *Pathol. Oncol. Res.* **2010**, *16*, 61–67. [CrossRef]
96. Ahmed, N.; Salsman, V.S.; Yvon, E.; Louis, C.U.; Perlaky, L.; Wels, W.S.; Dishop, M.K.; Kleinerman, E.E.; Pule, M.; Rooney, C.M.; et al. Immunotherapy for osteosarcoma: Genetic modification of T cells overcomes low levels of tumor antigen expression. *Mol. Ther.* **2009**, *17*, 1779–1787. [CrossRef]
97. Hegde, M.; Moll, A.J.; Byrd, T.T.; Louis, C.U.; Ahmed, N. Cellular immunotherapy for pediatric solid tumors. *Cytotherapy* **2015**, *17*, 3–17. [CrossRef]
98. Rainusso, N.; Brawley, V.S.; Ghazi, A.; Hicks, M.J.; Gottschalk, S.; Rosen, J.M.; Ahmed, N. Immunotherapy targeting HER2 with genetically modified T cells eliminates tumor-initiating cells in osteosarcoma. *Cancer Gene Ther.* **2012**, *19*, 212–217. [CrossRef]
99. Ahmed, N.; Brawley, V.S.; Hegde, M.; Robertson, C.; Ghazi, A.; Gerken, C.; Liu, E.; Dakhova, O.; Ashoori, A.; Corder, A.; et al. Human Epidermal Growth Factor Receptor 2 (HER2) -Specific Chimeric Antigen Receptor-Modified T Cells for the Immunotherapy of HER2-Positive Sarcoma. *J. Clin. Oncol.* **2015**, *33*, 1688–1696. [CrossRef]
100. Kawakami, M.; Kawakami, K.; Takahashi, S.; Abe, M.; Puri, R.K. Analysis of interleukin-13 receptor alpha2 expression in human pediatric brain tumors. *Cancer* **2004**, *101*, 1036–1042. [CrossRef]
101. Okada, H.; Low, K.L.; Kohanbash, G.; McDonald, H.A.; Hamilton, R.L.; Pollack, I.F. Expression of glioma-associated antigens in pediatric brain stem and non-brain stem gliomas. *J. Neurooncol.* **2008**, *88*, 245–250. [CrossRef] [PubMed]
102. Brown, C.E.; Starr, R.; Aguilar, B.; Shami, A.F.; Martinez, C.; D'Apuzzo, M.; Barish, M.E.; Forman, S.J.; Jensen, M.C. Stem-like tumor-initiating cells isolated from IL13Ralpha2 expressing gliomas are targeted and killed by IL13-zetakine-redirected T Cells. *Clin. Cancer Res.* **2012**, *18*, 2199–2209. [CrossRef] [PubMed]
103. Kahlon, K.S.; Brown, C.; Cooper, L.J.; Raubitschek, A.; Forman, S.J.; Jensen, M.C. Specific recognition and killing of glioblastoma multiforme by interleukin 13-zetakine redirected cytolytic T cells. *Cancer Res.* **2004**, *64*, 9160–9166. [CrossRef] [PubMed]
104. Brudno, J.N.; Kochenderfer, J.N. Recent advances in CAR T-cell toxicity: Mechanisms, manifestations and management. *Blood Rev.* **2019**, *34*, 45–55. [CrossRef] [PubMed]
105. Teachey, D.T.; Lacey, S.F.; Shaw, P.A.; Melenhorst, J.J.; Maude, S.L.; Frey, N.; Pequignot, E.; Gonzalez, V.E.; Chen, F.; Finklestein, J.; et al. Identification of Predictive Biomarkers for Cytokine Release Syndrome after Chimeric Antigen Receptor T-cell Therapy for Acute Lymphoblastic Leukemia. *Cancer Discov.* **2016**, *6*, 664–679. [CrossRef]
106. Maude, S.L.; Barrett, D.; Teachey, D.T.; Grupp, S.A. Managing cytokine release syndrome associated with novel T cell-engaging therapies. *Cancer J.* **2014**, *20*, 119–122. [CrossRef]
107. Straathof, K.C.; Pule, M.A.; Yotnda, P.; Dotti, G.; Vanin, E.F.; Brenner, M.K.; Heslop, H.E.; Spencer, D.M.; Rooney, C.M. An inducible caspase 9 safety switch for T-cell therapy. *Blood* **2005**, *105*, 4247–4254. [CrossRef]
108. Di Stasi, A.; Tey, S.K.; Dotti, G.; Fujita, Y.; Kennedy-Nasser, A.; Martinez, C.; Straathof, K.; Liu, E.; Durett, A.G.; Grilley, B.; et al. Inducible apoptosis as a safety switch for adoptive cell therapy. *N. Engl. J. Med.* **2011**, *365*, 1673–1683. [CrossRef]
109. Boyton, R.J.; Altmann, D.M. Natural killer cells, killer immunoglobulin-like receptors and human leucocyte antigen class I in disease. *Clin. Exp. Immunol.* **2007**, *149*, 1–8. [CrossRef]
110. Leung, W.; Iyengar, R.; Turner, V.; Lang, P.; Bader, P.; Conn, P.; Niethammer, D.; Handgretinger, R. Determinants of antileukemia effects of allogeneic NK cells. *J. Immunol.* **2004**, *172*, 644–650. [CrossRef]

111. Koscielniak, E.; Gross-Wieltsch, U.; Treuner, J.; Winkler, P.; Klingebiel, T.; Lang, P.; Bader, P.; Niethammer, D.; Handgretinger, R. Graft-versus-Ewing sarcoma effect and long-term remission induced by haploidentical stem-cell transplantation in a patient with relapse of metastatic disease. *J. Clin. Oncol.* **2005**, *23*, 242–244. [CrossRef] [PubMed]
112. Lang, P.; Pfeiffer, M.; Muller, I.; Schumm, M.; Ebinger, M.; Koscielniak, E.; Feuchtinger, T.; Foll, J.; Martin, D.; Handgretinger, R. Haploidentical stem cell transplantation in patients with pediatric solid tumors: Preliminary results of a pilot study and analysis of graft versus tumor effects. *Klin. Padiatr.* **2006**, *218*, 321–326. [CrossRef] [PubMed]
113. Kasow, K.A.; Handgretinger, R.; Krasin, M.J.; Pappo, A.S.; Leung, W. Possible allogeneic graft-versus-tumor effect in childhood melanoma. *J. Pediatr. Hematol. Oncol.* **2003**, *25*, 982–986. [CrossRef] [PubMed]
114. Inaba, H.; Handgretinger, R.; Furman, W.; Hale, G.; Leung, W. Allogeneic graft-versus-hepatoblastoma effect. *Pediatr. Blood Cancer* **2006**, *46*, 501–505. [CrossRef]
115. Perez-Martinez, A.; Leung, W.; Munoz, E.; Iyengar, R.; Ramirez, M.; Vicario, J.L.; Lassaletta, A.; Sevilla, J.; Gonzalez-Vicent, M.; Madero, L.; et al. KIR-HLA receptor-ligand mismatch associated with a graft-versus-tumor effect in haploidentical stem cell transplantation for pediatric metastatic solid tumors. *Pediatr. Blood Cancer* **2009**, *53*, 120–124. [CrossRef]
116. Ibrahim, E.C.; Guerra, N.; Lacombe, M.J.; Angevin, E.; Chouaib, S.; Carosella, E.D.; Caignard, A.; Paul, P. Tumor-specific up-regulation of the nonclassical class I HLA-G antigen expression in renal carcinoma. *Cancer Res.* **2001**, *61*, 6838–6845.
117. Wan, R.; Wang, Z.W.; Li, H.; Peng, X.D.; Liu, G.Y.; Ou, J.M.; Cheng, A.Q. Human Leukocyte Antigen-G Inhibits the Anti-Tumor Effect of Natural Killer Cells via Immunoglobulin-Like Transcript 2 in Gastric Cancer. *Cell. Physiol. Biochem.* **2017**, *44*, 1828–1841. [CrossRef]
118. Kailayangiri, S.; Altvater, B.; Spurny, C.; Jamitzky, S.; Schelhaas, S.; Jacobs, A.H.; Wiek, C.; Roellecke, K.; Hanenberg, H.; Hartmann, W.; et al. Targeting Ewing sarcoma with activated and GD2-specific chimeric antigen receptor-engineered human NK cells induces upregulation of immune-inhibitory HLA-G. *Oncoimmunology* **2017**, *6*, e1250050. [CrossRef]
119. Maki, G.; Hayes, G.M.; Naji, A.; Tyler, T.; Carosella, E.D.; Rouas-Freiss, N. Gregory SANK resistance of tumor cells from multiple myeloma chronic lymphocytic leukemia patients: Implication of, H.L.A.-G. *Leukemia* **2008**, *22*, 998–1006. [CrossRef]
120. Hutzen, B.; Ghonime, M.; Lee, J.; Mardis, E.R.; Wang, R.; Lee, D.A.; Cairo, M.S.; Roberts, R.D.; Cripe, T.P.; Cassady, K.A. Immunotherapeutic Challenges for Pediatric Cancers. *Mol. Ther. Oncolytics* **2019**, *15*, 38–48. [CrossRef]
121. Elster, J.D.; Krishnadas, D.K.; Lucas, K.G. Dendritic cell vaccines: A review of recent developments and their potential pediatric application. *Hum. Vaccin. Immunother.* **2016**, *12*, 2232–2239. [CrossRef] [PubMed]
122. Jarnjak-Jankovic, S.; Hammerstad, H.; Saeboe-Larssen, S.; Kvalheim, G.; Gaudernack, G. A full scale comparative study of methods for generation of functional Dendritic cells for use as cancer vaccines. *BMC Cancer* **2007**, *7*, 119. [CrossRef] [PubMed]
123. Fields, R.C.; Shimizu, K.; Mule, J.J. Murine dendritic cells pulsed with whole tumor lysates mediate potent antitumor immune responses in vitro and in vivo. *Proc. Natl. Acad. Sci. USA* **1998**, *95*, 9482–9487. [CrossRef] [PubMed]
124. Meadors, J.L.; Cui, Y.; Chen, Q.R.; Song, Y.K.; Khan, J.; Merlino, G.; Tsokos, M.; Orentas, R.J.; Mackall, C.L. Murine rhabdomyosarcoma is immunogenic and responsive to T-cell-based immunotherapy. *Pediatr. Blood Cancer* **2011**, *57*, 921–929. [CrossRef]
125. Geiger, J.D.; Hutchinson, R.J.; Hohenkirk, L.F.; McKenna, E.A.; Yanik, G.A.; Levine, J.E.; Chang, A.E.; Braun, T.M.; Mule, J.J. Vaccination of pediatric solid tumor patients with tumor lysate-pulsed dendritic cells can expand specific T cells and mediate tumor regression. *Cancer Res.* **2001**, *61*, 8513–8519.
126. Krishnadas, D.K.; Shapiro, T.; Lucas, K. Complete remission following decitabine/dendritic cell vaccine for relapsed neuroblastoma. *Pediatrics* **2013**, *131*, e336–e341. [CrossRef]
127. Krishnadas, D.K.; Shusterman, S.; Bai, F.; Diller, L.; Sullivan, J.E.; Cheerva, A.C.; George, R.E.; Lucas, K.G. A phase I trial combining decitabine/dendritic cell vaccine targeting MAGE-A1, MAGE-A3 and NY-ESO-1 for children with relapsed or therapy-refractory neuroblastoma and sarcoma. *Cancer Immunol. Immunother.* **2015**, *64*, 1251–1260. [CrossRef]

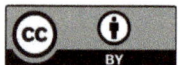

© 2019 by the authors. Licensee MDPI, Basel, Switzerland. This article is an open access article distributed under the terms and conditions of the Creative Commons Attribution (CC BY) license (http://creativecommons.org/licenses/by/4.0/).

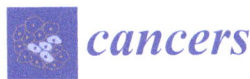

Review

Immune Dysfunctions and Immunotherapy in Colorectal Cancer: The Role of Dendritic Cells

Sandra Gessani [1,*] and Filippo Belardelli [2]

[1] Center for Gender-Specific Medicine, Istituto Superiore di Sanità, 00161 Rome, Italy
[2] Institute of Translational Pharmacology, CNR, 00131 Rome, Italy; filippo.belardelli@ift.cnr.it
* Correspondence: sandra.gessani@iss.it; Tel.: +38-0649903169

Received: 13 September 2019; Accepted: 27 September 2019; Published: 3 October 2019

Abstract: Colorectal cancer (CRC), a multi-step malignancy showing increasing incidence in today's societies, represents an important worldwide health issue. Exogenous factors, such as lifestyle, diet, nutrition, environment and microbiota, contribute to CRC pathogenesis, also influencing non neoplastic cells, including immune cells. Several immune dysfunctions were described in CRC patients at different disease stages. Many studies underline the role of microbiota, obesity-related inflammation, diet and host reactive cells, including dendritic cells (DC), in CRC pathogenesis. Here, we focused on DC, the main cells linking innate and adaptive anti-cancer immunity. Variations in the number and phenotype of circulating and tumor-infiltrating DC have been found in CRC patients and correlated with disease stages and progression. A critical review of DC-based clinical studies and of recent advances in cancer immunotherapy leads to consider new strategies for combining DC vaccination strategies with check-point inhibitors, thus opening perspectives for a more effective management of this neoplastic disease.

Keywords: colorectal cancer; dendritic cells; immunotherapy; pathogenesis; risk factors

---

1. Introduction

Colorectal cancer (CRC) is one of the major leading cause of cancer-associated mortality worldwide, thus representing an important public health issue, with a great impact in terms of human suffering and costs for the clinical management of patients [1]. The rate of CRC incidence is particularly high in populations living a Western lifestyle, but it is currently increasing in other geographic areas, including low income countries, thus representing a global health challenge [2].

The pathogenesis of CRC exhibits a great level of complexity, being characterized by several multi-step disease events, associated with the accumulation of both genetic and epigenetic alterations of the genome. In fact, the development of CRC is a long process taking several years to progress from barely detectable small neoplastic foci to adenomas and subsequently to malignant carcinomas endowed with metastatic behavior [3].

CRC is characterized by a high heterogeneity given the remarkable genomic instability [4]. Moreover, there is evidence that exogenous factors, such as lifestyle, diet, nutrition, environment and microbiota, contribute to the pathogenesis of CRC, also influencing non neoplastic cells, including immune cells, and leading to further heterogeneity [5,6].

Host immune dysfunctions are important factors contributing to CRC development. Indeed, a significant impairment of the host anti-tumor immunity has been reported during initiation of CRC mostly relying on escape mechanisms adopted by transformed cells to create a favorable growth environment [7–9]. During the initial stages of neoplastic transformation and progression, several changes occur within the tumor microenvironment to initially promote neoplastic cell proliferation, subsequently leading either to tumor progression and metastasis or to an immune-mediated cancer inhibition. In particular, the tumor microenvironment can dictate the recruitment of inflammatory and immune cells playing complex roles in either controlling tumor growth or inducing a chronic inflammation status, thus promoting CRC progression by induction of immune suppressive mechanisms [10,11].

Today, an ensemble of data support the statement that inflammation plays an important role in CRC pathogenesis and progression [10]. The low-grade chronic inflammation characterizing obesity, a major risk factor for CRC development, and the anti-inflammatory drug benefits in lowering CRC risk and retarding intestinal tumors in ulcerative colitis patients provide compelling evidence for a link between inflammation and cancer [12]. In this regard, diet is nowadays recognized to play a key role in CRC initiation and progression due to its potential to contribute to a chronic inflammatory condition, either locally in the adipose tissue (AT) or systemically by regulating a variety of immune and inflammatory pathways. In addition, diet strongly controls the composition of the intestinal microbiota that not only maintains the immune homeostasis but can also be involved in colorectal carcinogenesis [13–15].

Information stemming from both mouse models and studies in patients points to a key role of immune cells and soluble factors with immunosuppressive activity in the CRC disease process [11]. Among the many cells of the immune system exerting important functions in the host response to neoplastic transformation, dendritic cells (DC) deserve a special attention, since these cells, which are an highly heterogeneous cell population present in the blood, in the lymphoid organs as well as in the tumor microenvironment, represent the major actors in linking innate and adaptive anti-cancer immunity [16].

The clinical management of CRC is firstly based on surgical resection, but the optimal treatments in patients with advanced metastatic disease is still matter of debate. Different protocols of chemotherapy and immunotherapy, including combination therapies, have been used in metastatic patients with variable success [17]. Of note, CRC is one of the first human cancer where a stringent correlation was found between tumor infiltrating $CD8^+$ T cells and clinical outcome [18], thus supporting the rationale for evaluating the efficacy of immunotherapy protocols in this neoplastic disease. In fact, the clinical research for implementing the management of CRC patients in an advanced disease stage often included the use of cytokines (i.e., IFN, IL-2), adoptive cell therapy and DC-based vaccines, but variable and inconclusive results were obtained so far. Today, we are facing a momentum of enthusiasm on cancer immunotherapy in the light of the emerging great clinical impact of check-point inhibitors (CPI) [19]. However, major research challenges are to fully understand the mechanisms of the response and to obtain clinical efficacy in non-responding and poorly responding patients by designing more sounded combination therapies. While the role of immunosurveillance in the control of CRC growth and progression is assumed to be of great importance [17,18], patients appear to be resistant to the blockade of immunological checkpoints with monoclonal antibodies (mAbs) specific for cytotoxic T lymphocyte-associated protein 4 (CTLA4), programmed cell death 1 (PDCD1, best known as PD-1) and the PD-1 ligand CD274 (best known as PD-L1), with the exception of a minority of subjects characterized by microsatellite instability (MSI) lesions [20,21]. This has been considered as an apparent paradox and an intriguing issue demanding further research efforts for fully understanding the mechanisms of the resistance to CPI and developing new and more effective therapeutic strategies [22]. In this review, we intend to specifically address the role of DC in the pathogenesis and progression of CRC as well as in the response to immunotherapy. A special attention will be given to the role of microbiota, obesity-related inflammation, diet and host reactive cells, including DC, in CRC pathogenesis, then discussing how we can translate the research progress in this field in strategies of prevention and management of CRC. Likewise, we will review the ensemble of studies reporting the variations of different DC subsets in CRC patients and their correlation with disease stages and clinical outcome. Lastly, we will provide a brief critical overview of the results of DC-based clinical trials in CRC patients, discussing new perspectives for their combination with CPI and some current research challenges for the management of this neoplastic disease.

2. Diet, Inflammation and Microbiota in the Pathogenesis of CRC

2.1. Diet and Obesity as Important Factors in the Pathogenesis of CRC

Excess adiposity is associated with increased incidence of several cancers and represents an important indicator of survival, prognosis, recurrence and response to therapy in CRC. Notably, patterns and trends in CRC incidence and mortality correlate with geographical location, societal and economic changes and their increase may reflect the obesity epidemic and the adoption of more Western lifestyles. Both genetic and a range of environmental, largely modifiable, lifestyle factors play an important role in CRC etiology. Among these, the links between body weight, dietary patterns and CRC risk are some of the strongest for any type of cancer with profound implications for prevention strategies. It is now well-recognized that CRC risk is highly modifiable through lifestyle, particularly diet and physical activity; recent reports suggest that up to 47% of CRC cases could be prevented by staying physically active, maintaining a healthy body weight and eating a healthy diet (available at https://www.wcrf.org continuous-update-project 2017). Obese subjects have a 1.5–3.5-fold increased risk of developing CRC compared with lean individuals, and epidemiologic evidence indicates that abdominal rather than overall obesity may be more predictive of CRC risk [23]. Multiple changes arising in condition of chronic positive energy balance are likely to contribute to the increased CRC risk and worse outcomes in obesity. In particular, during the progression to obesity, the AT undergoes profound structural and functional modifications [24] tightly coupled with dramatic changes in the immune cell repertoire and functions [25,26], that shift the balance of cell subsets and soluble mediators toward a pro-inflammatory profile. Growing evidence indicates that the chronic low-grade inflammatory state characterizing obesity contributes to the impairment of immune functions, thus representing a key determinant in the development of obesity-related morbidities including cancer [27]. Furthermore, lipids, especially fatty acids (FA), the main components of AT, are recognized to play an important role not only in obesity development but also in the interplay between excessive adiposity and development of associated diseases [28]. In this regard, qualitative changes, rather than quantitative, in the FA composition of AT have been reported to influence tissue dysfunctions and are associated with an enhanced STAT3 activation and concomitant down-regulation of anti-inflammatory pathways such as PPARγ and its downstream target adiponectin [29].

The metabolic disturbances characterizing obesity lead to chronic immune activation as unraveled by the presence of elevated levels of plasmatic inflammatory markers in obese subjects [30]. The bulk of immune alterations observed in obesity may provide an explanation for the higher rate of vaccine failure and infectious disease [31]. In this regard, the white AT, particularly visceral fat, is now well-recognized as a complex immunocompetent organ, homing adipocytes and resident immune cells exhibiting secretory as well as immunological, metabolic and endocrine regulatory activities. Furthermore, AT is a medium- to long-term indicator of FA dietary intake. Among the different factors potentially influencing visceral AT microenvironment and immune cell distribution, the relative composition of ω3/ω6 polyunsaturated fatty acid (PUFA) might play a pivotal role, since these molecules are capable to markedly modulate inflammation and to influence immune functions [32,33]. In this regard, visceral fat adipocytes from obese and CRC subjects exhibit distinct secretory and ω6 PUFA profiles characterized by a prevalence of pro-inflammatory factors and inflammation-promoting FA [34]. Of note, we recently reported that obese and CRC subjects share inadequate dietary habits and altered lipid metabolism, suggesting that the quality of the diet consumed, regardless the quantity of energy intake, is an important aspect to preserve human health [35]. CRC and obese subjects were found to be more prone to follow a saturated fatty acid (SFA)-rich diet and exhibit a reduced content of monounsaturated fatty acids (MUFA) (especially in oleic acid). The composition of AT, in particular in FA, may thus represent an important determinant in shaping the immune cell phenotype and in influencing processes/events occurring in distal tissues that may set the basis for CRC carcinogenesis.

2.2. Relationships Between Diet, Microbiota and Immune Dysfunctions in CRC Pathogenesis

The key role of diet in CRC initiation and progression as well as in prevention is not only linked to the capacity of some nutritional components to contribute to a chronic inflammatory condition by regulating a variety of immune and inflammatory pathways, but also to strongly control the composition of the intestinal microbiota. The human microbiota, a collection of commensal microorganisms colonizing gastro-intestinal, genitourinary, oral, respiratory and cutaneous tracts, interacts with the host in different ways and contribute to many important processes such as nutrient absorption, metabolism, tissue development, immunity and tumorigenesis [13–15]. It is now well-known that microbiota is influenced by several factors of genetic, dietary and environmental nature. Likewise, some of the metabolic effects of diet rely on gut microbiota. Examples of how diet can influence microbiota emerged from studies in populations consuming different diets, leading to the conclusion that dietary patterns defined as "healthy" (e.g. Mediterranean diet) are associated with higher microbial richness [36]. Among the best associations between diet and gut microbiota are dietary fibers, polyphenols and fats. In particular, different dietary fats may exert different effects on gut microbiota (diversity, alterations of specific microorganisms and their functions) with metabolic consequences such as regulation of systemic low-grade inflammation [37].

In obesity, the gut microbiota displays distinctive features and most studies have demonstrated a reduction in diversity and richness—termed dysbiosis—which has been associated with low-grade inflammation, increased body weight and fat mass, as well as type 2 diabetes (T2D). Nevertheless, the exact microbial signature of a healthy or an obese gut microbiota is still matter of debate. Dysbiosis is associated with a large array of diseases including cancer, where it is implicated in different ways [6]. In addition, microbiota can be directly oncogenic by favoring local mucosal inflammation or systemic metabolic/immune dysregulation or can act indirectly by virtue of its capacity to modulate anti-tumor immunity or the efficacy of anti-cancer therapy. In this regard it is of interest that the abundance of *Akkermansia muciniphila* has been positively associated with the antitumor effect of PD-1 blockade in epithelial tumors [38] and hepatocellular carcinoma [39]. Interestingly, decreased amounts of this bacterium have been linked to obesity, insulin resistance, T2D and other cardiometabolic disorders in rodents and in humans [40]. In addition, alterations of fecal and mucosal microbiota with reduction of bacterial diversity have been reported in CRC patients at different cancer stages [41,42].

In the following chapters, we provide a brief overview of the role of DC in the regulation of inflammatory and immune responses, of their functional changes in CRC patients and of their exploitation in immunotherapy protocols against CRC.

3. The Role of DC in the Regulation of the Inflammatory and Immune Responses in CRC

DC represent a heterogeneous group of innate immune cells endowed with the unique capacity to initiate and coordinate the immune response. They are professional antigen presenting cells (APC) and comprise a variety of subsets, of both myeloid and lymphoid origin, as either resident or migrating cells, in lymphoid and non-lymphoid organs. They are able to recognize, capture and process antigens and to present them to naïve T lymphocytes. DC are nowadays recognized as a family comprising several subtypes that differ in ontogeny, gene expression profile, anatomical location, phenotypic and functional features [43]. In this regard, consensus has been recently achieved on the recognition of five major DC types: plasmacytoid DC (pDC), type 1 conventional DC (cDC1), type 2 cDC (cDC2), Langerhans cells and monocyte-derived DC (MoDC). In the steady state, DC are largely present as immature cells exhibiting a high capacity to capture antigen, and a low expression of co-stimulatory molecules and secretion of effector cytokines. The exposure to different stimuli including microorganisms or damaged cells/tissues promotes DC activation, a functional state characterized by a decreased capacity to capture antigen, enhanced expression of MHC class I and II antigens as well as costimulatory molecules, active production of effector cytokines and migration to lymph nodes, where they interact with naïve $CD4^+$ and $CD8^+$ T lymphocytes.

It is currently thought that DC play an important role in presenting tumor antigens to T cells and in shaping an antitumor immune response, which may result in an effective control of tumor growth [13,14]. However, many studies have revealed how the phenotype and functions of these cells can markedly be affected by several molecular and cellular actors playing complex and even opposite roles within the tumor microenvironment. As an example, there is plenty of evidence indicating that tumors can not only suppress DC maturation, but can also induce the generation of DC endowed with immunosuppressive activities [45,46].

Dietary habits and excessive adiposity can not only influence cancer growth but also shape host immune response [47]. Myeloid DC, but not pDC, have been described to accumulate in the subcutaneous AT of obese subjects. While the number of CD11c$^+$/CD141$^+$DC is the same in lean with respect to obese subjects, the number of CD11c$^+$/CD1c$^+$ cells positively correlates with the body mass index (BMI). This accumulation parallels an enhanced presence of Th17 lymphocytes in AT, suggesting a role of DC infiltrating AT in the regulation of tissue inflammation and Th17 cell expansion [31]. Of note, studies carried out in mouse models of obesity suggest that the presence of CD131$^+$ DC in the AT of lean mice can be important for the local expansion of T regulatory cells providing anti-inflammatory signals to maintain AT homeostasis [31]. Interestingly, the exposure of immune cells to visceral adipocyte conditioned media from obese and CRC affected subjects favors IL-10 production, reduces the immunostimulatory activity of DC and hampers their capacity to generate γδ T cell-mediated responses induced ex vivo, further highlighting the existence of a regulatory/suppressive AT microenvironment in both obesity and CRC [34]. Furthermore, distinct alterations of the immune cell repertoire in the periphery with respect to the AT uniquely characterize or are shared by obesity and CRC [48].

4. Changes in the Phenotype and Function of DC in CRC Patients

Several groups have described qualitative as well as quantitative changes of DC in the blood as well as in the tumor microenvironment of CRC patients at different stages of disease and their possible correlation with the clinical response of patients [46]. The interpretation of the overall results is not always easy, since contradictory data were reported in some cases, possibly due to differences in the clinical settings as well and in the methodologies used to identify specific DC subsets. Here, we will restrict our review to the discussion of only some studies, selected in view of their special potential clinical relevance. The possible correlations between the presence and maturation phenotype of tumor-infiltrating DC with the patient prognosis and clinical response have been investigated by Gulubova and colleagues [49]. These authors found that the presence of CD83$^+$ mature DC was lower in the tumor stroma of patients in an advanced disease stage. In general, we can state that negative correlations between the detection of these tumor infiltrating DC and the number of lymph node metastases as well as the survival time of CRC patients were frequently documented [49–51]. Notably, by comparing human primary CRC specimens with respect to normal colon mucosa, Schwaab and co-workers found that the number of infiltrating mature DC was higher in the CRC samples, while the DC density in metastases was markedly lower than in CRC primary tumors [52]. Of interest, Michielsen and colleagues reported that tumor conditioned-media from cultured human CRC tissue can impair DC maturation process, possibly by releasing chemokines and other soluble factors capable of inhibiting IL-12p70 secretion by DC [53,54]. Of note, Bauer and colleagues [55] reported that infiltration with mature DC was more elevated in MSI-high (MSI-H) tumors as compared to microsatellite-stable CRC. This observation is interesting since it can provide an explanation for the preferential clinical response of MSI-H CRC patients to novel immunotherapies, including CPI [20,21]. Some groups have also investigated the number and phenotype of DC in the peripheral blood of CRC patients with respect to healthy individuals as well to the disease stage and progression [56–59]. In particular, it has been found that the number and functions of different blood DC subsets were impaired in CRC patients, demonstrating that the magnitude of these effects positively correlated with the disease stage and prognosis [59]. Similar results were obtained by Orsini et al. [57], who described a significant reduction of the DC number in total and advanced stage-CRC patients compared to healthy controls, and reported that this reduction was totally recovered after complete tumor resection, further supporting the concept of the importance of systemic immunosuppressive effects exerted by the tumor toward circulating blood immune cells. Of interest, some authors have also reported that the reduction in DC was mostly due to changes in pDC population [57].

A useful in vitro model to investigate the biology of DC and the mediators and mechanisms important in shaping their functions is represented by MoDC, generated from monocytes by in vitro treatments with GM-CSF and various cytokines, such as IL-4, IFN and other activation/maturation factors. Thus, some published studies where the phenotype and functions of MoDC from CRC patients were compared to those detectable in control subjects are available [56,60–62]. In particular, Orsini and colleagues showed an impaired in vitro differentiation of CRC patients' monocytes into immature DC, compared to healthy subjects [57]. Of note, CRC MoDC exhibited a reduced expression of costimulatory molecules and an impaired ability to present antigens to allogenic T lymphocytes and to stimulate proliferation, together with an immunosuppressive cytokine profile, mostly characterized by increased IL-10 and reduced IL-12 secretion [57]. Of interest, it was reported that the maturation status of the MoDC from CRC patients was phenotypically and functionally superior to the in vivo blood DC recovered from the same individuals. This observation somehow supported the potential value of using MoDC from CRC patients for clinical studies of cancer immunotherapy [63].

5. DC and Immunotherapy of CRC

Since the early study by William Coley in cancer patients treated with killed bacterial vaccine in 1891, for more than 120 years, the history of cancer immunotherapy has been characterized by alternate cycles of optimism and discouragement. The clinical use of certain cytokines (i.e., IFN-α and IL-2), the subsequent identification of the first set of human tumor antigens, the progress on cancer vaccines and in the development of protocols based on adoptive cell therapy have all represented important milestones in the field of cancer immunotherapy. However, it is only in recent years that we have registered a fundamental progress, which today leads to consider cancer immunotherapy as the latest revolution in cancer therapy. This is mainly due to the impressive results achieved in patients with different type of malignancies after treatment with CPI [19]. With regard to CRC, however, only modest clinical effects have been observed so far in patients treated with these new immunotherapy drugs (including anti-CTLA-4, anti-PD1 and anti-PD-L1 antibodies) [64], which instead proved to be highly effective in other human malignancies (including melanoma, Hodgkin lymphoma and non-small lung cell cancer).

In view of their crucial role in linking innate and adaptive antitumor immunity, DC have extensively been used in cancer immunotherapy clinical trials over the last two decades [44,65]. Notably, the large majority of DC-based studies involved the use of patient-derived DC generated from peripheral blood monocytes differentiated in vitro by the addition of cytokines (generally GM-CSF and IL-4), loaded with tumor-derived antigens by different experimental procedures and subjected to a further step of in vitro maturation, before their injection in therapeutic vaccination protocols [65]. In 2011, the registration of the DC-based Provenge vaccine for patients with prostate cancer led to a transient momentum of special optimism for the clinical development of DC-based cancer vaccines. However, in the following years, this cancer vaccine was not further developed and, in view of the limited response observed in hundreds of clinical trials, the clinical development of DC-based vaccines was regarded with a lower attention with respect to that devoted to new emerging tools in cancer immunotherapy, such as CPI and CAR-T adoptive cell transfer. There are recent and comprehensive reviews reporting the results of DC-based clinical trials, which also critically discuss the major challenges for their clinical development [44,65]. While the lack of any relevant toxicity represents a good starting point, there are still several critical issues to be addressed, including identification of the optimal DC to be used, reliable criteria to characterize the quality and potency of these cell products, the source/loading of tumor antigens, the modalities of injection and the possible combinations with other drugs/treatments to increase their clinical efficacy. Today, we are facing a renovated interest in the development of new generation DC-based vaccines, as a result of a better understanding of the DC biology and of the discovery of new immunomodulatory molecules expected to enforce cancer immunotherapies [66–68].

In considering new and potentially more effective DC types to be used in cancer immunotherapy protocols, we may consider to use DC generated by monocytes by a short-term in vitro exposure to IFN-α and GM-CSF [69]. In fact, these DC (named as IFN-DC) exhibit a unique attitude to take-up tumor apoptotic bodies and induce a potent tumor specific T cell immunity in preclinical models [70] as well as in cancer patients, as suggested by results in pilot clinical trials where IFN-DC have been inoculated intratumorally in patients with metastatic melanoma [71] and indolent lymphomas [72].

Table 1 reports the main published data of clinical trials based on the use of DC in CRC patients. The general messages stemming from an overview of the main results published so far can be summarized as follows: (i) the large majority of studies reported results of pilot phase I-II trials in metastatic CRC patients with a relatively small number of patients; (ii) different methodologies were used for the in vitro generation of DC-based vaccines from monocytes, including the use of various cytokines and other activation/maturation factors, rendering difficult the comparison of the results; (iii) different methods of tumor antigen loading of DC were utilized and, in a few cases, unloaded DC were used; (iv) the regimen and route of DC administration as well as the number of DC injected markedly differed among the published studies; (v) in some cases, the patients were also treated with either conventional (for instance chemotherapy) or additional experimental cell therapies; (vi) there were marked differences in the protocol design as well as in the immunomonitoring methods to evaluate DC-induced immunogenicity. All this suggests that, even though some of these trials have represented important proof-of-principles for the lack of toxicity and potential efficacy of DC-based vaccines in inducing antitumor immune responses in CRC, the translation of the possible use of DC for the development of new-generation strategies of CRC immunotherapy needs further and coordinated research efforts.

Table 1. Main clinical studies aimed at evaluating DC-based therapies in CRC patients.

Patients	DC generation	Ag loading	DC administration	N	Major findings	Ref.
Metastatic, CEA$^+$, HLA-*0201; Phase I	GM-CSF/IL-4, + TNFα, PGE2, IL-1β	CEA altered peptide	$1–5 \times 10^7$, i.v.; 4 times, every 2nd week	7	In vivo expansion of peptide-specific CD8$^+$ T cells	[73]
Metastatic, CEA$^+$; Phase I	GM-CSF/IL-4	Fowl-pox vector encoding rCEA and costimulatory molecules	5×10^5; s.c./i.d; 1 or 2 cycles of 4 weekly injections	11	Induction of CEA-specific T cells; trend of correlation with clinical response	[74]
Metastatic, HLA-A2$^+$, Phase I	IL-13/GM-CSF, maturation factors	6 CEA peptides	35×10^6, i.d., 4 injections every 3 weeks	11	Progressive disease in spite of T cell response to tumor associated antigens	[75]
Metastatic, after resection of metastases; Phase I-II	GM-CSF/IL-4	Autologous tumor lysate, KLH	5×10^6 into 2 inguinal lymph nodes under ultrasound guidance; week 1, 3 and 6	26	Tumor specific T cell response (63%); correlation with recurrence-free survival; no difference if DC were further treated or not with CD40L	[76]
Metastatic, CEA$^+$, HLA-A*2402; Phase I-II	IL-4/GM-CSF/IFNα, streptococcus pyrogenes	CEA peptide	$11–115 \times 10^6$, s.c., 2-8 injections	8	Trend of correlation between CEA-specific cytotoxic T cells and clinical efficacy	[77]
Metastatic, after metastasis resection; Phase II	IL-4/GM-CSF	Poxvectors encoding CEA, MUC-1 and costimulatory molecules	10^7, s.c./i.d. 3 times per month/3 months; comparison with patients injected with poxvectors + GM-CSF	37	Both DC-poxCEA and poxCEA +GM-CSF treatments showed similar response; longer survival time compared to contemporary unvaccinated group	[78]
Stage Dukes B2 and Dukes C; Phase I-II	IL-4/GM-CSF	TCL, rCEA protein	$5 \times 10^6 – 2 \times 10^7$, s.c.; days 1, 14, 28, 56	12	Suggestion of clinical effect with TCL-DC, but no effect with CEA-DC	[79]
Metastatic, after resection of metastases; pretreatment with low dose chemotherapy; Phase I-II	IL-4/GM-CSF	TCL	Average DC dosage: 188×10^6, s.c.; 3–5 injections in 2 weeks; patients also received i.v. injections of CIK cells	13	Reduction of post-operative disease risk; increase of overall survival	[80]
Metastatic, unresectable; Phase II	IL-4/GM-CSF/TNFα	TCL	10^7, i.v, for the first 3 weeks; i.d. for the last 3 weeks; i.v. CIK cell infusions for 4 days	100	DC/CIK therapy can induce anti-CRC immune response (DTH) with a potential impact on survival and quality life with respect to control group	[81]

Table 1. Cont.

Patients	DC generation	Ag loading	DC administration	N	Major findings	Ref.
Metastatic, resistant to standard therapies; Phase I-II	IL-4/GM-CSF; + maturation factors	rCEA protein	10^6, s.c., mixed with tetanus toxoid; 3 other s.c. injections of the same DC number	12	T cell reactive against CEA in 2 patients; 2 patients with stable disease; 10 patients showed progression; need to enhance antitumor T cell response	[82]
Metastatic, phase II; DC vaccine + best supportive care versus best supportive care	IL-4/GM-CSF + maturation factors	Autologous TCL	5×10^6 (1, 10, 20, 40, 120 days), s.c.	28	Induction of tumor specific T cell response; no increase of overall survival with respect to the "best supportive care" group	[83]
Metastatic, resistant to standard therapies; Phase I-II	GM-CSF + killed BCG mycobacteria + IFNα	No in vitro antigen loading	$2-15 \times 10^6$; 2-6 injections, i.t. using image guidance	7	Cytokines produced by DC (IL-8 and IL-12p40) correlate with clinical outcome	[84]

Abbreviations: N: Patients' number; TCL: tumor cell lysate; rCEA: recombinant CEA; s.c.: subcutaneous; i.d.: intradermal; i.v.: intravenous; i.t.: intratumoral; CIK: cytokine-induced killer cell. * 6 out of 12 patients injected with DC-loaded TCL, 6 with CEA.

One of the major reason for the limited response of CRC to the immunotherapy is thought to be represented by the immunosuppressive tumor microenvironment which generally occurs in patients with advanced disease. As a matter of fact, the major challenge for developing an effective protocol of cancer immunotherapy is indeed to counteract the several and complex immunosuppressive mechanisms activated in the tumor microenvironment of cancer patients. The role of several cancer-induced immunosuppressive mediators in CRC prognosis and treatment response has been reviewed elsewhere [9–11]. These mediators include cells endowed with immunosuppressive activity, such as regulatory T cells and certain macrophage populations, as well as soluble factors. Notably, modulations of the local production of certain cytokines as well as in their response can play a role in shaping the type of antitumor response [85]. Of interest, loss of type I IFN receptor has recently been identified as an important key factor linked to tumor microenvironment immunosuppression in CRC patients [86]. Thus, we may assume that a local production of and response to cytokines such as type I IFN can exhibit a beneficial role in shaping the response towards an effective immune control of CRC.

Today, in the new era of CPI, major research challenges are to fully understand the mechanisms of the response and how to increase the clinical efficacy in poorly responding patients by designing more sounded combination therapies, which may also include DC. Of interest, a recent study showed that an effective antitumor response to anti-PD1 mAbs strictly requires the occurrence of intratumoral DC [68]. Likewise, some recent studies have added further evidence underscoring a previously underestimated role of intratumoral DC in the tumor microenvironment in mediating the clinical response to immunotherapy regimens in cancer patients [87,88]. Of interest, the intratumoral DC involved in the generation of an antitumor response to anti-PD1 mAbs were characterized as mature DC producing high levels of IL-12 [68]. Notably, IFN-DC, which undergo a rapid and complete maturation after peripheral blood lymphocyte co-cultivation, are high producers of IL-12 [89] and therefore may represent good candidates for potentiating anti-PD1-based therapies. Of interest, we had previously shown that IFN-DC are highly efficient APC in inducing both $CD8^+$ and $CD4^+$ T-cell-mediated responses against the colon tumor antigen-1 in CRC patients at different stages of the disease [90]. Thus, on the basis of the overall preclinical and clinical data on IFN-DC obtained by our group [69–72,89,90], we consider these DC as valuable autologous cell products for the development of new-generation DC products to be used in clinical trials in CRC patients. For these DC-based therapies, we may envisage therapeutic scenarios where CRC patients are treated with autologous DC, either as unloaded APC injected intratumorally (endogenous tumor vaccination) in combination with agents either inducing or enhancing tumor cell death [71,72], or as in vitro antigen loaded DC, and subsequently injected with anti-PD1 antibodies or other CPI to increase the antitumor response in selected combination therapies.

6. Conclusions

CRC represents one of the human malignancies where promotion of prevention strategies can play a major role in reducing cancer development and tumor burden and progression. In fact, primary prevention, based on special attention to reduce exposure to environmental and lifestyle risk factors (including diet and physical exercise) is indeed of great importance for reducing CRC incidence, with enormous impact in terms of public health and reduction of costs for the national health services. In addition, in view of the long and multi-step processes involved in CRC development, strategies of secondary prevention, including the promotion of the use of early diagnostic platforms, can be very important for prevention and control of CRC. In spite of all this, the optimal therapeutic management of patients with metastatic CRC remains an important issue in clinical oncology. While surgery and chemo-radiotherapy interventions continue to represent essential therapeutic options depending on the stage of the disease and the clinical settings, immunotherapy has recently emerged as a powerful tool for tertiary immune prevention.

Recently, we have learned new rationales and modalities for combining different immunotherapy regimens with both conventional and target therapies. Likewise, we have recently started to understand the importance of sex- and gender-specific differences in several pathologies including cancer. In fact, gender disparities have been reported in different aspects that can collectively influence CRC pathogenesis and therapy [91]. Thus, CRC incidence, outcome and survival as well as microbiota composition exhibit a different trend in men and women [92]. Likewise, some of the main risk factors for CRC, such as obesity and lifestyle-related aspects (i.e. diet and physical activity), are strongly linked to gender [93,94]. Worth of note, differences in the immune response have also been reported in women and men [95]. However, at the moment there are no studies describing gender differences in DC functions in CRC patients. Studies on gender related immune dysfunctions in CRC taking into consideration the DC biology are expected to contribute to our understanding of the pathogenesis and to the clinical management of this neoplastic disease.

Figure 1 summarizes the main DC dysfunctions observed in a specific non-neoplastic tissue relevant for CRC pathogenesis (i.e., AT), blood and tumor microenvironment of CRC patients, along with the risk factors playing a role in the disease process. It also depicts some main strategies and challenges for the development of DC-based immunotherapy strategies in CRC patients. Such strategies are aimed at considering DC either as in vivo targets for tumor antigen delivery and/or for recruiting and activating DC within the tumor microenvironment, or as autologous cell products generated from monocytes by different in vitro manipulations and then reinfused into the patients. In any case, new generation immunotherapy strategies should consider what is the impact and possible role of DC, which represent important cell actors in CRC pathogenesis and antitumor immune-based control.

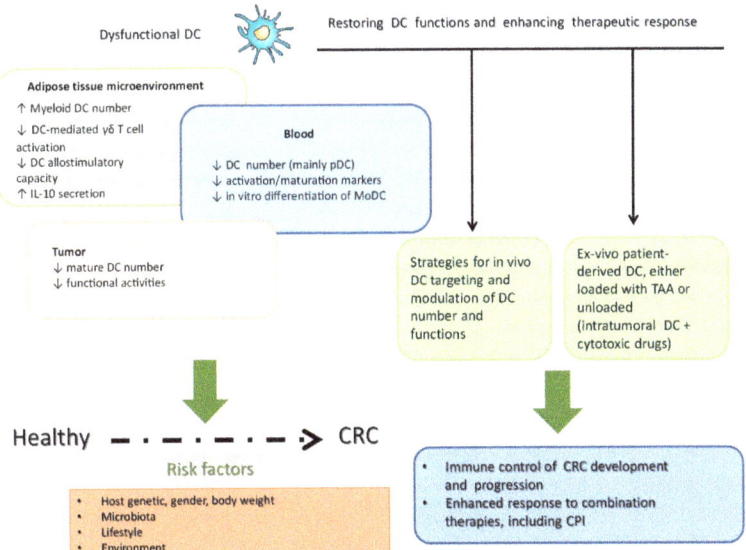

Figure 1. A schematic representation of the main DC dysfunction in adipose tissue, peripheral blood and tumor tissue highlighting the main strategies to restore DC functions and to enhance anticancer immune response.

How to reverse DC dysfunctions occurring at different disease stages and in various tissues in CRC patients still remains a complex issue deserving further research efforts. In principle, intervention strategies for restoring DC functions in the very early stages of the disease could also be considered, but we need to reach a better knowledge of the role of this highly heterogeneous cell population in the pathogenesis and progression of CRC. The recent advances on the cross-talk between gut microbiota and human health and on the potential of lifestyle, food components and/or dietary patterns to modulate this functional interplay has opened new perspectives for diet-based interventions in the modulation of the antitumor immune response [96].

With regard to the still critical issue of implementing the management of advanced metastatic CRC, a great importance is currently given to combination therapies, since we now have a much better knowledge on how different therapeutic tools and strategies should be associated. With the advent of next-generation sequencing methodologies, we have now the unprecedented ability to identify tumor, host, and microbial genomes. The growing application of these novel technologies to finely characterize patient's tumor and driver mutations as well as the immune repertoire for evaluating genetic responses to current immunotherapies has opened new ways to maximize patient benefits through cancer precision medicine strategies. We conclude by stating that, taking into account some recent findings [68,87,88], new generation DC-based strategies can represent a promising added value for enhancing the response to the new therapeutic regimens, including CPI, in CRC patients.

Author Contributions: S.G. and F.B. conceived, designed and wrote the review article.

Funding: This research was funded in part by Italian Association for Cancer Research (AIRC), grants 14185 (SG) and 16891 (FB).

Conflicts of Interest: The authors declare no conflict of interest.

References

1. Bray, F.; Ferlay, J.; Soerjomataram, I.; Siegel, R.L.; Torre, L.A.; Jemal, A. Global Cancer Statistics 2018: GLOBOCAN Estimates of Incidence and Mortality Worldwide for 36 Cancers in 185 Countries. *CA A Cancer J. Clin.* **2018**, *68*, 394–424. [CrossRef] [PubMed]
2. Van der Geest, L.L.; Lam-Boer, J.; Koopman, M.; Verhoef, C.; Elferink, M.M.; de Wilt, J.J. Nationwide Trends in Incidence, Treatment and Survival of Colorectal Cancer Patients with Synchronous Metastases. *Clin. Exp. Metastasis* **2015**, *32*, 457–465. [CrossRef] [PubMed]
3. Pandurangan, A.A.; Divya, T.; Kumar, K.; Dineshbabu, V.; Velavan, B.; Sudhandiran, G. Colorectal Carcinogenesis: Insights into the Cell Death and Signal Transduction Pathways: A review. *World J. Gastrointest. Oncol.* **2018**, *10*, 244–259. [CrossRef] [PubMed]
4. Vogelstein, B.; Papadopoulos, N.; Velculescu, V.V.; Zhou, S.; Diaz, L.L., Jr.; Kinzler, K.K. Cancer Genome Landscapes. *Science* **2013**, *339*, 1546–1558. [CrossRef] [PubMed]
5. Ogino, S.; Nowak, J.J.; Hamada, T.; Phipps, A.A.; Peters, U.; Milner, D.D., Jr.; Giovannucci, E.E.; Nishihara, R.; Giannakis, M.; Garrett, W.W.; et al. Integrative Analysis of Exogenous, Endogenous, Tumour and Immune Factors for Precision Medicine. *Gut* **2018**, *67*, 1168–1180. [CrossRef]
6. Kosumi, K.; Mima, K.; Baba, H.; Ogino, S. Dysbiosis of the Gut Microbiota and Colorectal Cancer: The Key Target of Molecular Pathological Epidemiology. *J. Lab. Precis. Med.* **2018**, *3*. [CrossRef]
7. Shi, Y.; Li, Z.; Zheng, W.; Liu, X.; Sun, C.; Laugsand, J.J.; Liu, Z.; Cui, G. Changes of Immunocytic Phenotypes and Functions from Human Colorectal Adenomatous Stage to Cancerous Stage: Update. *Immunobiology* **2015**, *220*, 1186–1196. [CrossRef]
8. McLean, M.M.; Murray, G.G.; Stewart, K.K.; Norrie, G.; Mayer, C.; Hold, G.G.; Thomson, J.; Fyfe, N.; Hope, M.; Mowat, N.N.; et al. The Inflammatory Microenvironment in Colorectal Neoplasia. *PLoS ONE* **2011**, *6*, e15366. [CrossRef]
9. Croci, D.D.; Zacarias, F.M.M.; Rico, M.M.; Matar, P.; Rabinovich, G.G.; Scharovsky, O.O. Dynamic Cross-Talk between Tumor and Immune Cells in Orchestrating the Immunosuppressive Network at the Tumor Microenvironment. *Cancer Immunol. Immunother.* **2007**, *56*, 1687–1700. [CrossRef]
10. Lasry, A.; Zinger, A.; Ben-Neriah, Y. Inflammatory Networks Underlying Colorectal Cancer. *Nat. Immunol.* **2016**, *17*, 230–240. [CrossRef]
11. West, N.N.; McCuaig, S.; Franchini, F.; Powrie, F. Emerging Cytokine Networks in Colorectal Cancer. *Nat. Rev. Immunol.* **2015**, *15*, 615–629. [CrossRef] [PubMed]
12. Gregor, M.M.; Hotamisligil, G.G. Inflammatory Mechanisms in Obesity. *Annu. Rev. Immunol.* **2011**, *29*, 415–445. [CrossRef] [PubMed]
13. Lin, C.; Cai, X.; Zhang, J.; Wang, W.; Sheng, Q.; Hua, H.; Zhou, X. Role of Gut Microbiota in the Development and Treatment of Colorectal Cancer. *Digestion* **2019**, *100*, 72–78. [CrossRef] [PubMed]

14. Chen, J.; Pitmon, E.; Wang, K. Microbiome, Inflammation and Colorectal Cancer. *Semin. Immunol.* **2017**, *32*, 43–53. [CrossRef]
15. De Almeida, C.C.; de Camargo, M.M.; Russo, E.; Amedei, A. Role of Diet and Gut Microbiota on Colorectal Cancer Immunomodulation. *World J. Gastroenterol.* **2019**, *25*, 151–162. [CrossRef]
16. Fu, C.; Jiang, A. Dendritic Cells and CC8 T Cell Immunity in Tumor Microenvironment. *Front. Immunol.* **2018**, *9*, 3059. [CrossRef]
17. Wrobel, P.; Ahmed, S. Current Status of Immunotherapy in Metastatic Colorectal Cancer. *Int. J. Colorectal Dis.* **2019**, *34*, 13–25. [CrossRef]
18. Galon, J.; Costes, A.; Sanchez-Cabo, F.; Kirilovsky, A.; Mlecnik, B.; Lagorce-Pages, C.; Tosolini, M.; Camus, M.; Berger, A.; Wind, P.; et al. Type, Density and Location of Immune Cells within Human Colorectal Tumors Predict Clinical Outcome. *Science* **2006**, *313*, 1960–1964. [CrossRef]
19. Diesendruck, Y.; Benhar, I. Novel Immune Check Point Inhibiting Antibodies in Cancer Therapy-Opportunities and Challenges. *Drug Resist. Updates* **2017**, *30*, 39–47. [CrossRef]
20. Gutting, T.; Burgermeister, E.; Hartel, N.; Ebert, M.M. Checkpoints and Beyond—Immunotherapy in Colorectal Cancer. *Semin. Cancer. Biol.* **2019**, *55*, 78–89. [CrossRef]
21. Westdorp, H.; Fennemann, F.F.; Weren, R.R.; Bisseling, T.T.; Ligtenberg, M.M.; Figdor, C.C.; Schreibelt, G.; Hoogerbrugge, N.; Wimmers, F.; de Vries, I.I. Opportunities for Immunotherapy in Microsatellite Instable Colorectal Cancer. *Cancer. Immunol. Immunother.* **2016**, *65*, 1249–1259. [CrossRef] [PubMed]
22. Kroemer, G.; Galluzzi, L.; Zitvogel, L.; Fridman, W.W. Colorectal cancer: The First Neoplasia Found to be under Immunosurveillance and the Last One to Respond to Immunotherapy? *Oncoimmunology* **2015**, *4*, e1058597. [CrossRef] [PubMed]
23. Cozzo, A.A.; Fuller, A.A.; Makowski, L. Contribution of Adipose Tissue to Development of Cancer. *Compr. Physiol.* **2018**, *8*, 237–282. [CrossRef]
24. Longo, M.; Zatterale, F.; Naderi, J.; Parrillo, L.; Formisano, P.; Raciti, G.G.; Beguinot, F.; Miele, C. Adipose Tissue Dysfunction as Determinant of Obesity-Associated Metabolic Complications. *Int. J. Mol. Sci.* **2019**, *20*, 2358. [CrossRef]
25. Guzik, T.T.; Skiba, D.D.; Touyz, R.R.; Harrison, D.D. The Role of Infiltrating Immune Cells in Dysfunctional Adipose Tissue. *Cardiovasc. Res.* **2017**, *113*, 1009–1023. [CrossRef]
26. Del Corno, M.; Conti, L.; Gessani, S. Innate Lymphocytes in Adipose Tissue Homeostasis and Their Alterations in Obesity and Colorectal Cancer. *Front. Immunol.* **2018**, *9*, 2556. [CrossRef]
27. Meiliana, A.; Dewi, N.N.; Wijaya, A. Adipose Tissue Inlammation (Meta-inlammation) and Obesity Management. *Indones. Biomed. J.* **2015**, *7*, 129–146. [CrossRef]
28. Masoodi, M.; Kuda, O.; Rossmeisl, M.; Flachs, P.; Kopecky, J. Lipid Signaling in Adipose Tissue: Connecting Inflammation & Metabolism. *Biochim. Biophys. Acta* **2015**, *1851*, 503–518. [CrossRef]
29. D'Archivio, M.; Scazzocchio, B.; Giammarioli, S.; Fiani, M.M.; Vari, R.; Santangelo, C.; Veneziani, A.; Iacovelli, A.; Giovannini, C.; Gessani, S.; et al. omega3-PUFAs Exert Anti-Inflammatory Activity in Visceral Adipocytes from Colorectal Cancer Patients. *PLoS ONE* **2013**, *8*, e77432. [CrossRef]
30. Andersen, C.C.; Murphy, K.K.; Fernandez, M.M. Impact of Obesity and Metabolic Syndrome on Immunity. *Adv. Nutr.* **2016**, *7*, 66–75. [CrossRef]
31. Bertola, A.; Ciucci, T.; Rousseau, D.; Bourlier, V.; Duffaut, C.; Bonnafous, S.; Blin-Wakkach, C.; Anty, R.; Iannelli, A.; Gugenheim, J.; et al. Identification of Adipose Tissue Dendritic Cells Correlated with Obesity-Associated Insulin-resistance and Inducing, Th17 Responses in Mice and Patients. *Diabetes* **2012**, *61*, 2238–2247. [CrossRef] [PubMed]
32. Yessoufou, A.; Ategbo, J.J.; Attakpa, E.; Hichami, A.; Moutairou, K.; Dramane, K.K.; Khan, N.N. Peroxisome Proliferator-Activated Receptor-Alpha Modulates Insulin Gene Transcription Factors and Inflammation in Adipose Tissues in Mice. *Mol. Cell. Biochem.* **2009**, *323*, 101–111. [CrossRef] [PubMed]
33. Kim, W.; Khan, N.N.; McMurray, D.D.; Prior, I.I.; Wang, N.; Chapkin, R.R. Regulatory Activity of Polyunsaturated Fatty Acids in T.-cell Signaling. *Prog. Lipid Res.* **2010**, *49*, 250–261. [CrossRef] [PubMed]
34. Del Corno, M.; D'Archivio, M.; Conti, L.; Scazzocchio, B.; Vari, R.; Donninelli, G.; Varano, B.; Giammarioli, S.; De Meo, S.; Silecchia, G.; et al. Visceral Fat Adipocytes From Obese and Colorectal Cancer Subjects Exhibit Distinct Secretory and Omega6 Polyunsaturated Fatty Acid Profiles and Deliver Immunosuppressive Signals to Innate Immunity Cells. *Oncotarget* **2016**, *7*, 63093–63105. [CrossRef] [PubMed]

35. Scazzocchio, B.; Vari, R.; Silenzi, A.; Giammarioli, S.; Masotti, A.; Baldassarre, A.; Santangelo, C.; D'Archivio, M.; Giovannini, C.; Del Corno, M.; et al. Dietary Habits Affect Fatty Acid Composition of Visceral Adipose Tissue in Subjects with Colorectal Cancer or Obesity. *Eur. J. Nutr.* 2019. [CrossRef] [PubMed]

36. Kong, L.L.; Holmes, B.B.; Cotillard, A.; Habi-Rachedi, F.; Brazeilles, R.; Gougis, S.; Gausseres, N.; Cani, P.P.; Fellahi, S.; Bastard, J.J.; et al. Dietary Patterns Differently Associate with Inflammation and Gut Microbiota in Overweight and Obese Subjects. *PLoS ONE* 2014, *9*, e109434. [CrossRef]

37. Mokkala, K.; Houttu, N.; Cansev, T.; Laitinen, K. Interactions of Dietary Fat with the Gut Microbiota: Evaluation of Mechanisms and Metabolic Consequences. *Clin. Nutr.* 2019. [CrossRef]

38. Routy, B.; Le Chatelier, E.; Derosa, L.; Duong, C.C.M.; Alou, M.M.; Daillere, R.; Fluckiger, A.; Messaoudene, M.; Rauber, C.; Roberti, M.M.; et al. Gut Microbiome Influences Efficacy of PP-1-based Immunotherapy Against Epithelial Tumors. *Science* 2018, *359*, 91–97. [CrossRef]

39. Zheng, Y.; Wang, T.; Tu, X.; Huang, Y.; Zhang, H.; Tan, D.; Jiang, W.; Cai, S.; Zhao, P.; Song, R.; et al. Gut Microbiome Affects the Response To Anti-PD-1 Immunotherapy in Patients with Hepatocellular Carcinoma. *J. Immunother. Cancer* 2019, *7*, 193. [CrossRef]

40. Debedat, J.; Clement, K.; Aron-Wisnewsky, J. Gut Microbiota Dysbiosis in Human Obesity: Impact of Bariatric Surgery. *Curr. Obes. Rep.* 2019, *8*, 229–242. [CrossRef]

41. Ahn, J.; Sinha, R.; Pei, Z.; Dominianni, C.; Wu, J.; Shi, J.; Goedert, J.J.; Hayes, R.R.; Yang, L. Human Gut Microbiome and Risk for Colorectal Cancer. *J. Natl. Cancer Inst.* 2013, *105*, 1907–1911. [CrossRef] [PubMed]

42. Huipeng, W.; Lifeng, G.; Chuang, G.; Jiaying, Z.; Yuankun, C. The Differences in Colonic Mucosal Microbiota between Normal Individual and Colon Cancer Patients by Polymerase Chain Reaction-Denaturing Gradient Gel Electrophoresis. *J. Clin. Gastroenterol.* 2014, *48*, 138–144. [CrossRef] [PubMed]

43. Solano-Galvez, S.S.; Tovar-Torres, S.S.; Tron-Gomez, M.M.; Weiser-Smeke, A.A.; Alvarez-Hernandez, D.D.; Franyuti-Kelly, G.G.; Tapia-Moreno, M.; Ibarra, A.; Gutierrez-Kobeh, L.; Vazquez-Lopez, R. Human Dendritic Cells: Ontogeny and Their Subsets in Health and Disease. *Med. Sci.* 2018, *6*, 88. [CrossRef] [PubMed]

44. Palucka, K.; Banchereau, J. Cancer Immunotherapy via Dendritic Cells. *Nat. Rev. Cancer* 2012, *12*, 265–277. [CrossRef]

45. Gabrilovich, D. Mechanisms and Functional Significance of Tumour-Induced Dendritic-Cell Defects. *Nat. Rev. Immunol.* 2004, *4*, 941–952. [CrossRef]

46. Legitimo, A.; Consolini, R.; Failli, A.; Orsini, G.; Spisni, R. Dendritic Cell Defects in the Colorectal Cancer. *Hum. Vaccines Immunother.* 2014, *10*, 3224–3235. [CrossRef]

47. Alwarawrah, Y.; Kiernan, K.; MacIver, N.N. Changes in Nutritional Status Impact Immune Cell Metabolism and Function. *Front. Immunol.* 2018, *9*, 1055. [CrossRef]

48. Donninelli, G.; Del Corno, M.; Pierdominici, M.; Scazzocchio, B.; Vari, R.; Varano, B.; Pacella, I.; Piconese, S.; Barnaba, V.; D'Archivio, M.; et al. Distinct Blood and Visceral Adipose Tissue Regulatory T Cell and Innate Lymphocyte Profiles Characterize Obesity and Colorectal Cancer. *Front. Immunol.* 2017, *8*, 643. [CrossRef]

49. Gulubova, M.M.; Ananiev, J.J.; Vlaykova, T.T.; Yovchev, Y.; Tsoneva, V.; Manolova, I.I. Role of Dendritic Cells in Progression and Clinical Outcome of Colon Cancer. *Int. J. Colorectal Dis.* 2012, *27*, 159–169. [CrossRef]

50. Nagorsen, D.; Voigt, S.; Berg, E.; Stein, H.; Thiel, E.; Loddenkemper, C. Tumor-Infiltrating Macrophages and Dendritic Cells in Human Colorectal Cancer: Relation to Local Regulatory T Cells, Systemic T-Cell Response Against Tumor-Associated Antigens and Survival. *J. Transl. Med.* 2007, *5*, 62. [CrossRef]

51. Dadabayev, A.A.; Sandel, M.M.; Menon, A.A.; Morreau, H.; Melief, C.C.; Offringa, R.; van der Burg, S.S.; Janssen-van Rhijn, C.; Ensink, N.N.; Tollenaar, R.R.; et al. Dendritic Cells in Colorectal Cancer Correlate with Other Tumor-Infiltrating Immune Cells. *Cancer Immunol. Immunother.* 2004, *53*, 978–986. [CrossRef] [PubMed]

52. Schwaab, T.; Weiss, J.J.; Schned, A.A.; Barth, R.R., Jr. Dendritic Cell Infiltration in Colon Cancer. *J. Immunother.* 2001, *24*, 130–137. [CrossRef] [PubMed]

53. Michielsen, A.A.; Hogan, A.A.; Marry, J.; Tosetto, M.; Cox, F.; Hyland, J.J.; Sheahan, K.K.; O'Donoghue, D.D.; Mulcahy, H.H.; Ryan, E.E.; et al. Tumour Tissue Microenvironment can Inhibit Dendritic Cell Maturation in Colorectal Cancer. *PLoS ONE* 2011, *6*, e27944. [CrossRef] [PubMed]

54. Michielsen, A.A.; Noonan, S.; Martin, P.; Tosetto, M.; Marry, J.; Biniecka, M.; Maguire, A.A.; Hyland, J.J.; Sheahan, K.K.; O'Donoghue, D.D.; et al. Inhibition of Dendritic Cell Maturation by the Tumor Microenvironment Correlates with the Survival of Colorectal Cancer Patients Following Bevacizumab Treatment. *Mol. Cancer Ther.* **2012**, *11*, 1829–1837. [CrossRef]
55. Bauer, K.; Michel, S.; Reuschenbach, M.; Nelius, N.; von Knebel Doeberitz, M.; Kloor, M. Dendritic Cell and Macrophage Infiltration in Microsatellite-Unstable and Microsatellite-Stable Colorectal Cancer. *Fam. Cancer* **2011**, *10*, 557–565. [CrossRef]
56. Bellik, L.; Gerlini, G.; Parenti, A.; Ledda, F.; Pimpinelli, N.; Neri, B.; Pantalone, D. Role of Conventional Treatments on Circulating and Monocyte-Derived Dendritic Cells in Colorectal Cancer. *Clin. Immunol.* **2006**, *121*, 74–80. [CrossRef]
57. Orsini, G.; Legitimo, A.; Failli, A.; Ferrari, P.; Nicolini, A.; Spisni, R.; Miccoli, P.; Consolini, R. Defective generation and maturation of dendritic cells from monocytes in Colorectal Cancer Patients During the Course of Disease. *Int. J. Mol. Sci.* **2013**, *14*, 22022–22041. [CrossRef]
58. Huang, A.; Gilmour, J.J.; Imami, N.; Amjadi, P.; Henderson, D.D.; Allen-Mersh, T.T. Increased Serum Transforming Growth Factor-Beta1 in Human Colorectal Cancer Correlates with Reduced Circulating Dendritic Cells and Increased Colonic, Langerhans Cell Infiltration. *Clin. Exp. Immunol.* **2003**, *134*, 270–278. [CrossRef]
59. Porta, M.D.; Danova, M.; Rigolin, G.G.; Brugnatelli, S.; Rovati, B.; Tronconi, C.; Fraulini, C.; Rossi, A.R.; Riccardi, A.; Castoldi, G. Dendritic Cells and Vascular Endothelial Growth Factor in Colorectal Cancer: Correlations with Clinicobiological Findings. *Oncology* **2005**, *68*, 276–284. [CrossRef]
60. Orsini, G.; Legitimo, A.; Failli, A.; Ferrari, P.; Nicolini, A.; Spisni, R.; Miccoli, P.; Consolini, R. Quantification of Blood Dendritic Cells in Colorectal Cancer Patients During the Course of Disease. *Pathol. Oncol. Res. Por.* **2014**, *20*, 267–276. [CrossRef]
61. Onishi, H.; Morisaki, T.; Baba, E.; Kuga, H.; Kuroki, H.; Matsumoto, K.; Tanaka, M.; Katano, M. Dysfunctional and Short-Lived Subsets in Monocyte-Derived Dendritic Cells from Patients with Advanced Cancer. *Clin. Immunol.* **2002**, *105*, 286–295. [CrossRef] [PubMed]
62. Hasebe, H.; Nagayama, H.; Sato, K.; Enomoto, M.; Takeda, Y.; Takahashi, T.T.; Hasumi, K.; Eriguchi, M. Dysfunctional Regulation of the Development of Monocyte-Derived Dendritic Cells in Cancer Patients. *Biomed. Pharmacother.* **2000**, *54*, 291–298. [CrossRef]
63. Kvistborg, P.; Bechmann, C.C.; Pedersen, A.A.; Toh, H.H.; Claesson, M.M.; Zocca, M.M. Comparison of Monocyte-Derived Dendritic Cells from Colorectal Cancer Patients, Non-Small-Cell-Lung-Cancer patients and Healthy Donors. *Vaccine* **2009**, *28*, 542–547. [CrossRef] [PubMed]
64. Yaghoubi, N.; Soltani, A.; Ghazvini, K.; Hassanian, S.S.; Hashemy, S.S. PD-1/PD-L1 Blockade As a Novel Treatment for Colorectal Cancer. *Biomed. Pharmacother.* **2019**, *110*, 312–318. [CrossRef]
65. Garg, A.A.; Vara, P.M.; Schaaf, M.; Agostinis, P.; Zitvogel, L.; Kroemer, G.; Galluzzi, L. Trial Watch: Dendritic Cell-Based Anticancer Immunotherapy. *Oncoimmunology* **2017**, *6*, e1328341. [CrossRef]
66. Garg, A.A.; Coulie, P.P.; Van den Eynde, B.B.; Agostinis, P. Integrating Next-Generation Dendritic Cell Vaccines into the Current Cancer Immunotherapy Landscape. *Trends Immunol.* **2017**, *38*, 577–593. [CrossRef]
67. Karaki, S.; Anson, M.; Tran, T.; Giusti, D.; Blanc, C.; Oudard, S.; Tartour, E. Is There Still Room for Cancer Vaccines at the Era of Checkpoint Inhibitors. *Vaccines* **2016**, *4*, 37. [CrossRef]
68. Garris, C.C.; Arlauckas, S.S.; Kohler, R.R.; Trefny, M.M.; Garren, S.; Piot, C.; Engblom, C.; Pfirschke, C.; Siwicki, M.; Gungabeesoon, J.; et al. Successful, Anti-PD-1 Cancer Immunotherapy Requires T Cell-Dendritic Cell Crosstalk Involving the Cytokines IIN-gamma and Il-12. *Immunity* **2018**, *49*, 1148–1161 e1147. [CrossRef]
69. Santini, S.S.; Lapenta, C.; Logozzi, M.; Parlato, S.; Spada, M.; Di Pucchio, T.; Belardelli, F. Type I Interferon As a Powerful Adjuvant for Monocyte-Derived Dendritic Cell Development and Activity in vitro and in Hu-PBL-SCID Mice. *J. Exp. Med.* **2000**, *191*, 1777–1788. [CrossRef]
70. Lapenta, C.; Donati, S.; Spadaro, F.; Castaldo, P.; Belardelli, F.; Cox, M.M.; Santini, S.S. NK Cell Activation in the Antitumor Response Induced by IIN-alpha Dendritic Cells Loaded with Apoptotic Cells from Follicular Lymphoma Patients. *J. Immunol.* **2016**, *197*, 795–806. [CrossRef]
71. Rozera, C.; Cappellini, G.G.; D'Agostino, G.; Santodonato, L.; Castiello, L.; Urbani, F.; Macchia, I.; Arico, E.; Casorelli, I.; Sestili, P.; et al. Intratumoral Injection of IIN-Alpha Dendritic Cells after Dacarbazine Activates Anti-Tumor Immunity: Results from a Phase I Trial in Advanced Melanoma. *J. Transl. Med.* **2015**, *13*, 139. [CrossRef] [PubMed]

72. Cox, M.M.; Castiello, L.; Mattei, M.; Santodonato, L.; D'Agostino, G.; Muraro, E.; Martorelli, D.; Lapenta, C.; Di Napoli, A.; Di Landro, F.; et al. Clinical and Antitumor Immune Responses in Relapsed/Refractory Follicular Lymphoma Patients after Intranodal Injections of IINalpha-Dendritic Cells and Rituximab. *Clin. Cancer Res.* **2019**. [CrossRef]
73. Babatz, J.; Rollig, C.; Lobel, B.; Folprecht, G.; Haack, M.; Gunther, H.; Kohne, C.C.; Ehninger, G.; Schmitz, M.; Bornhauser, M. Induction of Cellular Immune Responses Against Carcinoembryonic Antigen in Patients with Metastatic Tumors after Vaccination with Altered Peptide Ligand-Loaded Dendritic Cells. *Cancer Immunol. Immunother.* **2006**, *55*, 268–276. [CrossRef] [PubMed]
74. Morse, M.M.; Clay, T.T.; Hobeika, A.A.; Osada, T.; Khan, S.; Chui, S.; Niedzwiecki, D.; Panicali, D.; Schlom, J.; Lyerly, H.H. Phase I Study of Immunization with Dendritic Cells Modified with Fowlpox Encoding Carcinoembryonic Antigen and Costimulatory Molecules. *Clin. Cancer Res.* **2005**, *11*, 3017–3024. [CrossRef] [PubMed]
75. Kavanagh, B.; Ko, A.; Venook, A.; Margolin, K.; Zeh, H.; Lotze, M.; Schillinger, B.; Liu, W.; Lu, Y.; Mitsky, P.; et al. Vaccination of Metastatic Colorectal Cancer Patients with Matured Dendritic Cells Loaded with Multiple Major Histocompatibility Complex Class I Peptides. *J Immunother* **2007**, *30*, 762–772. [CrossRef] [PubMed]
76. Barth, R.R., Jr.; Fisher, D.D.; Wallace, P.P.; Channon, J.J.; Noelle, R.R.; Gui, J.; Ernstoff, M.M. A Randomized Trial of ex vivo CC40L Activation of a Dendritic Cell Vaccine in Colorectal Cancer Patients: Tumor-Specific Immune Responses are Associated with Improved Survival. *Clin. Cancer Res.* **2010**, *16*, 5548–5556. [CrossRef]
77. Sakakibara, M.; Kanto, T.; Hayakawa, M.; Kuroda, S.; Miyatake, H.; Itose, I.; Miyazaki, M.; Kakita, N.; Higashitani, K.; Matsubara, T.; et al. Comprehensive Immunological Analyses of Colorectal Cancer Patients in the Phase I/II Study of Quickly Matured Dendritic Cell Vaccine Pulsed with Carcinoembryonic Antigen Peptide. *Cancer Immunol. Immunother.* **2011**, *60*, 1565–1575. [CrossRef]
78. Morse, M.M.; Niedzwiecki, D.; Marshall, J.J.; Garrett, C.; Chang, D.D.; Aklilu, M.; Crocenzi, T.T.; Cole, D.D.; Dessureault, S.; Hobeika, A.A.; et al. A Randomized Phase II Study of Immunization with Dendritic Cells Modified with Poxvectors Encoding CCA and MMC1 Compared with the Same Poxvectors Plus GG-CSF for Resected Metastatic Colorectal Cancer. *Ann. Surg.* **2013**, *258*, 879–886. [CrossRef]
79. Hunyadi, J.; Andras, C.; Szabo, I.; Szanto, J.; Szluha, K.; Sipka, S.; Kovacs, P.; Kiss, A.; Szegedi, G.; Altorjay, I.; et al. Autologous dendritic cell based adoptive immunotherapy of patients with colorectal cancer-A phase I-II study. *Pathol. Oncol. Res. Por.* **2014**, *20*, 357–365. [CrossRef]
80. Gao, D.; Li, C.; Xie, X.; Zhao, P.; Wei, X.; Sun, W.; Liu, H.H.; Alexandrou, A.A.; Jones, J.; Zhao, R.; et al. Autologous Tumor Lysate-Pulsed Dendritic Cell Immunotherapy with Cytokine-Induced Killer Cells Improves Survival in Gastric and Colorectal Cancer Patients. *PLoS ONE* **2014**, *9*, e93886. [CrossRef]
81. Zhu, H.; Yang, X.; Li, J.; Ren, Y.; Zhang, T.; Zhang, C.; Zhang, J.; Pang, Y. Immune Response Safety and Survival and Quality of Life Outcomes for Advanced Colorectal Cancer Patients Treated with Dendritic Cell Vaccine and Cytokine-Induced Killer Cell Therapy. *Biomed. Res. Int.* **2014**, *2014*, 603871. [CrossRef]
82. Liu, K.K.; Chao, T.T.; Chang, J.J.; Cheng, A.A.; Chang, H.H.; Kao, W.W.; Wu, Y.Y.; Yu, W.W.; Chung, T.T.; Whang-Peng, J. A Phase I Clinical Study of Immunotherapy for Advanced Colorectal Cancers Using Carcinoembryonic Antigen-Pulsed Dendritic Cells Mixed with Tetanus Toxoid and Subsequent II-2 Treatment. *J. Biomed. Sci.* **2016**, *23*, 64. [CrossRef] [PubMed]
83. Caballero-Banos, M.; Benitez-Ribas, D.; Tabera, J.; Varea, S.; Vilana, R.; Bianchi, L.; Ayuso, J.J.; Pages, M.; Carrera, G.; Cuatrecasas, M.; et al. Phase II Randomised Trial of Autologous Tumour Lysate Dendritic Cell Plus Best Supportive Care Compared with Best Supportive Care in Pre-Treated Advanced Colorectal Cancer Patients. *Eur. J. Cancer* **2016**, *64*, 167–174. [CrossRef] [PubMed]
84. Subbiah, V.; Murthy, R.; Hong, D.D.; Prins, R.R.; Hosing, C.; Hendricks, K.; Kolli, D.; Noffsinger, L.; Brown, R.; McGuire, M.; et al. Cytokines Produced by Dendritic Cells Administered Intratumorally Correlate with Clinical Outcome in Patients with Diverse Cancers. *Clin. Cancer Res.* **2018**, *24*, 3845–3856. [CrossRef] [PubMed]
85. Mager, L.L.; Wasmer, M.M.; Rau, T.T.; Krebs, P. Cytokine-Induced Modulation of Colorectal Cancer. *Front. Oncol.* **2016**, *6*, 96. [CrossRef] [PubMed]
86. Katlinski, K.K.; Gui, J.; Katlinskaya, Y.Y.; Ortiz, A.; Chakraborty, R.; Bhattacharya, S.; Carbone, C.C.; Beiting, D.D.; Girondo, M.M.; Peck, A.A.; et al. Inactivation of Interferon Receptor Promotes the Establishment of Immune Privileged Tumor Microenvironment. *Cancer Cell* **2017**, *31*, 194–207. [CrossRef]

87. Barry, K.K.; Hsu, J.; Broz, M.M.; Cueto, F.F.; Binnewies, M.; Combes, A.A.; Nelson, A.A.; Loo, K.; Kumar, R.; Rosenblum, M.M.; et al. A Natural Killer-Dendritic Cell Axis Defines Checkpoint Therapy-Responsive Tumor Microenvironments. *Nat. Med.* **2018**, *24*, 1178–1191. [CrossRef]
88. Binnewies, M.; Mujal, A.A.; Pollack, J.J.; Combes, A.A.; Hardison, E.E.; Barry, K.K.; Tsui, J.; Ruhland, M.M.; Kersten, K.; Abushawish, M.M.; et al. Unleashing Type-2 Dendritic Cells to Drive Protective Antitumor CC4(+) T Cell Immunity. *Cell* **2019**, *177*, 556–571 e516. [CrossRef]
89. Lapenta, C.; Santini, S.S.; Spada, M.; Donati, S.; Urbani, F.; Accapezzato, D.; Franceschini, D.; Andreotti, M.; Barnaba, V.; Belardelli, F. IFN-Alpha-Conditioned Dendritic Cells are Highly Efficient in Inducing Cross-Priming CC8(+) T Cells Against Exogenous Viral Antigens. *Eur. J. Immunol.* **2006**, *36*, 2046–2060. [CrossRef]
90. Maccalli, C.; Di Cristanziano, V.; Fodale, V.; Corsi, D.; D'Agostino, G.; Petrangeli, V.; Laurenti, L.; Guida, S.; Mazzocchi, A.; Arienti, F.; et al. Induction of Both CC8+ and CC4+ T-Cell-Mediated Responses in Colorectal Cancer Patients by Colon Antigen-1. *Clin. Cancer Res.* **2008**, *14*, 7292–7303. [CrossRef]
91. Kim, S.S.; Paik, H.H.; Yoon, H.; Lee, J.J.; Kim, N.; Sung, M.M. Sex- and Gender-Specific Disparities in Colorectal Cancer Risk. *World J. Gastroenterol.* **2015**, *21*, 5167–5175. [CrossRef] [PubMed]
92. Kim, Y.Y.; Unno, T.; Kim, B.B.; Park, M.M. Sex Differences in Gut Microbiota. *World J. Men's Health* **2019**. [CrossRef] [PubMed]
93. Mauvais-Jarvis, F. Epidemiology of Gender Differences in Diabetes and Obesity. *Adv. Exp. Med. Biol.* **2017**, *1043*, 3–8. [CrossRef] [PubMed]
94. Vari, R.; Scazzocchio, B.; D'Amore, A.; Giovannini, C.; Gessani, S.; Masella, R. Gender-Related Differences in Lifestyle May Affect Health Status. *Ann. Dell'istituto Super. Di Sanita* **2016**, *52*, 158–166. [CrossRef]
95. Capone, I.; Marchetti, P.; Ascierto, P.P.; Malorni, W.; Gabriele, L. Sexual Dimorphism of Immune Responses: A New Perspective in Cancer Immunotherapy. *Front. Immunol.* **2018**, *9*, 552. [CrossRef] [PubMed]
96. Soldati, L.; Di Renzo, L.; Jirillo, E.; Ascierto, P.P.; Marincola, F.F.; De Lorenzo, A. The Influence of Diet on Anti-Cancer Immune Responsiveness. *J. Transl. Med.* **2018**, *16*. [CrossRef] [PubMed]

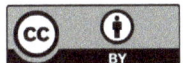

© 2019 by the authors. Licensee MDPI, Basel, Switzerland. This article is an open access article distributed under the terms and conditions of the Creative Commons Attribution (CC BY) license (http://creativecommons.org/licenses/by/4.0/).

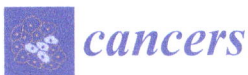

Review

The Interplay of Autophagy and Tumor Microenvironment in Colorectal Cancer—Ways of Enhancing Immunotherapy Action

Evangelos Koustas [1], Panagiotis Sarantis [1], Georgia Kyriakopoulou [1], Athanasios G. Papavassiliou [1] and Michalis V. Karamouzis [1,2,*]

[1] Molecular Oncology Unit, Department of Biological Chemistry, Medical School, National and Kapodistrian University of Athens, 11527 Athens, Greece; vang.koustas@gmail.com (E.K.); psarantis@bioacademy.gr (P.S.); gpkyriakopoulou@yahoo.com (G.K.); papavas@med.uoa.gr (A.G.P.)
[2] First Department of Internal Medicine, 'Laiko' General Hospital, Medical School, National and Kapodistrian University of Athens, 11527 Athens, Greece
* Correspondence: mkaramouz@med.uoa.gr; Tel.: +30-21-0746-2508 or +30-21-0746-2509; Fax: +30-21-0746-2703

Received: 25 March 2019; Accepted: 11 April 2019; Published: 14 April 2019

Abstract: Autophagy as a primary homeostatic and catabolic process is responsible for the degradation and recycling of proteins and cellular components. The mechanism of autophagy has a crucial role in several cellular functions and its dysregulation is associated with tumorigenesis, tumor–stroma interactions, and resistance to cancer therapy. A growing body of evidence suggests that autophagy is also a key regulator of the tumor microenvironment and cellular immune response in different types of cancer, including colorectal cancer (CRC). Furthermore, autophagy is responsible for initiating the immune response especially when it precedes cell death. However, the role of autophagy in CRC and the tumor microenvironment remains controversial. In this review, we identify the role of autophagy in tumor microenvironment regulation and the specific mechanism by which autophagy is implicated in immune responses during CRC tumorigenesis and the context of anticancer therapy.

Keywords: Autophagy; colorectal cancer; immunotherapy; tumor stroma; tumor microenvironment

1. Introduction

Colorectal cancer (CRC) is the third most frequently diagnosed malignancy and the second leading cause of cancer-related deaths in the U.S.A. and worldwide [1]. By 2030, the estimated global burden of CRC is expected to reach more than 2.2 million new cases and 1.1 million deaths [2]. Despite significant advances in standard of care therapies, the 5-year survival rate for patients diagnosed with metastatic CRC remains very poor, at approximately 12% [1]. Among others, autophagy is a major mechanism which is strongly associated with tumorigenesis in different types of cancer, including CRC.

The mechanism of autophagy has been identified as a catabolic process with an essential role to digest proteins and dysfunctional cellular organelles [3]. Numerous steps related to autophagy include membrane trafficking vesicles, essential autophagy proteins, a double membrane organelle, which is called an autophagosome, and fusion with lysosomes to create the autophagolysosome. Autophagolysosome is a fundamental structure responsible for degrading the luminal content [4]. The role of autophagy is extended from cellular homeostasis to tumor development [5,6].

Many genes and proteins are crucial for the initiation and progression of autophagy. Genes, like *Beclin-1*, *LC3*, *ATG5*, and *ATG6*, have a crucial role for autophagy from normal function to CRC, where these genes have been reported with high expression. Furthermore, these autophagy gene-markers are associated with a more aggressive CRC phenotype [7].

Various morphological changes characterize the autophagy process. In the first step of autophagy, which is called initiation or nucleation, the phagophore, a double membrane structure, is formed through the activation of the class-III PI3K-Beclin-1 complex. Elongation is the next step in the autophagy process. This step is characterized by the arising of the phagophore from different double membrane organelles, such as the Endoplasmic Reticulum (ER), Golgi, and mitochondria. The phagophore starts to enclose the cytosolic cargos, leading to the formation of the autophagosome. The formation of the phagophore is highlighted by different Atgs, p62/ SQSTM1 (an adaptor protein responsible for the docking of specific cargoes), and the lipid-modification of LC3I to LC3II. The maturation step and the following fuse step include the autophagosome formation, which eventually fuses with lysosomes to form autolysosomes. Finally, during the degradation step, lysosomal/vacuolar hydrolases digest autolysosomal products and release them in the cytosol [4].

Over the last years, many studies have been conducted that support the dual role of autophagy in CRC. Autophagy appears to be responsible for maintaining the energy homeostasis in cells, which is required for several cellular functions, such as proliferation [8], angiogenesis, migration [9], and EMT (epithelial-mesenchymal transition) phenotype [10]. Autophagy is identified to be upregulated in a hypoxic region of already established tumors, where the energy demands are increased [11]. Moreover, cancer cells of high graded tumors appear to be addicted to autophagy to maintain their energy balance [12,13]. Numerous studies report the impact of autophagy in cancer patients' response to chemotherapy. Increasing levels of autophagy are linked with inadequate response to chemotherapeutic drugs and dismal survival rates [14].

In different cancer types, such as CRC, a single-nucleotide polymorphism, in autophagy-related genes, like *ATG16L1*, is associated with a reduction of autophagy and a significant negative predictive value for patients' survival with metastatic disease [15,16]. Besides, monoallelic deletion of other crucial autophagy genes, such as *Beclin-1*, which leads to autophagy reduction, has been identified in several diseases, such as cancer and Alzheimer's [17–19]. Other studies highlight the positive impact of monoallelic deletion or total loss of other genes, such as *ATG5*, *ATG7*, and *ATG4C*, in cancer development [20]. In addition, *KRAS*, an essential oncogene in CRC development, is strongly associated with autophagy [21]. Cancer cells of *KRAS*-dependent tumors use autophagy in order to support the growth of cancer cells under stressful conditions in hypoxic regions of tumors [8]. All these studies highlight the dual role of autophagy as a tumor promoter or tumor suppressor mechanism. The accumulation of dysfunctional proteins and cellular organelles through the reduction of autophagy increases the risk for malignant transformation. Furthermore, low basic levels of autophagy are required for cell survival as was identified through experiments with a knockout of different autophagy genes, such as *ATG* genes, *Beclin-1*, or *AMBRA1* [22,23]. Autophagy is responsible for recycling cellular components and producing energy and pro-oncogenic factors [24]. Different stage of tumors, anti-cancer treatment, mutations in *ATGs*, and oncogenes are closely associated with autophagy and its controversial role in tumorigenesis. Further study is required in order to address the link between autophagy and hallmarks of cancer.

Furthermore, the increasing levels of autophagy, in these regions, are strongly associated with the regulation of the immune response in the tumor microenvironment [11,25]. The microenvironment of different malignant tumors, including CRC, is characterized by numerous cell types (including immune, tumor, and other types of cells). All these stroma cell types utilize a different extent of autophagy. Therefore, focusing on autophagy and its role in the tumor microenvironment for the discovery of novel anti-cancer therapeutic targets should be further elucidated [11,26]. The role of autophagy in developing an immune response against tumor cells is far more complex. Therefore, autophagy may be a promising therapeutic target in combination with other anti-neoplastic drugs and immunotherapy in the context of this unique cellular composition of the tumor microenvironment.

2. The Major Players in the Tumor Microenvironment

For years, solid cancers were considered as a mass of homogenous cancer cells [27]. Cancer evolution and resistance to treatment is caused by tumor heterogeneity. Over the past decade, it has become increasingly clear that there is a wild diversity of cells with tangled and branching pedigrees in the same tumor. One section of a tumor might be dense with cells containing a particular oncogene mutation, whereas another section might have vastly different mutation backgrounds driving their growth [28]. Tumors should be perceived as separate tissues with a different and more complex cellular network with specialized or dedifferentiated malignant cell types, fibroblasts, tumor stem cells, immune, and endothelial cells. This complex network is characterized as a tumor stroma with unique potential for anticancer therapy [29].

2.1. The Heterogeneity of the Tumor Microenvironment

The vast majority of solid tumors are composed of not only malignant cells, but also of fibroblasts. It is widely accepted that tumorigenesis is a multistep process, the progression of which depends on a sequential accumulation of mutations within tissue cells. Moreover, tumor initiation is associated with the activation of different stromal, endothelial and mesenchymal cells, fibroblasts, and immunogenic cells [30,31]. It is well known that tumor heterogeneity is associated with the more aggressive phenotype and a lack of response against anti-cancer therapy in different types of cancer, including CRC [32].

2.2. The Role of T-Lymphocytes

The major effectors of the immune response against tumor cells are the cytotoxic CD8+ T-lymphocytes or T-cells (CTL). The abundance of T-cells is a decisive prognostic factor for the response of chemotherapy and immunotherapy in cancer patients especially at early stages of the disease, where patients have a strong effector T cell response and more frequently present a high Immunoscore [33,34]. CTLs are responsible for killing hostile cells, such as tumor cells [35]. Type 1 of T-helper cells (Th-1) regulates the activation of CTL and Th-2 initiates humoral immunity [36]. In many studies, the activation of the immune system and tumor-infiltrating lymphocytes (TILs) are used for the grading of the tumor and as a putative prognostic marker for CRC patients. The characterization is based on TILs, tumor invasion, spread to the lymph nodes, and the tumor staging system [33,35].

Many studies have identified that the activation of CTL is inhibited by the PD-L1/PD1 axis interaction in CRC tumors with the Mismatch repair deficiency/Microsatellite instability -high MMRd/MSI-H phenotype [37–39]. The clinical effectiveness of anti-PD1 monoclonal antibodies is beneficial for this subgroup of patients [40]. In contrast, with MSI-H CRC tumors, in almost all MSS CRC tumors, inhibition of the PD-L1/PD1 axis has no significant clinical effect, thus underlining the complexity of this immunosuppressive mechanism [41].

A particular group of lymphocytes that are strongly associated with tumors is the regulatory T-cells [42]. The role of Tregs (regulatory T cells) is controversial because of the genetic and phenotypic differentiation of T-cells. The Treg-specific DNA hypo-methylated regions contribute to the stable expression of Treg function-associated key genes, including *Foxp3*. Accordingly, FoxP3 robustly represses different genes, including *Il2*, contributing to Treg suppressive activity. In tumors, it is critical to deplete *FOXP3* high CD45RA_CD25 high effector Treg cells, which are firmly installed with the Treg-type hypo-methylation and are most suppressive [43]. The origin of Tregs can be either directly from the thymus (tTreg) or by peripheral differentiation (pTreg) of conventional T lymphocytes [44]. The majority of Tregs are characterized by a high expression of specific biomarkers such as FOXP3, IL-2 receptor alpha chain, CD25 IL-10, TGF-β, and IL-35. Also, proteins, like CTLA-4 (cytotoxic T-lymphocyte–associated antigen 4), PD-1 (programmed death 1), and GITR (the receptor of glucocorticoid-induced tumor necrosis factor), have been identified in the surface of Tregs [45–47]. It is well known that molecules, like IL-27 and IL-33, are stimulators of Tregs in CRC through TGF-β-mediated differentiation of Tregs [44].

The primary role of Tregs is to control inflammation and maintain peripheral tolerance in immune homeostasis. Furthermore, FOXP3+ Tregs are crucial in the inhibition of the cytotoxic effect of T-cells in many cancer types, including CRC [42]. The lack of FOXP3+ Tregs and the ratio of CD3+/FOXP3+ T cell may be a prognostic marker for clinical outcomes in patients with CRC [48].

2.3. The Role of Tumor-Associated Myeloid Cells

Different cell types, such as cancer-associated fibroblasts (CAFs) and tumor-associated macrophages (TAMs), in the tumor microenvironment, regulate tumor growth, invasion, and the metastatic phenotype of cancer cells [49,50]. Many studies support the hypothesis that bone marrow-derived cells (TANs, TAMs, and myeloid-derived suppressor cells or MDSCs) are closely associated with the progression of the tumor [50,51].

Two different sub-populations of TAMs, the anti-tumorigenic and pro-tumorigenic or M1 and M2 phenotype, respectively, with high plasticity, have already been identified [52,53]. The most common myeloid infiltrate in solid tumors is composed of myeloid-derived suppressor cells (MDSCs) and tumor-associated macrophages (TAMs). These cells promote tumor growth through their inherent immunosuppressive activity, neoangiogenesis, and mediation of epithelial-mesenchymal transition. Several small molecules are already used in order to inhibit the tumorigenic action of these cells [52]. It is well known that neutrophils regulate the tumor microenvironment through the production of several immunogenic, angiogenic, and inflammatory factors, such as matrix metalloproteinases (MMPs), Vascular endothelial growth factor (VEGF), neutrophil elastase, and hepatocyte growth factor [54–56]. The number of neutrophils in peripheral blood is already evaluated as a negative clinical progression marker in various malignant tumors, including CRC [57]. The two different types of neutrophils, N1 and N2 neutrophils, have been associated with tumor progression. N1 neutrophils reduce tumor immunosuppression through the production of several molecules, such as TNF-α, ROS (Reactive oxygen species), ICAM-1 (Intercellular Adhesion Molecule 1), and Fas. In contrast, N2 neutrophils, increase tumorigenicity through the production of MMP-9, VEGF, and several chemokines [58].

Myeloid-derived suppressor cells or MDSCs have an immunosuppressive ability that is triggered by inflammation. MDSCs are abundant in different tumors types with a critical role in tumor progression [56]. Tumors produce several chemokines, such as CCL2 and CCL5, which regulate the migration of MDSCs in tumors [59]. Several studies support the idea that tumors attract MDSCs in the tumor microenvironment. MDSCs suppress the anti-tumor activity of the immune system through the activation of different genes associated with arg1 (Arginase 1), fatty acid oxidation (FAO), and ROS [60]. Furthermore, MDSCs seem to inhibit both antigen-specific and nonspecific (CD3/CD28) proliferative responses in the tumor microenvironment in both ROS-dependent and independent ways. Also, MDSCs inhibit the stimulation of CD3/CD28 T-cells through the production of NO (Nitric Oxide) and Arg1 [61]. In the tumor microenvironment, MDSCs are converted into nonspecific suppressor cells through the up-regulation of iNOS (inducible nitric oxide synthase) and arginase I. These enzymes are known to be actively involved in T cell suppression in a way that does not require antigen-specific contact between MDSC and T cells to inhibit their function [62].

Several studies over the last years highlight the impact of autophagy in MDSCs' survival in the tumor microenvironment. Glycolytic metabolism is strongly associated with the metabolism of MDSCs [63]. Glycolysis prevents the AMPK-ULK1, a key player in autophagy regulation, which increases the GM-CSF (granulocyte macrophage colony-stimulating factor) expression and supports the development of MDSCs in the tumor microenvironment [64]. Furthermore, MDSCs activate autophagy through phosphorylation of AMPK. The initiation of autophagy increases several anti-apoptotic factors, such as BCL-2 (B-cell lymphoma 2) and MCL-1 (Myeloid cell leukemia 1), which promotes multiple myeloma (MM) progression [65].

2.4. Cancer-Associated Fibroblasts (CAFs)

Cancer-associated fibroblasts or CAFs represent a heterogeneous group of cells. They are responsible for the remodeling of the extracellular matrix (ECM) and support the invasion and metastasis of cancer cells [66]. Different molecules, such as FAP (fibroblast activation protein) and alpha-smooth muscle actin (a-SMA), have been already used as markers of activated CAFs and other fibroblasts [67]. CRC transcriptome studies associate the presence of CAFs with poor outcomes of patients, thus underlining the clinical significance of CAFs as a prognostic marker. Furthermore, the differentiation of CAFs and induction of the fibrogenic phenotype is regulated by the signaling pathway of TGF-β, mechanical stress, and fibronectin [68–70].

2.5. Angiogenesis and Neo-Vascularization Process in Tumor Stroma

It is well known that the stroma of CRC is also the scaffold for the development of tumor-associated blood vessels. Mesenchymal cell type, such as fibroblasts and immune cells, are responsible for supplying the VEGF with tumors cells [71]. Other molecules, like MMPs and associated proteases, that are expressed by immunosuppressive myeloid cells (IMCs) and CAFs appear to be increased in the tumor microenvironment. These enzymes help neo-angiogenesis by altering the ECM and proteolytic activation of embedded angiogenic factors (FGF and VEGF) [72].

2.6. Other Immune Cell Types in the Tumor Microenvironment

Several studies identified many other immune cell types in the tumor microenvironment of CRC. Immune cell types that appear in CRC microenvironment, like neutrophils, mast cells, natural killer (NK) cells, or eosinophils, did not appear to have a significant role in the impact of the clinical progression of CRC patients [73,74].

3. The Role of Autophagy in Stroma Development, Inflammation, and the Immunity Response

It has been proven that autophagy affects the microenvironment of the tumor and vice versa. These microenvironmental factors include cytokines, hypoxia, and inflammation in the tumor environment [75]. In response to stress conditions in the tumor microenvironment, autophagy is activated to maintain and supply energy. Additionally, digestion of intracellular components prevents the accumulation of toxic cellular remnants.

Cancer cells coexist with their microenvironment and the role of autophagy in modulating their interactions with other cell types may be a target for the modulation of autophagy, as a potential anti-cancerous treatment [76]. Autophagy is also a key factor in the function of APCs and T-cells. Autophagy is implicated in the presentation of antigens in both MHC-I and MHC-II in Dendritic cells (DCs). Finally, autophagy contributes to the functional activity of immune cells by creating T-cell memory, depending on autophagy [77].

3.1. The Role of Inflammation in Colorectal Cancer Development

Chronic inflammation is a high-risk factor for cancer. Patients with inflammatory bowel disease (IBD), including Crohn's disease (CD) and ulcerative colitis (UC), have a three-fold increased risk of developing CRC. This type of cancer is known as "colitis-associated colorectal cancer (CAC)" [78]. Activation of Toll-like receptor 4 (TLR4) promotes the development of colitis-associated cancer through activation of the Cox-2 and EGFR signaling pathway [79]. Cancer development is due to the non-neoplastic inflammatory epithelium. Mutations in essential genes (*c-src*, *p53*, *K-RAS*, *β-catenin*, and *APC*) are caused by inflammation as well as DNA damage, which then leads to CAC onset in patients with IBD. Moreover, inflammation triggers signaling pathways, such as STAT3 (Signal transducer and activator of transcription 3) and β-catenin, which causes proliferation and remodeling of epithelial cells and then promotes tumor growth [80]. The CAC microenvironment is a complex system of various types of cells, cytokines, and signaling molecules that play a significant role in tumorigenesis. Immune cells develop many individual functions in the CAC microenvironment. Macrophages promote CAC tumorigenesis and the development of reactive oxygen species (ROS), IL-5, and nitric oxide synthase (NOS) [80]. Tregs and Th17 cells have tumor-promoting activity during CAC [81,82] formation while CD8+ T cells serve a protective role against CAC oncogenesis [83]. TAMs and CADs regulate the production of cytokines, such as IL-6, IL-8, IL-10, and IFN-γ, in the tumor microenvironment. Cytokines are key molecules to the development of inflammation during tumor progression [84]. Several studies support that autophagy is triggered via inflammation. In addition, NLRP3 (NLR Family Pyrin Domain Containing 3) inflammasome (a mitochondrion that is damaged depending on the structure) is negatively regulated by autophagy with IL-1b and IL-18 production and subsequent inflammation response under control [25].

3.2. Hypoxia-Induced Autophagy in the Tumor Microenvironment

Many studies have shown that many types of tumors are found under hypoxic conditions [4,26]. Autophagy in a hypoxic environment in tumors depends on the duration and percentage of hypoxia. Under moderate and chronic hypoxia, hypoxia-induced factor-1 (HIF-1a) and PKC-JNK regulate autophagy [85]. Since hypoxia results in BNIP3 or REDD1 being dependent on autophagy, the question arises as to whether there is an association between BNIP3, HIF-1, and/or REDD1. Many published data support the notion that HIF-1α can up-regulate BNIP3 transcription. Enhanced BNIP3 then interferes with the Beclin1 and BCL2-forming complex and further suppresses Rheb-mTOR [86,87]. Hypoxia raises the levels of REDD1, which then separates the 14-3-3 proteins from the TSC2 complex and finally reduces mTOR [87]. Also, a stress sensor, Ataxia Telangiectasia Mutated (ATM), was verified as being involved in the REDD1-modulated mTOR signaling. Under the hypoxic environment, ATM (Ataxia Telangiectasia Mutated) (-/-) MEFs perform decreased expressions of HIF-1α and REDD1. Overall, it is suggested that hypoxia-induced ATM activation results in increased HIF-1α-BNIP3 and REDD1 to increase autophagy through the inhibition of mTOR [87,88].

3.3. The Cross-Talk between Autophagy and Antigen Presenting Cells

Activation of the anticancer T-cell is induced by identifying the antigenic tumor peptides present on the cell surface of professional APCs, like DCs. However, autophagy through DCs and macrophages affects the surface expression of the MHC-I and peptide complex. For example, the expression of MHC-I in embryo mice DCs and macrophages was upregulated during inhibition of autophagy using chemical inhibitors or downregulation of the main autophagy genes [89,90]. This adjustment was attributed to the slower internalization of classical MHC class I molecules, leading to increased CD8+ T cell stimulation [90]. Hence, in the absence of autophagy, MHC-I molecules appear more consistently expressed and less degenerated [91]. Equally, DCs from mice lacking VPS34 (vacuolar protein sorting-associated protein 34) expressed more MHC-I on the cell surface as well as MHC-II [92]. In contrast, surface expression of MHC-II in macrophages was downregulated when inhibiting autophagy using 3-Methyladenine (3-MA) [91]. Autophagy is associated with the cross-presentation of antigens in DCs. Cross-presentation is a process that permits the loading of MHC-I into DCs with extracellular antigens, which is essential for activating, for example, CTL responses in melanoma [91,93–95]. The cross-presentation capability of bone marrow-derived dendritic cells (DCs) is characterized by increased levels of autophagy [90,96].

Antigen presentation in MHC-II was similarly altered in the inhibition of autophagy with reduced DC treatment mediated by an immunodominant mycobacterial peptide with the reduced presentation of vaccinia virus Ankara antigens and herpes simplex virus (HSV) antigens [97,98]. Accordingly, antigen-specific T-cell responses were down-regulated. Thus, inhibition of autophagy modified the peptide pool presented in MHC and reducing the presentation of immunodominant epitopes [99]. Although, inhibition of autophagy up-regulates surface expression of MHC-I, it also changes the group of immunogenic peptides presented on MHC. Thus, the effect on surface expression of MHC-I and II is less well-confirmed, which has been best determined in the context of the so-called cross-presentation in DCs [93,100,101]. As it was mentioned before, increased levels of autophagy characterize the cross-presentation capability of DCs compared with DCs that do not cross-present antigens, and the autoimmune inhibition that reduces the cross-presentation of MHC-I mediated MHC-I [102,103]. Inhibition of autophagy modified the presentation of the different peptides in MHC and appeared to change the pool of immunodominant epitopes of these peptides. Further mechanistic studies are needed to define how autophagy serves as a target for MHC class I cross-presentation. The central role of autophagy in antigen-presenting cells (APCs) is presented in Figure 1.

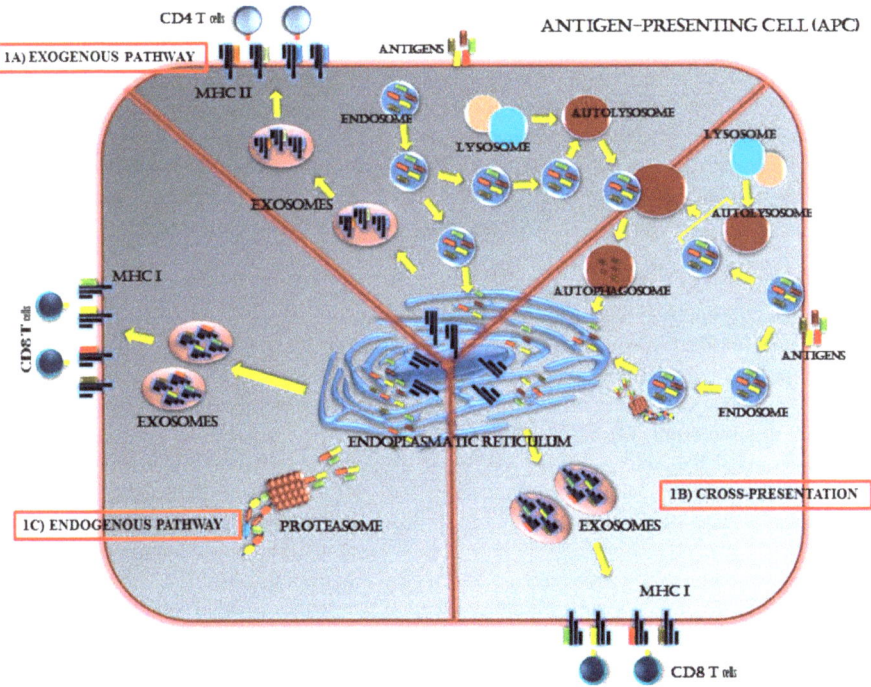

Figure 1. The role of autophagy in the presentation of immunogenic peptides in antigen-presenting cells (APCs). Autophagy has a vital role in the degradation of proteins in order for APCs to use them as antigenic peptides on Major Histocompatibility Complex (MHC)-I and II. Three distinct pathways of antigen processing by the APC have been identified: Exogenous (1A), cross-presentation (1B), and endogenous (1C) pathway. In the exogenous pathway, different antigens and peptides are produced outside the APC and placed on the MHC class II for recognition by CD4+ T cells. The exogenous pathway occurs in macrophages, dendritic cells, and B cells. The endogenous pathway loads cell-produced antigenic peptides onto MHC class I for recognition by CD8+ T cells. The endogenous pathway is responsible for immune recognition of peptides from the virus or self-digested peptides. The endogenous pathway characterizes many cell types, not just APCs, allowing for sensing of viral infection in all cell types. In the cross-presentation pathway, different peptides, from endocytosis and the autophagy degradation pathway, are loaded on MHC class I for recognition by CD8+ T cells. The peptides originate from the surrounding cell environment of tumor apoptotic bodies. This pathway targets virus-infected cells other than APCs and the tumor. The cross-presentation pathway is identified as the most efficient in dendritic cells.

In general, peptides are cleaved and digest from proteins through proteasome in the endogenous pathway. In the exogenous and cross-presentation pathway, the endocytotic peptides are closely associated with autophagy. Endosomes fuse with the autolysosomes in order to digest the peptides and the neo-antigens are loaded onto MHC I and II in the endoplasmic reticulum (ER).

In the already developed tumor microenvironment, M2-phenotype tumor-associated macrophages (TAMs) promote angiogenesis, growth, and metastasis of tumor and cancer cells [104]. However, different studies support that M1 macrophages inhibit tumor growth [58]. The latest reports have shown that autophagy plays a crucial role in the production and polarization of macrophages. Deficiency of TLR2 strongly inhibits autophagy and leads to the biosynthesis of the M2 macrophage, which in turn promotes oncogenesis [58,105]. Moreover, the initiation of autophagy in TAM can increase the radiosensitivity of CRC, inhibit proliferation, and trigger apoptotic cell death [106].

Thus, autophagy in TAM can play a crucial role in cancer suppression. Also, the role of other native immune cells, such as NK cells and neutrophils, plays a vital role in the tumorigenesis of CRC. For example, tumor-associated neutrophils (TANs) facilitate the onset and development of CAC and increase autophagy in neutrophils, which are associated with increased migration of cancer cells [91]. Several in vivo studies suggest that inhibition of autophagy in tumor cells reduces the development of tumors by facilitating the removal of cancer cells via NK cells [107]. Analogous results have also been observed in other types of cancers, such as renal cell carcinoma and melanoma [81].

3.4. Autophagy—A Key Regulator of T-Cell Activation

The adaptive immune system includes the identification of pathogen or tumor proteins and their presence in MHC molecules by antigen-presenting cells (APCs). For this aim, MHC class I molecules are recognized by T cell receptors (TCRs) in CD8+ T cells. Subsequently, MHC class II molecules are recognized by TCRs in CD4+ T cells [90–92]. T cells are activated and differentiated into various types of effector T cells, including Tregs, Th cells, and cytotoxic T cells. Tregs produce anti-inflammatory cytokines, like IL-10 and TGF-β. Also, Th-cells can produce pro-inflammatory cytokines, such as IL-2, IL-5, IL-13, and IL-17A, and interferon gamma (INF-γ). Cytotoxic T cells cause the apoptosis of infected or malignant cells with the release of perforin and granzymes [81,108].

It has been reported that autophagy enhances the adaptive immune response by facilitating APC recognition and preserving the function, survival, and homeostasis of T cells among others [77]. T cell homeostasis involves the clearance of T cells deficient in autophagy [109]. For example, the loss of VPS34 accumulates ROS, which causes an increase in pre-apoptotic protein expression and robust apoptosis of these T cells [110]. Also, depletion of VPS34 also prevents the normal operation of Tregs. Moreover, the deletion of ATG5 and Beclin 1 results in inefficient proliferation and disordered function of CD8+ and CD4+ T cells, respectively, following TCR stimulation [111,112]. On the contrary, autophagy contributes to the maintenance of the survival and function of T cell lymphocytes CD8+ [113].

4. The Current State of Immunotherapy in CRC Patients

The treatment for CRC patients with early-stage disease is surgical removal of tumors. Chemotherapy usually follows the surgery for more advanced disease [114]. Recently, it has been shown that immunotherapy amplifies the immune responses against tumors and it has already been used for patients with solid tumors [115].

In the last few years, many immunomodulating agents have been developed that show significant efficacy. The FDA (Food and Drug Administration) has already approved immune checkpoint inhibitors, such as ipilimumab (an anti-CTLA-4 MoAbs), nivolumab, and pembrolizumab (anti-PD-1 MoAbs) or atezolizumab, avelumab, and durvalumab (anti-PD-L1 MoAbs) for different types of cancer, like melanoma, lung cancer, and renal cell carcinoma. They have recently shown promising activity as a treatment for CRC, although efficacy is reserved for a specific subset of patients [116,117].

It is well known that PD-L1, on tumor and stromal cells, suppresses the antitumor activity of the immune system through stabilization of TNF-α [118]. Furthermore, the PD-1/PD-L1 axis regulates inhibition of the immune response and leads T-cells to exhaustion and apoptotic cell death [119,120].

Wang et al. have shown that metastatic colorectal cancer (mCRC) has higher levels of PD-L1 [121]. Furthermore, dysregulation of signaling pathways, like PI3K-AKT, or chromosomal amplification of the 9q24.1 locus regulates the expression of PD-L1 and PD-L2 in different types of gastrointestinal cancers [120,122].

It is well known that the MSI phenotype in CRC varies according to the stage of the disease. CRC patients with mismatch repair (MMR) deficiency (15% to 20% of stage II/III CRCs) have a better prognosis. Metastatic CRC with deficient MMR represent around 5% and is associated with a poor prognosis [123]. Predictive biomarkers, like MMR and microsatellite status, a mutation in proto-oncogenes, and the expression of PD-L1 have already been used to classify patients in whom immunotherapy might be more beneficial [116,124]. Unfortunately, the percentage of patients with gastrointestinal cancer who will acquire durable clinical responses remains limited. The response rate for CRC patients with mismatch repair deficiency is less than 50% [125] and less than 30% for gastroesophageal cancer [125,126].

In many types of cancer, immunotherapy has been proven as a prominent therapeutic approach. Moreover, in the last few years, significant advances have also been made in CRC. An anti-CTLA-4 monoclonal antibody (tremelimumab) has proven useful for CRC patients, obtaining one 6-month strong response [127]. In a phase II trial, three groups of patients were formed according to their microsatellite status—MSI-H, non-MSI-H, and MSS CRC—in order to test the clinical activity of anti-PD1 MoAb, Pembrolizumab. The immune-related objective response rate (ORR) and immune-related 6-month PFS progression-free survival (PFS) rate were 40% and 78%, respectively, for mismatch repair–deficient (dMMR) colorectal cancers and 0% and 11% for mismatch repair-proficient colorectal cancers patients. The KEYNOTE-177 phase III trial evaluated the above results in patients with dMMR mCRC after treatment with Pembrolizumab versus standard therapy. In Checkmate 142, treatment with Nivolumab alone or in combination with Ipilimumab was tested in metastatic CRC patients according to the microsatellite status. In the update published on Lancet, 31% of CRC patients who were treated with Nivolumab had an objective response, with a disease control rate of 69% for 12 weeks or longer [123]. The combinatorial treatment of Nivolumab and Ipilimumab showed a 55% ORR, while the disease control rate for 12 weeks or longer was 80% [128,129].

The first anti-PD-L1 monoclonal antibody with FDA approval is atezolizumab. This is a fully humanized antibody which targets explicitly PD-L1. It is currently approved for patients with metastatic NSCLC and metastatic urothelial carcinoma with disease progression after treatment of platinum-based chemotherapy [130,131]. Atezolizumab shows response rates higher for patients with PD-L1 positive tumors [132,133]. A similar antibody is durvalumab. The safety and tolerability of durvalumab alone or in combination with tremelimumab have already been tested in a phase I trial for patients with CRC. Promising results have been presented in patients with PD-L1-expressing tumors with microsatellite instability [120,133,134]. These kinds of tumors are characterized by a higher number of infiltrated immune cells.

Furthermore, anti-PD-L1 therapy is more efficient in combination because of the differential expression of PD-1 and PD-L1 in the tumor microenvironment. On the other hand, several types of cancers, such as melanoma and breast cancer, are characterized by PD-L1 expression in both tumors and infiltrating immune cells [120]. The other, a less studied ligand of PD-1 is PD-L2. PD-L2 has been identified to be expressed in macrophages, B-cells, and dendritic cells [124,135]. In CRC, the expression of PD-L2 is approximately 40% and it is regulated by glycosylation and IFNγ [136]. Further, ongoing studies are evaluating the combinations of PD-1, PD-L1, and/or CTLA-4 monoclonal antibodies with other chemotherapeutic molecules, which will re-activate the immune system against CRC tumors (Table 1).

Table 1. Clinical studies with immunotherapy for patients with Please define this term if appropriate.

Number of Study	Immune Target	Agent/Compound	Phase of Study
NCT01876511	PD-1	Pembrolizumab	II
NCT02981524	PD-1	Cyclophosphamide followed by Pembrolizumab	II
NCT03657641	PD-1	Pembrolizumab + Vicriviroc	I/II
NCT03631407	PD-1	Pembrolizumab + Regorafenib	II
NCT03475004	PD-1	Pembrolizumab, Bevacizumab, and Binimetinib	II
NCT03658772	PD-1	Pembrolizumab + grapiprant	I
NCT03519412	PD-1	Pembrolizumab + temozolomide	II
NCT02713373	PD-1	Pembrolizumab + cetuximab	I/II
NCT02375672	PD-1	Pembrolizumab + FOLFOX	II
NCT03332498	PD-1	Pembrolizumab + Ibrutinib	I/II
NCT02851004	PD-1	Pembrolizumab + SBRT	I/II
NCT02837263	PD-1	Pembrolizumab + BBI609	I
NCT02992912	PD-1	Atezolizumab + stereotactic ablative radiotherapy	II
NCT03712943	PD-1	Nivolumab + Regorafenib	I
NCT03711058	PD-1	Nivolumab + Copanlisib	I/II
NCT03414983	PD-1	Nivolumab, Oxaliplatin, Leucovorin, Fluorouracil, Bevacizumab	II/III
NCT02860546	PD-1	Nivolumab + TAS-102	II
NCT03026140	PD-1 and CTLA-4	Nivolumab + Ipilimumab +/− celecoxib	I/III
NCT03693846	PD-1 and CTLA-4	Nivolumab + Ipilimumab	II
NCT03104439	PD-1 and CTLA-4	Nivolumab + Ipilimumab + radiotherapy	II
NCT03377361	PD-1 and CTLA-4	Nivolumab + Ipilimumab + Trametinib	I/II
NCT03832621	PD-1 and CTLA-4	Nivolumab, Ipilimumab, Temozolomide	II
NCT02327078	PD-1 and IDO	Nivolumab + Epacadostat	VII
NCT02983578	PD-L1	AZD9150 + MEDI4736	II
NCT02982694	PD-L1	Atezolizumab + Bevacizumab	II
NCT02777710	PD-L1	Durvalumab + Pexidartinib	I
NCT03827044	PD-L1	Avelumab	III
NCT02669914	PD-L1	Durvalumab	II
NCT02754856	PD-L1 and CTLA-4	MEDI4736 + Tremelimumab	I
NCT03202758	PD-L1 and CTLA-4	Durvalumab, Tremelimumab, and FOLFOX	I/II

NCT, national clinical trial; PD-1, programmed cell death-1; PD-1, programmed cell death-1 ligand; CTLA-4, cytotoxic T-lymphocyte-associated protein 4; IDO, indoleamine-pyrrole 2,3-dioxygenase.

Several studies associate the expression of PD-L1 with PD-L2 and with the geographical association of different types of immune cells. The protein levels of PD-L1 and PD-L2 are associated with the response of anti-PD1 MoAbs. Thus, PD-L2 may be a promising target in immunotherapeutic schemes for CRC [137,138]. It is well known that increasing levels of CD73 block the activation of lymphocytes via increasing adenosine levels. Thus, inhibition of CD73 enhances the therapeutic effect of anti-PD1 and anti-CTL4 monoclonal antibodies [139]. Furthermore, several studies, have explored the relationship between the inhibition of PD-1/CTLA-4 and the increasing levels of CD8+ and CD4+ T cells and cytokines, Tregs inhibition, and other molecules essential for T-cell function [120,140].

5. Targeting Autophagy—A Promising Anti-Cancer Strategy

5.1. The Main Autophagy Inhibitors in Cancer Therapy

Different studies in the last years support the concept of the protective role of autophagy against a different type of cancer therapy, like radiotherapy, chemotherapy, and immunotherapy [141]. The crucial role of autophagy is to regulate the energy and metabolic balance of cancer cells [17] and through the impairment of cell death [142]. Years of efforts have led to the development of molecules that inhibit autophagy. Because of the crucial role of autophagy in cancer cell initiation and progression, the inhibition of autophagy has been shown to be beneficial in anticancer treatment.

Chloroquine (CQ) and its derivative, hydroxychloroquine (HCQ), is one of the most well-known inhibitors that target the fusion of the autophagosome with a lysosome. Over the last years, different clinical trials have attempted to evaluate the clinical significance of autophagy inhibition with CQ or HCQ in several types of cancers [76]. Unfortunately, these clinical trials failed to provide clinically significant benefits because of a lack of consistent inhibition of autophagy with CQ and its derivative, HCQ [143]. However, the combination of autophagy inhibition with other agents provides some encouraging results [76,144]. The combination of HCQ with chemotherapy, like gemcitabine, in pancreatic adenocarcinoma reduced the level of tumor marker 19-9 around 60% [145]. Furthermore, inhibition of autophagy may also have benefits in immunotherapy. The combination of CQ with IL-2 has proven effective with limited toxicity in a preclinical murine hepatic metastasis model. Moreover, this combinatorial scheme increases long term survival and the proliferation and infiltration of immune cells in the liver and spleen [141].

The clinical response of CQ and HCQ appears to vary widely. CQ and its derivative, CHQ, are not specific inhibitors of autophagy [141] and this appears to affect the bioavailability of other drugs by altering the tumor pH [143,146]. Also, the lack of a specific biomarker, which evaluates the inhibition of autophagy, add to the difficulties of these autophagy inhibitors to provide clinically significant results. New, more specific autophagy inhibitors may provide benefits for patients [76,141].

A more potent autophagy inhibitor is Lys05, a dimeric for of Chloroquine. Lys05 alters the acidification of the lysosomes and causes impairment of lysosomal enzymes. It can be used in lower doses. Thus, it is more tolerated and associated with stronger anti-tumor activity [147]. Another autophagy inhibitor is SAR405. SAR405 is a specific kinase inhibitor of Vps18 and Vps34. Vps34 and Beclin-1 regulate the initiation of the autophagy process. Inhibition of Vps34 leads to dysfunctional lysosome and vesicle trafficking activity [148]. Several studies support that inhibition of Beclin-1 reduces tumor growth and enhances anti-tumor NK cell activity. Decreasing levels of Beclin-1 leads tumor cells to overexpress CCL5 cytokine, which regulates the trafficking of NK cells to the tumors [141]. SBI-0206965 is a highly selective, small molecule inhibitor for ULK1 (Unc-51 like kinase-1). This molecule inhibits autophagy through the reduction of ULK1-mediated phosphorylation events in cells. In vivo experiments support the antitumor activity of SBI-0206965 via inhibition of autophagy in different types of cancer [149]. Several other drugs, such as verteporfin, clomipramine, and desmethylclomipramine (DCMI), have been FDA-approved for use in therapy. All these agents alter the acidification of lysosomes or block autophagosome-lysosome fusion [150]. Specifically, autophagy inhibition through DCMI enhances the efficacy of doxorybicin in in vitro studies [151]. Another potent autophagy inhibitor is spautin-1. The mechanism by which spautin-1 inhibits autophagy has already been identified. It inhibits two ubiquitin-specific peptidases, USP10 and USP13, which regulate the deubiquitination of Beclin-1 in Vps34 complexes. Thus, autophagy initiation is inhibited [152]. Due to the strong association of autophagy with the tumor microenvironment and the immune response against tumors, autophagy inhibition may have a negative effect on the adaptive antitumor immunity against tumors. Starobinets et al. (2016) identified that adaptive antitumor immunity is not adversely associated with autophagy inhibition in breast and melanoma cancer models. Thus, autophagy inhibitors can be safely combined with other chemotherapeutic drugs, such as anthracyclines, and still trigger a productive antitumor T cell response against tumors [153].

5.2. Activators of Autophagy for Cancer Therapy

The current review attempts to extensively analyze the role of autophagy in the development of the tumor microenvironment and anti-cancer immunotherapy. In many cases, it is well understood that autophagy has a crucial role in the anti-tumor immune response in CRC. Autophagy not only regulates the antigen presentation in MHC I and II, but it has also been associated with apoptotic cell death in some cases. Due to the multifaceted role of autophagy in cancer, several molecules that induce autophagy have been developed in order to have benefits in anti-cancer therapy.

The most well-known autophagy activators are rapamycin and rapalogs (everolimus, temsirolimus, and deforolimus—analogs of rapamycin). They are inhibitors of mTOR and mTORC1, respectively, and consequently activate autophagy [154]. In endometrial cancer cells, everolimus has been identified as a suppressor of proliferation, especially when it is combined with paclitaxel [155]. Rapamycin was reported to enhance radiation therapy in A549 lung cancer cells through the induction of autophagy and delaying of DNA damage repair [156]. Rapamycin and rapalogs are putative therapeutic molecules that act through autophagy induction, especially when combined with other anti-neoplastic drugs. The clinical application of autophagy activators requires further investigation [155].

Another compound which reduces cell proliferation through the induction of autophagy is metformin. Inhibition of autophagy with specific autophagy inhibitors or knockdown of Beclin-1 reversed the cytotoxic effects of metformin. Furthermore, metformin was identified to increase TNF-related apoptosis-inducing ligand (TRAIL)-dependent apoptosis in lung adenocarcinoma cells through the induction of autophagy machinery [152]. In a BRCA1-deficient mammary tumor model, the combination of metformin with spautin-1 sensitizes BRCA1-deficient breast tumors to mitochondrial disruptors. It is well known that these two agents target different aspects of mitochondrial function and thus it may partially explain the contradictory observation of an autophagy inhibitor (spautin-1) with an autophagy inducer (metformin) in the reduction of cell viability [157].

Obatoclax, a molecule that specifically targets the Bcl-2 family, has been identified as an anti-cancer agent against hematologic malignancies [158]. The main anticancer mechanism of Obatoclax is strongly associated with autophagy induction. Furthermore, Obatoclax stimulates the assembly of necrosomes in the membranes of autophagosomes and consequently induces necroptosis [154]. Several studies have established natural alkaloids, such as isoliensinine, cepharanthine, and liensinine, as inducers of autophagy in cancer [159]. Alkaloids regulate autophagy through phosphorylation of AMPK and inhibition of mTOR. These kinds of alkaloids have been reported to induce apoptotic cell death in apoptosis-resistant MEFs [154].

Herein, we provide two summarized tables about small molecules that inhibit or activate autophagy. Regulation of autophagy is already used in research to develop new chemotherapeutic strategies with immunotherapy for different types of cancer, including CRC (Tables 2 and 3).

Table 2. Commonly used molecules inhibiting autophagy. Small molecules that have been identified as inhibitors of autophagy and the main mechanism of action.

Compound	Autophagy Inhibitors
	Mechanism of Action
Bafilomycin A1	Inhibitor of v-ATPase, inhibition of lysosomal acidification
Concanamycin A	Inhibitor of v-ATPase, inhibition of lysosomal acidification
Azithromycin	Inhibitor of v-ATPase, inhibition of lysosomal acidification
3-Methyladenine (3-MA)	Inhibitor of class III PI3K
Chloroquine (CQ)	Neutralizes the acidic pH of intracellular vesicles
Hydroxy-chloroquine (HCQ)	CQ derivative-Neutralizes the acidic pH of intracellular vesicles
Lys05	CQ derivative-alter the acidification of the lysosomes
SAR405	Kinase inhibitor of Vps18 and Vps34
SBI-0206965	Inhibitor of ULK1
Verteporfin	Inhibit acidification of lysosomes
Clomipramine	Inhibit acidification of lysosomes
desmethylclomipramine (DCMI)	Inhibit Autophagosome-Lysosome fusion
Paclitaxel	Microtubule stabilizer- inhibits phosphorylation of VPS34 at T159
SAHA	Interact in autophagosome-lysosome fusion
Monensin	Inhibit autophagosome-lysosome fusion
Sputin-1	Inhibits the activity of ubiquitin-specific peptidases, USP10 and USP13
SP600125	Inhibition of JNK—reduction of Beclin-1
U0126	Inhibitor of MEK1 and MEK2
Wortmannin	PI3K inhibitor
LY294002	PI3K inhibitor
SB202190	Cross-inhibition of the PI3K/mTOR and MAPKs pathway
SB203580	Inhibit autophagy by interfering with the trafficking of Atg9
MHY1485	mTOR activator

Table 3. Commonly used molecules to induce autophagy. Small molecules that have been identified as autophagy inducers and the primary mechanism of action.

Compound/Molecule	Autophagy Inducers
	Mechanism of Action
Rapamycin	mTORC1 inhibitor
Temsirolimus	mTORC1 inhibitor
Deforolimus	mTORC1 inhibitor
Everolimus	mTORC1 inhibitor
Metformin	AMPK activator
Obatoclax	Inhibitor of Bcl-2 family proteins
isoliensinine	Natural alkaloid
cepharanthine	Natural alkaloid
liensinine	Natural alkaloid
Perifosine	AKT inhibitor
Tat–Beclin-1 peptide	Releases beclin-1 into cytoplasm-regulate autophagosome formation
Lithium	Increase the levels of Beclin-1/VPS34 complexes
GDC-0980	Dual inhibitor of PI3K and mTORC1
GDC-0941	Inhibitor of class I PI3K
fluspirilene	Antagonists of L-type Ca2+ channels
verapamil	Antagonists of L-type Ca2+ channels
loperamide	Antagonists of L-type Ca2+ channels
nimodipine	Antagonists of L-type Ca2+ channels
amiodarone	Antagonists of L-type Ca2+ channels

6. Conclusions

In the last decade, autophagy has been strongly associated with tumorigenesis in colorectal cancer. The dual role of autophagy as survival and a pro-death mechanism has become a field of research in order to develop more effective therapeutic schemes against cancer. In established tumors, autophagy has a vital role as a survival mechanism, especially in the hypoxic regions of tumors. It is well known that tumors are characterized by a highly heterogeneous population of cancer, mesenchymal, immune, and stromal cells in a complex structure, which is identified as the tumor microenvironment. A growing body of evidence supports the hypothesis that autophagy regulates not only the metabolic function of cancer cells, but also other types of cells in the tumor microenvironment. Autophagy has a crucial role as a regulator of immune responses by sustaining the activation, homeostasis, and biological functions of different immune cells, such as T-cells, macrophages, and antigen presenting cells. Moreover, the impact of autophagy on tumor cells has also been observed in the active participation in intracellular and extracellular antigen processing for MHC-I and/or MHC-II presentation. Besides, autophagy has also been reported to associate with the cross-presentation of neo-antigens for MHC-I presentation and the internalization process. Several studies support autophagy as a potential target to strengthen or attenuate the effects of immunotherapy against different types of cancer, including CRC. In the future, efforts should be focused on how to regulate autophagy in the tumor microenvironment in order to strengthen the response of the immune system and overcome anti-tumor immune resistance in immunotherapy for colorectal cancer.

Author Contributions: E.K., P.S. and G.K. made substantial contributions to acquisition, analysis and interpretation of data. A.G.P. and M.V.K. made substantial contributions in the conception, design and interpretation of the data as well as in drafting the manuscript and revising it critically for important intellectual content.

Funding: This research received no external funding.

Conflicts of Interest: The authors declare that they have no competing interests.

Abbreviations

ATGs	Autophagy-related genes
CAFs	Cancer-associated fibroblasts
CRC	Colorectal cancer
CTLs	Cytotoxic T lymphocytes
CTLA-4	cytotoxic T-lymphocyte-associated antigen-4
CQ	Chloroquine
PD-1	Programmed cell death protein 1
PD-L1	Programmed death-ligand 1
HCQ	Hydroxyl-chloroquine
mCRC	metastatic Colorectal cancer
MDSCs	Myeloid-derived suppressor cell
MHC I and II	Major histocompatibility complex I and II
MoAbs	Monoclonal antibodies
NSCLC	Non-small cell lung cancer
MMRd	Mismatch repair deficiency
MSI-H	Microsatellite instability-High
MSS	Microsatellite stable
TANs	Tumor-associated neutrophils
TAMs	Tumor-associated macrophages
TCR	T-cell receptor
TILs	Tumor-infiltrating lymphocytes
Tregs	Regulatory T cells
3-MA	3-Methyladenine

References

1. Siegel, R.L.; Miller, K.D.; Jemal, A. Cancer statistics, 2019. *CA Cancer J. Clin.* **2019**, *69*, 7–34. [CrossRef] [PubMed]
2. Arnold, M.; Sierra, M.S.; Laversanne, M.; Soerjomataram, I.; Jemal, A.; Bray, F. Global patterns and trends in colorectal cancer incidence and mortality. *Gut* **2017**, *66*, 683–691. [CrossRef]
3. Mizushima, N.; Ohsumi, Y.; Yoshimori, T. Autophagosome Formation in Mammalian Cells. *Cell Struct. Funct.* **2002**, *27*, 421–429. [CrossRef]
4. Koustas, E.; Karamouzis, M.V.; Mihailidou, C.; Schizas, D.; Papavassiliou, A.G. Co-targeting of EGFR and autophagy signaling is an emerging treatment strategy in metastatic colorectal cancer. *Cancer Lett.* **2017**, *396*, 94–102. [CrossRef] [PubMed]
5. Pandurangan, A.K.; Divya, T.; Kumar, K.; Dineshbabu, V.; Velavan, B.; Sudhandiran, G.; AshokKumar, P. Colorectal carcinogenesis: Insights into the cell death and signal transduction pathways: A review. *J. Gastrointest. Oncol.* **2018**, *10*, 244–259.
6. Kroemer, G.; Mariño, G.; Levine, B. Autophagy and the integrated stress response. *Mol. Cell* **2010**, *40*, 280–293. [CrossRef]
7. Burada, F.; Nicoli, E.R.; Ciurea, M.E.; Uscatu, D.C.; Ioana, M.; Gheonea, D.I. Autophagy in colorectal cancer: An important switch from physiology to pathology. *World J. Gastrointest. Oncol.* **2015**, *7*, 271–284. [CrossRef] [PubMed]
8. Koustas, E.; Sarantis, P.; Papavassiliou, A.G.; Karamouzis, M. V Upgraded role of autophagy in colorectal carcinomas. *World J. Gastrointest. Oncol.* **2018**, *10*, 367–369. [CrossRef]
9. Schaaf, M.B.; Houbaert, D.; Meçe, O.; Agostinis, P. Autophagy in endothelial cells and tumor angiogenesis. *Cell Death Differ.* **2019**, *26*, 665–679. [CrossRef]
10. Colella, B.; Faienza, F.; Di Bartolomeo, S. EMT Regulation by Autophagy: A New Perspective in Glioblastoma Biology. *Cancers* **2019**, *11*, 312. [CrossRef] [PubMed]
11. Yang, X.; Yu, D.-D.; Yan, F.; Jing, Y.-Y.; Han, Z.-P.; Sun, K.; Liang, L.; Hou, J.; Wei, L.-X. The role of autophagy induced by tumor microenvironment in different cells and stages of cancer. *Cell Biosci.* **2015**, *5*, 14. [CrossRef] [PubMed]
12. White, E. Deconvoluting the context-dependent role for autophagy in cancer. *Nat. Rev. Cancer* **2012**, *12*, 401–410. [CrossRef] [PubMed]
13. Guo, J.Y.; White, E. Autophagy, metabolism, and cancer. *Cold Spring Harb. Symp. Quant. Biol.* **2016**, *81*, 73–78. [CrossRef] [PubMed]
14. Mellor, H.R.; Harris, A.L. The role of the hypoxia-inducible BH3-only proteins BNIP3 and BNIP3L in cancer. *Cancer Metastasis Rev.* **2007**, *26*, 553–566. [CrossRef] [PubMed]
15. Huijbers, A.; Plantinga, T.S.; Joosten, L.A.B.; Aben, K.K.H.; Gudmundsson, J.; Heijer, M.D.; Kiemeney, L.A.L.M.; Netea, M.G.; Hermus, A.R.M.M.; Netea-Maier, R.T. The effect of the ATG16L1 Thr300Ala polymorphism on susceptibility and outcome of patients with epithelial cell-derived thyroid carcinoma. *Endocr. Relat. Cancer* **2012**, *19*, L15–L18. [CrossRef] [PubMed]
16. Huang, C.-Y.; Huang, S.-P.; Lin, V.C.; Yu, C.-C.; Chang, T.-Y.; Lu, T.-L.; Chiang, H.-C.; Bao, B.-Y. Genetic variants of the autophagy pathway as prognostic indicators for prostate cancer. *Sci. Rep.* **2015**, *5*, 14045. [CrossRef] [PubMed]
17. Yun, C.W.; Lee, S.H. The Roles of Autophagy in Cancer. *Int. J. Mol. Sci.* **2018**, *19*, 3466. [CrossRef]
18. Miracco, C.; Cosci, E.; Oliveri, G.; Luzi, P.; Pacenti, L.; Monciatti, I.; Mannucci, S.; De Nisi, M.C.; Toscano, M.; Malagnino, V.; et al. Protein and mRNA expression of autophagy gene Beclin 1 in human brain tumours. *Int. J. Oncol.* **2007**, *30*, 429–436. [PubMed]
19. Pickford, F.; Masliah, E.; Britschgi, M.; Lucin, K.; Narasimhan, R.; Jaeger, P.A.; Small, S.; Spencer, B.; Rockenstein, E.; Levine, B.; et al. The autophagy-related protein beclin 1 shows reduced expression in early Alzheimer disease and regulates amyloid β accumulation in mice. *J. Clin. Investig.* **2008**, *118*, 2190–2199. [CrossRef]
20. Mariño, G.; Salvador-Montoliu, N.; Fueyo, A.; Knecht, E.; Mizushima, N.; López-Otín, C. Tissue-specific Autophagy Alterations and Increased Tumorigenesis in Mice Deficient in Atg4C/Autophagin-3. *J. Biol. Chem.* **2007**, *282*, 18573–18583. [CrossRef]

21. Oikonomou, E.; Koustas, E.; Goulielmaki, M.; Pintzas, A. BRAF vs. RAS oncogenes: Are mutations of the same pathway equal? Differential signalling and therapeutic implications. *Oncotarget* **2015**, *5*, 11752–11777. [CrossRef]
22. Cianfanelli, V.; D'Orazio, M.; Cecconi, F. AMBRA1 and BECLIN 1 interplay in the crosstalk between autophagy and cell proliferation. *Cell Cycle* **2015**, *14*, 959–963. [CrossRef]
23. Yue, Z.; Jin, S.; Yang, C.; Levine, A.J.; Heintz, N. Beclin 1, an autophagy gene essential for early embryonic development, is a haploinsufficient tumor suppressor. *Proc. Natl. Acad. Sci. USA* **2003**, *100*, 15077–15082. [CrossRef]
24. Guo, J.Y.; Chen, H.-Y.; Mathew, R.; Fan, J.; Strohecker, A.M.; Karsli-Uzunbas, G.; Kamphorst, J.J.; Chen, G.; Lemons, J.M.; Karantza, V.; et al. Activated Ras requires autophagy to maintain oxidative metabolism and tumorigenesis. *Genes Dev.* **2011**, *25*, 460–470. [CrossRef]
25. Zhong, Z.; Sanchez-Lopez, E.; Karin, M. Autophagy, Inflammation and Immunity: A Troika Governing Cancer and Its Treatment. *Cell* **2016**, *166*, 288–298. [CrossRef]
26. Degenhardt, K.; Mathew, R.; Beaudoin, B.; Bray, K.; Anderson, D.; Chen, G.; Mukherjee, C.; Shi, Y.; Gélinas, C.; Fan, Y.; et al. Autophagy promotes tumor cell survival and restricts necrosis, inflammation, and tumorigenesis. *Cancer Cell* **2006**, *10*, 51–64. [CrossRef]
27. Gerlinger, M.; Rowan, A.J.; Horswell, S.; Math, M.; Larkin, J.; Endesfelder, D.; Gronroos, E.; Martinez, P.; Matthews, N.; Stewart, A.; et al. Intratumor heterogeneity and branched evolution revealed by multiregion sequencing. *N. Engl. J. Med.* **2012**, *366*, 883–892. [CrossRef]
28. Molinari, C.; Marisi, G.; Passardi, A.; Matteucci, L.; De Maio, G.; Ulivi, P. Heterogeneity in Colorectal Cancer: A Challenge for Personalized Medicine? *Int. J. Mol. Sci.* **2018**, *19*, 3733. [CrossRef]
29. Pietras, K.; Östman, A. Hallmarks of cancer: Interactions with the tumor stroma. *Exp. Cell Res.* **2010**, *316*, 1324–1331. [CrossRef]
30. Tape, C.J. The Heterocellular Emergence of Colorectal Cancer. *Trends Cancer* **2017**, *3*, 79–88. [CrossRef]
31. Fridman, W.H.; Zitvogel, L.; Sautès-Fridman, C.; Kroemer, G. The immune contexture in cancer prognosis and treatment. *Nat. Rev. Clin. Oncol.* **2017**, *14*, 717–734. [CrossRef]
32. Kather, J.N.; Halama, N.; Jaeger, D. Genomics and emerging biomarkers for immunotherapy of colorectal cancer. *Semin. Cancer Biol.* **2018**, *52*, 189–197. [CrossRef]
33. Bupathi, M.; Wu, C. Biomarkers for immune therapy in colorectal cancer: Mismatch-repair deficiency and others. *J. Gastrointest. Oncol.* **2016**, *7*, 713–720. [CrossRef]
34. Mlecnik, B.; Bindea, G.; Kirilovsky, A.; Angell, H.K.; Obenauf, A.C.; Tosolini, M.; Church, S.E.; Maby, P.; Vasaturo, A.; Angelova, M.; et al. The tumor microenvironment and Immunoscore are critical determinants of dissemination to distant metastasis. *Sci. Transl. Med.* **2016**, *8*, 327. [CrossRef]
35. Nakagawa, K.; Tanaka, K.; Homma, Y.; Nojiri, K.; Kumamoto, T.; Takeda, K.; Endo, I. Low Infiltration of Peritumoral Regulatory T Cells Predicts Worse Outcome Following Resection of Colorectal Liver Metastases. *Ann. Surg. Oncol.* **2015**, *22*, 180–186. [CrossRef]
36. Yu, P.; Fu, Y.X. Tumor-infiltrating T lymphocytes: Friends or foes? *Lab. Investig.* **2006**, *86*, 231–245. [CrossRef]
37. Hu, Z.; Ma, Y.; Shang, Z.; Hu, S.; Liang, K.; Liang, W.; Xing, X.; Wang, Y.; Du, X. Improving immunotherapy for colorectal cancer using dendritic cells combined with anti-programmed death-ligand in vitro. *Oncol. Lett.* **2018**, *15*, 5345–5351. [CrossRef]
38. Pauken, K.E.; Wherry, E.J. Overcoming T cell exhaustion in infection and cancer. *Trends Immunol.* **2015**, *36*, 265–276. [CrossRef]
39. Singh, P.P.; Sharma, P.K.; Krishnan, G.; Lockhart, A.C. Immune checkpoints and immunotherapy for colorectal cancer. *Gastroenterol. Rep.* **2015**, *3*, 289–297. [CrossRef]
40. Derhovanessian, E.; Maier, A.B.; Beck, R.; Jahn, G.; Hähnel, K.; Slagboom, P.; De Craen, A.J.M.; Westendorp, R.G.J.; Pawelec, G. Hallmark Features of Immunosenescence Are Absent in Familial Longevity. *J. Immunol.* **2010**, *185*, 4618–4624. [CrossRef]
41. Koustas, E.; Papavassiliou, A.G.; Karamouzis, M.V. The role of autophagy in the treatment of BRAF mutant colorectal carcinomas differs based on microsatellite instability status. *PLoS ONE* **2018**, *13*, e0207227. [CrossRef]
42. Chen, Y.; Colello, J.; Jarjour, W.; Zheng, S.G. Cellular Metabolic Regulation in the Differentiation and Function of Regulatory T Cells. *Cells* **2019**, *8*, 188. [CrossRef]

43. Morikawa, H.; Sakaguchi, S. Genetic and epigenetic basis of Treg cell development and function: From a FoxP3-centered view to an epigenome-defined view of natural Treg cells. *Immunol. Rev.* **2014**, *259*, 192–205. [CrossRef]
44. Herk, E.H.; Velde, A.A. Treg subsets in inflammatory bowel disease and colorectal carcinoma. Characteristics, role and therapeutic targets. *J. Gastroenterol. Hepatol.* **2016**, *31*, 1393–1404. [CrossRef]
45. Hori, S.; Nomura, T.; Sakaguchi, S. Control of Regulatory T Cell Development by the Transcription Factor Foxp3. *Science* **2003**, *299*, 1057–1061. [CrossRef]
46. Fontenot, J.D.; Gavin, M.A.; Rudensky, A.Y. Foxp3 programs the development and function of CD4+CD25+ regulatory T cells. *Nat. Immunol.* **2003**, *4*, 330–336. [CrossRef]
47. Salama, P.; Phillips, M.; Grieu, F.; Morris, M.; Zeps, N.; Joseph, D.; Platell, C.; Iacopetta, B. Tumor-infiltrating FOXP3+ T regulatory cells show strong prognostic significance in colorectal cancer. *J. Clin. Oncol.* **2009**, *27*, 186–192. [CrossRef]
48. Sinicrope, F.A.; Rego, R.L.; Ansell, S.M.; Knutson, K.L.; Foster, N.R.; Sargent, D.J. Intraepithelial Effector (CD3+)/Regulatory (FoxP3+) T-Cell Ratio Predicts a Clinical Outcome of Human Colon Carcinoma. *Gastroenterology* **2009**, *137*, 1270–1279. [CrossRef]
49. Gao, D.; Mittal, V. The role of bone-marrow-derived cells in tumor growth, metastasis initiation and progression. *Trends Mol. Med.* **2009**, *15*, 333–343. [CrossRef]
50. Gabrilovich, D.I.; Ostrand-Rosenberg, S.; Bronte, V. Coordinated regulation of myeloid cells by tumours. *Nat. Rev. Immunol.* **2012**, *12*, 253–268. [CrossRef]
51. Mantovani, A.; Cassatella, M.A.; Costantini, C.; Jaillon, S. Neutrophils in the activation and regulation of innate and adaptive immunity. *Nat. Rev. Immunol.* **2011**, *11*, 519–531. [CrossRef] [PubMed]
52. Szebeni, G.J.; Vizler, C.; Nagy, L.I.; Kitajka, K.; Puskas, L.G.; Tanaka, T.; Shimizu, M. Pro-Tumoral Inflammatory Myeloid Cells as Emerging Therapeutic Targets. *Int. J. Mol. Sci.* **2016**, *17*, 1958. [CrossRef]
53. Shaul, M.E.; Fridlender, Z.G. Neutrophils as active regulators of the immune system in the tumor microenvironment. *J. Leukoc. Biol.* **2017**, *102*, 343–349. [CrossRef] [PubMed]
54. Houghton, A.M.; Rzymkiewicz, D.M.; Ji, H.; Gregory, A.D.; Egea, E.E.; Metz, H.E.; Stolz, D.B.; Land, S.R.; Marconcini, L.A.; Kliment, C.R.; et al. Neutrophil Elastase-Mediated Degradation of IRS-1 Accelerates Lung Tumor Growth. *Nat. Med.* **2010**, *16*, 219–223. [CrossRef]
55. Galdiero, M.R.; Varricchi, G.; Loffredo, S.; Mantovani, A.; Marone, G. Roles of neutrophils in cancer growth and progression. *J. Leukoc. Biol.* **2018**, *103*, 457–464. [CrossRef] [PubMed]
56. Wislez, M.; Rabbe, N.; Marchal, J.; Milleron, B.; Crestani, B.; Mayaud, C.; Antoine, M.; Soler, P.; Cadranel, J. Hepatocyte growth factor production by neutrophils infiltrating bronchioloalveolar subtype pulmonary adenocarcinoma: Role in tumor progression and death. *Cancer Res.* **2003**, *63*, 1405–1412. [PubMed]
57. Li, Z.; Zhao, R.; Cui, Y.; Zhou, Y.; Wu, X. The dynamic change of neutrophil to lymphocyte ratio can predict clinical outcome in stage I–III colon cancer. *Sci. Rep.* **2018**, *8*, 9453. [CrossRef] [PubMed]
58. Mizuno, R.; Kawada, K.; Itatani, Y.; Ogawa, R.; Kiyasu, Y.; Sakai, Y. The Role of Tumor-Associated Neutrophils in Colorectal Cancer. *Int. J. Mol. Sci.* **2019**, *20*, 529. [CrossRef] [PubMed]
59. Qian, B.Z.; Li, J.; Zhang, H.; Kitamura, T.; Zhang, J.; Campion, L.R.; Kaiser, E.A.; Snyder, L.A.; Pollard, J.W. CCL2 recruits inflammatory monocytes to facilitate breast-tumour metastasis. *Nature* **2011**, *475*, 222–225. [CrossRef]
60. Kumar, V.; Patel, S.; Tcyganov, E.; Gabrilovich, D.I. The nature of myeloid-derived suppressor cells in the tumor microenvironment. *Trends Immunol.* **2016**, *37*, 208–220. [CrossRef]
61. Haverkamp, J.M.; Crist, S.A.; Elzey, B.D.; Cimen, C.; Ratliff, T.L. In vivo suppressive function of myeloid-derived suppressor cells is limited to the inflammatory site. *Eur. J. Immunol.* **2011**, *41*, 749–759. [CrossRef] [PubMed]
62. Corzo, C.A.; Condamine, T.; Lu, L.; Cotter, M.J.; Youn, J.-I.; Cheng, P.; Cho, H.-I.; Celis, E.; Quiceno, D.G.; Padhya, T.; et al. HIF-1α regulates function and differentiation of myeloid-derived suppressor cells in the tumor microenvironment. *J. Exp. Med.* **2010**, *207*, 2439–2453. [CrossRef]
63. Jiang, G.M.; Tan, Y.; Wang, H.; Peng, L.; Chen, H.T.; Meng, X.J.; Li, L.L.; Liu, Y.; Li, W.F.; Shan, H. The relationship between autophagy and the immune system and its applications for tumor immunotherapy. *Mol. Cancer* **2019**, *18*, 17. [CrossRef]

64. Li, W.; Tanikawa, T.; Kryczek, I.; Xia, H.; Li, G.; Wu, K.; Wei, S.; Zhao, L.; Vatan, L.; Wen, B.; et al. Aerobic Glycolysis Controls Myeloid-Derived Suppressor Cells and Tumor Immunity via a Specific CEBPB Isoform in Triple-Negative Breast Cancer. *Cell Metab.* **2018**, *28*, 87–103.e6. [CrossRef] [PubMed]

65. De Veirman, K.; Menu, E.; Maes, K.; De Beule, N.; De Smedt, E.; Maes, A.; Vlummens, P.; Fostier, K.; Kassambara, A.; Moreaux, J.; et al. Myeloid-derived suppressor cells induce multiple myeloma cell survival by activating the AMPK pathway. *Cancer Lett.* **2019**, *442*, 233–241. [CrossRef] [PubMed]

66. Xing, F. Cancer associated fibroblasts (CAFs) in tumor microenvironment. *Front. Biosci.* **2010**, *15*, 166. [CrossRef]

67. Koliaraki, V.; Pallangyo, C.K.; Greten, F.R.; Kollias, G. Mesenchymal Cells in Colon Cancer. *Gastroenterology* **2017**, *152*, 964–979. [CrossRef]

68. Grillo, A.R.; Scarpa, M.; D'Inca, R.; Brun, P.; Scarpa, M.; Porzionato, A.; De Caro, R.; Martines, D.; Buda, A.; Angriman, I.; et al. TAK1 is a key modulator of the profibrogenic phenotype of human ileal myofibroblasts in Crohn's disease. *Am. J. Physiol. Gastrointest. Liver Physiol.* **2015**, *309*, 443–454. [CrossRef]

69. Hawinkels, L.J.A.C.; Paauwe, M.; Verspaget, H.W.; Wiercinska, E.; Van Der Zon, J.M.; Van Der Ploeg, K.; Koelink, P.J.; Lindeman, J.H.N.; Mesker, W.; Ten Dijke, P.; et al. Interaction with colon cancer cells hyperactivates TGF-β signaling in cancer-associated fibroblasts. *Oncogene* **2014**, *33*, 97–107. [CrossRef]

70. Calon, A.; Espinet, E.; Palomo-Ponce, S.; Tauriello, D.V.F.; Iglesias, M.; Céspedes, M.V.; Sevillano, M.; Nadal, C.; Jung, P.; Zhang, X.H.F.; et al. Dependency of Colorectal Cancer on a TGF-β-Driven Program in Stromal Cells for Metastasis Initiation. *Cancer Cell* **2012**, *22*, 571–584. [CrossRef]

71. O'Connell, J.T.; Sugimoto, H.; Cooke, V.G.; MacDonald, B.A.; Mehta, A.I.; LeBleu, V.S.; Dewar, R.; Rocha, R.M.; Brentani, R.R.; Resnick, M.B.; et al. VEGF-A and Tenascin-C produced by S100A4+ stromal cells are important for metastatic colonization. *Proc. Natl. Acad. Sci. USA* **2011**, *108*, 16002–16007. [CrossRef]

72. Bonnans, C.; Chou, J.; Werb, Z. Remodelling the extracellular matrix in development and disease. *Nat. Rev. Mol. Cell Biol.* **2014**, *15*, 786–801. [CrossRef]

73. Charoentong, P.; Finotello, F.; Angelova, M.; Mayer, C.; Efremova, M.; Rieder, D.; Hackl, H.; Trajanoski, Z. Pan-cancer Immunogenomic Analyses Reveal Genotype-Immunophenotype Relationships and Predictors of Response to Checkpoint Blockade. *Cell Rep.* **2017**, *18*, 248–262. [CrossRef]

74. Halama, N.; Braun, M.; Kahlert, C.; Spille, A.; Quack, C.; Rahbari, N.; Koch, M.; Weitz, J.; Kloor, M.; Zoernig, I.; et al. Natural Killer Cells are Scarce in Colorectal Carcinoma Tissue Despite High Levels of Chemokines and Cytokines. *Clin. Cancer Res.* **2011**, *17*, 678–689. [CrossRef]

75. Vaupel, P.; Mayer, A. Hypoxia and anemia: Effects on tumor biology and treatment resistance. *Transfus. Clin. Biol.* **2005**, *12*, 5–10. [CrossRef]

76. Levy, J.M.M.; Towers, C.G.; Thorburn, A. Targeting Autophagy in Cancer Therapy. *Nat. Rev. Cancer* **2016**, *17*, 528–542. [CrossRef]

77. Durães, F.V.; Niven, J.; Dubrot, J.; Hugues, S.; Gannagé, M. Macroautophagy in Endogenous Processing of Self- and Pathogen-Derived Antigens for MHC Class II Presentation. *Front. Immunol.* **2015**, *6*, 79. [CrossRef]

78. Bernstein, C.N.; Blanchard, J.F.; Kliewer, E.; Wajda, A. Cancer risk in patients with inflammatory bowel disease: A population-based study. *Cancer* **2001**, *91*, 854–862. [CrossRef]

79. Fukata, M.; Chen, A.; Vamadevan, A.S.; Cohen, J.; Breglio, K.; Krishnareddy, S.; Hsu, D.; Xu, R.; Harpaz, N.; Dannenberg, A.J.; et al. Toll-like receptor-4 promotes the development of colitis-associated colorectal tumors. *Gastroenterology* **2007**, *133*, 1869–1881. [CrossRef]

80. Chaturvedi, M.M.; Sung, B.; Yadav, V.R.; Kannappan, R.; Aggarwal, B.B. NF-κB addiction and its role in cancer: One size does not fit all. *Oncogene* **2011**, *30*, 1615–1630. [CrossRef]

81. Wu, Y.; Yao, J.; Xie, J.; Liu, Z.; Zhou, Y.; Pan, H.; Han, W. The role of autophagy in colitis-associated colorectal cancer. *Signal Transduct. Target. Ther.* **2018**, *3*, 31. [CrossRef]

82. Ning, C.; Li, Y.-Y.; Wang, Y.; Han, G.-C.; Wang, R.-X.; Xiao, H.; Li, X.-Y.; Hou, C.-M.; Ma, Y.-F.; Sheng, D.-S.; et al. Complement activation promotes colitis-associated carcinogenesis through activating intestinal IL-1β/IL-17A axis. *Mucosal Immunol.* **2015**, *8*, 1275–1284. [CrossRef]

83. Olguín, J.E.; Medina-Andrade, I.; Molina, E.; Vázquez, A.; Pacheco-Fernández, T.; Saavedra, R.; Pérez-Plasencia, C.; Chirino, Y.I.; Vaca-Paniagua, F.; Arias-Romero, L.E.; et al. Early and partial reduction in CD4+Foxp3+ regulatory T cells during colitis-associated colon cancer induces CD4+ and CD8+ T cell activation inhibiting tumorigenesis. *J. Cancer* **2018**, *9*, 239–249. [CrossRef]

84. Ngabire, D.; Kim, G.-D. Autophagy and Inflammatory Response in the Tumor Microenvironment. *Int. J. Mol. Sci.* **2017**, *18*, 2016. [CrossRef]
85. Bellot, G.; Garcia-Medina, R.; Gounon, P.; Chiche, J.; Roux, D.; Pouysségur, J.; Mazure, N.M. Hypoxia-Induced Autophagy Is Mediated through Hypoxia-Inducible Factor Induction of BNIP3 and BNIP3L via Their BH3 Domains. *Mol. Cell. Biol.* **2009**, *29*, 2570–2581. [CrossRef]
86. Lin, A.; Yao, J.; Zhuang, L.; Wang, D.; Han, J.; Lam, E.W.; Network, T.R.; Gan, B. The Foxo-BNIP3 axis exerts a unique regulation of mTORC1 and cell survival under energy stress. *Oncogene* **2014**, *33*, 3183–3194. [CrossRef]
87. Li, Y.-Y.; Feun, L.G.; Thongkum, A.; Tu, C.-H.; Chen, S.-M.; Wangpaichitr, M.; Wu, C.; Kuo, M.T.; Savaraj, N. Autophagic Mechanism in Anti-Cancer Immunity: Its Pros and Cons for Cancer Therapy. *Int. J. Mol. Sci.* **2017**, *18*, 1297. [CrossRef]
88. Çam, H.; Easton, J.B.; High, A.; Houghton, P.J. mTORC1 signaling under hypoxic conditions is controlled by ATM-dependent phosphorylation of HIF-1α. *Mol. Cell* **2010**, *40*, 509–520. [CrossRef]
89. Valečka, J.; Almeida, C.R.; Su, B.; Pierre, P.; Gatti, E. Autophagy and MHC-restricted antigen presentation. *Mol. Immunol.* **2018**, *99*, 163–170. [CrossRef]
90. Keller, C.W.; Loi, M.; Ligeon, L.-A.; Gannage, M.; Lunemann, J.D.; Münz, C. Endocytosis regulation by autophagy proteins in MHC restricted antigen presentation. *Curr. Opin. Immunol.* **2018**, *52*, 68–73. [CrossRef]
91. Folkerts, H.; Hilgendorf, S.; Vellenga, E.; Bremer, E.; Wiersma, V.R. The multifaceted role of autophagy in cancer and the microenvironment. *Med. Res. Rev.* **2019**, *39*, 517–560. [CrossRef] [PubMed]
92. Parekh, V.V.; Wu, L.; Boyd, K.L.; Williams, J.A.; Gaddy, J.A.; Olivares-Villagómez, D.; Cover, T.L.; Zong, W.-X.; Zhang, J.; Van Kaer, L. Impaired autophagy, defective T cell homeostasis and a wasting syndrome in mice with a T cell-specific deletion of Vps34. *J. Immunol.* **2013**, *190*, 5086–5101. [CrossRef] [PubMed]
93. Loi, M.; Müller, A.; Steinbach, K.; Niven, J.; Barreira da Silva, R.; Paul, P.; Ligeon, L.A.; Caruso, A.; Albrecht, R.A.; Becker, A.C.; et al. Macroautophagy Proteins Control MHC Class I Levels on Dendritic Cells and Shape Anti-viral CD8+ T Cell Responses. *Cell Rep.* **2016**, *15*, 1076–1087. [CrossRef] [PubMed]
94. Germic, N.; Frangez, Z.; Yousefi, S.; Simon, H.-U. Regulation of the innate immune system by autophagy: Monocytes, macrophages, dendritic cells and antigen presentation. *Cell Death Differ.* **2019**, *26*, 715–727. [CrossRef] [PubMed]
95. Münz, C. Autophagy proteins in antigen processing for presentation on MHC molecules. *Immunol. Rev.* **2016**, *272*, 17–27. [CrossRef]
96. Mintern, J.D.; Macri, C.; Chin, W.J.; Panozza, S.E.; Segura, E.; Patterson, N.L.; Zeller, P.; Bourges, D.; Bedoui, S.; McMillan, P.J.; et al. Differential use of autophagy by primary dendritic cells specialized in cross-presentation. *Autophagy* **2015**, *11*, 906–917. [CrossRef] [PubMed]
97. Loi, M.; Ligeon, L.-A.; Münz, C. MHC Class I Internalization via Autophagy Proteins. *Methods Mol. Biol.* **2019**, *1880*, 455–477.
98. Thiele, F.; Tao, S.; Zhang, Y.; Muschaweckh, A.; Zollmann, T.; Protzer, U.; Abele, R.; Drexler, I. Modified vaccinia virus Ankara-infected dendritic cells present CD4+ T-cell epitopes by endogenous major histocompatibility complex class II presentation pathways. *J. Virol.* **2015**, *89*, 2698–2709. [CrossRef] [PubMed]
99. Bronietzki, A.W.; Schuster, M.; Schmitz, I. Autophagy in T-cell development, activation and differentiation. *Immunol. Cell Biol.* **2015**, *93*, 25–34. [CrossRef]
100. Nedjic, J.; Aichinger, M.; Mizushima, N.; Klein, L. Macroautophagy, endogenous MHC II loading and T cell selection: The benefits of breaking the rules. *Curr. Opin. Immunol.* **2009**, *21*, 92–97. [CrossRef]
101. Khan, N.; Vidyarthi, A.; Pahari, S.; Negi, S.; Aqdas, M.; Nadeem, S.; Agnihotri, T.; Agrewala, J.N. Signaling through NOD-2 and TLR-4 Bolsters the T cell Priming Capability of Dendritic cells by Inducing Autophagy. *Sci. Rep.* **2016**, *6*, 19084. [CrossRef]
102. Tey, S.-K.; Khanna, R. Autophagy mediates transporter associated with antigen processing-independent presentation of viral epitopes through MHC class I pathway. *Blood* **2012**, *120*, 994–1004. [CrossRef]
103. Lee, H.K.; Mattei, L.M.; Steinberg, B.E.; Alberts, P.; Lee, Y.H.; Chervonsky, A.; Mizushima, N.; Grinstein, S.; Iwasaki, A. In Vivo Requirement for Atg5 in Antigen Presentation by Dendritic Cells. *Immunity* **2010**, *32*, 227–239. [CrossRef]
104. Galdiero, M.R.; Bonavita, E.; Barajon, I.; Garlanda, C.; Mantovani, A.; Jaillon, S. Tumor associated macrophages and neutrophils in cancer. *Immunobiology* **2013**, *218*, 1402–1410. [CrossRef]

105. Yang, M.; Liu, J.; Shao, J.; Qin, Y.; Ji, Q.; Zhang, X.; Du, J. Cathepsin S-mediated autophagic flux in tumor-associated macrophages accelerate tumor development by promoting M2 polarization. *Mol. Cancer* **2014**, *13*, 43. [CrossRef]
106. Shao, L.-N.; Xing, C.-G.; Yang, X.-D.; Young, W.; Zhu, B.-S.; Cao, J.-P. Effects of autophagy regulation of tumor-associated macrophages on radiosensitivity of colorectal cancer cells. *Mol. Med. Rep.* **2016**, *13*, 2661–2670. [CrossRef]
107. Viry, E.; Baginska, J.; Berchem, G.; Noman, M.Z.; Medves, S.; Chouaib, S.; Janji, B. Autophagic degradation of GZMB/granzyme B: A new mechanism of hypoxic tumor cell escape from natural killer cell-mediated lysis. *Autophagy* **2014**, *10*, 173–175. [CrossRef]
108. Shibutani, S.T.; Saitoh, T.; Nowag, H.; Münz, C.; Yoshimori, T. Autophagy and autophagy-related proteins in the immune system. *Nat. Immunol.* **2015**, *16*, 1014–1024. [CrossRef]
109. Oral, O.; Yedier, O.; Kilic, S.; Gozuacik, D. Involvement of autophagy in T cellbiology. *Histol. Histopathol.* **2017**, *32*, 11–20.
110. Willinger, T.; Flavell, R.A. Canonical autophagy dependent on the class III phosphoinositide-3 kinase Vps34 is required for naive T-cell homeostasis. *Proc. Natl. Acad. Sci. USA* **2012**, *109*, 8670–8675. [CrossRef]
111. Xu, X.; Araki, K.; Li, S.; Han, J.H.; Ye, L.; Tan, W.G.; Konieczny, B.T.; Bruinsma, M.W.; Martinez, J.; Pearce, E.L.; et al. Autophagy is essential for effector CD8(+) T cell survival and memory formation. *Nat. Immunol.* **2014**, *15*, 1152–1161. [CrossRef] [PubMed]
112. Reed, M.; Morris, S.H.; Jang, S.; Mukherjee, S.; Yue, Z.; Lukacs, N.W. Autophagy-inducing protein beclin-1 in dendritic cells regulates CD4 T cell responses and disease severity during respiratory syncytial virus infection. *J. Immunol.* **2013**, *191*, 2526–2537. [CrossRef] [PubMed]
113. Henson, S.M.; Lanna, A.; Riddel, N.E.; Franzese, O.; Macaulay, R.; Griffiths, S.J.; Puleston, D.J.; Watson, A.S.; Simon, A.K.; Tooze, S.A.; et al. P38 signaling inhibits mTORC1-independent autophagy in senescent human CD8+ T cells. *J. Clin. Investig.* **2014**, *124*, 4004–4016. [CrossRef]
114. Venook, A. Critical Evaluation of Current Treatments in Metastatic Colorectal Cancer. *Oncologist* **2005**, *10*, 250–261. [CrossRef] [PubMed]
115. Le, D.T.; Durham, J.N.; Smith, K.N.; Wang, H.; Bartlett, B.R.; Aulakh, L.K.; Lu, S.; Kemberling, H.; Wilt, C.; Luber, B.S.; et al. Mismatch-repair deficiency predicts response of solid tumors to PD-1 blockade. *Science* **2017**, *357*, 409–413. [CrossRef]
116. Zhou, C.; Zhang, J. Immunotherapy-based combination strategies for treatment of gastrointestinal cancers: Current status and future prospects. *Front. Med.* **2019**, *13*, 12–23. [CrossRef]
117. Arora, S.P.; Mahalingam, D. Immunotherapy in colorectal cancer: For the select few or all? *J. Gastrointest. Oncol.* **2018**, *9*, 170–179. [CrossRef]
118. Lim, S.-O.; Li, C.-W.; Xia, W.; Cha, J.-H.; Chan, L.-C.; Wu, Y.; Chang, S.-S.; Lin, W.-C.; Hsu, J.-M.; Hsu, Y.-H.; et al. Deubiquitination and Stabilization of PD-L1 by CSN5. *Cancer Cell* **2016**, *30*, 925–939. [CrossRef]
119. Juneja, V.R.; McGuire, K.A.; Manguso, R.T.; LaFleur, M.W.; Collins, N.; Haining, W.N.; Freeman, G.J.; Sharpe, A.H. PD-L1 on tumor cells is sufficient for immune evasion in immunogenic tumors and inhibits CD8 T cell cytotoxicity. *J. Exp. Med.* **2017**, *214*, 895–904. [CrossRef]
120. Yaghoubi, N.; Soltani, A.; Ghazvini, K.; Hassanian, S.M.; Hashemy, S.I. PD-1/ PD-L1 blockade as a novel treatment for colorectal cancer. *Biomed. Pharmacother.* **2019**, *110*, 312–318. [CrossRef]
121. Bin Wang, H.; Yao, H.; Li, C.S.; Liang, L.X.; Zhang, Y.; Chen, Y.X.; Fang, J.-Y.; Xu, J.; Fang, J. Rise of PD-L1 expression during metastasis of colorectal cancer: Implications for immunotherapy. *J. Dig. Dis.* **2017**, *18*, 574–581. [CrossRef]
122. O'Donnell, J.S.; Massi, D.; Teng, M.W.; Mandala, M. PI3K-AKT-mTOR inhibition in cancer immunotherapy, redux. *Semin. Biol.* **2018**, *48*, 91–103. [CrossRef]
123. Battaglin, F.; Naseem, M.; Lenz, H.J.; Salem, M.E. Microsatellite instability in colorectal cancer: Overview of its clinical significance and novel perspectives. *Clin. Adv. Hematol. Oncol.* **2018**, *16*, 735–745.
124. Overman, M.J.; McDermott, R.; Leach, J.L.; Lonardi, S.; Lenz, H.J.; Morse, M.A.; Desai, J.; Hill, A.; Axelson, M.; Moss, R.A.; et al. Nivolumab in patients with metastatic DNA mismatch repair-deficient or microsatellite instability-high colorectal cancer (CheckMate 142): An open-label, multicentre, phase 2 study. *Lancet Oncol.* **2017**, *18*, 1182–1191. [CrossRef]

125. Kang, Y.K.; Boku, N.; Satoh, T.; Ryu, M.H.; Chao, Y.; Kato, K.; Chung, H.C.; Chen, J.S.; Muro, K.; Kang, W.K.; et al. Nivolumab in patients with advanced gastric or gastro-oesophageal junction cancer refractory to, or intolerant of, at least two previous chemotherapy regimens (ONO-4538-12, ATTRACTION-2): A randomised, double-blind, placebo-controlled, phase 3 trial. *Lancet* **2017**, *390*, 2461–2471. [CrossRef]
126. Fuchs, C.S.; Doi, T.; Jang, R.W.; Muro, K.; Satoh, T.; Machado, M.; Sun, W.; I Jalal, S.; A Shah, M.; Metges, J.-P.; et al. Safety and Efficacy of Pembrolizumab Monotherapy in Patients with Previously Treated Advanced Gastric and Gastroesophageal Junction Cancer: Phase 2 Clinical KEYNOTE-059 Trial. *JAMA Oncol.* **2018**, *4*, e180013. [CrossRef]
127. Chung, K.Y.; Fong, L.; Venook, A.; Beck, S.B.; Dorazio, P.; Criscitiello, P.J.; Healey, D.I.; Huang, B.; Gómez-Navarro, J.; Saltz, L.B.; et al. Phase II Study of the Anti-Cytotoxic T-Lymphocyte–Associated Antigen 4 Monoclonal Antibody, Tremelimumab, in Patients with Refractory Metastatic Colorectal Cancer. *J. Clin. Oncol.* **2010**, *28*, 3485–3490. [CrossRef]
128. Le, D.T.; Uram, J.N.; Wang, H.; Bartlett, B.; Kemberling, H.; Eyring, A.; Skora, A.; Azad, N.S.; Laheru, D.A.; Donehower, R.C.; et al. PD-1 blockade in tumors with mismatch repair deficiency. *N. Engl. J. Med.* **2015**, *372*, 2509–2520. [CrossRef]
129. Overman, M.J.; Lonardi, S.; Wong, K.Y.M.; Lenz, H.-J.; Gelsomino, F.; Aglietta, M.; Morse, M.A.; Van Cutsem, E.; McDermott, R.; Hill, A.; et al. Durable Clinical Benefit with Nivolumab Plus Ipilimumab in DNA Mismatch Repair-Deficient/Microsatellite Instability-High Metastatic Colorectal Cancer. *J. Clin. Oncol.* **2018**, *36*, 773–779. [CrossRef]
130. Rico, G.T.; Price, T.J. Atezolizumab for the treatment of colorectal cancer: The latest evidence and clinical potential. *Opin. Biol. Ther.* **2018**, *18*, 449–457. [CrossRef]
131. Calles, A.; Aguado, G.; Sandoval, C.; Álvarez, R. The role of immunotherapy in small cell lung cancer. *Clin. Transl. Oncol.* **2019**, 1–16. [CrossRef]
132. Herbst, R.S.; Soria, J.-C.; Kowanetz, M.; Fine, G.D.; Hamid, O.; Gordon, M.S.; Sosman, J.A.; McDermott, D.F.; Powderly, J.D.; Gettinger, S.N.; et al. Predictive correlates of response to the anti-PD-L1 antibody MPDL3280A in cancer patients. *Nature* **2014**, *515*, 563–567. [CrossRef]
133. Link, J.T.; Overman, M.J. Immunotherapy Progress in Mismatch Repair–Deficient Colorectal Cancer and Future Therapeutic Challenges. *Cancer J.* **2016**, *22*, 190–195. [CrossRef]
134. Emambux, S.; Tachon, G.; Junca, A.; Tougeron, D. Results and challenges of immune checkpoint inhibitors in colorectal cancer. *Expert Opin. Biol. Ther.* **2018**, *18*, 561–573. [CrossRef]
135. Zhong, X.; Tumang, J.R.; Gao, W.; Bai, C.; Rothstein, T.L. PD-L2 expression extends beyond dendritic cells/macrophages to B1 cells enriched for VH11/VH12 and phosphatidylcholine binding. *Eur. J. Immunol.* **2007**, *37*, 2405–2410. [CrossRef]
136. Wang, H.; Yao, H.; Li, C.; Liang, L.; Zhang, Y.; Shi, H.; Zhou, C.; Chen, Y.; Fang, J.-Y.; Xu, J. PD-L2 expression in colorectal cancer: Independent prognostic effect and targetability by deglycosylation. *Oncoimmunology* **2017**, *6*, e1327494. [CrossRef]
137. Guo, P.-D.; Sun, Z.-W.; Lai, H.-J.; Yang, J.; Wu, P.-P.; Guo, Y.-D.; Sun, J. Clinicopathological analysis of PD-L2 expression in colorectal cancer. *OncoTargets Ther.* **2018**, *11*, 7635–7642. [CrossRef]
138. Taube, J.M.; Klein, A.; Brahmer, J.R.; Xu, H.; Pan, X.; Kim, J.H.; Chen, L.; Pardoll, D.M.; Topalian, S.L.; Anders, R.A. Association of PD-1, PD-1 ligands, and other features of the tumor immune microenvironment with response to anti-PD-1 therapy. *Clin. Cancer Res.* **2014**, *20*, 5064–5074. [CrossRef]
139. Seto, T.; Sam, D.; Pan, M. Mechanisms of Primary and Secondary Resistance to Immune Checkpoint Inhibitors in Cancer. *Med. Sci.* **2019**, *7*, 14.
140. Curran, M.A.; Montalvo, W.; Yagita, H.; Allison, J.P. PD-1 and CTLA-4 combination blockade expands infiltrating T cells and reduces regulatory T and myeloid cells within B16 melanoma tumors. *Proc. Natl. Acad. Sci. USA* **2010**, *107*, 4275–4280. [CrossRef]
141. Janji, B.; Berchem, G.; Chouaib, S. Targeting Autophagy in the Tumor Microenvironment: New Challenges and Opportunities for Regulating Tumor Immunity. *Front. Immunol.* **2018**, *9*, 887. [CrossRef] [PubMed]
142. Qian, H.-R.; Shi, Z.-Q.; Zhu, H.-P.; Gu, L.-H.; Wang, X.-F.; Yang, Y. Interplay between apoptosis and autophagy in colorectal cancer. *Oncotarget* **2017**, *8*, 62759–62768. [CrossRef] [PubMed]

143. Rosenfeld, M.R.; Ye, X.; Supko, J.G.; Desideri, S.; A Grossman, S.; Brem, S.; Mikkelson, T.; Wang, D.; Chang, Y.C.; Hu, J.; et al. A phase I/II trial of hydroxychloroquine in conjunction with radiation therapy and concurrent and adjuvant temozolomide in patients with newly diagnosed glioblastoma multiforme. *Autophagy* **2014**, *10*, 1359–1368. [CrossRef] [PubMed]
144. Goulielmaki, M.; Koustas, E.; Moysidou, E.; Vlassi, M.; Sasazuki, T.; Shirasawa, S.; Zografos, G.; Oikonomou, E. BRAF associated autophagy exploitation: BRAF and autophagy inhibitors synergise to efficiently overcome resistance of BRAF mutant colorectal cancer cells. *Oncotarget* **2015**, *7*, 9188–9221. [CrossRef] [PubMed]
145. Boone, B.A.; Bahary, N.; Zureikat, A.H.; Moser, A.J.; Normolle, D.P.; Wu, W.C.; Singhi, A.D.; Bao, P.; Bartlett, D.L.; Liotta, L.A.; et al. Safety and Biologic Response of Pre-operative Autophagy Inhibition in Combination with Gemcitabine in Patients with Pancreatic Adenocarcinoma. *Ann. Surg. Oncol.* **2015**, *22*, 4402–4410. [CrossRef] [PubMed]
146. Pellegrini, P.; Strambi, A.; Zipoli, C.; Hägg-Olofsson, M.; Buoncervello, M.; Linder, S.; De Milito, A. Acidic extracellular pH neutralizes the autophagy-inhibiting activity of chloroquine: Implications for cancer therapies. *Autophagy* **2014**, *10*, 562–571. [CrossRef] [PubMed]
147. Amaravadi, R.K.; Winkler, J.D. Lys05: A new lysosomal autophagy inhibitor. *Autophagy* **2012**, *8*, 1383–1384. [CrossRef]
148. Ronan, B.; Flamand, O.; Vescovi, L.; Dureuil, C.; Durand, L.; Fassy, F.; Bachelot, M.-F.; Lamberton, A.; Mathieu, M.; Bertrand, T.; et al. A highly potent and selective Vps34 inhibitor alters vesicle trafficking and autophagy. *Nat. Chem. Biol.* **2014**, *10*, 1013–1019. [CrossRef] [PubMed]
149. Egan, D.F.; Chun, M.G.; Vamos, M.; Zou, H.; Rong, J.; Miller, C.J.; Lou, H.J.; Raveendra-Panickar, D.; Yang, C.-C.; Sheffler, D.J.; et al. Small Molecule Inhibition of the Autophagy Kinase ULK1 and Identification of ULK1 Substrates. *Mol. Cell* **2015**, *59*, 285–297. [CrossRef]
150. Vakifahmetoglu-Norberg, H.; Xia, H.-G.; Yuan, J. Pharmacologic agents targeting autophagy. *J. Clin. Investig.* **2015**, *125*, 5–13. [CrossRef]
151. Rossi, M.; Munarriz, E.R.; Bartesaghi, S.; Milanese, M.; Dinsdale, D.; Guerra-Martin, M.A.; Bampton, E.T.W.; Glynn, P.; Bonanno, G.; Knight, R.A.; et al. Desmethylclomipramine induces the accumulation of autophagy markers by blocking autophagic flux. *J. Cell Sci.* **2009**, *122*, 3330–3339. [CrossRef]
152. Liu, J.; Xia, H.; Kim, M.; Xu, L.; Li, Y.; Zhang, L.; Cai, Y.; Norberg, H.V.; Zhang, T.; Furuya, T.; et al. Beclin1 Controls the Levels of p53 by Regulating the Deubiquitination Activity of USP10 and USP13. *Cell* **2011**, *147*, 223–234. [CrossRef]
153. Starobinets, H.; Ye, J.; Broz, M.; Barry, K.; Goldsmith, J.; Marsh, T.; Rostker, F.; Krummel, M.; Debnath, J. Antitumor adaptive immunity remains intact following inhibition of autophagy and antimalarial treatment. *J. Clin. Investig.* **2016**, *126*, 4417–4429. [CrossRef]
154. Yang, Z.J.; Chee, C.E.; Huang, S.; Sinicrope, F.A. The Role of Autophagy in Cancer: Therapeutic Implications. *Mol. Cancer Ther.* **2011**, *10*, 1533–1541. [CrossRef]
155. Byun, S.; Lee, E.; Lee, K.W. Therapeutic Implications of Autophagy Inducers in Immunological Disorders, Infection, and Cancer. *Int. J. Mol. Sci.* **2017**, *18*, 1959. [CrossRef]
156. Wang, H.; Li, D.; Li, X.; Ou, X.; Liu, S.; Zhang, Y.; Ding, J.; Xie, B. Mammalian target of rapamycin inhibitor RAD001 sensitizes endometrial cancer cells to paclitaxel-induced apoptosis via the induction of autophagy. *Oncol. Lett.* **2016**, *12*, 5029–5035. [CrossRef]
157. Yeo, S.K.; Paul, R.; Haas, M.; Wang, C.; Guan, J.-L. Improved efficacy of mitochondrial disrupting agents upon inhibition of autophagy in a mouse model of BRCA1-deficient breast cancer. *Autophagy* **2018**, *14*, 1214–1225. [CrossRef]
158. Opydo-Chanek, M.; Gonzalo, O.; Marzo, I. Multifaceted anticancer activity of BH3 mimetics: Current evidence and future prospects. *Biochem. Pharmacol.* **2017**, *136*, 12–23. [CrossRef]
159. Law, B.Y.K.; Chan, W.K.; Xu, S.W.; Wang, J.R.; Bai, L.P.; Liu, L.; Wong, V.K.W. Natural small-molecule enhancers of autophagy induce autophagic cell death in apoptosis-defective cells. *Sci. Rep.* **2014**, *4*, 5510. [CrossRef]

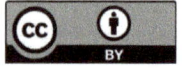 © 2019 by the authors. Licensee MDPI, Basel, Switzerland. This article is an open access article distributed under the terms and conditions of the Creative Commons Attribution (CC BY) license (http://creativecommons.org/licenses/by/4.0/).

MDPI
St. Alban-Anlage 66
4052 Basel
Switzerland
Tel. +41 61 683 77 34
Fax +41 61 302 89 18
www.mdpi.com

Cancers Editorial Office
E-mail: cancers@mdpi.com
www.mdpi.com/journal/cancers

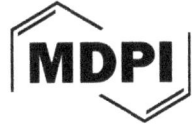

www.ingramcontent.com/pod-product-compliance
Lightning Source LLC
LaVergne TN
LVHW070241100526
838202LV00015B/2164